Immunological and
Clinical Aspects
of Allergy

Immunological and Clinical Aspects of Allergy

EDITED BY

M. H. Lessof

Professor of Medicine
Guy's Hospital Medical School
London

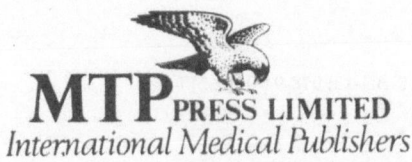

MTP PRESS LIMITED
International Medical Publishers

British Library Cataloguing in Publication Data

Immunological and clinical aspects of allergy.
  1. Allergy – Immunological aspects
  I. Lessof, Maurice Hart
  616.9'7'079   RC584

ISBN-13: 978-94-011-6219-7   e-ISBN-13: 978-94-011-6217-3
DOI: 10.1007/ 978-94-011-6217-3

Contents

List of Contributors

H. E. Amos
Medical Department,
ICI Pharmaceuticals Ltd,
Mereside,
Alderley Park,
Macclesfield, Cheshire SK10 4TG

P. D. Buisseret
Department of Medicine,
Louisiana State University Medical Center,
New Orleans, Louisiana, USA

M. G. C. Dahl
University Department of Dermatology,
Royal Victoria Infirmary,
Newcastle upon Tyne NE1 4LP

R. J. Davies
Academic Unit of Respiratory Medicine,
St Bartholomew's Hospital,
London EC1A 7BE

J. M. Dewdney
Beecham Pharmaceuticals Research Division,
Biosciences Research Centre,
Great Burgh, Epsom,
Surrey KT18 5XQ

D. L. Easty
Department of Ophthalmology,
University of Bristol
Bristol

A. W. Frankland
139 Harley Street,
London W1N 1DJ

M. H. Lessof
Department of Medicine,
Guy's Hospital Medical School,
London SE1 9RT

N. Mygind
Otopathological Laboratory,
Rigshospitalet,
Copenhagen, Denmark

T. A. E. Platts-Mills
Division of Immunological Medicine
MRC Clinical Research Centre,
Harrow, Middlesex HA1 3UJ

J. F. Price
Department of Child Health,
King's College Hospital,
London SE5 9RS

J. Thomsen
University ENT Department,
Rigshospitalet,
Copenhagen, Denmark

M. W. Turner
Department of Immunology,
Institute of Child Health,
London WC1N 1EH

D. Gwyn Williams
Renal Unit, Department of Medicine,
Guy's Hospital Medical School,
London SE1 9RT

L. J. F. Youlten
Department of Medicine,
Guy's Hospital Medical School,
London SE1 9RT

Preface

In the scientific aspects of immunology, the pace of advance has been almost overwhelming, but with some notable exceptions, clinical benefits have been slow. For those who are interested in allergy, the situation has been somewhat different. Here, the scientific aspects have lagged sadly behind other branches of immunology. There has, however, been a recent explosion of knowledge, which began with the discovery of immunoglobulin E, and a curious situation has come to light. The speculations of the older allergists, which had often been derided as mere inventions, now appear to be largely true. A number of 'preposterous' hypotheses have acquired the respectability that comes with scientific proof and the entire field is now full of excitement and challenge. It is no longer doubted that 'reaginic' antibody can sensitize cells that reside beneath the surface of the skin or mucous membranes. Skin prick tests with 'hair of the tail of the dog' have been legitimized by correlating them with the carefully validated results of radioallergosorbent tests. It has furthermore been shown beyond doubt that immunotherapy with increasing amounts of bee venom really can 'hyposensitize' patients who have previously suffered anaphylactic reactions to bee stings.

This book has been published in the hope that, in the field of allergy, it will bridge the gap between basic science and the clinical application. Like many another volume it has depended on the collaboration of a team of scientists and clinicians, on the help of an excellent secretary (Miss Sally Wood) and on the forbearance of the editor's wife and family. To all of these I extend my thanks.

MAURICE H. LESSOF

1
The Biological Role of Allergy

T. A. E. PLATTS-MILLS

INTRODUCTION

Allergy as known to lay persons ranges from mild rhinitis in dusty conditions to severe and even fatal anaphylactic reactions to bee stings or penicillin injections. However, in all its forms, allergy is known only as a disadvantage. It is therefore reasonable to ask why the tendency to allergy has persisted, or put another way, what the biological role of these reactions is. Before making any assessment of this kind it is essential to understand the underlying immunological events. Firstly, it is necessary to limit and define the groups of allergic conditions we are considering. Allergy or 'a state of altered reactivity' covers a wide range of clinical conditions. In many cases the underlying events are very poorly understood and the present discussion will be restricted to · three groups of conditions. Firstly, those conditions characterized by 'immediate' symptoms, positive weal and flare reactions to prick tests and in most cases evidence for specific IgE antibodies. Secondly, conditions characterized by reactions within a few hours and the presence of serum precipitins; farmer's lung is typical of this group. The third group is characterized by delayed responses, in particular the wide range of contact sensitivities of which nickel sensitivity is typical. In each of these groups there is good evidence that the patients have made an immune response to a protein or chemical compound. Other individuals who are not allergic either fail to make an immune response or make a response that does not lead to symptoms. However, the important feature in all these cases is that the substance that elicits the reaction does not appear to be harmful in the absence of the allergic responses. For example, pollen grains, hay dust and nickel are not considered

1

to be toxic materials. It is only in the presence of a particular type of immune response that they become so.

Although these allergies can be very troublesome to many people and dangerous to a few, it is not clear that they represent a biological disadvantage. There appear to be two possible explanations for the persistence of allergy. These responses might be an accidental result of an immune response to certain types of antigen or antigen exposure, which persists because it is biologically irrelevant. Alternatively, under different circumstances, these types of response may represent an important part of the immune reaction to harmful substances or organisms. This chapter will first summarize what is known about immune responses to allergens and then speculate about the importance of these reactions.

Allergens and purified allergens

The study of allergy is based on an understanding of the substances that cause the reactions. Before Blackley[1] and Wyman[2] demonstrated that grass pollen was responsible for summer hay fever the nature of the disease was obscure. Similarly the study of dust allergy has become much more interesting since Voorhorst et al.[3] established that many of the patients were allergic to the mites growing in the dust. For many years it was thought that allergens must be inherently toxic. Noon first justified injections of pollen extract as a method of raising immunity to pollen toxin[4]. More recently Berrens has again related allergenicity to non-specific irritant activity[5]. He also postulated that this was due to activation of complement by sugars linked through N-glycosides to protein[5]. Studies on purified allergens have generally led to different conclusions.

Table 1.1 Some purified allergens used as models in studying the antibody responses in allergic persons

Allergy	Source of allergen*	Purified allergen		Status	Molecular weight
Grass hay fever	rye grass pollen	group I protein;	Rye I†	major‡	27 000
Ragweed hay fever	short ragweed	antigen E;	AgE†	major	37 800
	pollen	antigen 3	Ra3	minor	11 000
		antigen 5	Ra5	minor	5000
House dust allergy	*Dermatophagoides*	*Dermatophagoides*			
	pteronyssinus	antigen P₁	P₁†	major	26 000
	culture				
Bee sting allergy	honey bee venom	phospholipase A;	PLA	major	19 500
Penicillin allergy	—	benzylpenicilloyl-			
		poly-L-lysine;	BPO	major	—

* Source from which allergen has been purified
† These purified antigens have been shown to account for a large proportion of the IgE antibody to the crude allergen, and a significant proportion of the total serum IgE
‡ Purified allergens have been judged 'major' because a high proportion (≈90%) of patients with this allergy have IgE antibody to the allergen

A major object of studies on allergen purification has been to understand what properties lead these substances to give rise to allergy. In most cases the major allergens have turned out to be freely soluble proteins which are neither toxic nor irritant to non-allergic persons (Table 1.1). Although the function (e.g. in the pollen grain or dust mite) of most of the purified allergens is not known, they do not appear to have special biochemical properties. Thus amino acid analysis and even sequencing have not revealed any distinctive features of the allergens (reviewed by T. P. King[6] and D. G. Marsh[7]). Although the chemical properties of allergens do not appear to be related to their 'allergenicity' the physical properties are distinctive. In addition to being water soluble they are generally stable and very similar in size. Thus all the major allergens (e.g. AgE, Rye I, Timothy B, PLA, *Dermatophagoides pteronyssinus* P_1, horse dander allergen b_2, cod allergen M, etc.) are between 10 000 and 40 000 daltons. The size appears to be limited because molecules larger than this will not pass freely through mucosal surfaces[8]. The lower limit is certainly not absolute, the minor ragweed antigen 5 is only 5000 daltons, however it is assumed that in general smaller molecules are less immunogenic. The reason for this might be a lack of repeating structures or simply too few determinants making it less likely that the molecule would be recognized by lymphocytes or macrophages. In addition to physical size it is probable that the rate at which proteins can elute from a pollen grain or dust particle is important. It has been estimated that under normal conditions a pollen grain which lands in the nose will be swallowed within 30 minutes[7]. Belin systematically studied the time course of elution of allergens from birch pollen[9]. Similar studies on ragweed pollen suggest that AgE elutes slowly ($< 50\%$ in 100 minutes) while other allergens including Ra5 elute rapidly (95% in 5 minutes)[7]. Thus in assessing an allergen it is necessary to know its size, solubility, rate of elution and quantity. It is worth sounding a note of caution because 'major' allergens are the substances to which immune responses have already occurred. *In vivo* these allergens are inhaled in pollen grains or dust which contains other substances. The observations about non-specific irritant activity have been predominantly made on unpurified extracts, and it is possible that other substances play a critical role in stimulating the initial response to an allergen[5]. Thus the 'irritant materials' might have an adjuvant effect for an antibody response to the non-irritant 'major' allergens. The critical experiment would be to show that allergic people can be sensitized by inhaling small quantities of a purified allergen (see page 13).

Most 'major' allergens represent only a small proportion of the crude material ($< 1\%$ by weight)[7]. However, much of the material in pollen grains is not soluble and would not pass through the mucous membrane. Indeed when aqueous extracts are studied it appears that 'major' allergens often represent a reasonable or even large proportion of the total protein. Certainly aqueous extract of rye grass pollen contains good quantities of Rye I (possibly as high as 15%). Our recent studies on *D. pteronyssinus* culture illustrate a similar point. The yield of P_1 from crude culture is less than 1%, however in aqueous extract proteins bearing the antigen P_1 appear to represent as much as 20% of the total protein[10]. This conclusion is derived from immunodiffusion studies, from radioimmunoassay for P_1 and finally from SDS polyacrylamide gel electrophoresis (PAGE). On SDS PAGE the purified P_1 gives a single homogeneous band (26 000 daltons) while the crude extract of *D. pteronyssinus* culture shows the heaviest band in exactly the same position[10]. Thus it appears that the major allergen from dust mites may well be the commonest dust antigen that crosses the nasal mucosa.

All allergens have been purified on the basis of skin reactivity, and a 'major' allergen is one to which a great majority of the groups of patients will respond. More recent studies have shown that in many cases IgE antibody to a purified allergen can represent a large proportion of the total IgE[10-13]. This idea was suggested by Ishizaka in his original studies on IgE antibodies[14]. Subsequently Gleich and Jacob showed that a high proportion of total serum IgE in ragweed allergic persons could be absorbed using sepharose beads coated with ragweed antigens (RAST absorption)[11]. In recent studies[10] on over 150 dust mite allergic patients we have estimated that on average 12% of total IgE is antibody against antigen P_1. Thus the studies on purified allergens lead to the conclusion that 'major' allergens represent a large proportion of the protein which would reach the lymphocytes in the nasal mucosa. In keeping with this, the bulk of the IgE antibody response is often directed against these proteins and they probably cause most of the symptoms. Nonetheless these conclusions will not apply to all patients in a group. It is therefore safer to regard studies using purified allergens as models of the response which occurs to several or even many different proteins present in the original allergen. Using purified allergens it is possible to measure antibodies against the allergen and in addition it becomes possible to measure the quantities of an allergen to which people are exposed *in vivo*. These estimates are interesting because the quantities of inhaled allergens turn out to be very low (often less than 1 µg of protein/season) (see reference 7). Some of these estimates are so low that it is surprising that the allergens are recognized at all.

IMMEDIATE HYPERSENSITIVITY

Allergic states characterized by immediate symptoms and immediate skin reactions

Immediate allergic reactions can be divided conveniently into inhalant and non-inhalant forms. Inhalant allergies are extremely common, affecting 10–15% of the population at some time. The commonest allergens are plant pollens, followed closely by dust allergens, animal danders and mould spores. The wind-born pollens responsible for hay fever vary from season to season and also from country to country. In general the most important plant allergens are those that give rise to a large number of suitably sized pollen grains in an area, e.g. birch trees in Sweden, ragweed in the United States and the mesquit tree in Kuwait. However, many pollen antigens are distributed evenly over wide areas, and it is reasonable to assume that all persons within an area have been exposed to similar quantities of pollen antigens. Thus hay fever may be regarded as a marker of the group of persons who are 'capable' of making this type of reaction. By contrast exposure to animal danders, mould spores and probably dust mite allergens varies greatly from one house to another. Therefore the population developing symptoms to these allergens will reflect both susceptibility and degree of exposure. It is worth distinguishing here between the quantities of allergen necessary to induce symptoms and the quantity necessary to sensitize the patient in the first place. The former can be studied by nasal or bronchial challenge. Very little is known about the quantities of allergens necessary to induce sensitivity. However, clinically patients are seen who appear to have become sensitized in an environment where they did not experience symptoms, while other persons fail to respond to an allergen for many years but subsequently have severe symptoms from exposure to the same concentrations of allergen. It is possible that sensitization depends not only on susceptibility and allergen dose but also on other factors such as intermittent viral infections[15].

There are three major groups of non-inhalant immediate allergens; these are foods, insect venoms and penicillin. Fish allergens have pride of place because the original Prausnitz–Küstner (P–K) passive transfer reactions were demonstrated with serum from a fish allergic patient[16] and because the cod fish allergens have been extensively purified[17]. On the other hand, exposure to egg or cow's milk proteins in young children is very widespread and allergies to these foods are relatively common. The problem with food allergens is that because of digestion it is very difficult to assess what the effective dose of an allergen is. In addition there has been much controversy about the use of RAST in the diagnosis of food allergy. Consequently it is often difficult to define a group of patients who are allergic to food. Nonetheless it seems likely that food allergies occur in children who show a high incidence of inhalant allergies later in life. Certainly Coca and Cooke included food allergy in their original description of families with a high incidence of allergies[18]. Our understanding of allergic reactions to bee venom has expanded rapidly since it became clear that positive skin tests and serum IgE antibody to phospholipase A (PLA) were present in most of the patients[19]. However, exposure to bee venom is only common among beekeepers and their families. Thus any observations about the immune response to phospholipase A must be related to other beekeepers. Penicillin allergy has contributed more to our understanding of the mechanisms of histamine release than to our understanding of the factors underlying allergy[20]. However a large proportion of the population is exposed to penicillin and the development of immediate reactions to penicillin might well indicate a difference in immune responsiveness.

It has been clear for many years that highly allergic persons tend to develop allergies to many different allergens[18]. And also that this tendency runs in families. It is this tendency that is referred to as atopy. The simplest and probably best working definition of an atopic person is that he will give a positive skin reaction to at least one common allergen (see Pepys[21]). However, all of the allergens that would be used in England, e.g. grass pollen, dust mites, cat dander, dog dander and tree pollens, are inhalant allergens. In addition almost all the evidence on the inheritance of allergies relates to inhalant allergens[7]. It seems that one could consider firstly the large group of 'atopic' persons who have an inherited tendency to become allergic to inhaled antigens and foods. Secondly, there are smaller numbers of people who become allergic to bee stings or penicillin where it is not clear that the response is dependent on any inherited tendency.

In the following discussion I will first outline what is known about inhalant allergies. The discussion of non-inhalant immediate allergies will then focus on evidence comparing these other allergies with inhalant allergy.

IgE and IgE-mediated reactions

Prausnitz and Küstner in 1921 established that immediate skin reactions could be transferred with an intradermal injection of serum from an allergic person[16]. However, it was not until 1967 that Ishizaka et al. demonstrated in studies on ragweed hay fever that this heat labile, 'reaginic' activity was mediated by antibody but was not IgG, IgA, IgM or IgD[22]. The new immunoglobulin class was named IgE and the findings were confirmed by Bennich et al.[23] with the identification of an IgE myeloma (ND). This discovery of IgE led rapidly in three directions. Firstly, it became possible to define the relationship between IgE and its specific receptor on mast cells and basophils[24]. Secondly, it became possible to measure total serum IgE and also to measure IgE antibodies in vitro using the radioallergosorbent technique (RAST). Thirdly, there was an enormous expansion of experimental interest in immediate hypersensitivity both in animals and man.

Briefly to explain what is now known about IgE; it is a monomeric immunoglobulin with light and heavy polypeptide chains. It has a slightly higher molecular weight that IgG and the ability to bind to a receptor on the surface of human mast cells and basophils. Because the antibody molecule is divalent it can cross-link IgE receptors on the surface of mast cells or basophils and it is now thought that antigen-mediated histamine release is a direct consequence of cross-linking. This has been shown with divalent haptens of penicillin[25]. More recently it has been shown that the Fab$'_2$ fragment of an antibody to the IgE receptor can cause histamine release by cross-linking receptors in the absence of IgE[26]. There is good evidence that the complement anaphylotoxins C3a and C5a can cause histamine release by direct reaction with basophils[27a]. This type of release may be involved in allergic reactions to some drugs and to X-ray contrast media[27b] but complement components are not thought to be involved in IgE-mediated histamine release. The actual mechanism of histamine release remains unclear. However the granules containing histamine appear to fuse with the external membrane, the histamine then dissolves rapidly and leaves the cell[28,29]. This process which has been filmed[28] does not damage the basophils, and they can probably regranulate.

IgE like other immunoglobulins is produced by plasma cells. These cells have been observed in nasal mucosa, tonsils, the gut and lymph nodes draining the nose[30]. IgE plasma cells are generally not found in lymph nodes in other parts of the body or in the spleen. Although IgE is associated with some secretions there does not appear to be a specific mechanism leading to the localization of IgE plasma cells or the secretion of IgE. Firstly, IgE in secretions is a monomer and is not modified by the addition of secretory piece[31] (Table 1.2). Secondly, although IgE may become intracellular in mast

Table 1.2 Immunoglobulin classes and the response to inhalant allergens

	IgE	IgG	IgA	IgM
*Total**				
Serum concentration	0.01–10 μg	6–12 mg	0.2–3.0 mg	0.2–2 mg
Nasal secretions	1.0–10 ng	45 μg	74 μg	< 1 μg
Saliva	< 1 ng	20 μg	40 μg	< 1 μg
Secretory piece	No	No	Yes	Yes or No
Specific antibodies to Rye I†				
Serum units/ml	200	800	50	< 10
(≃ng/ml)	(100)	(400)	(25)	< 5
Antibody to Rye I as a percentage of total	1–50	0.01	0.005	< 0.002
Nasal secretions				
units/ml	3–5	20	26	< 1
(≃ng/ml)	(2)	(10)	(13)	(< 1)
Antibody to Rye I as a percentage of total	30	0.2	0.1	—

* Total immunoglobulin levels were obtained by radioimmunoassay, except for serum IgG, IgA and IgM which were measured by Mancini technique. Total IgE values in serum and nasal secretions are higher in allergic persons. Total levels of the other classes are the same in allergic and non-allergic persons[36]
† Mean values for antibodies to Rye I are derived from a study on 45 untreated cases of hay fever[38]. The estimation of antibody levels in nanograms is based on RAST absorption and antigen binding techniques[13]. The calculation of antibody to Rye I as a percentage of the total immunoglobulin in each class can only be regarded as an approximate guide to the true values.

cells[32] there is no evidence to suggest that mast cells can act as a transport mechanism for IgE. In general IgE antibody which may well be produced locally tends to become distributed all over the body. That is, most patients will give positive skin tests wherever they are tested, they will also give positive bronchial and nasal provocation tests. In addition, patients with hay fever are susceptible to systemic anaphylaxis. Unfortunately there is no simple test of gastrointestinal sensitivity equivalent to a skin test or nasal provocation.

There are some patients with food allergy who develop diarrhoea or abdominal pain shortly after oral challenge. On the other hand there are many others who appear to be allergic to food but do not complain of abdominal symptoms. In these cases one has to assume either that the gut is not sensitized or that despite local release of histamine no identifiable symptoms occur. Jejunal biopsies taken after a food challenge do show some changes but the timing and the interpretation of these biopsies pose great problems[33]. There is some evidence that patients can be 'locally' sensitive to an allergen either in the nose or in the gut without having positive skin tests[34]. Certainly it is possible that locally produced IgE could sensitize local mast cells without sensitizing the whole body[34,35]. However, it seems more likely that these cases demonstrate the range of variations in the 'sensitivity' of different organs. Thus one would expect that quantitative skin tests using higher concentrations of allergen would reveal positive skin tests in the majority of cases. The older literature on immediate allergies used the term 'shock organ' to describe that part of a patient which selectively responded to allergen exposure. The clinical observations are still valid. For example many young dust mite allergic asthmatic children do not appear to get rhinitis, and many adult eczematous patients do not suffer from hay fever although they can be shown to have high levels of IgE antibody to grass pollen antigens. These variations are not well understood but they are more likely to be explained by variations in the distribution or sensitivity of mast cells than by the local production of IgE antibodies.

In summary, IgE antibody is produced in small quantities in response to a restricted group of antigens and is bound selectively to mast cells and basophils. Subsequent arrival of the allergen either by the same or other routes will cause immediate release of histamine and other mediators (see Chapter 2). At a biological level there are clearly two parts to this phenomenon. Firstly, the immune response of which IgE antibody is a part and, secondly, the consequences of mediator release from mast cells and basophils. Either of these could have biological advantages under certain circumstances.

The antibody response to inhalant allergens

Since it became clear that IgE antibodies were the major cause of immediate responses there has been a great tendency to consider only the factors that control IgE antibody production. For many years it was known that patients with hay fever or asthma did not have precipitating antibodies against pollen or dust allergens. In fact many authors doubted that 'atopic reagins' were antibodies at all. However, even before the discovery of IgE there was good evidence using radioactive techniques that allergic persons had serum IgG antibodies to pollen antigens while non-allergic persons did not[36,37]. More recently, using quantitative assays, it has become clear that patients with hay fever have IgG and IgA antibodies as well as IgE antibodies both in their serum and nasal secretions[38] (Figure 1.1). By contrast the majority of persons without hay fever have no detectable antibodies to grass pollen of any class either in their serum or their secretions[38]. This implies that the factors controlling the incidence of inhalant allergy control IgG and IgA antibody production as well as IgE antibody. Some earlier work had suggested that non-allergic persons had blocking activity[39] or IgA antibodies[40] in their nasal secretions. Further studies showed that the blocking activity in nasal

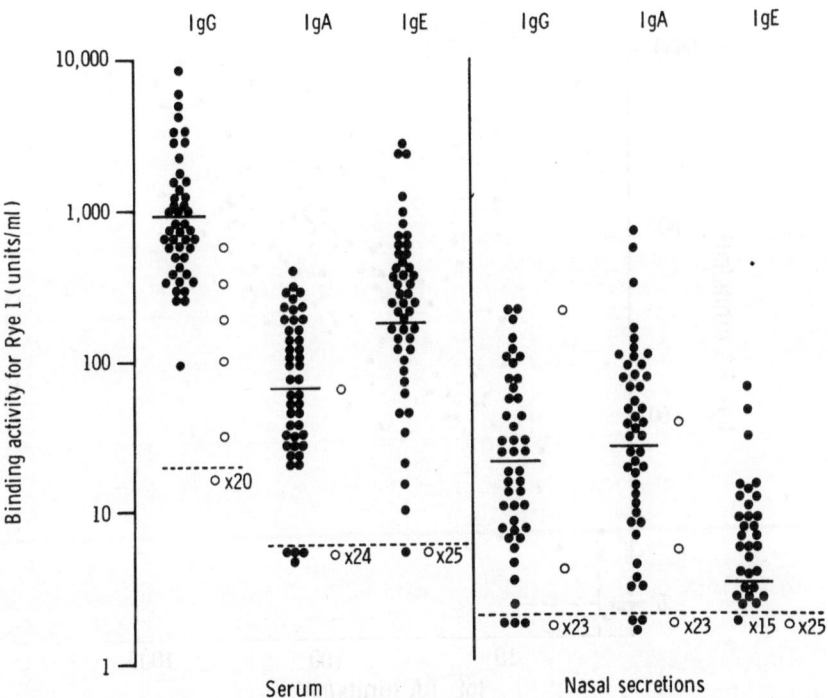

Figure 1.1 Class specific antibodies to a grass pollen antigen (Rye I) in patients with hay fever (●) and normal controls (○). Antibodies were measured by antigen binding radioimmunoassay[38] and are expressed in units of binding activity/ml of serum or concentrated nasal secretions

secretions of non-allergic persons was not due to specific antibody. In some of these studies RAST had been used to measure IgA antibodies and it is now clear that the background radioactivity was too high and too variable in those assays[40, 41]. Serum from most patients with hay fever or dust allergy contains both IgG and IgE antibodies, furthermore there is a good quantitative relationship between the two classes (Figure 1.2)[13, 42]. This correlation certainly suggests that the IgG antibody is part of the same response as the IgE antibody. It also suggests that if the antibody response is localized to one part of the body both classes are likely to be produced in the same place. Analysis of the IgG and IgA antibody to grass pollen found in nasal secretions showed that almost all the secreted antibody was produced locally[38]. Those studies suggested a model of the local antibody response in which the secreted antibody was produced in the mucosa while antibody entering the serum was derived predominantly from the local lymph nodes (Figure 1.3). The production of IgE antibody leads to allergic reactions in the nasal mucosa, and this local inflammation might act as a non-specific adjuvant for IgG antibody responses. Thus although it seems unlikely, it might be suggested

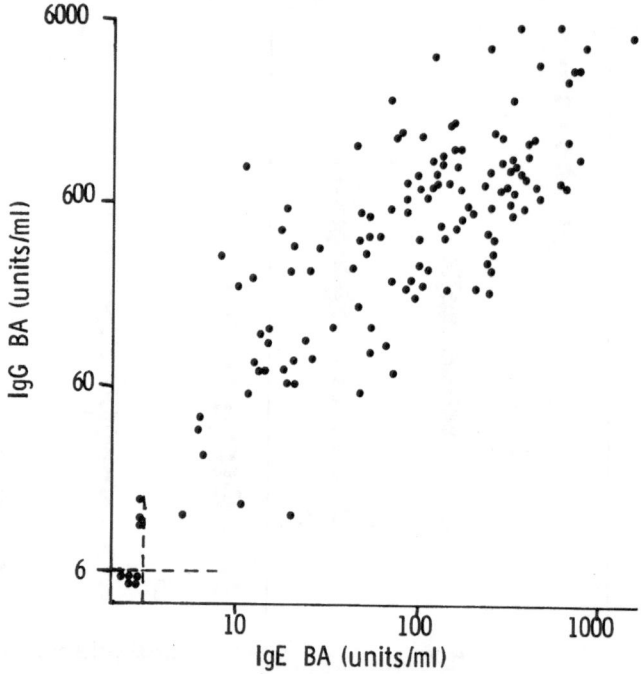

Figure 1.2   IgG and IgE antibodies to a house dust mite antigen (*D. pteronyssinus* – P₁) in patients with perennial rhinitis. Antibodies were measured by radioimmunoassay[10, 42], and are expressed as units of binding activity (BA)/ml of serum. Linear regression analysis of IgG BA against IgE BA showed a highly significant correlation ($r = 0.86$, $p < 0.001$)

that the high incidence and local production of IgG antibody to pollen was occurring secondary to IgE antibody production. Two pieces of direct evidence suggest that this is not so. Firstly, there are a few persons who have strongly positive skin tests to grass pollen but deny any symptoms and have normal nasal mucosa. These persons have both IgG and IgE antibodies to pollen in their serum. If IgG antibody was produced secondary to an IgE response one would expect the adjuvant effect to act on other proteins in the same pollen. However, patients who are allergic to the major ragweed antigen

AgE do not have IgG antibodies to the minor antigen Ra3 unless they are also allergic[43] to Ra3.

Symptoms and skin tests to inhalant allergens can occur within 10 minutes, so there seems little need to invoke a primary role for cell mediated immunity. Indeed patients with immediate hypersensitivity do not generally produce delayed skin reactions. On the other hand there is good evidence that allergic patients have lymphocytes in their peripheral blood which are capable of making proliferative responses to allergens[44–47]. It is generally assumed that the cells making these responses are T cells. Using antigen E denatured with urea, it has been found that the cells which proliferate *in vitro* will respond to antigenic determinants which are not recognized by specific antibodies[48]. This observation strongly suggests that the proliferating cells are T cells and also underlines the fact that these allergens can have multiple different antigenic determinants. Despite some reports to the contrary, most studies have found that lymphocytes from non-allergic persons do not respond to allergens *in vitro*[49].

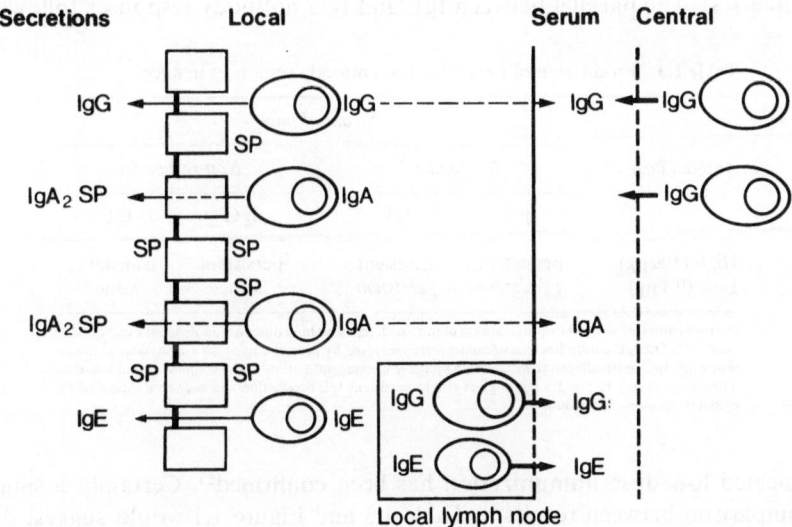

Figure 1.3 A model of the local immune response to pollen antigens. Antibodies produced in the mucosa are predominantly secreted whereas the local lymph nodes are the main site of production of serum IgG and IgE antibodies to pollen antigens. Injections of pollen extract will give rise to IgG antibodies produced predominantly in 'central' lymphoid tissue. SP = secretory piece[38]

It might appear that the presence of reactive T cells in the absence of delayed hypersensitivity is incongruous. However, in guinea-pigs it is lymphokine production and not proliferation which is an *in vitro* correlate of delayed hypersensitivity[50]. Strikingly the only reports of lymphokine production *in vitro* have used lymphocytes from patients who have had 'desensitizing' injections[45]. Similarly Slavin *et al.*[51] reported that only cells from immunized patients could transfer delayed reactivity. On balance it appears likely that patients with hay fever have sensitized T cells in their peripheral blood but that these T cells are helper cells for antibody production rather than mediators of delayed hypersensitivity. Whether the initial response to allergens is mediated by T cells, B cells or macrophages it seems clear that the response includes T cells as well as IgG, IgA and IgE antibodies. This suggests that the underlying difference between atopic and non-atopic individuals is likely to control the primary recognition of allergens and cannot be regarded as a specific control over IgE production.

Many experiments have been carried out to understand the conditions under which IgE antibody responses occur in mice. The first successful experiments were those of Levine and Vaz which showed that persistent IgE antibody responses could only be obtained by repeated low dose immunization in alum[52,53]. They also demonstrated that some strains of mice were much better at producing IgE responses. In addition, they observed that the persistent IgE responses were always accompanied by IgG antibody (see Table 1.3). The parallel between IgE and IgG antibody responses following

Table 1.3 Production of persistent IgE antibody responses in mice

	Strain of mice			
	Responder		*Non-responder*	
Antigen dose	IgG	IgE	IgG	IgE
High (100 µg)	persistent	transient	persistent	transient
Low (0.1 µg)	*persistent*	*persistent*	none	none

Derived from studies on the immunization of mice with repeated high doses or low doses of ovalbumin in alum[52-54]. The IgE antibodies to ovalbumin were measured by passive cutaneous anaphylaxis in mouse skin while IgG antibodies were measured by passive haemagglutination[54]. The combination of low dose immunization in a responder strain gives rise to persistent IgE production and may be a model of the events in an atopic individual

repeated low dose immunization has been confirmed[54]. Certainly a simple comparison between results in Table 1.3 and Figure 1.1 would suggest that allergic humans are equivalent to responder mice immunized with a repeated low dose immunization. The reason why IgE antibody responses following high dose immunization are transient has been shown to be due to suppressor T cells which act on IgE production. In many situations these suppressor T cells appear to be IgE specific[55-57]. However the results do not clearly distinguish whether the T cells are specific for IgE or whether IgE B cells can be 'turned off' by a combination of T-cell factors which has a positive effect on IgG production. Jarrett and her colleagues studying the effect of *Nippostrongylus brasiliensis* on IgE responses have defined a rat model where any dose of antigen over 10 ng would suppress IgE responses. In that system doses as low as 1 pg could boost an IgE response[58]. These doses of antigen used for boosting IgE are in the same range as the doses of inhalant allergens to which we are exposed *in vivo*. By contrast many experiments on IgE production in mice do not appear to be relevant to human inhalant allergy. Some mouse 'models' have used systemic immunization with 100 µg of antigen which gives rise to $\simeq$1000 µg IgG antibody/ml within a few weeks[59]. This should be compared with the human situation where 100 ng of pollen antigen is inhaled per season and produces $\leqslant$0.5 µg IgG antibody/ml over a period of several years. The animal studies suggest that under most circumstances IgE production is controlled very effectively by T cells. However, the unusual immunization regime with repeated low dose antigen in an atopic (i.e. responder) human appears to prime B cells and helper T cells under conditions where controlling or suppressor T cells are not primed.

Very few direct experiments have been carried out on humans. Repeated injections of ragweed or grass pollen in alum will produce transient reaginic sensitivity in non-atopic persons[60, 61]. Salvaggio and his colleagues immunized allergic and non-allergic persons nasally or systemically. They found that allergic persons responded better to nasal immunization but that there was no difference for systemic immunization[62, 63]. These results suggested the possibility that non-allergic persons had a nasal barrier preventing antigen entry. However, direct experiments to test this hypothesis demonstrated no difference in mucosal permeability between allergic and non-allergic individuals[64]. In retrospect those experiments are in keeping with the view that allergic persons have an increased ability to recognize and respond to low dose antigens at mucosal surfaces.

In summary. Direct experiments on allergic patients show that the antibody response to pollen is a local response and includes IgG and IgA antibodies as well as IgE antibodies. Experimental studies in man suggest that atopic individuals have an increased ability to respond to nasal immunization. Animal experiments have demonstrated that repeated low dose immunization is the most effective way of producing persistent IgE responses. It remains unclear whether atopic persons have increased immune responsiveness confined to mucosal surfaces, or whether the nose is the main site at which repeated low dose exposure occurs in man.

The genetics of inhalant allergy

The title of this chapter implies that because allergy has persisted in the community it must have some advantages to overcome the obvious disadvantages. This argument assumes that the tendency to become allergic is inherited, and indeed the familial nature of hay fever has been recognized for over 100 years[18] (see reference 7). Detailed analyses of the inheritance of hay fever have revealed two independent controls. Firstly, high total IgE levels appear to be inherited as an autosomal recessive characteristic unrelated to HLA[65,66]. Secondly, sensitivity to several allergens particularly the small 'minor' ragweed antigens Ra3 and Ra5 (Table 1.1) has been shown to be associated with certain HLA types[66-68a]. Very interestingly the HLA related controls appear to be masked in individuals with high total IgE[66]. In general these controls have been thought of as controls over IgE or IgE antibody production. However, as has been pointed out, the response to pollen antigens includes IgG, IgA and IgE antibodies (page 9). At present the results are most easily interpreted as showing that the HLA related controls influence the initial recognition of a given allergen. Once an immune response occurs to an allergen it will include IgG, IgA and IgE antibodies. It is probable that the site and nature of this immune response is controlled by the route of exposure and the dosage rather than by genetic factors.

The genetic controls over total IgE are more difficult to interpret. However, several points seem relevant. Firstly, it has been clear for some years that patients can be highly allergic without having a high total serum IgE. Secondly, in a series of 45 patients with grass pollen hay fever the incidence of and quantities of IgG and IgA antibody to Rye I in nasal secretions was not related[38] to total serum IgE. By contrast the quantities of serum IgG antibodies as well as serum IgE antibodies were correlated with total serum IgE. Thirdly, IgG antibody responses to inhalant allergens ($\leqslant 0.5\,\mu$g IgG/ml) would make no effect on total serum IgG ($\fallingdotseq 10$ mg/ml). On the other hand IgE antibody responses do contribute to total IgE (Table 1.2)[11-13]. Thus a genetic control that increased both IgE and IgG antibody responses might appear to be a genetic control[38] over total serum IgE. Combining the genetic studies with the studies on local production of antibodies suggests two possible explanations of what is inherited by patients with high total IgE. The first explanation is that these patients have an increased ability to recognize low dose antigens which may or may not be restricted to mucosal surfaces. These patients would make multiple IgE antibody responses which together would increase total serum IgE. The second explanation is that patients with high total serum IgE make larger quantities of IgG and IgE antibodies in their local lymph nodes (see Figure 1.3). It might throw some light on this problem if we knew whether antibodies measured against a purified allergen were directed against one or many different antigenic determinants. Some preliminary efforts have been made towards assessing the heterogeneity of IgE antibodies[68] but it is not yet possible to answer whether patients with high total IgE produce more heterogeneous IgE antibodies.

In summary, studies of the inheritance of hay fever have revealed two different types of inherited controls over allergy. It is possible that these controls all affect the initial recognition of allergens, but it is also possible that some of them might act by increasing rates of production of specific antibodies. At present there seems little reason to regard any of these controls as class-specific controls over IgE or IgE antibody production.

The non-allergic state

In studies on patients with immediate hypersensitivity the individuals in the non-allergic control group are usually chosen because they have never had allergic symptoms and they have negative skin tests. When studying hay fever it is assumed that the controls have been exposed to pollen and therefore that the non-allergic persons can be regarded as 'non-responders'. However, in the whole population there are several different types of persons who do not experience allergic symptoms. Firstly, there are individuals who have positive skin tests and detectable serum IgE antibody but deny any symptoms. These individuals have generally not been followed long enough to answer whether they are going to develop symptoms. Secondly, there are persons who have had allergic symptoms in the past but have been 'spontaneously' cured. Thirdly, there are people who have not been exposed to an allergen. This may be obvious for an industrial allergen such as platinum or a geographically-restricted plant such as North American ragweed. On the other hand for dust or mould allergens it may be extremely difficult to assess whether asymptomatic individuals have been exposed to the same quantities of allergen as the allergic patients. If truly unexposed individuals can be found then they can provide a reliable means of assessing negative background for studies on allergic individuals. Finally, there is a very interesting but unstudied group of persons who are going to develop symptoms in the future. While one could assume that infants are in the process of becoming sensitized, it is most unlikely that an individual could take more than 20 years to become sensitized to grass pollen and then develop hay fever at age 25. These prolonged 'incubations' pose many unanswered questions. Does sensitization occur at this late stage because of a new set of circumstances, e.g. a particular type of virus infection at the height of the pollen season? Is the unsensitized state maintained by a suppressor mechanism which breaks down? Is it possible that these patients have had IgE antibodies for many years but they develop symptoms because of a change in the sensitivity or distribution of their mast cells and basophils[69]? Clearly it is not possible to answer these questions at present but there are some clinical observations and a few laboratory tests which suggest answers. Firstly, delayed sensitization and spontaneous cure appear to be antigen specific. It is not uncommon to see patients who have had dust allergic asthma and rhinitis as children which improve only to be followed by the development of hay fever. Secondly, the phenomena are not directly age related. Many immigrants who come to England from Hong Kong or the West Indies develop severe hay fever although they are already in their thirties or forties. What limited results we have suggest that spontaneous cure involves a reduction in antibody levels of all classes. Certainly geriatric patients do not have high levels of antibodies to inhalant allergens. Indeed there is no evidence that 'spontaneous' cure of any inhalant allergy can occur because of the development of high levels of IgG 'blocking' antibody. A very speculative diagram of the time course of sensitivity to two allergens in an allergic patient is shown in Figure 1.4. There are several important features of this model. Firstly, spontaneous cure is antigen specific. Secondly, changes in IgG and IgE antibodies generally occur in parallel. Thirdly, spontaneous cure in not directly age related.

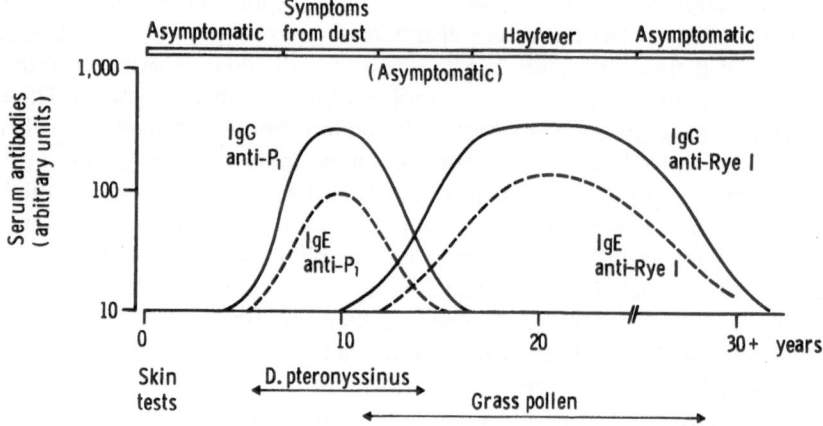

Figure 1.4 A possible model of the antibody response to a grass pollen antigen (Rye I) and a dust mite allergen (P_1). Both serum antibodies and positive skin tests would be present for longer than symptoms. It is suggested that IgG and IgE antibodies to these inhalant allergens would rise and fall in parallel. In addition it is suggested that spontaneous cure is antigen specific and is related to the time or extent of exposure rather than to the age of the patient

If recovery is not age related one assumes that it must in some way be related to cumulative antigen dose. It is very tempting to suggest that the length of allergic responses is inversely related to the antigen dose. Certainly IgE responses to the large quantities of cows' milk which are swallowed by infants may be transient, while IgE responses to pollen antigens ($\simeq$100 ng protein/ year) may last many years. However, there is no satisfactory way of comparing doses of absorbed protein with quantities of protein eluting from pollen grains on the nasal mucosa. At this point the question that seems most pertinent is: What is the cellular basis of spontaneous cure? Do B cells primed to a particular antigen have a limited number of divisions after which they die? If so, what prevents the priming of new B cells. Alternatively, is the antibody response to a particular antigen switched off by suppressor T cells? At present, despite considerable efforts, there are no reliable quantitative tests of T-cell sensitization. Certainly, no suitable *in vitro* assays to assess antigen specific suppression by human T cells are available.

If we now return to non-atopic asymptomatic individuals who have no detectable anti-allergen antibodies it is necessary to ask whether their non-allergic state is actively maintained. That is, are non-atopic individuals equivalent to unexposed persons, allergic persons who have (so far) failed to respond or to allergic persons who have been 'spontaneously' cured. At first sight the doses of inhalant allergens are so low that failure to recognize the antigens seems the most likely explanation for the non-allergic state. However, there are several animal studies which suggest that active suppression or tolerance can be induced by very low doses of antigens. For the present it seems that one should restrict interpretation to those results which are available on patients. These results suggest that the non-allergic individuals who have negative skin tests, no serum antibodies to allergens and no T-cell responses *in vitro* should be regarded as non-responders. As such they are probably immunologically similar to unexposed non-atopic individuals.

Immune deficiency and allergy

Direct studies on the antibody response to inhalant allergens have led to the conclusion that allergic patients are 'high responders'. Clearly these results do not suggest that immune deficiency would predispose patients to become allergic. In keeping with this, most studies have found that total serum IgG, IgA and IgM are normal in allergic patients[70, 71, 38]. However, several reports have suggested that allergic diseases occur with increased frequency among patients with certain immune deficiency diseases[72-75]. The idea that immune deficiency might predispose to allergy probably arose from the suggestion of Salvaggio *et al.*[63] that non-allergic persons had a block to nasal allergen entry. One possible explanation for 'nasal block' was that IgA antibody prevented antigen entry in non-allergic persons, and that allergic persons lacked this protective IgA antibody. In 1970 an increased incidence of IgA deficiency was reported among allergic patients[73], and it was also found that nasal secretions from non-allergic persons could block ragweed induced histamine release[39]. The following year a series of IgA deficient allergic patients was described[74]. In retrospect each of these studies has problems. Firstly, the patients with IgA deficiency reported by Kauffman and Hobbs had a wide range of allergic disorders including urticaria and migraine but they did not have documented allergy to inhalant allergens[73]. By contrast the series of patients reported by Schwartz and Buckley had well-defined inhalant allergy but they may not have had true IgA deficiency[74]. From earlier reports it appears that they found that 1% of the sera tested in their laboratory were IgA 'deficient'[76]. The generally accepted incidence of IgA deficiency is 1 person in 700 of the population (see reference 77 for further references). Certainly the definition of IgA deficiency should include low secretory IgA levels[78]. In a series of IgA-deficient patients with serum IgA < 0.05 mg/ml and salivary IgA < 0.01 mg/ml one does not find an increased incidence of allergy[77, 78]. The report by Turk *et al.* that nasal secretions from non-allergic persons could block *in vitro* histamine release[39] was initially supported by nasal antibody studies[40]. However, when antigen binding assays were used in the same laboratory it became clear that the blocking activity was not due to specific antibodies[79, 80]. An alternative explanation for the nasal 'block' was that non-allergic patients had a less permeable nasal mucosa; however, direct studies excluded this idea[64]. Indeed it now seems most unlikely that non-allergic persons have any mechanism that reduces allergen entry. It remains clear that allergy is common in the Wiskott–Aldrich syndrome[72] and probably in the Bruton type of sex-linked hypogammaglobulinaemia[75]. However, these conditions are rare and the raised incidence of allergy is more likely to reflect abnormalities of T-cell control than of antibody-mediated blocking mechanisms.

In their original paper Kauffman and Hobbs suggested that the production of IgE might be inversely related to IgA production[73]. Subsequently Hobbs reported that a few allergic children have markedly delayed maturation of *serum* IgA. Following this, Soothill and his group observed a correlation between low *serum* IgA in the first 6 months of life and the subsequent development of allergic disease[81]. The same finding has been reported from a different laboratory[82], but the reported levels of IgA were only modestly reduced and Kauffman and Frick in a detailed study could not confirm the observation[83]. In addition, it has not been shown that patients with 'delayed maturation' of serum IgA have low secretory IgA[84, 85]. Soothill has proposed that transient immune deficiency in infancy allows excess entry of allergens which in turn leads to increased IgE antibody production[85]. Clearly IgA deficiency during the first year of life would only be relevant to the development of allergy if sensitization occurred at this age. In addition, the theory depends on demonstrating that non-allergic patients produce specific IgA antibodies which are capable of blocking allergen entry[86]. As discussed previously (page 9) non-allergic adults do not appear to have specific IgA antibody in their nasal secretions. There seems little reason to believe that a modest reduction of total serum IgA implies a failure of local IgA production. Certainly the quantities of IgA antibody to inhalant allergens found in serum (approx. 20 ng/ml, see Table 1.2) would have no detectable effect[38] on serum IgA (approx. 1 mg/ml). At present there are no good studies available on the development of antibodies to inhalant allergens. It is very difficult to refute the idea that allergic infants generally become sensitized in their first year. However, it is clear that many adults arriving in England from Hong Kong or the West Indies develop grass pollen hay fever within a few years. The levels of grass pollen are very low in those areas so it seems likely that sensitization to pollen antigens can occur in adult life. Similarly many industrial allergens (e.g. castor beans and platinum salts) can induce IgE antibodies in adults.

In conclusion, there is an association between allergy and some rare types of immunodeficiency which may reflect the known role of T cells in controlling IgE responses. However, this does not appear to apply to IgA deficiency or common variable hypogammaglobulinaemia and there is no direct evidence that lack of serum or secretory antibodies can lead to overstimulation of IgE antibody production. Finally, it seems that the great majority of patients with hay fever are not immunologically deficient.

Injected allergens including bee stings and penicillin

Bee venom allergy will be discussed in full in Chapter 10; however the contrasts with inhalant allergy are worth considering here. The majority of persons who develop generalized or severe local reactions to bee stings can be shown to have IgE antibody to the enzyme phospholipase A (PLA)[19]. Phospholipase A represents approximately 15% of a bee sting and when purified is not irritant to non-allergic persons. Unlike pollen allergens, repeated exposure to bee venom is effectively restricted to beekeepers, many of whom receive 10 or more stings/week. This represents a much larger total dose than the maximum dose of pollen allergens. It is therefore not surprising that the antibody response to phospholipase A is very different from the antibody

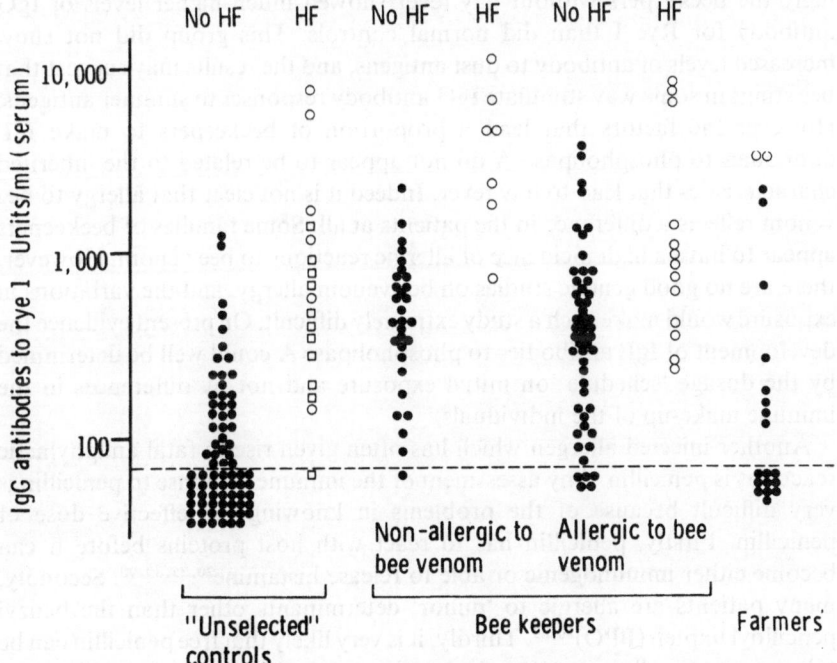

Figure 1.5 IgG antibodies to a grass pollen antigen (Rye I) in beekeepers and controls[87]. The beekeepers are divided into those who were allergic to bee venom and those who were not. In each group individuals with grass pollen hay fever (HF) are shown by open symbols (○ or □). The controls include 50 pregnant mothers where the diagnosis of hay fever was based on history alone. The hay fever subjects diagnosed without skin testing are indicated (□). A small group of farmers who averaged approximately 6 hours per day in the open air are included to show that being outside alone does not give rise to high levels of antibodies to grass pollen

response to pollen antigens. Most beekeepers, whether they are allergic to bee venom or not, have easily detectable serum IgG antibody to PLA. Furthermore, when IgG antibody was measured in nasal secretions from beekeepers there was no evidence for local production of antibodies to PLA[87]. Thus almost all beekeepers make IgG antibodies to PLA, while the allergic beekeepers make IgE antibodies as well as IgG antibodies.

Clearly it would be very interesting to know whether the beekeepers who make IgE antibody to PLA are those who make antibody responses to inhaled allergens. Previous studies have given equivocal results but there appeared to be an increased incidence of hay fever among the families of beekeepers who were allergic to bee venom[88]. In order to study this further we have measured antibodies to Rye I in sera from a large group of beekeepers[87]. The results show no significant difference in antibody to the pollen antigen between beekeepers who were allergic to bee venom and those who are not (Figure 1.5). Both groups of beekeepers with hay fever showed similar levels of IgG and IgE antibodies to Rye I to non-beekeepers with hay fever (Figure 1.5). Surprisingly the beekeepers without hay fever showed much higher levels of IgG antibody for Rye I than did normal controls. This group did not show increased levels of antibody to dust antigens, and the results may suggest that bee stings in some way stimulate IgG antibody responses to summer antigens. However the factors that lead a proportion of beekeepers to make IgE antibodies to phospholipase A do not appear to be related to the inherited characteristics that lead to hay fever. Indeed it is not clear that allergy to bee venom reflects a difference in the patients at all. Some families of beekeepers appear to have a high incidence of allergic reactions to bee venom. However, there are no good genetic studies on bee venom allergy, and the variations in exposure would make such a study extremely difficult. On present evidence the development of IgE antibodies to phospholipase A could well be determined by the dosage 'schedule' on initial exposure and not by differences in the immune make-up of the individuals.

Another injected allergen which has often given rise to fatal anaphylactic reactions is penicillin. Any assessment of the immune response to penicillin is very difficult because of the problems in knowing the effective dose of penicillin. Firstly, penicillin has to react with host proteins before it can become either immunogenic or able to release histamine[20, 25, 89, 90]. Secondly, many patients are allergic to 'minor' determinants other than the benzyl pencilloyl hapten (BPO)[20, 89]. Thirdly, it is very likely that free penicillin can be tolerogenic. Finally, most patients receive a complex mixture of tablets and injections, which are thought to influence the response[89]. However, despite these problems the antibody response to penicillin does appear to be similar to that to inhalant allergens. That is, allergic individuals have IgG and IgE antibodies, while patients who do not react to penicillin produce smaller quantities of IgG antibody alone or no detectable antibody[89, 90]. Several reports have shown a high incidence of atopy among penicillin allergic patients[89,90]. However, in some of these series it has not been clear how the patients were collected. In addition, allergic patients may receive more courses of penicillin for 'infections' and may also be more observant about the reactions. If antibody responses to penicillin (including IgG and IgE antibodies) are more common in atopic persons it might suggest that their increased responsiveness was general rather than being restricted to mucosal surfaces (see page 13).

The active and passive regimes for immunization against tetanus and diphtheria offer a striking contrast in the incidence of allergic reactions to injected foreign protein[91]. Toxoid preparations, with or without alum, give rise to very high levels of antitoxin and cause anaphylaxis very rarely. Indeed, many of the recorded reactions to toxoid were probably reactions to peptone broth[91]. Test injections with toxoid are not normally carried out even if the recipients are atopic and have been repeatedly immunized with toxoid in the past[91]. There is some in vitro evidence for IgE antibodies to diphtheria toxin in immunized persons[92], and it might be suggested that the lack of anaphylactic reactions is due to the high levels of IgG antibodies. However, the incidence of local immediate reactions to Schick testing is very low and these skin responses would not be dramatically reduced by serum IgG antibodies. On the other hand, horse antitoxin is a notorious cause of anaphylactic reactions and these can generally be predicted or avoided by test injections. In some cases these reactions are due to preceding sensitization with inhaled horse dander. Nonetheless antiserum injections often cause dangerous sensitization and it is possible that this occurs because horse serum proteins persist in the circulation for some time. Alternatively the IgE antibody response to horse serum proteins may be restricted to some part of the body where critical dosage occurs. The data for toxoids fit in very well with the results of animal experiments in showing that antigens or adjuvants that will give rise to high levels of IgG antibody will generally give rise to 'suppressor' T cells which terminate or prevent IgE antibody responses. By contrast the injection of freely soluble proteins or reactive haptens without adjuvant, e.g. phospholipase A, penicillin or horse serum carries a risk of inducing IgE antibody responses and is not an effective way of inducing precipitating levels of IgG antibody.

THE NON-IMMEDIATE ALLERGIES

Extrinsic allergic alveolitis (EAA)

Farmers' lung provides a very striking contrast to pollen allergy. Clinically, patients develop fever and a cough approximately 8 hours after exposure to mouldy hay dust. These symptoms are caused by the spores of thermophilic actinomycetes. Extract of these spores can reproduce the symptoms after bronchial challenge and give a skin reaction developing after about 6 hours.

Spores have to be less than 5 μm in diameter in order to enter the alveoli and very large numbers of these spores can be present in hay dust. Indeed Belin has estimated that the air in some sawmills where workers develop EAA can contain up to 10^9 fungal spores per cubic metre[93]. Even patients who are 'sensitive' still require relatively large quantities of dust to induce symptoms. Pepys and Jenkins[94] carried out bronchial challenge using partially purified extracts containing 10 mg protein/ml. This is, of course, an extremely large quantity of allergen by comparison with pollen allergens where concentrations < 1 ng/ml are often sufficient to induce skin reactions. In keeping with the large quantities of allergens involved these patients usually have easily demonstrable precipitins in their serum against several components of the dust which causes symptoms. In this respect the situation in EAA resembles immunization in the presence of a potent adjuvant. Thus in serum from patients with pigeon breeders' lung precipitins can be demonstrated against a variety of pigeon serum proteins[95]. It is possible that EAA develops because the inhaled substances have special properties. However under different circumstances serum proteins from birds (e.g. ovalbumin) are very effective at inducing anaphylactic sensitivity. Furthermore there are many different forms of EAA and it seems to occur in those situations where the largest quantities of fungal spores are inhaled. It seems unlikely that the disease reflects a special property shared by all the substances against which serum precipitins have been demonstrated[94, 95].

Recently Edwards and his colleagues have demonstrated that spores of *Micropolyspora faeni* are as active as Zymosan in consuming complement via the alternative pathway[97]. In addition they have shown that Zymosan or *M. faeni* spores will give rise to inflammatory lesions in the lungs of unsensitized rats or rabbits[98]. The lesions were very similar to the lesions seen in lung biopsies from patients with farmers' lung[98]. Those findings were related to the clinical observation that some patients appear to develop EAA on first exposure to mouldy hay and before they have demonstrable serum precipitins. Clearly, complement activation by *M. faeni* spores could be relevant in two ways. Firstly, it could be the cause of the symptoms and the immunopathology. Secondly, it might act as an adjuvant for the production of precipitins. Certainly the precipitins are demonstrated with soluble proteins that can be extracted; on the other hand the complement activation is only effective with whole spores[97]. If the alternative pathway activation was the cause of EAA then fungal spore inhalation might be regarded as a form of toxicity rather than allergy[99]. However, the time sequence and histology of both skin tests and lung lesions in farmer's lung and pigeon fancier's lung are similar to those of an Arthus reaction. Furthermore Wilkie *et al.* found that sensitized guinea-pigs gave much more severe lung reactions to *M. faeni* spores than non-sensitized animals[100]. Before attempting to purify an antigen responsible for extrinsic allergic alveolitis it is necessary to decide whether the antigen should be judged by its ability to:

(1) react with serum precipitins,
(2) activate complement,
(3) induce lung symptoms.

At present it seems most likely that complement activation or some other property of the spores causes local inflammation. This inflammation acts as an adjuvant for the production of serum precipitating antibodies directed against several different proteins present in the dust. On subsequent exposure the antibodies contribute to the symptoms by causing an Arthus reaction.

As stated previously, the conditions under which EAA develops involve the inhalation of large quantities of dust. In some diseases, e.g. bagassosis and byssinosis, it has been suggested that the inorganic matter in the dust is involved in the pathology. This is probably not so, because the inorganic dusts involved are not those that cause disease and, in addition, the lung disease in EAA is generally completely reversible. Nonetheless it is clear that quantities of dust involved are so high that they probably should not be regarded as non-toxic. Certainly in some types of EAA as many as 50% of the exposed population develop symptoms and there is no good evidence that susceptibility is controlled by an inherited trait. Traditionally, farmers have associated lung symptoms with mouldy hay and have avoided it. More recently the symptoms of bagassosis have prompted industrial changes which have dramatically reduced the inhalation of fungal spores[96]. The storage of bagasse was increased in the 1930s and the disease developed. Extensive investigation was then undertaken to discover the cause of the disease[96]. Partly as a result of those investigations bagasse is now used rapidly as a fuel or as a source of fibre and is stored under conditions where fungi do not grow well.

By definition, patients with EAA do not have active fungal infection of their lungs. However, similar symptoms and serum precipitins can occur with fungi which are capable of producing active infection in the lungs, e.g. *Aspergillus*. It is obvious that the ability to mount an immune response to potentially infective or toxic fungal spores in the lungs could be a biologically important part of the immune system.

Contact sensitivity

Patch testing has the great advantage that it is a direct model of the disease process which it is used to study. In diagnosing contact sensitivity the test substance is usually made up in a soft paraffin base and applied to undamaged skin. In order to penetrate, the test substance will have to be small and lipid soluble. It is thought that these substances then react with molecules in the skin and so give rise to an 'immunogenic' molecule. Certainly lymphocytes draining a patch of mouse skin painted with dinitrochlorobenzene (DNCB) can be very effective in actively immunizing another mouse to show contact sensitivity[101]. This suggests that skin sensitizing agents penetrate the skin and react with surface molecules (possibly HLA or H_2 antigens) on lymphocytes or macrophages. These modified cells then act as a potent stimulus to other lymphocytes, which become specifically sensitized. Certainly DNCB is small, chemically reactive and lipid soluble; it is thought that nickel and the industrial oils that cause many cases of clinical sensitivity are also chemically reactive. The cells that can transfer contact sensitivity in mice are T cells. Furthermore, many patients with hypogammaglobulinaemia and a severe deficiency of antibody production can be sensitized with DNCB. Thus there seems to be good evidence that a sensitive recognition system and effector T cells are involved in contact sensitivity. On this traditional view there would be little in common between the antibody response to inhaled pollen and the T-cell response to DNCB or poison ivy.

Recently the situation has become much more complicated, with evidence for a role for basophils and mast cells as well as serum antibodies in different types of delayed responses (recently reviewed by Askenase[102]). Firstly, there is evidence that many delayed responses including contact lesions in animals and man are heavily infiltrated with basophils[103]. Secondly, some delayed skin reactions can be blocked by inhibitors of vasoactive amines[102], suggesting that mast cell or basophil mediators are involved in the pathology of the lesion. Finally, it has become clear that contact sensitizing agents can induce an antibody response including reaginic antibodies[104]. While it is clear that many human skin lesions are infiltrated with basophils there is little evidence to suggest that IgE mediated hypersensitivity is involved in contact lesions in man. Intradermal injections of contact sensitizing agents generally produce a delayed response, not an immediate weal and flare. However, in many cases these agents are haptens and would not be expected to give an immediate response unless they were linked to a carrier (cf. penicillin). It is also generally thought that patients with contact hypersensitivity do not have serum antibodies. However, these antibodies have not been studied using the sensitive radioactive techniques that are currently available.

Approaching the problem from the other end, most inhalant allergens do not give rise to contact sensitivity. However, this does not answer whether the relevant T cells are sensitized. Clearly water-soluble pollen proteins with a molecular weight of $\simeq 30\,000$ would not easily penetrate the skin. When inhalant allergens are injected they give rise to an immediate weal and flare response, which may be followed by a late response but is not followed by a true delayed hypersensitivity response of tuberculin type. It may be that the immediate response by causing an influx of serum can 'block' or 'wash out' the antigen. Alternatively the immediate response may limit the dose to a level which is suboptimal for eliciting delayed sensitivity. In keeping with these possibilities it has been reported that immediate allergens injected together with an antihistamine will give rise to delayed responses[105].

In conclusion the nature of the substance causing contact sensitivity reflects primarily the physical and chemical properties necessary to penetrate the dermis and react with other molecules. The nature of the lesions similarly reflects the exact site in the skin at which the antigen interacts with sensitized cells, primarily T cells. The biological advantage of the system is not obvious; however, it may be that each component of the response is important under different circumstances. Thus sensitive recognition of surface alterations on lymphocytes or macrophages may be essential in developing many types of immune response. On the other hand T effector cells are probably responsible for controlling many virus infections. Contact sensitivity may well be an 'accidental' consequence of these systems. Sensitivity to *Primula obonica*, stinking mayweed, poison ivy or nickel may not carry a biological advantage but it would seem to be a small price to pay for good T-cell immunity.

THE BIOLOGICAL ROLE OF IMMEDIATE HYPERSENSITIVITY

The main conclusion of this brief discussion of underlying events is that allergies result from inappropriate or overactivity of many different parts of the immune system. Hay fever involves IgE antibodies, the mast cell/basophil system and local immunity. Extrinsic allergic alveolitis depends on the ability to produce large quantities of precipitating antibodies. Contact sensitivity represents an aspect of cellular immunity. If the question we are asking is 'What is the advantage of an immune system?' then the answer is clear. Without a system for responding specifically to pathogenic organisms humans do not survive. Infants with severe combined immune deficiency (SCID) can only survive in a pathogen-free environment. However, if the question is broken down into the different systems, then the answers become less simple. The biological advantage of a system may not be obvious over a short length of time or within a particular environment. The present population of Europe must still reflect those groups which have survived bubonic plague, smallpox, syphilis, tuberculosis and influenza. However, it would be very difficult today to study which aspects of the immune system were critical for resistance against the major causes of premature mortality in the past. With these problems in mind, the present discussion will focus on the factors involved in immediate hypersensitivity.

Mast cells and basophils

The anaphylactic release of histamine is a clearly defined process and has two important features. Firstly, it is very rapid, sneezing can develop within 30 seconds of intranasal challenge, skin tests can respond within 3 minutes, and histamine release from basophils *in vitro* may be complete within 2 minutes[29]. Secondly, the system can be extremely sensitive; intradermal skin responses can sometimes be produced with 0.05 ml of a $10^{-6} \mu g/ml$ dilution of purified allergen. This represents less than 1 pg of protein. the weal and flare response leads to a rapid influx of serum which contains antibodies. Furthermore, eosinophil chemotactic factor is released in parallel and many help to mobilize eosinophils to the same site[106].

The theory that mast cells act as a rapid method of mobilizing serum defences has been referred to as the gatekeeper hypothesis[107]. Early experiments demonstrated that if the skin was sensitized with IgE antibodies then a local injection of diphtheria toxin and allergen could be neutralized by IgG antitoxin present in the serum[107]. However, it seems likely that the system has more relevance to helminths than bacterial toxins. It is well established that schistosomules can be killed by eosinophils and that this killing is dependent on antibodies[108]. Thus an immediate skin response to a larval worm could lead to an influx of specific IgG antibody and eosinophils which together could kill the larva. In direct studies of infection of rats with schistosomules it has been difficult to prove that immediate responses are important in the undoubted protective immunity[109, 110]. However, the details of the experiments do not really matter to the present argument since we do not know with which parasites and under what conditions the system might have had its major advantage. The important principle is that an antibody response to a helminth could produce IgG and IgE antibodies which together with mast cells and eosinophils might give rapid protection against further larvae entering the skin.

Another site at which anaphylactic histamine release might prevent entry or passage of pathogens is in the lungs. Sneezing in response to allergens is certainly mediated by mast cells/basophils[111]. The mechanism of coughing induced by allergens is not completely clear but probably involves histamine or vasoamine release. Presumably coughing or sneezing could only act on pathogens in the airways. Previously it had been thought that mast cells were in the mucosa so that antigens would have to penetrate before causing histamine release. However, it is now clear that mast cells are present in the epithelium and that antigens or anti-IgE can cause histamine release without penetrating (see Mygind[111]). More recently Hastie et al.[69] have shown that there are basophils in the nasal mucus, so that it is clear that pathogens or allergens could react with these cells while they were still in the nasal passages. Mast cells and basophil responses are non-specific in their results. That is, the influx of serum and cells will not be restricted to the original antigen. A possible advantage of this non-specific response to a specific signal could occur with reactions to insect salivary proteins. After an insect bite mobilization of serum might well help to prevent entry of parasites present in the insect saliva. Clearly there are many insects which give rise to highly irritating local reactions. On the other hand it has not been established that insect bite reactions are IgE mediated or that local influx of serum can block entry of insect-borne pathogens. However, protozoan parasites generally do not give rise to IgE responses. Therefore, immediate responses to the insect saliva might be an effective way of achieving local protection against insect-borne protozoa.

The IgE-mediated anaphylactic release of histamine is not the only way in which mast cells and basophils can release histamine. Firstly, there are other ways of triggering anaphylactic release[27]. Secondly, there is considerable evidence that basophils can be mobilized to a site of antigen entry[69, 102]. Thirdly, it is probable that gradual release of mediators from granules can occur. The importance of these systems may not be clear but they probably represent ways in which mast cells and basophils evolved and were biologically important before the development of IgE antibodies. Histamine release can definitely be triggered[27] by C3a and C5a. *In vivo* these anaphylotoxins are rapidly destroyed by carboxypeptidases and would not normally persist in the circulation. However, local complement activation in an Arthus reaction or by direct activation of the alternative pathway (e.g. pneumococcus) could well cause local histamine release. Another trigger for mast cells could come from sensitized T cells. Among the tremendous array of lymphokines are factors that can increase vascular permeability and it is possible that these factors act via mast cells.

The realization that basophils can accumulate at a skin test site has revolutionized the interpretation of delayed hypersensitivity (reviewed in reference 102). The mechanism of accumulation almost certainly involves a basophil chemotactic factor[112]. The function of basophils in skin lesions has not been established. However they may act to amplify an existing response or they may act directly on a pathogen. It has been shown that basophils accumulating locally can degranulate in response to persisting or reintroduced antigens[102]. It has recently been shown that basophils can increase in the nasal secretions of allergic patients during the pollen season[69]. This accumulation may well be responsible for the progressive increase in symptoms that occurs during the season[69]. It has also been shown that an accumulation of basophils can have a direct toxic effect on a parasite[102]. In an elegant model Bagnall has shown that the tick *Ixodes holocychis* causes local basophil-rich reactions in guinea-pigs. Applying ticks to an immune guinea-pig can lead to a dramatic accumulation of basophils inside the ticks, which then fall off and die. There are good circumstantial reasons for believing that the basophils are responsible for the death of the parasites.

Histamine can also be released from mast cells or basophils gradually. This process is not easy to study. Clearly the local effects of gradual release may not resemble an immediate response, in particular the influx of cells might be much more pronounced than the influx of serum. At a more 'primitive' level it is possible that mast cells and basophils might have a role in influencing vascular tone and permeability.

In conclusion there seems to be good evidence that mast cells and basophils can degranulate in response to signals other than IgE. In addition these cells can accumulate locally and act in a variety of ways apart from causing a rapid accumulation of serum. It seems very likely that histamine containing cells have or have had a major role not dependent on IgE. If so it is likely that homocytotropic antibodies developed as a method of augmenting or accelerating mast cell mechanisms that were already available. Certainly there seems little reason to doubt that IgE on mast cells can act as a very rapid method either for mobilizing defence systems to the skin or for clearing pathogens from the airways.

IgE antibody responses

If IgE antibodies have a biological role it must be related to their ability to mediate degranulation of mast cells and basophils. It is very unlikely that IgE antibodies could have a significant role in any other way. The quantities of IgE produced do not appear to be sufficient to neutralize or agglutinate an antigen. Furthermore, IgE antibodies are accompanied in serum and secretions by larger quantities of IgG or IgA antibodies. The most striking feature of experimental IgE responses is the restricted conditions under which they occur (see page 12). In humans IgE responses occur predominantly against inhalant allergens or in the presence of helminth parasites.

It has been known for many years that infestation with some parasites can be associated with specific 'sensitization'. This may be restricted to local itching at the site of larval entry (swimmer's itch), but *Schistosoma japonicum* often gives rise to signs of systemic hypersensitivity including urticaria, generalized itching, cough and fever. As early as 1931 Taliafero and Taliafero demonstrated a positive PK test using serum from a patient with schistosomiasis[113]. Many different antigens have been used for skin testing these patients, but cercarial antigens will give positive weal and flare responses in as many as 95% of cases[114]. Clearly, the immune response to human pathogenic schistosomes is not very successful at preventing cercarial entry or the development of adult flukes. However humans also develop itching reactions to animal flukes which do not successfully parasitize man. It has been suggested that these itching (probably IgE mediated) reactions are important in preventing infection with 'non-pathogenic' flukes[115].

When IgE was discovered it was rapidly established that parasitic infections were associated with raised serum IgE levels[116]. Many experiments have been carried out in animals to understand the reasons why worms selectively stimulate IgE. It is now clear that infection of rats with *Nippostrongylus brasiliensis* leads to increases in all aspects of IgE production. The infected rats produce more IgE specific B cells[56], and increased quantities of specific IgE antibody both against the worms and against irrelevant antigens[58], in addition to having higher total serum IgE. These studies and the pattern of human diseases suggest that IgE responses occur because of special properties of the substances released by the worms. Thus the factors that give rise to IgE responses during worm infection may not relate to the conditions that give rise to IgE responses to allergens. If so one would not expect to find a direct advantage for atopic individuals in coping with parasites. Indeed the high incidence of positive skin tests in schistosomiasis would suggest that these worms can induce an IgE response in all humans.

Another example of a parasite which can give rise to 'sensitization' is the mite *Sarcoptes scabei* which causes scabies. The skin response to scabies includes urticaria and severe itching, both generalized and at the site of burrows[117]. In addition it is said that the itching response following reinfection of a sensitized person can occur 'within hours'[117]. More recently it has been reported that patients with scabies have raised serum IgE levels[118]. Mellanby found that the scratching of scabies was very effective in dislodging and killing the mites and he proposed that this was a direct protective mechanism[117]. Although many features suggest that the response to scabies is IgE mediated, the lesions around burrows typically develop vesicles and have many features of a delayed response. It seems that this may well represent another situation where a mast cell or basophil response is associated with a delayed skin lesion. Since adult female *Sarcoptes* appear to be able to continue burrowing in a 'sensitized' host it is likely that this mite is most vulnerable at the time when it first starts to enter the skin.

The scabies mite may represent a bridge between the two types of IgE response. House dust mites are an important cause of inhalant allergy and the major allergen appears to be a non-irritant protein which is repeatedly absorbed through the nasal mucosa[10]. On the other hand the scabies mite may induce an IgE response by burrowing in the skin. This suggests that the scabies mite may have a special ability to stimulate IgE responses similar to that of the helminths. However, the scabies mite does not appear to be irritant in a non-sensitized host. Most volunteers infected with scabies carry a small number of mites and experience no symptoms for the first 4 to 6 weeks[117]. Similarly the entry of cercaria through the skin of an unsensitized host is said to be asymptomatic. Thus both types of parasites appear to represent a source of antigen which does not create local inflammation and which persists for months.

Human IgE antibody responses occur in several different situations. However, there may be a connection in that the antigens are non-inflammatory, recur over a significant length of time, probably in low dose and are 'local'. Local here may mean simply that the main dose of antigen is in the nasal mucosa, the skin or the gastrointestinal tract rather than being in the circulation or the spleen. Certainly the conditions of a respiratory virus infection, cholera, staphylococcal infection or diphtheria toxoid immunization are all strikingly different from both helminth infection or natural exposure to grass pollen. It seems very likely that IgE responses are, or have been, biologically important in relation to those pathogens which are capable of inducing immediate hypersensitivity.

Sensitive local immunity

In the two previous sections we have considered the possible biological roles of the mast cell/basophil system and of IgE antibodies. However, non-allergic individuals have mast cells and basophils which can be sensitized; they also have IgE and the ability to make IgE antibody responses. On the other hand, the majority of non-allergic persons fail to make an immune response to inhalant allergens. It is the ability to make local immune responses to low dose antigens which is the essential characteristic of atopic persons and which needs explaining.

If the only antigens to which allergic persons responded differently were the inhalant allergens discussed here, then it would be very difficult to propose a biological advantage. On the other hand, having a sensitive recognition process for foreign antigens might have enormous importance in relation to micro-organisms. As we have said previously, immunization with high dosage ($>10\,\mu g$ antigen) generally does not produce persistent IgE responses. In most *in vivo* situations low dose antigens would only persist for a short time before either increasing or being eliminated. Thus under most naturally occurring conditions an antigen would not be present at low concentrations long enough to give rise to a persistent IgE antibody response. A sensitive recognition process might therefore be advantageous under conditions where it did not give rise to IgE antibodies. In order to identify these situations one would have to look for *negative* associations with atopy. That is, which diseases are less common in atopic patients? Although there are no important well-established negative associations with atopy, there are several reports in the literature and many apocryphal tales.

The most persistent reports of a negative association with allergy concern malignant tumours. Initially a report suggested that there was no association[119] but this was followed by four reports showing a low incidence of allergy in patients with cancer[120-123]. None of these studies documented 'allergy' very well but the report of Ure showing a negative association between allergy and gynaecological carcinomas is very striking[121]. McKee et al., in attempting to resolve the issue, found no difference in the allergic status of the cancer patients among a series of general surgical patients[124]. However they did not report a normal control group[124], and Augustin and Chandrassa[123] found that allergy was less common in all surgical patients than among normal controls. When it became possible to measure IgE several reports suggested that total IgE levels were low in patients with cancer[123, 125, 126]. In contrast, two recent reports have recorded normal levels of IgE in patients with cancer[127, 128]. However one of these was concerned predominantly with patients with sarcoma or melanoma[127], whereas the reports showing reduced incidence of allergy have predominantly concerned tumours of mucosal surfaces[120-122]. In Hodgkin's disease it has been reported repeatedly that the incidence of allergy is normal[129, 130] and that serum IgE is either high[126] or normal[131]. It appears possible that if there is a decreased incidence of allergy in patients with cancer this may not apply to lymphatic tissue tumours, sarcomas, melanomas[120] or ovarian carcinoma[132], and furthermore that the inverse correlation may be more marked in women[120, 121]. The finding of low levels of total IgE and of allergic symptoms in patients with cancer has often been interpreted as suggesting that IgE has some role in protection against cancer. However, if atopy is interpreted as a consequence of a high level of mucosal immunity, then a negative association between inhalant allergy and tumours of mucosal surfaces would be very interesting.

There are many other disease situations where increased local immunity might be advantageous but there are few good data. In order to study these situations it is essential to have a normal age matched control group, and an objective measure of allergy, preferably including both IgE and IgG antibodies. As well as defining the associated illness it is essential to define the type of allergy involved. Studies in which hay fever, urticaria, migraine and penicillin hypersensitivity are grouped together as 'allergy' are worse than useless. The proposition is that inhalant allergy is a consequence of a genetically determined 'increased' level of local immunity. It seems very likely that under some circumstances this would be advantageous, but that the advantage might be due to more rapid or better recognition rather than being related to IgE. If this is correct then an allergic response to harmless inhaled proteins would be seen as the price that atopic subjects pay for maintaining sensitive local immunity. The fact that the antibody response to inhaled proteins includes persistent IgE antibodies can be seen as a consequence of the unusual dosage schedule. The advantages of mast cells/basophils and IgE antibodies appear to relate to different circumstances including the defence against parasitic worms. Under primitive conditions it seems most unlikely that inhalant allergies would be an important disadvantage by comparison with the advantages of a rapid defence against worms or of generally increased local immunity.

References

1. Blackley. C. H. (1873). *Experiments and Researches on the Causes and Nature of 'Catarrhus Aestivus'.* (London: Baillière)
2. Wyman, M. (1872). *Autumnal Catarrh (Hay Fever).* (Cambridge, Mass.: Huro and Houghton)
3. Voorhorst, R., Spieksma, F. Th. M., Varekamp, M., Leupen, M. J. and Lyklema, A. W. (1967). The house dust mite (*Dermatophagoides pteronyssinus*) and the allergens it produces. Identity with the house dust allergen. *J. Allergy*, **39**, 325
4. Noon, L. (1911). Prophylactic inoculation against hay fever. *Lancet*, **1**, 1572
5. Berrens, L. (1974). Inhalant allergens in human atopic disease: their chemistry and modes of action. *Ann. NY Acad. Sci.*, **221**, 183

6. King, T. P. (1976). Chemical and biological properties of some atopic allergens. *Adv. Immunol.*, **23**, 77–105
7. Marsh, D. G. (1975). Allergens and the genetics of allergy. In Sela, M. (ed.) *The Antigens.* Vol. III, pp. 271–359. (New York: Academic Press)
8. Schneeberger, E. E. (1974). The permeability of the alveolar–capillary membrane to ultrastructural protein tracers. *Ann. N.Y. Acad. Sci.*, **221**, 238–243
9. Belin, L. (1972). Immunological analyses of birch pollen antigens with special reference to the allergenic components. *Int. Arch. Allergy Appl. Immunol.*, **42**, 300
10. Chapman, M. D. and Platts-Mills, T. A. E. (1980). Purification and characterization of the major allergen from *Dermatophagoides pteronyssinus* – antigen P_1. *J. Immunol.* (In press)
11. Gleich, G. J. and Jacob, G. L. (1975). Immunoglobulin E antibodies to pollen allergens account for high percentages of total immunoglobulin E protein. *Science*, **190**, 1106
12. Schellenberg, R. R. and Adkinson, N. F. (1975). Measurement of absolute amounts of antigen-specific human IgE by a radio allergosorbent test (RAST) elution technique. *J. Immunol.*, **115**, 1577 and Erratum 1976, **117**, 355
13. Platts-Mills, T. A. E., Snajdr, M. J., Ishizaka, K. and Frankland, A. W. (1978). Measurement of IgE antibody by an antigen binding assay: correlation with PK activity and IgG and IgA antibodies to allergens. *J. Immunol.*, **120**, 1201
14. Ishizaka, K., Ishizaka, T. and Hornbrook, M. M. (1967). Allergen binding activity of γE, γG and γA antibodies in sera from atopic patients: *in vitro* measurements of reaginic antibody. *J. Immunol.*, **98**, 490
15. Frick, O. L., German, D. F. and Mills, J. (1979). Development of allergy in children. I. Association with virus infections. *J. Allergy Clin. Immunol.*, **63**, 228
16. Prausnitz, C. and Küstner, H. (1921). Studien veber die verbering findlichkeit. *Zentrabl. Bakteriol., Parasitenkol. Infectionskr. Hyg. Abt.* 1. *Orig. Reihe A.*, **86**, 160
17. Aas, K. (1974). Allergol Proc. Int. Congr. 8th 1973. pp. 400–402. (Amsterdam: Excerpta Medica)
18. Coca, A. F. and Cooke, R. A. (1923). On the classification of the phenomena of hypersensitiveness. *J. Immunol.*, **8**, 163
19. Sobotka, A., Valentine, M., Leon, A. and Lichtenstein, L. M. (1974). Allergy to insect stings. Diagnosis of IgE mediated hymenoptera sensitivity by venom-induced histamine release. *J. Allergy. Clin. Immunol.*, **53**, 170
20. Levine, B. B. (1966). Immunological mechanisms of penicillin allergy. *N. Engl. J. Med.*, **275**, 1115
21. Pepys, J. (1974). Atopy. In Gell, P. G. M., Coombs, R. R. A. and Lachmann, P. J. (eds.) *Clinical Aspect of Immunology.* (Oxford: Blackwell)
22. Ishizaka, K., Ishizaka, T. and Hornbrook, M. M. (1966b). Physiochemical properties of human reaginic antibody. V. Correlation of reaginic activity with γE globulin antibody. *J. Immunol.*, **97**, 884
23. Bennich, H., Ishizaka, K., Ishizaka, T. and Johansson, S. G. O. (1969). Immunoglobulin E. A comparative study of γE globulin and myeloma IgND. *J. Immunol.*, **102**, 826
24. Ishizaka, T., DeBernardo, R., Tomioka, H., Lichtenstein, L. M. and Ishizaka, K. (1972). Identification of basophil granulocytes as a site of allergic histamine release. *J. Immunol.*, **108**, 1000
25. Siraganian, R. P., Hook, W. A. and Levine, B. B. (1975). Specific *in vitro* histamine release from basophils by bivalent haptens: Evidence for activation by simple bridging of membrane bound antibody. *Immunochemistry*, **12**, 149
26. Ishizaka, T. and Ishizaka, K. (1978). Triggering of histamine release from rat mast cells by divalent antibodies against IgE receptors. *J. Immunol.*, **120**, 800
27a. Hugli, T. E. and Müller-Eberhard, H. J. (1978). Anaphylotoxins: C3a and C5a. *Adv. Immunol.*, **26**, 1
27b. Simon, R. A., Schatz, M., Stevenson, D. P., Curry, N., Yamamoto, F., Plow, E., Ring, J.

and Arroyave, C. (1979). Radiographic contrast media infusions. Measurement of histamine, complement and fibrin split products and correlation with clinical parameters. *J. Allergy Clin. Immunol.*, **63**, 281

28. Hastie, R. (1971). The antigen-induced degranulation of basophil leucocytes from atopic subjects. studied by phase contrast microscopy. *Clin. Exp. Immunol.*, **8**, 45

29. Hastie, R., Levy, D. A. and Weiss, L. (1977). The antigen-induced degranulation of basophil leucocytes from atopic subjects studied by electron microscopy. *Lab. Invest.*, **36**, 173

30. Tada, T. and Ishizaka, K. (1970). Distribution of γE forming cells in lymphoid tissues of the human and monkey. *J. Immunol.*, **104**, 377

31. Newcomb, R. W. and Ishizaka, K. (1970). Physiochemical and antigenic studies on human γE in respiratory fluid. *J. Immunol.*, **105**, 85

32. Mayrhoffer, G., Bazin, H. and Gowans, J. L. (1976). Nature of cells binding anti-IgE in rats immunized with *Nippostrongylus brasiliensis*: IgE synthesis in regional nodes and concentration in mucosal mast cells. *Eur. J. Immunol.*, **6**, 537

33. Shiner, M., Ballard, J. and Smith, M. E. (1975). The small-intestinal mucosa in cow's milk allergy. *Lancet*, **1**, 136

34. Huggins. K. J. and Brostoff. J. (1975). Local production of specific IgE antibodies in allergic-rhinitis patients with negative skin tests. *Lancet*, **2**, 48

35. Merrett, T. G., Houri, M., Mayer, A. L. R., Merrett, J. (1976). Measurement of specific IgE antibodies in nasal secretion – evidence for local production. *Clin. Allergy*, **6**, 69

36. Yagi, Y., Maier, O., Pressman, D., Arbesman, C. E. and Reisman, R. E. (1963). The presence of the ragweed-binding antibodies in the β_2A–β_2M and globulins of the sensitive individuals. *J. Immunol.*, **91**, 83

37. Lichtenstein, L. M., Norman, P. S., Osler, A. G. and Winkenwerder, W. L. (1966). *In vitro* studies of human ragweed allergy: changes in cellular and humoral activity associated with specific desensitization. *J. Clin. Invest.*, **45**, 1126

38. Platts-Mills, T. A. E. (1979). Local production of IgG, IgA and IgE antibodies in grass pollen hay fever. *J. Immunol.*, **122**, 2218

39. Turk, A., Lichtenstein, L. M. and Norman, P. S. (1970). Nasal secretory antibody to inhalant allergens in allergic and non-allergic individuals. *Immunology*, **19**, 85

40. Taylor, G. (1974). The nose as a model for the study of respiratory tract allergic disease. *Ann. N.Y. Acad. Sci.*, **221**, 117

41. Stokes, C. R., Taylor, B. and Turner, M. W. (1974). Association of house-dust and grass-pollen allergies with specific IgA antibody deficiency. *Lancet*, **2**, 485

42. Chapman, M. D. and Platts-Mills. T. A. E. (1978). Measurement of IgG, IgA and IgE antibodies to *Dermatophagoides pteronyssinus* by antigen-binding assay, using a partially purified fraction of mite extract (F_4P_1). *Clin. Exp. Immunol.*, **34**, 126

43. Platts-Mills, T. A. E., Chapman, M. D. and Marsh, D. G. (1979). Human IgE and IgG antibody responses to the 'minor' ragweed allergen Ra3: correlation with skin tests and comparison with other allergens. (Manuscript in preparation)

44. Girard, J. P., Rose, N. R., Kunz, M., Kobayashi, S. and Arbesman, C. E. (1967). *In vitro* lymphocyte transformation in atopic patients: induced by antigens. *J. Allergy*, **39**, 65

45. Maini, R. N., Dumonde, D. C., Faux, J. A., Hargreave, F. E. and Pepys, J. (1971). The production of lymphocyte mitogenic factor and migration-inhibition factor by antigen stimulated lymphocytes of subjects with grass pollen allergy. *Clin. Exp. Immunol.*, **9**, 449

46. Black, P. L., Marsh, D. G., Jarrett, E., Delespesse, G. J. and Bias, W. B. (1976). Family studies of association between HLA and specific immune responses to highly purified pollen allergens. *Immunogenetics*, **3**, 349

47. Gatien, J. G., Merler, E. and Colten, H. R. (1975). Allergy to ragweed antigen E: effect of specific immunotherapy on the reactivity of human T lymphocytes *in vitro*. *Clin. Immunol. Immunopathol.*, **4**, 32

48. Ishizaka, K., Kishimoto, T., Delespesse, G. and King, T. P. (1974). Immunogenic properties of modified antigen E. I. Presence of specific determinants for T cells in denaturea antigen and polypeptide chains. *J. Immunol.*, **113**, 70

49. Ownby, D. R. and Buckley, R. H. (1979). Lymphocyte responses to ragweed antigens from different sources. *J. Allergy Clin. Immunol.*, **63**, 65 and correspondence pages 67–69 same vol.

50. Ashworth, L. A. E. and Ford, W. H. (1976). Mitogenic factor as an *in vitro* correlate of delayed hypersensitivity in the guinea-pig. *Int. Arch. Allergy Appl. Immunol.*, **50**, 583

51. Slavin, R. G., Tennenbaum, J. I., Becker, R. J., Feinberg, A. R. and Feinberg, S. M. (1963). Cell transfer of delayed hypersensitivity to ragweed from atopic subjects treated with emulsified ragweed extracts. *J. Allergy*, **34**, 368

52. Levine, B. B. and Vaz, N. M. (1970). Effect of combinations of inbred strain, antigen and antigen dose on immune responsiveness and reagin production in the mouse. A potential mouse model for immune aspects of human atopic allergy. *Int. Arch. Allergy Appl. Immunol.*, **39**, 156

53. Vaz, E. M., Vaz, N. M. and Levine, B. B. (1971). Persistent formation of reagins in mice injected with low doses of ovalbumin. *Immunology*, **21**, 11

54. Provvost-Danon, A., Mouton, D., Abadie, A., Mevel, J. C. and Biozzi, G. (1977). Genetic regulation of IgE and agglutinating antibody synthesis in lines of mice selected for high and low immune responsiveness. *Eur. J. Immunol.*, **7**, 342

55. Tada, T., Okumura, K. and Tanigouchi, M. (1973). In Goodfriend, L., Sehon, A. H. and Orange, R. P. (eds.) *Mechanisms in Allergy: Reagin Mediated Hypersensitivity*, pp. 43–61. (New York: Marcel Dekker)

56. Ishizaka, K. and Ishizaka, T. (1978). Mechanisms of reaginic hypersensitivity and IgE antibody response. *Immunol. Rev.*, **41**, 109

57. Hamaoka, T., Newburger, P. E., Katz, D. H. and Benacerraf, B. (1974). Hapten-specific IgE antibody responses in mice. III. Establishment of parameters for generation of helper T cell function regulating the primary and secondary responses of IgE and IgG B lymphocytes. *J. Immunol.*, **113**, 958

58. Jarrett, E. E. E. (1978). Stimuli for the production and control of IgE in rats. *Immunol. Rev.*, **41**, 52

59. Katz, D. M., Bargatze, R. F. Bogowitz, C. A. and Katz, L. R. (1979). Regulation of IgE antibody production by serum molecules. V. Evidence that coincidental sensitization and imbalance in the normal dumping mechanism results in 'Allergic Breakthrough'. *J. Immunol.*, **122**, 2191

60. Sparks, D. B., Feinberg, S. H. and Becker, R. J. (1962). Immediate skin reactivity induced in atopic and non-atopic individuals following injection of emulsified pollen extracts. *J. Allergy*, **33**, 245

61. Marsh, D. G., Lichtenstein, L. M. and Norman, P. S. (1972). Induction of IgE-mediated immediate hypersensitivity to group I rye grass pollen allergen and allergoids in non-allergic man. *Immunology*, **22**, 1013

62. Salvaggio, J. E., Cavanaugh, J. J. A., Lowell, F. C. and Leskowitz, S. (1964). A comparison of the immunological responses of normal and atopic individuals to intranasally administered antigen. *J. Allergy*, **35**, 62

63. Salvaggio, J. E., Kayman, H. and Leskovitz, S. (1966). Immunologic responses of normal and atopic individuals to aerosolized dextran. *J. Allergy*, **38**, 31

64. Kontou-Karakitsos, K., Salvaggio, J. E. and Mathews, K. P. (1975). Comparative nasal absorption of allergens in atopic and non-atopic subjects. *J. Allergy Clin. Immunol.*, **55**, 241

65. Hamburger, R. N., Orgel, H. A. and Bazaral, M. (1973). In Goodfriend, L. (ed.) *Mechanisms in Allergy: Reagin Mediated Hypersensitivity*, pp. 131. (New York: Marcel Dekker)

66. Marsh, D. G., Bias, W. B. and Ishizaka, K. (1974). Genetic control of basal serum

immunoglobulin E level and its effect of specific reaginic sensitivity. *Proc. Natl. Acad. Sci. USA*, **71**, 3588

67. Levine, B. B., Stember, R. H. and Fotino, M. (1972). Ragweed hay fever: genetic control and linkage to HLA-Haplotypes. *Science*, **178**, 1201

68a. Marsh, D. G., Goodfriend, L. and Bias, W. B. (1977). Basal serum IgE levels and HLA antigen frequencies in allergic subjects. I. Studies with ragweed allergen Ra3. *Immunogenetics*, **5**, 217

68b. Sprouji, A. H. and Marsh, D. G. (1979). Heterogeneity of IgE and IgG antibodies to allergens. (Abstr.) *J. Allergy Clin. Immunol.*, **63**, 139

69. Hastie, R., Heroy, J. H. and Levy, D. A. (1979). Basophil leukocytes and mast cells in human nasal secretions and scrapings studied by light microscopy. *Lab. Invest.*, **40**, 554

70. Huntley, C. C. and Lyerly, A. (1963). Immune globulin determinations in allergic children. *Am. J. Dis. Child.*, **106**, 545

71. Buckley, R. H., Dees, S. C. and O'Fallon, W. M. (1968). Serum immunoglobulins: levels in normal children and in uncomplicated childhood allergy. *Paediatrics*, **41**, 600

72. Berglund, G., Finnström, O., Johansson, S. G. O. and Möller, K. L. (1968). Wiskott–Aldrich Syndrome. *Acta Paediatr. Scand.*, **57**, 89

73. Kauffman, H. S. and Hobbs, J. R. (1970). Immunoglobulin deficiencies in an atopic population. *Lancet*, **2**, 1061

74. Schwartz, D. P. and Buckley, R. H. (1971). Serum IgE concentrations and skin reactivity to anti-IgE antibody in IgA-deficient patients. *N. Engl. J. Med.*, **284**, 513

75. Gail-Peczalska, K. J., Ballow, M., Hansen, J. A. and Good, R. A. (1973). IgE-bearing lymphocytes and atopy in a patient with X-linked infantile agammaglobulinaemia. *Lancet*, **1**, 1254

76. Buckley, R. M. and Dees, S. C. (1969). Correlation of milk precipitins with IgA deficiency. *N. Engl. J. Med.*, **281**, 465

77. Cassidy, J. T., Oldham, G. and Platts-Mills, T. A. E. (1979). Functional assessment of a B cell defect in patients with selective IgA deficiency. *Clin. Exp. Immunol.*, **35**, 296

78. Ammann, A. J. and Hong, R. (1971). Selective IgA deficiency: presentation of 30 cases and a review of the literature. *Medicine*, **50**, 223

79. Platts-Mills, T. A. E., von Maur, R. K., Ishizaka, K., Norman, P. S. and Lichtenstein, L. M. (1976). IgA and IgG anti-ragweed antibodies in nasal secretions: quantitative measurements of antibodies and correlation with inhibition of histamine release. *J. Clin. Invest.*, **57**, 1041

80. Tse, K. S., Wicher, K. and Arbesman, C. E. (1973). Effect of immunotherapy on the appearance of antibodies to ragweed in external secretions. *J. Allergy Clin. Immunol.*, **51**, 208

81. Taylor, B., Norman, A. P., Orgel, M. A., Stokes, C. R., Turner, M. W. and Soothill, J. F. (1973). Transient IgA deficiency and pathogenesis of infantile atopy. *Lancet*, **2**, 111

82. Orgel, H. A., Hamburger, R. N., Bazaral, M., Gorrin, H., Groshong, T., Lenoir, M., Miller, J. R. and Wallace, W. W. (1975). Development of IgE and allergy in infancy. *J. Allergy Clin. Immunol.*, **56**, 296

83. Kauffman, H. S. and Frick, O. L. (1976). Immunological development in infants of allergic parents. *Clin. Allergy*, **6**, 321

84. Ezeoke, A. J. C. (1975). Measurements of serum IgE. *PhD Thesis*, London

85. Soothill, J. F., Stokes, C. R., Turner, M. W., Norman, A. P. and Taylor, B. (1976). Predisposing factors and the development of reaginic allergy in infancy. *Clin. Allergy*, **6**, 305

86. Soothill, J. F. (1976). Some intrinsic and extrinsic factors predisposing to allergy. *Proc. R. Soc. Med.*, **69**, 439

87. Kemeny, D. M., Miyachi, S., Platts-Mills, T. A. E., Wilkins, S. and Lessof, M. (1981). Antibody responses to bee-venom and grass pollen antigens in beekeepers. (Manuscript in preparation)

88. Miyachi, S., Lessof, M. H., Kemeny, D. M. and Green, L. A. (1979). Comparison of the atopic background between allergic and non-allergic beekeepers. *Int. Arch. Allergy Appl. Immunol.*, **58**, 160

89. De Weck, A. L. (1971). Drug reactions. In Samter, M. (ed.) *Immunological Diseases*, p. 415. (Boston: Little Brown & Co.)

90. Levine, B. B., Redmond, A. P., Fellner, M. J., Voss, H. E. and Levytska, V. (1966). Immune responses of man to benzylpenicillin and penicillin allergy. *J. Clin. Invest.*, **45**, 1895

91. Wilson, G. S. (1967). *The Hazards of Immunization*, pp. 205–223. (London: Athlone Press)

92. Delespesse, G., Mauberge, J., De Kennes, B., Nicaise, R. and Govaerts, A. (1977). IgE mediated hypersensitivity in ageing. *Clin. Allergy*, **7**, 155

93. Belin, L. (1979). Wood trimmers disease – an allergic reaction to moulds in Swedish saw mills. Annual meeting of the European Academy of Allergology and Clinical Immunology

94. Pepys, J. and Jenkins, P. A. (1965). Precipitin (F.L.H.) test in farmer's lung. *Thorax*, **20**, 21

95. Hargreave, F. E. and Pepys, J. (1972). Allergic respiratory reactions in bird fanciers provoked by allergen inhalation provocation tests. *J. Allergy Clin. Immunol.*, **50**, 157

96. Salvaggio, J. E., Buechner, H. A., Seabury, J. H. and Arquembourg, P. (1966). Bagassosis. I. Precipitins against extracts of crude bagasse in the serum of patients. *Ann. Intern. Med.*, **64**, 748

97. Edwards, J. H. (1976). A quantitative study on the activation of the alternative pathway of complement by mouldy hay dust and thermophilic actinomycetes. *Clin. Allergy*, **6**, 19

98. Edwards, J. H., Wagner, J. C. and Seal, R. M. E. (1976). Pulmonary responses to particulate materials capable of activating the alternate pathway of complement. *Clin. Allergy*, **6**, 155

99. Emanuel, D. A., Wenzel, F. J. and Lawton, B. R. (1975). Massive fungal inhalation giving a toxic reaction. Pulmonary mycotoxicosis. *Chest*, **67**, 293

100. Wilkie, B., Pauli, B. and Gygax, M. (1973). Hypersensitivity pneumonitis experimental production in guinea-pigs with antigens of *Micropolyspora faeni*. *Pathol. Microbiol.*, **39**, 393

101. Asherson, G. L., Zembala, M. and Mayhew, B. (1977). Analysis of the induction phase of contact sensitivity of footpad transfer of regional lymph node cells. Macrophages and radioresistant T lymphocytes induce immunity. *Immunology*, **32**, 81

102. Askenase, P. (1977). Role of basophils, mast cells and vasoamines in hypersensitivity reactions with a delayed time course. *Prog. Allergy*, **23**, 199

103. Dvorak, H. F., Mimm, M. C. and Dvorak, A. M. (1976). Morphology of delayed-type hypersensitivity reactions in man. *J. Invest. Dermatol.*, **67**, 391

104. Thomas, W. R., Asherson, G. L. and Watkins, M. C. (1976). Reaginic antibody produced in mice with contact sensitivity. *J. Exp. Med.*, **144**, 1386

105. Brostoff, J. and Roitt, I. M. (1969). Cell mediated (delayed) hypersensitivity in patients with summer hay fever. *Lancet*, **2**, 1269

106. Kay, A. B. and Austen, K. F. (1971). The IgE mediated release of an eosinophil chemotactic factor from human lung. *J. Immunol.*, **107**, 899

107. Steinberg, P., Ishizaka, K. and Norman, P. S. (1974). Possible role of IgE-mediated reaction in immunity. *J. Allergy*, **54**, 359

108. Butterworth, A. E. (1976). The eosinophil and its role in immunity to helminth infection. *Curr. Top. Microb. Immunol.*, **75**, 127

109. Ogilvie, B. M. and Jones, V. E. (1973). Immunity in the parasitic relationship between helminths and hosts. *Prog. Allergy*, **17**, 94

110. Hsu, S. Y. L., Hsu, H. F., Penick, J. D., Lust, G. L. and Osborne, J. W. (1974). Dermal hypersensitivity to schistosome cercariae in rhesus monkeys during immunization and challenge. *J. Allergy Clin. Immunol.*, **54**, 339

111. Mygind, N. (1979). *Nasal Allergy*. (Oxford: Blackwell)

112. Boetcher, D. A. and Leonard, E. J. (1973). Basophil chemotaxis: augmentation by a factor from stimulated lymphocyte cultures. *Immunol. Commun.*, **2**, 421

113. Taliafero, W. H. and Taliafero, L. G. (1931). Skin reaction in persons infected with *Schistosoma mansoni*. *Puerto Rico J. Publ. Health Trop. Med.*, **7**, 23

114. Oliver-Gonzalez, J., Banman, P. M. and Benenson, A. S. (1955). Immunological aspects of infections with *Schistosoma mansoni*. *Am. J. Trop. Med. Hyg.*, **4**, 443

115. Lapage, G. (1957). *Animals Parasitic in Man*. (London: Penguin Books)

116. Johansson, S. G. O., Melbin, T. and Vahlquist, B. (1968). Immunoglobulin levels in Ethiopian pre-school children with special reference to high concentrations of immunoglobulin E (Ig ND). *Lancet*, **1**, 1118

117. Mellanby, K. (1943). *Scabies*. (Oxford: Oxford University Press)

118. Falk, E. S. (1979). Serum immunoglobulin values in patients with scabies. *Br. J. Dermatol.* (In press)

119. Logan, J. and Saker, D. N. (1953). The incidence of allergic disorders and cancer. *N. Zealand J. Med.*, **52**, 210

120. MacKay, W. D. (1966). The incidence of allergic disorders and cancer. *Br. J. Cancer*, **20**, 434

121. Ure, D. M. J. (1969). Negative association between allergy and cancer. *Scott. Med. J.*, **14**, 51

122. Gabriel, R., Dudley, B. M. and Alexander, W. D. (1972). Lung cancer and allergy. *Br. J. Clin. Pract.*, **26**, 202

123. Augustin, R. and Chandrassa, K. D. (1971). IgE levels and allergic skin reactions in cancer and non-cancer patients. *Int. Arch. Allergy*, **41**, 141

124. McKee, W. D., Arnold, C. A. and Perlman, M. D. (1967). A double blind study of the comparative incidence of malignancy and allergy. *J. Allergy*, **39**, 294

125. Jacobs, D., Houri, M., Landon, J. and Merrett, T. G. (1972). Circulating levels of IgE in patients with cancer. *Lancet*, **2**, 1059

126. Waldmann, T. A., Bull, J. M., Bruce, R. M., Broder, S., Jost, M. C., Balestra, S. T. and Suer, M. E. (1974). Serum immunoglobulin E levels in patients with neoplastic diseases. *J. Immunol.*, **113**, 379

127. Winters, W. W. and Heiner, D. C. (1976). IgE levels in the sera of cancer patients. *J. Allergy*, **57**, 181

128. McLaughlan, P. and Stanworth, D. R. (1975). A critical search for evidence of changes in levels of circulating IgE in patients with cancer. *Lancet*, **1**, 64

129. Dworkin, M., Diamond, H. D. and Craver, L. F. (1955). Hodgkin's disease and allergy. *Cancer*, **8**, 128

130. Shier, W. W. (1954). Cutaneous anergy and Hodgkin's disease. *N. Engl. J. Med.*, **250**, 353

131. Steinberg, P., Ross Thomas, M., Vataw, M. L. and Bayne, N. K. (1976). IgE levels in Hodgkin's disease. *J. Allergy*, **57**, 255

132. Fisherman, E. W. (1959). Does the allergic diathesis influence malignancy? *J. Allergy*, **31**, 74

2
Pharmacological Mediators of Allergy

L. J. F. YOULTEN

INTRODUCTION

In allergic reactions a more or less stereotyped response follows contact of a sensitive tissue with a specific substance – the allergen. Allergens are not always chemically defined compounds, consisting as they do of either proteins or other macromolecules, foreign to the body, or modified by acting as haptens. An almost infinite variety of substances can, in susceptible individuals, act as allergens; the response of these individuals is relatively limited, consisting as it usually does of a recognizable clinical syndrome such as asthma, rhinitis, eczema, other rashes or anaphylactic shock. It is a fundamental feature of allergic disease that the nature of the clinical manifestation is not specific to the allergen. The common response can be mimicked in certain respects by administration of endogenous pharmacological agents to normal subjects. Histamine pricked into the skin, for example, causes a weal and flare reaction very similar to that seen in allergic individuals responding to prick tests with appropriate allergens. Such observations led to the idea that histamine and other endogenously released chemical mediators may be involved in various types of allergic reaction[1]. This has proved a quite fruitful approach, particularly in the case of Type I, anaphylactic reactions. It has thrown some light on the action of drugs effective in allergy.

Many of the substances which have been implicated as possible mediators of allergic reactions also appear to be involved in other inflammatory lesions, and similarities between the triple response to skin trauma, the early stages of thermal injury or pyogenic infection, the response to a bee sting or to a

39

positive diagnostic prick test suggest that an immunological mechanism is only one among many different stimuli which may lead to a common response.

The mediator theory may not fully explain the phenomenon of allergy and other mechanisms may have been unduly neglected, for example the possibility that vascular or bronchial smooth muscle or other cells could have specific immunoglobulins bound to their cell membranes, and that contraction or relaxation could then follow interaction of antigen and cell-bound antibody, without the involvement of chemical mediation. Another rather neglected aspect of this subject is the study of possible endogenous factors involved in limiting or reversing the changes seen in allergy.

Because of the non-specific nature of the response of tissues to a wide variety of irritant substances, certain strict criteria should be met before a proposed chemical mediator can be accepted as an essential element in any pathological process.

(1) The putative mediator or the biochemical capacity to synthesize it should be detectable in the affected tissues, preferably in larger amounts than in normal areas.

(2) The mediator should produce, on application to normal tissues, some or all of the effects observed in the natural pathological process, and no others.

(3) Measures known to be effective in preventing the release or inhibiting the relevant action of the mediators should reduce the intensity of the pathological process.

(4) Measures enhancing the action of the mediator by, for example, inhibiting its enzymic breakdown, or increasing target organ sensitivity should enhance the pathological process.

In practice these criteria are usually only partially met. If only evidence from man were acceptable, there is no chemical mediator so far proposed whose involvement in any allergic or inflammatory process has been firmly demonstrated by all four of the above criteria.

Briefly, among the reasons for this state of affairs are artifacts and other difficulties in the measurement of tissue mediator levels, differences in the effects of exogenous application and endogenous release, and the lack of specificity of blocking or enhancing agents. The probable involvement of more than one mediator, and interactions between such mediators further complicate the picture. There is consequently still much uncertainty about the exact role of the various mediators proposed. In the following paragraphs, individual mediators, some chemically defined, others not, will be discussed, with particular reference to the evidence that they are involved in allergic diseases in man. Satisfactory animal models of allergy are rare, and the known species differences in dominant mediators of acute inflammation make it difficult to extrapolate the findings directly to human disease. For obvious reasons more work has been done in the more serious Type I reactions and in the more accessible tissues such as the respiratory tract and skin, than in other areas.

For many years, vascular effects such as hyperaemia, oedema and decreased selectivity of the vascular barrier to macromolecules ('increased capillary plasma protein permeability') have been emphasized in experimental studies in this field. More recently the importance of other aspects, such as cellular migration and modulation of cellular function has been realized, and with it has come the knowledge that some mediators may in fact have dual roles, having at different times or at different concentrations both pro- and anti-allergic roles.

One important aspect of the mediator question is that of the relative contribution to disease of allergic basis of increased release of mediator and increased sensitivity of target tissues to mediators. This question can be illustrated by reference to allergic asthma. Mediator release is held responsible for the weal and flare reaction seen in skin testing with allergens, the immediate reaction corresponding closely in appearance and time course to that seen on injection of histamine into an allergic or normal subject's skin Many individuals have positive skin test responses to common inhaled allergens without clinical evidence of allergic rhinitis or asthma. It has been shown clearly in the case of lung responses that asthmatics' lungs are more sensitive than those of normal subjects to applied mediators, including histamine, methacholine[2] and prostaglandins[3]. In some cases there is a many-fold difference in sensitivity, and in the case of prostaglandins there may even be a reversal of the normal response, the asthmatic subjects showing a bronchoconstrictor response to inhalation of a prostaglandin (E_2) which in a normal individual may be bronchodilator. These clear-cut differences have not been seen in the nose[4]. They do however illustrate that the importance of mediator release in allergic disease may be difficult to assess precisely.

It has been widely assumed that mediators released from mast cells by the interaction of antigen with cell-bound specific immunoglobulins play an important role in producing the observed phenomenon of allergy. Such mediators have been widely studied, and much theorizing has been based on *in vitro* experiments, which may be quite misleading if their findings are extrapolated too readily to clinical manifestation of allergy in man. To mention only one aspect of this problem, it is the immediate or Type I reaction which has received the largest amount of attention, whereas, apart from the diagnostic use of skin or other provocation testing, and the relatively rare generalized anaphylactic reactions to foods, drugs or venoms seen in very sensitive individuals, much of the clinical picture is more likely to be associated with other types of reaction such as, in the case of respiratory tract allergy, the late reaction. Much less is known about mediator involvement in such reactions, and it may even be that some mediators have proallergic or inflammatory effects in immediate, but opposing effects in late reactions.

MEDIATORS

The mediators of allergy so far defined fall into three main categories, namely amines, peptides and lipids. These groups will be briefly dealt with in turn.

Amines

Catecholamines

Catecholamines may induce some of the features of the allergic response, such as vasodilatation and bronchospasm, and it has recently been suggested that increased sensitivity to such effects of, for example, adrenaline may be a feature of the allergic patient[5]. In general, however, it is the antiallergic properties of such compounds which are of most practical interest.

Histamine

Probably the most important, and certainly the most widely studied of the mediators, histamine, has potent biological activity in man. Applied to normal tissues it causes vascular changes (dilatation and increased permeability to plasma proteins) and other smooth muscle effects, such as bronchoconstriction. Its additional role as a physiological mediator of gastric secretion has been defined in recent years by the introduction of the H_2 receptor antagonists. It is found not only in mast cells and basophils but also in many other tissues[6]. Its levels are relatively easy to measure in body fluids or tissues, but since tissues have the capacity to synthesize and degrade it, such estimates are difficult to interpret in terms of likely levels found in lesions. Two classes of effect have been identified by the use of blockers. The older, H_1 receptor antagonist or classical antihistamine drugs, many of which have been extensively used in the therapy of allergic and other conditions, block most of the histamine effects associated with the immediate hypersensitivity reaction, for example the weal and flare reaction in the skin, and bronchoconstriction *in vivo*. More recently the H_2 receptor antagonists such as cimetidine have been used to define other possible roles of histamine.

Normally histamine can be considered a local mediator, but there are situations where it may reach levels in the circulating blood sufficient to have effects distant from the site of release. Venous blood from a cooled limb in a patient with cold-induced urticaria has been shown to contain increased amounts of histamine[7]. It is possible in some conditions for damaging effects to occur, either because of overproduction or release of histamine or because of deficiencies in the normal breakdown. Cardiomyopathy related to increased histamine levels has been reported, and it is possible that the gastric ulceration associated with severe burns may be a response to histamine overstimulation. Histamine challenge produces a brisk and short-lasting reaction in skin (itch, weal and flare), lungs (cough, dyspnoea and wheeze) and nose (sneezing, obstruction, rhinorrhoea). These effects however are seen in normal subjects only at applied concentrations which are very much higher than those measured in secretions or tissues during allergic reactions. Several possible reasons have been proposed for this. Histamine may cause some of its effects by stimulation of sensory nerve endings, thus eliciting reflex responses.

In recent years, an extension of interest beyond the immediate, mainly vascular, inflammatory effects has caused some revision of the traditional view of histamine as a purely proinflammatory mediator. Cellular effects, which may well be of greater relevance in the majority of allergic disorders, are in many cases found to be anti-inflammatory[8,9]. Such effects include inhibition of further histamine release from human basophils (a convincing example of negative feedback which is a feature of so many cell control mechanisms), chemotactic attraction of eosinophils and suppression of various lymphocyte functions. Even the acute vascular effects may lead to both pro- and anti-inflammatory consequences, since histamine-induced increases in vascular permeability have a number of possible consequences, including the deposition of immune complexes and delivering of neutralizing antibody.

Use of blocking drugs to define the role of histamine in allergic disease in man has been unable to give very clear-cut answers in many cases. On the other hand, many studies in which antihistamines were shown to be ineffective were carried out before the importance of H_2 receptors was realized and before H_2 antagonists were available. Another problem is that the H_1 antihistamine drugs have other actions, including central sedative and peripheral anticholinergic (atropine-like) effects. Consequently, the effectiveness of such drugs in certain conditions, such as rhinitis, may be due in part at least to such other actions. It would be useful in this area to have drugs which inhibited the breakdown of histamine, so that their ability to potentiate or inhibit allergic responses could be used as an index of histamine involvement. It is unlikely that such drugs will be readily discovered, however, except perhaps by accident, for they have at present no obvious therapeutic role, and since there is more than one enzymic pathway for the breakdown of histamine, there would be correspondingly less chance of a single inhibitor being effective against them all. The cumulative evidence from studies using histamine challenge and the antihistamines of both classes available at present does not support the concept that histamine is of overriding importance in the genesis of clinically significant allergic syndromes. A case in point is allergic asthma, where antihistamines have been generally found to have little useful therapeutic role, although there is a recent resurgence of interest in this subject due to the demonstration that inhaled antihistamines may in fact be effective in relieving asthma[10]. One possible explanation of the general lack of efficiency of antihistamines in asthma is the existence of a third type of histamine receptor, but this is not supported by studies showing that in fact existing antihistamines are quite effective against asthma induced by histamine administration. Though differences in the effect of locally released, locally acting histamines have been proposed to account for this, a more straightforward explanation is of course that other mediators are more important than histamine, and there are several candidates to be considered under this heading.

5-Hydroxytryptamine

5-Hydroxytryptamine, which appears to play a role equivalent to that of histamine in certain mammalian species, notably rat and rabbit, is probably not a significant mediator of allergic reactions in man in the respiratory tract or skin. In the gastrointestinal tract, which is rich in 5-HT, it may sometimes be involved.

Peptides

A variety of peptides have been described which are released from, or more usually generated by, cells or tissues during allergen challenge. Some of these have potent biological activity of a type suggesting that they may play a role in the allergic response. For none of them, however, has this role been clearly defined since specific blockers of release or antagonists are not yet available. Among them are ECF-A (eosinophil chemotactic factor of anaphylaxis), kinins and complement products.

Bradykinin

Prominent among the peptides endogenously produced and having a potent acute inflammatory effect is bradykinin which is generated from a plasma protein precursor (bradykininogen) by an enzyme (kallikrein) and possibly by other routes also. Difficulties in isolating and measuring this rather labile substance have delayed the definition of its role, if any, in allergic disease. Kallikrein activation is effected by an enzyme cascade beginning with factor XII (Hageman factor). Apart from its vasodilator and permeability-increasing actions, actions of bradykinin which may be relevant to allergic responses include smooth muscle contraction, hypotension and pain. Stimulation of prostaglandin release in various systems has also been described, and this is thought to occur through activation of phospholipase A_2 and consequent release of arachidonic acid, a prostaglandin precursor[11].

No specific blocking agents for bradykinin are known, although there is an experimental technique for diminishing generation of bradykinin, namely depletion of precursor by systemic cellulose sulphate treatment. This is not a technique which can be used to elucidate the possible role of bradykinin in human disease. Bradykinin however is unusual among mediators in that a pharmacological means of preventing its breakdown, and thus potentiating its action, is available. A 'bradykinin potentiating peptide' has been described[12] which works by inhibiting a kininase which in the lung is also the enzyme responsible for converting angiotensin I to active angiotensin II. Such enzyme inhibitors are at present finding their way into clinical practice as antihypertensive agents. It is interesting that both the known actions of converting enzyme inhibitors, namely reduction of circulating angiotensin II and increase of bradykinin, work in the direction of reducing blood pressure. It remains to be seen whether the use of such drugs will uncover bradykinin involvement in other disease, including allergy, by causing exacerbations. An interesting parallel could be drawn here with the exacerbations of asthma induced by another group of drugs, of totally different mode of action, already widely used in the treatment of hypertension, namely the adrenergic β-blockers.

Some evidence has been provided that bradykinin may be involved in Type I allergic reactions. A kallikrein-like enzyme, BK-A has been found in human lung and leukocytes[13]. Both kallikrein (in the cat)[14] and a bradykinin-like compound (in man)[15] have been detected in nasal secretions.

Asthmatics have been shown to have raised blood levels of bradykinin[16] as well as being more sensitive than normal subjects to bradykinin inhalation[17]. In skin perfusate, increased levels of bradykinin have been demonstrated along with the mediators in patients challenged locally with allergens[18].

Other peptides

ECF-A, the eosinophil chemotactic factor of anaphylaxis, is released, along with histamine and slow reacting substance of anaphylaxis (SRS-A), from antigenically or chemically stimulated human leukocytes or sensitized lung. Two tetrapeptides have been shown to have chemotactic activity for eosinophils and may play a role *in vivo* causing the migration of eosinophils into tissues involved in allergic responses[19].

Other peptides with vascular effects associated with acute inflammation are the complement products[20], including C3a and C5a, and a 'neurogenic peptide' demonstrated in rat skin inflamed by antidromic stimulation of its sensory nerves[21]. The role of such peptides in human allergic disease is at present unknown.

Lipid mediators

Prostaglandins and other cyclo-oxygenase products

Prostaglandins have been extensively investigated in the past 10 years for their possible role in almost every known disease process. The field of allergy is no exception, and controversy still exists about the importance of this ubiquitous group of fatty acid derivatives. To understand the debate, it is necessary to know a little about the metabolic pathways for production of prostaglandins and related compounds, as well as their effects in normal and diseased individuals.

Arachidonic acid, a 20:4 unsaturated essential fatty acid, is the precursor of the '2' series of prostaglandins, which is the most abundant and most studied group. This precursor is derived from cell membranes, and probably other sources, by the action of phospholipase A_2, an enzyme whose activation in perfused animal lungs has been recently shown to be prevented by anti-inflammatory steroids[22]. Once formed, two main metabolic pathways, cyclo-oxygenase and lipogenase, can lead to the formation of biologically active compounds from arachidonic acid. A cyclo-oxygenase reaction (potently inhibited by aspirin and many other non-steroid anti-inflammatory drugs) converts arachidonic acid to the cyclic endoperoxides PGG_2 and PGH_2. These compounds are relatively unstable, and apart from having some biological activity themselves, are soon converted, spontaneously or by enzymic pathways, to either the 'parent' prostaglandins PGD_2, PGE_2 and $PGF_{2\alpha}$ or thromboxane A_2 (a potent vasoconstrictor and platelet aggregating agent) or prostacyclin (PGI_2) a thromboxane antagonist. Lipoxygenase, resistant to inhibition by aspirin-like drugs, generates from arachidonic acid a different group of compounds including HETE (hydroxyarachidonic acid) which is a chemotactic agent, and, it now seems likely, another compound which may be the immediate precursor of the slow reacting substance of anaphylaxis (SRS-A) whose structure seems to have yielded its secrets at last (see below). The critical point is that, in this system, anti-inflammatory steroids and aspirin act at different points. Steroids with anti-inflammatory potency will inhibit all production of both lipoxygenase and cyclo-oxygenase products, unless a steroid-resistant mode of activating phospholipase A_2 is involved. (Bradykinin may be an example of this, as may the phagocytosis-associated events in polymorphonuclear leukocytes[23]). Aspirin-like drugs however, although able to prevent generation of prostaglandins, thromboxane and prostacyclin, may actually enhance the generation of lipoxygenase products by leaving more arachidonic acid available. This may be relevant to the phenomenon of aspirin-induced asthma.

Phospholipase A_2 activation, and the subsequent release of a mixture of potent compounds, is seen on antigen challenge of perfused lung, both animal and human. Almost any tissue perturbation, mechanical, chemical, pharmacological or immunological, may lead to increased prostaglandin levels, and this makes the interpretation of their significance difficult.

Turning to the effects of prostaglandins and related compounds which may be relevant to allergy, the situation is complicated, not only by the multiplicity of compounds concerned, some with opposing actions, but by their apparent effectiveness in more than one relevant system. In general, the acute, vascular effects are proinflammatory, including vasodilatation and the potentiation of the vascular and pain-producing effects of histamine and bradykinin. The 'chronic', cellular part of the response may be predominantly antiallergic, since PGE_2, like many other compounds with antiallergic activity, raises intracellular cyclic AMP levels[24]. This aspect, now widely appreciated in relation to chronic inflammatory disease, is so far largely unexplored.

The question of the importance of cyclo-oxygenase products in the genesis of any pathological process must depend largely on the effect of aspirin and the other potent cyclo-oxygenase inhibitors. The failure of adequate doses of indomethacin or aspirin to modify a process makes it highly unlikely that prostaglandins, thromboxane or prostacyclin play an essential role in it. In circumstances where such drugs do have an effect, of course, reduction in cyclo-oxygenase products is only one possible explanation; among others which must now be included is an increase in SRS-A and other lipoxygenase products. In fact, aspirin-like drugs have little consistent effect in most allergic conditions. There are, however, some interesting exceptions. An appreciable number of asthmatics notice that aspirin causes exacerbations, which also follow administration of other non-steroid anti-inflammatory drugs[25]. There is an association between this sensitivity and development of nasal polypi. Identification of a biochemical abnormality common to this subgroup of asthmatics, who may also be sensitive to tartrazine, could possibly throw light on the mechanisms of other forms of asthma. A much smaller proportion of asthmatics report relief by aspirin, and this group too should repay further study.

The ability of tissue to produce prostaglandins when stimulated is so universal and non-specific that it is hard to draw any firm conclusion about their occurrence in blood or tissues during allergic reactions. In some patients with specific food intolerance which may or may not have an immunological basis, cyclo-oxygenase inhibitors have been remarkably effective in preventing gastrointestinal symptoms, and sometimes also manifestations in other areas, such as headache, rhinitis or asthma[26]. Unprotected challenge in these subjects was associated with an increase in circulating prostaglandins and metabolites.

Asthmatics' airways are very much more sensitive than normal to the bronchoconstrictor effects of inhaled or injected $PGF_{2\alpha}$, and may even respond by bronchoconstriction to the normally bronchodilator PGE_2. The bronchodilator and nasal decongestant effects[27] of PGE_2 are not likely to have direct practical therapeutic applications, since this compound is also irritant, causing coughing and sneezing.

Lipoxygenase products – SRS-A

The structure of a SRS has recently been identified as that of a lipoxygenase product with a cysteine side-chain[28]. This will doubtless lead to an advance in our understanding of the role of slow reacting substance of anaphylaxis in allergic reactions. It is of particular interest in asthma, where histamine effects seem inadequate to explain Type I reactions and their relative resistance to antihistamines.

SRS-A is produced by neutrophils as well as by basophils and mast cells. It contracts smooth muscle, is resistant to antihistamine block and has been reported to slow mucus transport in humans. Antagonists have been described[29], for example FPL 55712, but they are not yet sufficiently specific to give very clear answers to the obvious questions about SRS-A involvement in human disease processes. The relationship of corticosteroid treatment to SRS-A production has not yet been settled in man. In some animal preparations corticosteroids block SRS-A release, which is consistent with the postulated anti-inflammatory role of steroids being at least partly mediated through the prevention of phospholipase A_2 activation.

Other lipoxygenase products may also have a role in allergy, which remains to be defined. Some, like HETE, may be chemotactic factors.

MODE OF ACTION OF ANTIALLERGIC DRUGS

A variety of pharmacological approaches have been made to the treatment of allergic disease, some of which also apply to non-allergic conditions which may share common mediators, such as intrinsic asthma and urticaria. In addition to the obvious practical benefits of providing effective therapy, the efficacy of such drugs helps in the understanding of the basic mechanisms involved in allergic disease. Some drugs have apparently more than one site of action, and the rationale for the introduction of a particular drug may not in fact account for its efficacy. Attempts have been made to define a common intracellular pathway which would explain the different mode of action of antiallergic drugs. Many of them cause rises in cyclic AMP either by stimulation of adenylcyclase or by inhibition of phosphodiesterase. Cyclic AMP has been proposed as a key substance in allergy and inflammation, as well as in many other cell functions. The two cell types mainly studied in the immediate hypersensitivity response are the mediator-releasing cell (mast cell or blood basophil leukocyte) and the smooth muscle cell. It should be remembered, however, that others are also involved, such as mucus secreting cells, neurons both sensory and autonomic, endothelial cells and migrating leukocytes.

Disodium cromoglycate and related compounds

A new compound for the treatment, or rather prevention, of asthma was introduced in 1965[30]. This was disodium cromoglycate, and it had properties unlike those of any of the existing drugs effective in asthma. It did not block the effects on smooth muscle of histamine or other mediators, nor was it a bronchodilator. Lacking also anti-inflammatory properties, its mode of action appeared to be to prevent degranulation and mediator release from mast cells. It was poorly absorbed and for this and other reasons had no demonstrable systemic effects when applied topically or injected. It is effective in many patients in preventing, but not in reversing, experimentally induced allergic or exercise-associated asthma. Similar protection occurs in the nose and eyes but, as in the lung, the drug must be given before the challenge to be effective. In some studies, benefits have been claimed in intrinsic or non-allergic asthma, but there is as yet no way, apart from a therapeutic trial, of identifying which patients will benefit from it. Blockage of mediator release may not be the only, or even the main, basis of the therapeutic action of this compound. It has been reported to block sulphur dioxide provoked asthma in some individuals and this may well contribute to its effect in asthma. Several other compounds with similar activity have been described, and some have been clinically evaluated. There is particular interest in finding an equivalent compound which is effective when taken by the oral route, since the mode of administration (the 'Spinhaler') is, on balance, an awkward feature of cromoglycate treatment. It is somewhat puzzling, and casts some doubt on the stated mechanism of action of cromoglycate, that other compounds with marked mast-cell stabilizing properties have been found ineffective in controlling allergic reactions *in vivo*. Interestingly, even cromoglycate itself has not been shown to block histamine release from human basophils *in vitro*.

Anti-inflammatory corticosteroids

Anti-inflammatory corticosteroids, whether topical or systemic, do not effect the immediate response to allergen challenge in skin or the respiratory tract. Such drugs however are outstandingly successful in preventing allergic rhinitis and asthma. This is presumably because they are effective against the late reactions which are more clinically relevant manifestations of respiratory allergy than is the immediate action. There is however no *in vitro* model of the late reaction, and little is known of its mechanism or mediators, except that it usually depends on a preceding immediate reaction. The implication is that some of the experimental work on immediate reactions may be largely irrelevant to clinical practice.

Discussion

The effects of the various groups of drugs used in the treatment and prevention of allergic reactions, and those which may share some common features such as non-allergic urticaria, rhinitis or asthma might be expected to elucidate the mechanisms involved. In fact, the picture that emerges from the study of such drug effects is often far from clear, and in many cases throws some doubt on our understanding of the mode of action of the drugs as well as the involvement of particular mediators. Almost every type of agent effective in therapy has more than one biochemical site of action. The agents raising cyclic AMP levels such as β-adrenergic agonists and theophylline, for example, are

50   IMMUNOLOGICAL ASPECTS OF ALLERGY

thought to relax smooth muscle or reduce its response to constrictor substances, and also to inhibit mediator release from mast cells. Antihistamines of the H_1 type as well as antagonizing the H_1 effects of histamine, may also act as 5-hydroxytryptamine antagonists, and many of them share atropine-like properties which may be relevant to their therapeutic effect. There are difficulties in accounting for the efficacy of cromoglycate by the single action of suppressing mast cell mediator release.

The mediators too may have dual actions. Some, like histamine and prostaglandin may be proinflammatory in the early vascular phase and anti-inflammatory in the later, cellular phase. The actions of antagonists may be correspondingly different in the different phases of the allergic response. Mediators may interact by enhancing the effects of one another, as prostaglandins and histamine, or by one releasing or activating others in a sequential pattern, such as bradykinin and prostaglandins.

Apart from this, we have little detailed knowledge of the *in vivo* significance of the various mediators, such as lymphokines, which may be implicated in responses other than Type I reactions. There is still, therefore, much to learn about mediators of allergy.

It is probably hopelessly optimistic to think that there is waiting to be discovered a single definitive biochemical route to the allergic manifestations seen in disease. It is probably significant that the most commonly effective drugs such as the β-adrenergic agonists act at a late phase in the sequence, namely on the smooth muscle response. Undoubtedly, however, there is more than one pathway to asthma and other allergy-related disease. There are many variables to consider, such as an unpredictable individual responsiveness to mediators, and to drugs, so that the treatment of every patient becomes a therapeutic trial.

References

1. Lewis, T. (1927). *The Blood Vessels of the Human Skin and their Responses.* (London: Shaw)
2. Itkin, I. H. (1967). Bronchial hypersensitivity to mecholyl and histamine in asthma subjects. *J. Allergy*, **40**, 245
3. Mathé, A. and Hedqvist, P. (1975). Effect of prostaglandins $F_{2\alpha}$ and E_2 on airway conductance in healthy subjects and asthmatic patients. *Am. Rev. Resp. Dis.*, **111**, 313
4. McLean, J. A., Mathews, K. P., Solomon, W. R., Brayton, P. R. and Ciarkowski, A. A. (1977). Effect of histamine and methacholine on nasal airway resistance in atopic and non-atopic subjects. *J. Allergy Clin. Immunol.*, **59**, 165
5. Henderson, W. R., Shelhamer, J. H., Reingold, D. B., Smith, L. J., Evans, R. and Kaliner, M. (1979). Alpha adrenergic hyper-responsiveness in asthma. Analysis of vascular and pupillary responses. *N. Engl. J. Med.*, **300**, 642
6. Vugman, I. and Rocha e Silva, M. (1966). Biological determination of histamine in living tissues and body fluid. In Rocha e Silva, M. (ed.) *Handbook of Experimental Pharmacology*, Vol. XVIII/1, p. 81

7. Kaplan, A. P., Gray, L., Staff, R. E., Horakowa, Z. and Beaven, M. A. (1975). *In vivo* studies of mediator release in cold urticaria and cholinergic urticaria. *J. Allergy Clin. Immunol.*, **55**, 394

8. Lichtenstein, L. M. and Gillespie, E. (1973). Inhibition of histamine release by histamine is controlled by an H_2 receptor. *Nature (London)*, **244**, 287

9. Lichtenstein, L. M. and Gillespie, E. (1975). The effects of the H_1 and H_2 antihistamines on 'allergic' histamine release and its inhibition by histamine. *J. Pharmacol. Exper. Ther.*, **192**, 441

10. Nogrady, S. G. and Bevan, C. (1978). Inhaled antihistamines – bronchodilatation and effects on histamine – and methacholine-induced bronchoconstriction. *Thorax*, **33**, 700

11. Blackwell, G. J., Flower, R. J., Nijkamp, F. P. and Vane, J. R. (1978). Phospholipase A_2 activity of guinea-pig isolated perfused lungs: stimulation and inhibition by anti-inflammatory steroids. *Br. J. Pharmacol.*, **62**, 79

12. Greene, L. J., Camargo, A. C. M., Kreiger, E. M., Stewart, J. M. and Ferreira, S. H. (1972). Inhibition of the conversion of angiotensin I to II and potentiation of bradykinin by small peptides present in *Bothrops jacaraca* venom. *Circ. Res.*, **30** (Suppl. II), 62

13. Newball, H. H., Talamo, R. C. and Lichtenstein, L. M. (1975). Release of leucocyte kallikrein mediated by IgE. *Nature (London)*, **254**, 635

14. Eccles, R. and Wilson, H. (1973). A kallikrein-like substance in cat nasal secretion. *Br. J. Pharmacol.*, **49**, 711

15. Dolovich, J., Bach, N. and Arbesman, C. E. (1970). Kinin-like activity in nasal secretions of allergic patients. *Int. Arch. Allergy*, **38**, 337

16. Abe, K., Watanabe, N., Kumagai, N., Mouri, T., Seki, T. and Yoshinaga, K. (1967). Circulating plasma kinin in patients with bronchial asthma. *Experienttia (Basel)*, **23**, 626

17. Herxheimer, H. and Streseman, E. (1963). Bradykinin and ethanol in bronchial asthma. *Arch. Int. Pharmacodyn.*, **144**, 315

18. Black, A. K., Greaves, M. W., Hensby, C. N. and Plummer, N. A. (1977). A method of obtaining human skin inflammatory exudate for pharmacological analysis. *Br. J. Pharmacol.*, **58**, 317

19. Goetzl, E. J. and Austen, K. F. (1975). Purification and synthesis of eosinophilotactic tetrapeptides of human lung tissue: identification as eosinophil chemotactic factor of anaphylaxis. *Proc. Natl. Acad. Sci. USA*, **72**, 4123

20. Siraganian, R. P. and Hook, W. A. (1976). Complement-induced release from human basophils II. Mechanism of the histamine release reaction. *J. Immunol.*, **116**, 639

21. Garcia-Laem, J. and Hamamura, L. (1974). Formation of a factor increasing vascular permeability during electrical stimulation of the saphenous nerve in rats. *Br. J. Pharmacol.*, **51**, 383

22. Flower, R. J. and Blackwell, G. J. (1979). Anti inflammatory steroids induce biosynthesis of a phospholipase A_2 inhibitor which prevents prostaglandin generation. *Nature (London)*, **278**, 456

23. Dray, F., McCall, E. and Youlten, L. J. F. (1980). Failure of anti inflammatory steroids to inhibit the production of prostaglandins by rat polymorphonuclear leucocytes. *Br. J. Pharmacol.* (In press)

24. Lichtenstein, L. M., Gillespie, E., Bourne, H. R. and Henney, C. S. (1972). The effects of a series of prostaglandins on *in vitro* models of the allergic response and cellular immunity. *Prostaglandins*, **2**, 579

25. Szczeklik, A., Gryglewski, R. J. and Czerniawska-Mysik, G. (1975). Relationship of inhibition of prostaglandin biosynthesis by analgesics to asthma attacks in aspirin-sensitive patients. *Br. Med. J.*, **1**, 67

26. Buisseret, P. D., Youlten, L. J. F., Heinzelmann, D. I. and Lessof, M. H. (1978). Prostaglandin-synthesis inhibitors in prophylaxis of food intolerance. *Lancet*, **1**, 906

27. Änggard, A. (1969). The effect of prostaglandins on nasal airway resistance in man. *Ann. Otol. Rhinol. Laryngol.*, **78**, 657
28. Murphy, R. C., Hammarström, S. and Samuelsson, B. (1979). Leuktriene C: a slow reacting substance from mouse mastocytoma cells. *Proc. Natl. Acad. Sci. USA*, **76**, 4275
29. Augstein, J., Farmer, J. B., Lee, T. B., Sheard, P. and Tattersall, M. L. (1973). Selective inhibition of slow reacting substance of anaphylaxis. *Nature (London) New Biol.*, **245**, 215
30. Howell, J. B. L. and Altounyan, R. E. C. (1967). A double blind trial of disodium cromoglycate in the treatment of allergic bronchial asthma. *Lancet*, **2**, 539

3
Diagnostic Tests

PART I:
Prick, Scratch and Intradermal Tests

M. H. LESSOF

INTRODUCTION

The use of diagnostic tests for allergy is beset with difficulties. As a reminder of the complexity of the immunological response, skin tests with an allergenic extract can provoke not only an immediate (Type I) response, with a weal which develops within minutes and subsides within 1–2 hours. Late reactions (including Type III) may reach a maximum after 5–7 hours. In addition, a firm, lymphocyte-infiltrated nodule of delayed hypersensitivity (Type IV) can arise after an interval of 24–48 hours. Apart from the difficulty in devising methods for the analysis of such complex reactions, allergy tests can never be any better than the test materials which they employ. For the most part, these allergenic materials are poorly standardized and of variable composition.

In practice, when the reaction is not of the immediate kind, IgE-mediated tests such as skin tests or radioallergosorbent technique (RAST) are unhelpful. Tests for IgG antibodies are no more encouraging in such cases and do not appear to discriminate reliably between asymptomatic individuals who have antibodies and those with symptoms who also have (or may not have) IgG antibodies. Challenge tests come nearest to fulfilling the clinical aim of identifying those who react adversely. Bronchial challenge tests, however, also carry an element of risk.

The general problem of standardizing test materials has been highlighted by recent developments in bee sting allergy[1]. For many years, extracts prepared from the bodies of bees were used both for skin tests and for treating patients with this condition. The large majority of patients are sensitized to bee venom alone and are capable of reacting adversely to injections of the more crude bee body extracts[2]. It has nevertheless taken some years to overcome administrative objections and to establish bee venom as the appropriate material both for skin tests and for treating patients with this condition.

In this relatively simple and well studied allergy to bee venom, the nature and quantity of allergen which penetrates into the body is precisely known. The standardization of testing material is nevertheless far from being satisfactory. However carefully it may be collected and stored, freeze-dried bee venom is a chemical mixture that has a highly variable composition. If it is standardized in terms of the main allergenic component, phospholipase A, this will not provide a satisfactory standard material in those cases where hyaluronidase, mellitin, or other allergens are responsible for the patient's reaction.

Not surprisingly, the problems of defining the allergenic components of dust mites, pollens and animal fur or other materials are even greater. The difficulty does not concern only the production of a satisfactory test extract, but also the different types of sensitization that affect different individuals. Laboratory workers who are sensitized to experimental animals are more likely to produce skin reactions to sera of these animals than to the commercial animal dander or skin extracts. The reverse is true of atopic subjects who keep animals as pets, who have more frequent and stronger reactions to commercial preparations than to animal serum[3].

In cases such as allergy to animals, where the range of potential allergenic proteins is very wide, there appear to be advantages in using relatively crude extracts for skin test purposes. In studying allergy to dog dander, Meriney et al.[4] have drawn attention to the importance of considering the breed specificity of dander extracts. In a study of 20 patients who were sensitive to dogs it was noted, however, that testing with three individual-breed extracts was no better than using the most potent mixed epidermal antigen. For diagnostic purposes this mixed extract performed considerably better than RAST and did not give any positive reactions in control subjects.

Despite the empiricism that surrounds the preparation and standardization of test extracts there is, in fact, a good correlation between the results of skin tests and a history of allergy to grass pollens, dust mites and animal dander. Tests with *Aspergillus fumigatus* and other moulds have also been reported as giving clinically helpful results[5]. Food extracts, however, appear to be less reliable, partly because of the difficulty in excluding non-specific irritants while obtaining undenatured allergen-rich preparations. The histamine content of spinach and tomato may give false positives, and similar reactions have been thought to result from the bacterial decomposition of histidine in cheese and wine[6]. Nevertheless, extracts of some foods, such as egg, fish, and nuts appear to give very useful results, and a combination of skin test and RAST may have advantages over either method alone[7,8].

SKIN TEST TECHNIQUES

In spite of the problems of standardization and the variability implicit in a biological test, skin tests provide a simple and convenient screening method and have been estimated by Eriksson[9] to provide a 77% agreement with provocation tests. The results, when combined with the case history, will often give a clear-cut result which renders a provocation test unnecessary[10]. The most appropriate technique has, however, been the subject of some discussion. Prick tests, when carried out by the method of Pepys[3], are sensitive, quick and simple. It has been estimated that they introduce a volume of 10^{-6} ml into the epidermis[11]. Scratch tests are even simpler but introduce a more variable amount of antigen and are therefore more difficult to standardize. Intradermal tests, involving the injection of 0.01–0.02 ml of the extract, have the advantage of even greater sensitivity but are not necessarily more reproducible[12]. They are more difficult to perform, more painful, and more expensive.

When considering the possible advantages of the intradermal test, in terms of the accurate knowledge it provides of the amount of allergen injected, it is perhaps worth considering the quality and the clinical relevance of the information which can be obtained. When Hagy and Settipane[13] carried out scratch tests in 1836 college students, they recorded numerous positive reactions to pollens which were unaccompanied by symptoms. These positive tests were not without significance, for on follow-up the frequency with which new cases of hay fever developed among those with positive tests (18.2%) was 10 times higher than in those with negative results (1.7%). However accurate the method of carrying out such tests, the interpretation of their clinical significance is thus subject to limitations unless this evidence is combined with the history or with challenge test results, indicating a clinically significant allergy at the time the test is carried out.

The skin prick has been compared with the intradermal method in an exhaustive study by Woorhorst and van Kriskin[14]. Both tests depend to some extent on the skill of the operator, but these investigators found a greater scatter in the size of reactions provoked by skin pricks than in the intracutaneous test. The extracts used for the prick test were 1000 times more concentrated than for the intracutaneous technique and for either method – but especially for prick tests – these authors suggested that replicate tests should be carried out, preferably in three separate dilutions. When testing children or screening with a number of different allergens, such advice may appear to be counsel of perfection.

Despite criticisms, Pepys[3] has emphasized that the skin prick test is highly sensitive and reliable. In platinum-allergic subjects, reactions occur to platinum salt at 10^{-9} g dilutions, which taken together with the amount of solution introduced suggests that approximately 100 000 molecules are sufficient to produce a skin weal. Indeed, stenius et al.[15] found a better correlation between skin prick tests and the presence of specific IgE antibody to *D. farinae* and grass pollen than was found with intracutaneous tests. Some variability must be accepted, however. In general, reactions are greatest on the trunk, greater near the cubital fossa than near the wrist, and greater on the ulnar side than on the radial side of the forearm[6]. Age also influences the reaction, and a child under the age of 2 years produces much less reaction than older children or adults. There is some evidence that atopic subjects tend to acquire an increasing number of positive reactions as they get older[16].

For either the skin prick or the intradermal method, the reaction develops within minutes and is usually read after 10–15 minutes. It subsides within 1–2 hours and mimics perfectly the reaction to histamine which the American Committee on Standardization[17] have recommended as a control whenever skin tests are performed. Whether this type of reaction always indicates an IgE response is another matter. It has been found by Parish[18] that certain IgG antibodies can induce short-term sensitization in mast cells and so can induce immediate skin test reactions.

A second, late skin reaction may develop as an ill-defined oedematous swelling that is usually maximal after about 5 or 6 hours and resolves within 24 hours or so. There may be an area of induration in the centre, and it is usually assumed that immune complexes are involved, just as they may be in the late reactions in the bronchus which are seen in patients giving a 'dual response' to a bronchial challenge test. These differ again from the delayed hypersensitivity reaction which occurs after 2 or 3 days, as in the classical tuberculin reaction.

Antihistamines should be discontinued for at least 24–48 hours before skin testing in order to avoid the false negative reactions which may otherwise occur[19]. Whereas antihistamines may reduce the reaction, it has been suggested that β-adrenergic blocking agents such as propranolol can significantly increase skin reactivity[20].

In a few situations, skin prick tests are of particular value. In patients with asthma and pulmonary eosinophilia, there is a high incidence of allergy to *Aspergillus fumigatus*. In these circumstances, a positive skin prick test to *A. fumigatus* is virtually diagnostic of bronchopulmonary aspergillosis[21]. It should be noted, however, that positive reactions to *A. fumigatus* may also be obtained in patients with uncomplicated asthma, so that in the absence of pulmonary eosinophilia, this test is less useful.

Another use for skin tests is in considering immunization against tetanus in patients who are suspected of being sensitive to horse serum. A positive skin test is a contraindication of the use of material containing antitoxin raised in horses. Alternatively, skin testing may be carried out with the antiserum itself. A similar principle applies when using antisera, or antilymphocyte globulin, which is raised in other animals.

Skin tests are also of value in assessing the atopic status of those who are exposed to industrial sensitizing agents. For example, skin tests with a battery of relatively common environmental allergens have been used to assess the liability of an individual to become sensitized to the enzymes of *Bacillus* *subtilis* which are produced in the manufacture of biological detergents. Those who have positive skin tests – even in the absence of symptoms – become sensitized to the enzymes twice as frequently as non-atopic individuals[22].

LATE SKIN REACTIONS

In respiratory disorders such as allergic bronchopulmonary aspergillosis, both IgE and IgG antibodies are a feature and both an early and late skin reaction may be seen. However, in order to elicit the late reaction it may be necessary to use higher concentrations of allergen (or intracutaneous injection). In various types of extrinsic alveolitis such as bird breeder's lung, most of the subjects who are non-atopic have IgG but not IgE antibodies[23]. In such cases, late skin reactions can occur on prick testing, but intradermal tests with higher concentrations of the antigen are usually needed to elicit both an immediate and then a late skin response of the Arthus type, in which the deposition of immunoglobulins and complement can be demonstrated[3]. In such patients, serological tests for IgG antibodies are probably of greater diagnostic value.

DISCREPANCIES BETWEEN DIFFERENT TEST METHODS

Local sensitization appears to occur in certain tissues without any detectable sensitivity in the skin. Of nasal reactors to grass pollen, 13–17% give negative prick tests or RAST[3]. Challenge tests can demonstrate local allergic reactions in the nasal mucosa or lungs in patients with negative findings on skin prick tests[24] or RAST[25]. Gastrointestinal reactions, despite suggestive evidence of a local IgE reaction[26] may appear, in some cases, to be sufficiently localized within the gut to remain undetectable by serological or skin test methods[27].

MODIFIED SKIN TESTS

The Prausnitz–Küstner (P–K) test is an indirect intradermal test, first introduced in 1921. The serum of an allergic patient is injected into the skin of a non-allergic recipient; 2–4 days later the area of skin that has been passively sensitized in this way is challenged with an intradermal injection of allergen. A positive result is indicated by a weal and flare. As a demonstration of the ability of reaginic antibody to bind to the skin, this test remains remarkably impressive. As in various animal models of passive cutaneous anaphylaxis, the actual mechanism for the release of mediators from sensitized mast cells appears to be non-specific. Like animal species, all healthy human subjects are capable of releasing histamine and of developing a weal and flare reaction once the sensitization step has been completed.

As a diagnostic method, P–K testing is often regarded as being ingenious rather than useful, and the potential risk of transferring viral infection has discouraged its use. Two intriguing modifications have, however, been described. Kontou-Karakitsos et al.[28] injected the serum of a peanut-allergic individual into the skin of volunteers and showed that when the challenge material – in this case peanut – was given by nasal insufflation, the test could still be made to work. In this experiment, oral administration gave negative results. As a method of assessing the extent to which allergenically intact molecules can be absorbed across mucous membranes the method has a number of possible applications. As far as Kontou-Karakitsos's own study was concerned, the findings were essentially negative, since no change in mucosal permeability could be demonstrated in hay fever.

Cooke and his colleagues[29] developed the P–K test in a different way, in order to study the serological changes which take place after immunotherapy for hay fever. They noted that, when injected into the skin of a volunteer, a mixture of pollen extract and the serum of a hay fever sufferer was capable of inducing a skin reaction. However, up to 20 times more allergen is required when it is mixed with serum taken from the same subject after a course of immunotherapy. The development of the patient self (P–S) test has solved the problem of the use of volunteers in this kind of study[30]. Stored serum, taken from the patient at various stages of immunotherapy for hay fever, is incubated overnight with different concentrations of grass pollen extract. The allergen-neutralizing capacity of the post-treatment serum is taken as an indication of the rise in blocking antibody. The method is cumbersome as compared to direct laboratory measurements of IgG antibody. It also has the same defect that both effective and ineffective vaccines can provoke antibody production, but the presence of antibody may not necessarily reflect the patient's clinical progress.

References

1. Hunt, K. J., Valentine, M. D., Sobotka, A. K., Benton, A. W., Amodio, F. J. and Lichtenstein, L. M. (1978). A controlled trial of immunotherapy in insect hypersensitivity. N. Engl. J. Med., 299, 157
2. Hunt, K. J., Sobotka, A. K., Valentine, M. D., Yunginger, J. W. and Lichtenstein, L. M. (1978). Sensitization following hymenoptera whole body extract therapy. J. Allergy Clin. Immunol., 61, 48
3. Pepys, J. (1975). Skin testing. Br. J. Hosp. Med., 14, 412
4. Meriney, D. K., Wallace, D., Miller, J., Goel, Z. A. and Grieco, M. H. (1979). Clinical comparison of skin testing and the radioallergosorbent test in dog-sensitive patients using mixed and breed-specific antigens. Int. Arch. Allergy Appl. Immunol., 58, 453
5. Hendrick, D. J., Davies, R. J., D'Souza, M. F. and Pepys, J. (1975). An analysis of skin prick test reactions in 656 asthmatic patients. Thorax, 30, 2

6. Tapay, N. (1973). Diagnostic tests for allergy. In Speer, F. and Dockhorn, R. J. (eds.) *Allergy and Immunology in Children*, pp. 358–370. (Springfield, Ill.: Charles C. Thomas)

7. Chua, Y. Y., Brenner, K., Llobet, J. L., Kokubu, H. L. and Collins-Williams, C. (1976). Diagnosis of food allergy by the radioallergosorbent test. *J. Allergy Clin. Immunol.*, **58**, 477

8. Lessof, M. H., Buisseret, P. D., Merrett, J., Merrett, T. G. and Wraith, D. G. (1980). Assessing the value of skin prick tests. *Clin. Allergy*, **10**, 115

9. Eriksson, N. E. (1977). Diagnosis of reaginic allergy with house dust, animal dander and pollen allergens in adult patients. *Int. Arch. Allergy*, **53**, 341

10. Eriksson, N. E. (1977). Diagnosis of reaginic allergy with house dust, animal dander and pollen allergens in adult patients. III. Case histories and combinations with skin test, RAST and provocation tests. *Int. Arch. Allergy*, **53**, 441

11. Squire, J. R. (1952). Tissue reactions to protein sensitization. *Br. Med. J.*, **1**, 1

12. Pascual, H. C., Reddy, P. M., Nagaya, H., Lee, S. K., Lauridsen, J., Gupta, S. and Jerome, D. (1977). Agreement between radioallergosorbent test and skin test. *Ann. Allergy*, **39**, 325

13. Hagy, G. W. and Settipane, G. A. (1972). Prognosis of positive allergy skin tests in an asymptomatic population. *J. Allergy Clin. Immunol.*, **43**, 200

14. Woorhorst, R. and van Kriskin, H. (1973). Atopic skin tests re-evaluated. II. Variability in result of skin testing done in octuplicates. *Ann. Allergy*, **31**, 499

15. Stenius, B., Wide, L., Seymour, W. M., Holford-Stevens, V. and Pepys, J. (1971). Clinical significance of specific IgE to common allergens. *Clin. Allergy*, **1**, 37

16. Morrison Smith, J. (1973). Skin tests and atopic allergy in children. *Clin. Allergy*, **3**, 269

17. Scherr, M. S., Grater, W. C., Baer, H., Berman, B. A., Center, J. G. and Hale, R. (1971). Report of the Committee on Standardization: 1. A method of evaluating skin test response. *Ann. Allergy*, **29**, 30

18. Parish, W. E. (1970). Short-term anaphylactic IgG antibodies in human sera. *Lancet*, **2**, 591

19. Slavin, R. G. (1974). Skin tests in the diagnosis of allergies of the immediate type. *Med. Clin. N. Am.*, **58**, 65

20. Schereff, R., Harwell, W., Lieberman, P., Rosenberg, W. and Robinson, H. (1973). Effect of beta adrenergic stimulation and blockade on immediate hypersensitivity skin test reactions. *J. Allergy Clin. Immunol.*, **52**, 328

21. McCarthy, D. S. and Pepys, J. (1971). Allergic broncho-pulmonary aspergillosis: clinical immunology (i) clinical features (i) skin, nasal and bronchial tests. *Clin. Allergy*, **1**, 261, 415

22. Greenberg, M., Milne, J. F. and Watt, A. (1970). Survey of workers exposed to dusts containing derivatives of *Bacillus subtilis*. *Br. Med. J.*, **2**, 629

23. Hargreave, F. E. and Pepys, J. (1972). Allergic respiratory reactions in bird fanciers provoked by allergen inhalation provocation tests. Relation to clinical features and allergic mechanisms. *J. Allergy Clin. Immunol.*, **50**, 157

24. Huggins, K. G. and Brostoff, J. (1975). Local production of specific IgE antibodies in allergic-rhinitis patients with negative skin tests. *Lancet*, **2**, 148

25. Merrett, T. G., Houri, M. and Merrett, J. (1975). The measurement of IgE antibodies in nasal secretion as an aid to allergy diagnosis. *Clin. Allergy*, **5**, 458

26. Shiner, M., Ballard, J. and Smith, M. E. (1975). The small-intestinal mucosa in cow's milk allergy. *Lancet*, **1**, 136

27. Lessof, M. H., Wraith, D. G., Merrett, T. G., Merrett, J. and Buisseret, P. D. (1980). Food allergy and intolerance in 100 patients – local and systemic effects. *Q. J. Med.*, **49**, 259

28. Kontou-Karakitsos, K., Salvaggio, J. E. and Mathews, K. P. (1975). Comparative nasal absorption of allergens in atopic and non-atopic subjects. *J. Allergy Clin. Immunol.*, **55**, 241

29. Cooke, P. A., Bernard, J. H., Herald, S. and Stull, A. (1935). Serological evidence of immunity with co-existing sensitization in type of human allergy (hay fever). *J. Exp. Med.*, **62**, 733

30. Munro-Ashman, D., McEwen, H. and Feinberg, J. G. (1971). The Patient Self (P–S) Test. *Int. Arch. Allergy*, **40**, 448

3
Diagnostic Tests

PART II:
Patch Tests

M. G. C. DAHL

PATCH TESTING

Allergic contact eczema can be confirmed clinically by patch testing. This involves applying the suspected allergen to intact skin and observing the development of a delayed eczematous reaction usually over a period of 48–96 hours.

TECHNIQUES

In the open method of patch testing the allergen is applied to normal skin which is left uncovered. This method is suitable for testing volatile substances, strong potential sensitizing agents and substances which may be irritant under occluded conditions. Photo-patch tests which require light exposure are also performed by an open method. However, the majority of common contact allergens encountered in clinical practice penetrate intact skin relatively poorly and some form of occlusive or closed patch test is required for reliable elicitation of positive reactions.

In the closed patch test, allergens are applied under some form of occlusive dressing. A variety of methods has been devised[1,2]. The most widely adopted method in the United Kingdom involves the use of cellulose paper discs mounted on polythene covered aluminium foil (A1-test, Imeco, Sweden)[3]. Allergens in a suitable vehicle are placed on the cellulose discs and the patches are applied to the skin with adhesive tape. The time before reading is chosen empirically and is usually 48 hours. The upper back is the most convenient site on which to test multiple allergens.

Most common contact allergens can be prepared in soft paraffin. This is a convenient base which is almost totally inert and in which most allergens will remain stable. Moreover it is easy to apply small amounts to the patch test discs and the vehicle ensures good contact with the skin. Many common contact allergens are commercially available in standard concentrations in soft paraffin and are packed in disposable polypropylene syringes for ease of handling. The cellulose discs are absorbent and are also convenient for other allergens which may require a fluid vehicle such as water, oil or organic solvent.

The time course of the development of positive reactions varies with different allergens and is a function of the rate of percutaneous absorption. The latter is dependent on the concentration of applied allergen among other factors. The majority of reactions are already unequivocally positive after 2 days, when the patches are usually removed, but in one study[4] there were 21% more positive reactions on day 7 compared with day 2. For convenience many clinicians employ a single reading on day 3 or 4. Although this represents a reasonable compromise in terms of patient attendance and clinician's time, it is inevitable that some positive reactions, for example to neomycin[5], will be missed by this practice.

Some method is required of marking the sites of allergen application. This can be conveniently done by applying a 20% solution of dihydroxyacetone to the skin adjacent to each patch test site at the time of application. This produces a local brown discoloration of skin which fades after a few days. For more fastidious patients and for those with deeply pigmented skin fluorescent marking agents can be used which require ultraviolet irradiation for visualization.

CHOICE OF ALLERGENS

The choice of patch test allergens will of course depend on the suspected cause of the eczema. However, in practice it is both convenient and wise to employ a battery of common allergens even if the cause appears obvious. Multiple sensitivity is common and will not be detected unless multiple allergens are routinely tested. Standard contact allergen batteries have been developed to cover the most common causes of allergic eczema. Such allergen batteries differ slightly in different areas of the world, but usually include metallic ions, e.g. nickel, cobalt and chromate; a variety of rubber accelerators and antioxidants; constituents of topical drugs, creams and ointments and miscellaneous sensitizers such as formaldehyde and epoxy resins. While the number of possible contact sensitizing agents is immense such relatively small standard batteries will detect a very high percentage of allergic contact dermatitis reactions.

The concentration of allergen used for patch testing must be determined empirically. The use of too high concentrations may result in false positive toxic or irritant reactions or may produce unacceptably vigorous allergic reactions. Moreover the risk of primary sensitization by patch testing will be increased if very high concentrations of allergens are used. On the other hand if too low concentrations are used there may be inadequate penetration through the skin and false negative results.

It is important to remember that factors other than concentration may affect the rate of percutaneous absorption of an allergen. Absorption may be affected by the physicochemical state of the allergen and by the vehicle or solvent in which it is applied. For instance, absorption of hexavalent chromate greatly exceeds that of the trivalent ion and is also higher under alkaline conditions[6]. Moreover the state of the skin itself is important in determining allergen absorption. The skin of the back is normally intact and undamaged and covered with a protective layer of sebum. By contrast the hands of an industrial or building worker may be damaged by minor abrasions and cuts due to his work or to nail biting, or by an irritant dermatitis, thus destroying natural barrier function and allowing greater allergen penetration. For these reasons it is often necessary for test allergen concentrations to be higher than the usual environmental concentration in order to give reliable and reproducible positive reactions on normal back skin in allergic subjects. Suitable concentrations for many allergens for patch testing can be found in standard texts[7] and many of the common ones are commercially available in suitable concentrations. However, when investigating a new contact allergen it is often necessary to employ a range of test concentrations in several sensitive subjects and in control in order to determine the threshold concentration which will elicit positive reactions reproducibly and thus be suitable for reliable screening thereafter.

PATCH TEST REACTIONS

Positive allergic reactions exhibit redness, infiltration and oedema, vesiculation and in extreme reactions pustule formation and ulceration. Positive reactions frequently itch, but severe reactions may be sore. Unfortunately, positive reactions are not easily quantified and reactions are usually scored by subjective grading. The International Contact Dermatitis Research Group has suggested the following scoring system[8]:

?+ doubtful reaction
+ weak (non-vesicular reaction)
++ strong (oedematous or vesicular reaction)
+++ extreme reaction

Another method which attempts to quantify sensitivity involves the use of different concentrations of allergen and determination of the threshold concentration for a positive reaction. However such a method depends critically on the rates of percutaneous absorption and it has not been established that the threshold concentration for positive reactions in a group of sensitive patients reliably reflects immunological sensitivity rather than other physical non-immune variables. Such limitations in both standardizing and quantifying data from patch tests has greatly hindered research in contact dermatitis.

The distinction between allergic and irritant reactions is not always easy. Mild erythema due to local irritation is sometimes present immediately after removal of the patches. This reaction rapidly fades and is not accompanied by oedema or infiltration. A petechial reaction commonly occurs with cobalt chloride and is considered to be non-allergic[9]. More extreme irritant reactions may exhibit a uniform macular erythema with a rather shiny glazed or wrinkled appearance and sometimes epidermal necrosis with sloughing and ulceration. Such reactions are often strictly limited to the area beneath the occlusive patch test without much oedema, whereas strongly positive allergic reactions accompanied by ulceration invariably spread well beyond the margins of the original patch test disc and show vesiculation around the margins. Irritant reactions seldom itch but may be sore if they are severe. Some irritant reactions show a predominantly neutrophilic infiltration and can be distinguished histologically in skin biopsies from the typical mononuclear infiltrate of the true allergic reaction. However this feature is not reliable and a mononuclear infiltrate may also predominate in some irritant reactions[9]. In suspected allergic reactions to unusual allergens which may not previously have been studied it is important to use various allergen concentrations and to test a number of control subjects to exclude non-specific irritant reactions.

INTERPRETATION AND RELEVANCE OF POSITIVE REACTIONS

Like other types of positive skin test reactions, a truly allergic positive patch test reaction indicates only that the patient has been previously sensitized to that particular allergen or to a related cross-reacting substance. It does not indicate that the allergen is necessarily the cause of the eczema which is being investigated. Finding a positive patch test reaction is clinically most useful when it either confirms an already suspected allergy or when it reveals a previously unsuspected allergy whose relevance can be subsequently established. Unfortunately many patients exhibit positive patch test reactions which may explain their eczema only partially or not at all. For instance patients with chronic hand eczema quite commonly exhibit positive reactions to nickel. Many such patients will give a past history of typical nickel allergy due to metal earrings or a watch strap, but the relevance of nickel sensitivity to their hand eczema remains unclear.

Ideal criteria to establish the relevance of a positive patch test to an episode of eczematous dermatitis would include the following:

(1) Evidence of exposure to the relevant allergen.
(2) Onset of eczema in relation to allergen exposure and on areas of skin in contact with the allergen.
(3) Clearance of dermatitis following cessation of allergen exposure.

In practice such ideal criteria are frequently not satisfied.

References

1. Magnusson, B. and Hersle, K. (1966). Patch test methods. III. Influence of adhesive tape on test response. *Acta Dermatovenereol.*, **46**, 275
2. Pirila, V. (1975). Chamber test versus patch test for epicutaneous testing. *Contact Derm.*, **1**, 48
3. Calnan, C. D. and Turk, J. L. (1975). Allergic contact dermatitis. In Gell, P. G. H., Coombs, R. R. A. and Lachmann, P. J. (eds.) *Clinical Aspects of Immunology*, p. 1019. (Oxford: Blackwell)
4. Mitchell, J. C. (1978). Day 7 (D7) patch test reading – valuable or not? *Contact Derm.*, **4**, 139
5. Hjorth, N. and Thomsen, K. (1966). Patch tests with neomycin. Time of reaction patch test sensitization. *Acta Allergol.*, **21**, 487
6. Skog, E. and Wahlberg, J. E. (1969). Patch testing with potassium dichromate in different vehicles. *Arch. Dermatol.*, **99**, 697
7. Fisher, A. A. (1973). *Contact Dermatitis.* (Philadelphia: Lea and Febiger)
8. Wilkinson, D. S., Fregert, S., Magnusson, B., Bandmann, H. J., Calnan, C. D., Cronin, E., Hjorth, N., Maibach, H. J., Malten, K. E., Meneghini, C. L. and Pirila, V. (1970). Terminology of contact dermatitis. *Acta Dermatovenereol.*, **50**, 287
9. Schmidt, H., Larsen, F. S., Larsen, P. Ø. and Søgaard, H. (1980). Petechial reaction following patch testing with cobalt. *Contact Derm.*, **6**, 91

3
Diagnostic Tests

PART III:
Challenge Tests – Oral Nasal and Bronchial

R. J. DAVIES

PROVOCATION TESTS

Provocation tests with allergens in one form or another have been widely used for many years. In 1873 Charles Harrison Blackley published the results of provocation tests with grass pollen on his conjunctiva, soft palate and by scarification of his skin. He also performed bronchial provocation testing by inhalation of pollen grains. These early studies were of paramount importance in identifying the relationship between contact with allergens and the development of symptoms. Since that time provocation tests have been widely used in attempts to identify agents causing allergic disease: they remain invaluable as research techniques not only for identifying new allergens causing disease, particularly in occupational asthma or extrinsic allergic bronchio-alveolitis, but also because they provide a convenient method for comparing and evaluating new treatments for allergic disease in man. Further, the reproduction of the disease under controlled conditions allows careful study of its physiology, immunology and pharmacology. However, the role of provocation tests in clinical practice is more limited: all are potentially hazardous and must be performed by trained personnel, preferably in the hospital environment.

ORAL PROVOCATION TESTS

Food allergy may present with a wide range of symptoms varying from vomiting, abdominal pain and diarrhoea, to rashes and urticaria. Sometimes allergy to food may give rise to respiratory symptoms such as rhinitis and wheezing and occasionally, in very sensitive individuals, to anaphylaxis. Much of the symptomatology of food allergy is subjective, and it is important to have a carefully controlled method of deciding whether such symptoms are in fact due to allergy to foods.

The diagnosis of food allergy can often be difficult and although it has been suggested that significant food allergy, particularly in children, is frequently associated with the demonstration of skin-sensitizing antibody or the presence of specific IgE antibodies in serum[1], it is usually necessary to perform a provocation test with the food thought to cause the patient's symptoms. All foods that have been suspected of causing adverse reactions should be excluded from the diet for a period of 2 weeks prior to the challenge and the patient taken off drugs such as antihistamines which may inhibit the reaction. Small amounts of the dried food or placebo should be placed in opaque colourless capsules, which should be fed to the patient on the day of the test. If the patient is thought to have a high degree of allergy then small amounts of the food (20 mg) should be given initially. A history of an anaphylactic response to a food precludes oral provocation testing. The capsules should be administered in a double-blind fashion so that neither patient nor observer is aware of which is being given. Subsequent subjective symptoms should be noted as well as the development of diarrhoea or urticaria, and any changes in respiratory function measured. Symptoms may occur within minutes but rarely after 24 hours. If the test is negative the amount of food given in the capsule should be increased 10-fold on subsequent days until a maximum of 8 g is reached. If this dose is tolerated then it is less likely that this particular food is causing symptoms and it can be reintroduced into the diet, though it is still wise to watch for the development of any adverse reactions. This type of double-blind oral provocation test allows a realistic assessment of the role of various foods in the development of symptoms. Further, it is possible to test the effect of drugs such as sodium cromoglycate, which may inhibit the allergic reaction to foods, by prior administration of the pharmacological agent up to 30 minutes before the provocation test with the food or placebo capsule[2].

This type of oral provocation test can only be used satisfactorily for symptoms and signs which develop soon after ingestion of food and which may be related to Type I allergy. Foods may, however, cause diseases such as eczema which can take days or weeks to develop and under these circumstances it is not possible to carry out this type of provocation test. If a particular food is suspected as a cause of such a disease then it is necessary to withdraw it completely from the diet and observe the symptoms and signs over the subsequent days or weeks. The food should then be reintroduced and the patient watched for recrudescence of symptoms. This type of elimination or allergen avoidance diet may be difficult to perform since it is often hard to exclude the food completely and such tests may require careful control, at least in the first instance, to obtain acceptable results[3].

NASAL PROVOCATION TESTS

Nasal provocation tests have been widely used for many years. While they have proved valuable in the experimental investigation of allergic rhinitis and in determining the effect of drugs, the role of this technique in clinical practice is not as clear. Generally, the clinical history together with a concordant skin test is all that is required for a diagnosis of seasonal allergic rhinitis due to contact with grass pollen. However, with other allergens, in particular the house dust mite, the patient's history may be far from conclusive and it may be necessary to perform nasal provocation testing with the allergens giving rise to positive skin tests. Further, it has been reported that allergic rhinitis due to allergens from the house dust mite may occur in patients who have both negative skin tests and a negative serum RAST for this allergen[4]. In this situation, the only method of diagnosis is a nasal provocation test.

Application of allergens

Allergen solutions should not be dropped into the nose since this is potentially dangerous. The fluid may run over the floor of the nose on to the larynx and in allergic people give rise to laryngeal oedema. The allergen extract usually in a volume of $100–200 \mu l$ should be sprayed into the nostril and the patient instructed to inspire and then breath-hold during the manoeuvre. This should be followed by exhalation 30 seconds later. It is only possible to test a patent nostril since if the nose is blocked little of the allergen solution will reach the mucosa. In general the starting concentration of allergen for nasal provocation testing should be that which causes a weal of less than 3 mm on skin prick testing. However, no quantitative correlation has been shown to exist between weal diameters on skin testing and the changes in nasal airway resistance following administration of varying doses of allergen in patients with allergic rhinitis[5].

Sneezing and rhinorrhoea

There are a number of ways of assessing the results of nasal provocation tests. It is possible to count the number of sneezes that occur during the 15 minutes after the provocation test, and if the patient sits forward to measure the nasal discharge. This 'sneeze drip score' can be used for semiquantitation of nasal reactions when different allergen doses are compared to placebo[6].

Rhinomanometry

The most quantitative and objective assessment of the results of nasal provocation testing is the measurement of changes in nasal airway resistance by the technique of rhinomanometry. The technique measures both pressure and flow and so in fact is rhinorheomanometry. A number of methods have been developed to measure changes in nasal airway resistance. The majority involve the measurement of changes in both nostrils in parallel and this often produces results which are difficult to interpret. Reflex changes may occur in one nostril when the other responds to provocation with an allergen. Recently a modification of the technique of anterior rhinometry has been developed which allows nasal airway resistance to be measured in each nostril separately[7]. This technique is illustrated in Figure 3.III.1. The cuff of an

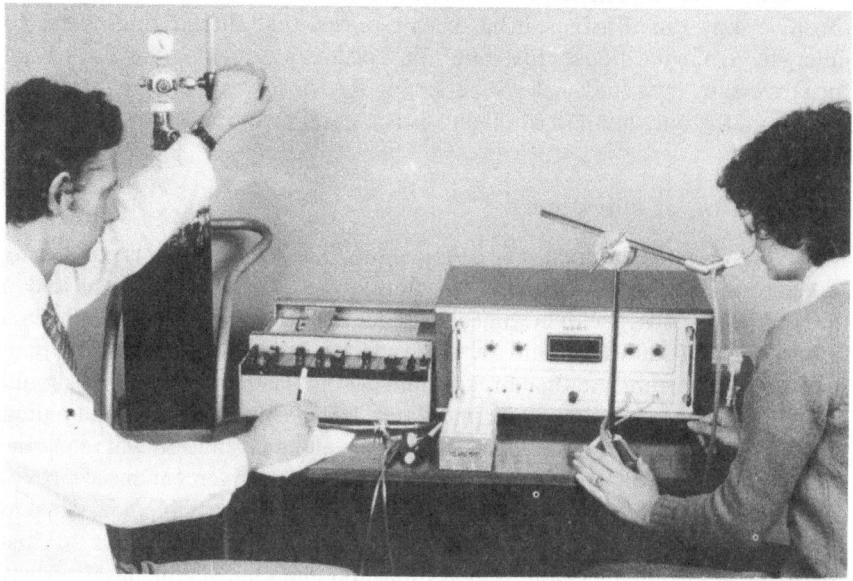

Figure 3.III.1 The technique of anterior rhinomanometry using the nasal airway resistance tester

infant's endotracheal tube is inflated in one nostril to produce an airtight seal. Air is then blown into the nostril at a rate of 3 l/min and the pressure recorded. The nasal airway resistance tester (NART[R] P. K. Morgan, Chatham, Kent) will compute the resistance directly or the pressure flow trace can be recorded on an X–Y recorder. This technique is non-invasive and extremely quick, each recording taking only a few seconds. The advantages of recording the pressure change in each nostril independently is clearly shown in Figure 3.III.2. This shows the results of nasal provocation tests with a control solution of phenol saline, and with two concentrations of an extract of *Dermatophagoides pteronyssinus*. The increase in nasal airway resistance in the challenged nostril is related to the dose of allergen. However, due to approximately equal but opposite reflex changes in the unchallenged nostril, only small increases are seen in total nasal resistance. This technique allows the evaluation of the effect of various drugs on allergen nasal airways' resistance dose–response relationships. The pharmacological agents can be given either orally before the tests or sprayed into the nose in a similar fashion to the administration of the allergen[8].

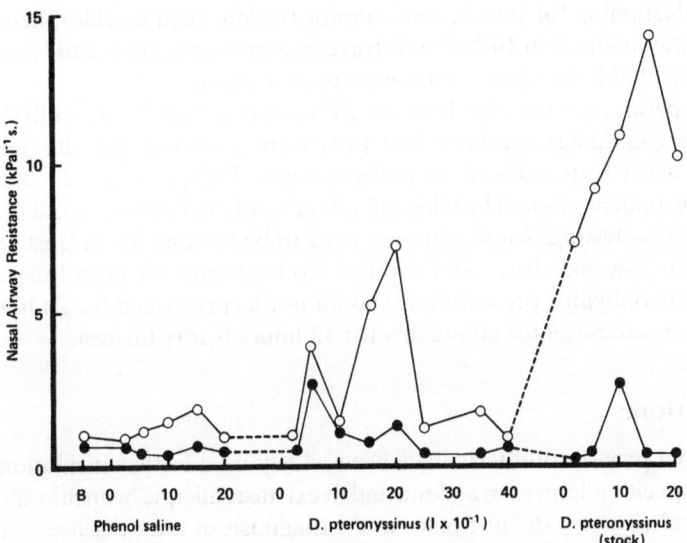

Figure 3.III.2   Allergen dose–response relationships. Changes in nasal airway resistance in each nostril following instillation into one nostril of a control solution (phenol saline), a *D. pteronyssinus* extract diluted 1:10, and the·undiluted extract of *D. pteronyssinus*.
○-○ Challenged nostril; ● ● unchallenged nostril; B = baseline nasal airway resistance. Horizontal axis = time after provocation test in minutes

The exact place of improved techniques of rhinomanometry in the clinical evaluation of patients has still to be evaluated. However, these techniques are likely to be particularly valuable in providing useful information about nasal allergy in patients with perennial rhinitis, where the correlation between nasal and skin tests has previously been found to be relatively poor[9].

BRONCHIAL PROVOCATION TESTS

In 1947 Lowell and Schiller[10] showed that the inhalation of aerosols of pollen extract provoked a fall in the vital capacity of the lungs in asthmatic patients. Since that time bronchial provocation tests, in which the reaction has been monitored with lung function tests, have been extensively used in the investigation of patients with asthma and extrinsic allergic bronchio-alveolitis due to identifiable extrinsic agents. Overall the techniques are safe, indeed in one series no anaphylactic or other severe reactions were noted in over 9000 bronchial provocation tests performed with a wide variety of allergens in 1035 children[11]. Nevertheless these tests should only be performed in the hospital environment with appropriate resuscitation facilities readily at hand. These include a β_2-adrenoceptor stimulant such as salbutamol in aerosolized form, an antihistamine for intravenous administration, such as chlorpheniramine 10 mg, adrenaline 1 in 10 000 for intravenous administration and appropriate mechanical aids for cardiopulmonary resuscitation.

In general, patients who have an FEV_1 of less than 2 l are unlikely to be suitable candidates for bronchial provocation testing and this technique should never be performed on patients whose FEV_1 is below 1 l. Whenever possible, patients should be taken off all forms of medication before bronchial provocation testing. Antihistamines need to be omitted for at least 48 hours and corticosteroid drugs and sodium cromoglycate for even longer. Slow release theophylline preparations should not be prescribed for 24 hours and inhaled β-adrenoceptor stimulants for 12 hours before the test.

Indications

Bronchial provocation tests have been widely used in the elucidation of the role of specific allergens in asthma and in extrinsic allergic bronchio-alveolitis. This test has a very definite place in the diagnosis of these diseases caused by previously unrecognized allergens but its role in everyday clinical practice is disputed. With many allergens, for example grass pollen, the appropriate history together with a positive skin test to grass pollen allergens is usually sufficient for diagnosis. With other allergens, in particular the house dust mite, the situation is not as clear-cut. It is frequently difficult to be convinced about a history of contact with house dust mite leading to asthma, and bronchial provocation testing under these circumstances may well be a useful adjunct to diagnosis particularly when specific therapy such as allergen avoidance or hyposensitization could result. In one study up to 30% of patients with a history suggestive of house dust allergy yet with negative skin tests to this allergen had positive bronchial provocation tests[12]. In general the greater the size of the skin prick test reaction to the allergen the more likely it is that the bronchial provocation test with the same allergen will be positive. However, it is important to realize that it is possible to have false positive bronchial provocation tests, that is the patient may have no history of asthma and yet develop reversible airflow obstruction on bronchial provocation testing, particularly when a high dose of allergen is used[13].

Bronchial provocation tests can be used to monitor the effects of immunotherapy or the effectiveness of drugs[14]. but it is important to remember that although a drug may diminish the bronchial response to allergen on provocation testing, it may not be effective clinically[15]. Similarly these techniques have been of great value in assessing the physiology, immunology and pharmacology of the different types of asthmatic reaction[16, 17]. At the present time bronchial provocation tests play a fundamental role in the evaluation of dusts, gases, vapours and fumes involved in the aetiology of occupational asthma and until these diseases are better characterized the inhalation challenge test remains an essential diagnostic test[18].

The American Thoracic Society includes bronchial hyper-reactivity in its definition of asthma, and this feature of patients with this disease can be demonstrated by bronchial provocation testing with a number of agents particularly methacholine and histamine. Both agents give very similar results, and studies by Townley and co-workers have shown that the respiratory tract of patients with asthma is 100- to 1000-fold more sensitive to methacholine than that of subjects without the disease[19]. They also showed that patients with rhinitis were not significantly different, in terms of bronchial response to inhaled methacholine, from control subjects from families with atopic diseases. This is important, since studies using bronchial provocation tests with allergens have suggested that there may be little difference in the bronchial response, at least in the large airways, between patients with asthma and hay fever[20]. For this reason inhalation challenge tests with methacholine or histamine may be useful diagnostically to distinguish patients with asthma from those with rhinitis alone.

Apart from causing asthma, inhaled allergens may lead to development of respiratory disease which affects not only the large and small airways but also the interstitial tissue of the lung. A wide variety of inhaled organic agents are known to cause this disease, best called extrinsic allergic bronchio-alveolitis, and much of the understanding of this disease has come from studies following bronchial provocation tests[21]. Now that the causes of this disease are well recognized, the appropriate history, radiographic and physiological changes coupled with a history of exposure to the particular agent and the presence of specific precipitating antibody against the agent in the serum is all that is required for the diagnosis. Nevertheless bronchial provocation testing may still have a role when one or more of these factors is absent or appears contradictory. As with asthma, bronchial provocation testing has an invaluable role in the initial assessment of new materials thought to give rise to extrinsic allergic bronchio-alveolitis.

Methods

The traditional method for performing bronchial provocation tests is to use a nebulized extract of allergen or pharmacological agent. This method of administration bears little resemblance to natural exposure, particularly to those agents which normally occur in particulate form. Further, there is little similarity in terms of dose, rate of administration, presentation of allergen or site of deposition within the respiratory tract. Indeed studies in patients with ragweed hay fever and asthma showed no pulmonary function changes when these patients inhaled whole pollen. It was only when the pollen was fragmented to a particle size of 5μm or smaller that asthmatic reactions resulted[22]. For these reasons many investigators question the adequacy of much of the methodology used for bronchial provocation testing and attention has been increasingly focused on a number of factors which influence the respiratory reaction. These include the method of delivery of the provoking agent and the most appropriate method for measuring the respiratory reaction.

Studies of occupational asthma have led to the development of a different type of bronchial provocation test. Pepys and co-workers have developed simple and safe techniques for simulating work exposure within the hospital environment[17, 23]. The patient is exposed to the industrial dust. gas. vapour or fume in the form in which it is encountered in the factory. Since it is now frequently possible to assess factory exposure accurately this 'occupational' type of bronchial provocation test can be refined to allow the subject to be tested with the particular industrial material in the same form and in the same concentration, though for a shorter duration, as that encountered at work. Further, on-site observations in industry have allowed correlation between the types of respiratory reaction seen at work and those that can be reproduced in the hospital laboratory[24].

Delivery system

There is no system currently available which will allow the dose of material reaching the respiratory tract during a bronchial provocation test to be determined accurately. Much of the material inhaled is deposited in the nose, mouth and oropharynx. The proportion reaching the respiratory tract and its site of deposition depends upon a number of variables: these include the particle size of the aerosol or dust, the rate and depth of breathing and, where aerosols are being generated by a nebulizer, by its output. Studies using radiolabelled aerosols (99m-technetium) have shown the importance of the rate of breathing. Rapid inspiration leads to impaction of most of the material above the glottis while tidal breathing and slow vital capacity inspirations give diffuse airway deposition[25, 26].

Where the aim of a bronchial provocation test is simply to induce an identifiable reaction, standardization of the conditions of bronchial provocation testing is less critical. However, where repeated tests need to be compared as in the assessment of pharmacological agents or the effects of immunotherapy, the accuracy and reproducibility with which particular doses of allergen or pharmacological agent are administered becomes of considerable importance. It is vital to test individual methods for uniformity of delivery and particle size, and the same equipment should be used for each patient throughout the investigation.

At the present time, there are two basic procedures for bronchial provocation testing which have been intensively investigated with solutions of allergens, histamine and methacholine. Figure 3.III.3 illustrates the use of a Wright's nebulizer driven by oxygen at 8 l/min. This is connected to a face mask and rebreathing bag. The patient is instructed to breathe naturally around his functional residual capacity (FRC) during the inhalation test which is continued for 2 minutes[26, 27]. The Wright's nebulizer is known to

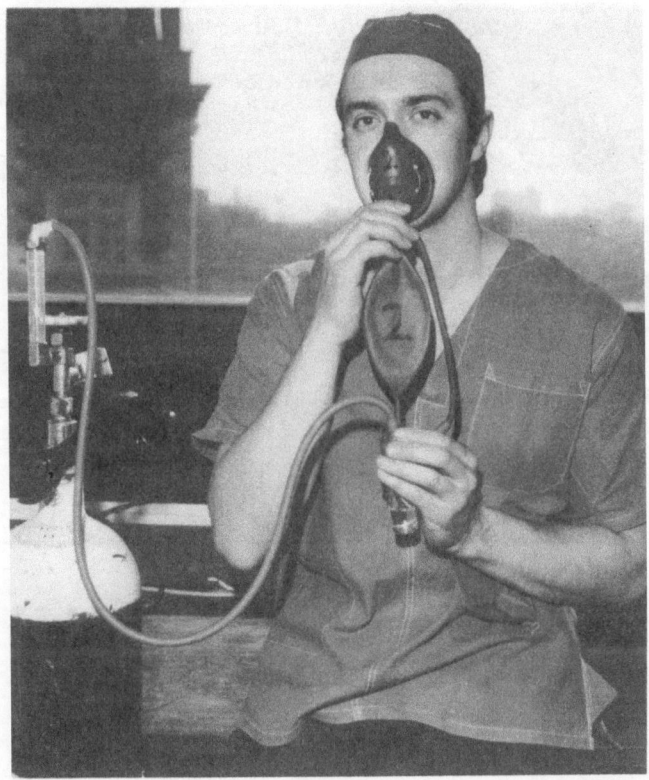

Figure 3.III.3   An allergen bronchial provocation test using a Wright's nebulizer

produce particles of mass median diameter 3 μm[28]. The second method is illustrated in Figure 3.III.4 and shows a bronchial provocation test with a Johns Hopkins dosimeter connected to a de Vilbiss 646 nebulizer. This equipment allows the nebulizer to be triggered when the patient inspires and the device delivers the aerosol for a predetermined time, usually 0.6 s. Five slow vital capacity breaths are taken from FRC. It is known that the de Vilbiss 646 nebulizer produces particles of a mass median diameter of 1.3 μm. This method has been incorporated in a standardization procedure for bronchial provocation testing in the United States of America[29].

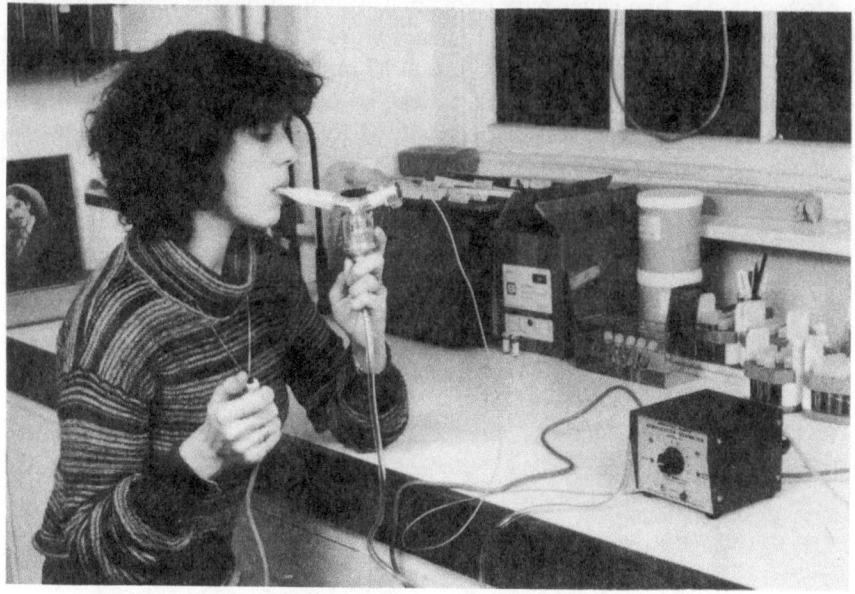

Figure 3.III.4 An allergen bronchial provocation test with a de Vilbiss 646 nebulizer and Johns Hopkins dosimeter

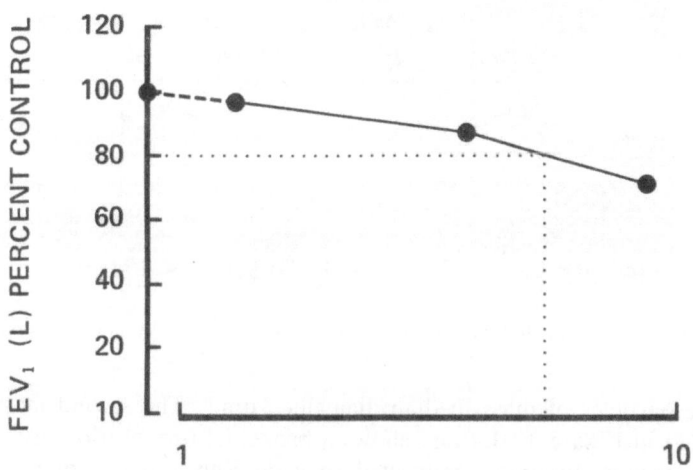

HISTAMINE ACID PHOSPHATE – BREATH UNITS

Figure 3.III.5 Results of a bronchial provocation test with histamine: a cumulative dose–response curve. Per cent change in forced expiratory volume (FEV_1) on the vertical axis and the cumulative dose of histamine expressed in breath units on a logarithmic scale on the horizontal axis. The provocation dose needed to cause a 20% fall in the FEV_1 (PD_{20} FEV_1) is illustrated

Figure 3.III.5 shows the results of a bronchial provocation test with histamine expressed in the way suggested by Chai and co-workers[29]. A cumulative dose–response curve has been produced with the forced expiratory volume in 1 s (FEV_1) expressed on the vertical axis and the dose of histamine on a logarithmic scale on the horizontal axis. The histamine dose has been expressed in terms of breath units, where one breath unit is equivalent to one inhalation of a concentration of 1 mg/ml. The histamine dose required to produce a 20% fall in FEV_1 can then be determined and is expressed as the provocation dose for a 20% fall in FEV_1 ($PD_{20} FEV_1$). Allergen dose–response curves can be expressed in the same way where one breath unit is the equivalent of one inhalation of 1 µg protein nitrogen solution or one inhalation of 1/5000 weight/volume concentration. Comparisons between the use of the Wright's nebulizer and the Johns Hopkins dosimeter have shown dissimilar results[30] and this underlines the need for standardization of techniques for bronchial provocation tests on a worldwide basis which would allow direct comparison between different laboratories.

Occupational materials

The occupation type of bronchial provocation test should be carried out in an exposure chamber with adequate extraction facilities. Care should be taken to prevent the escape of any of the test materials into the atmosphere of the laboratory, not only for the protection of staff but also because of the exquisitely high degree of sensitivity of some patients which may result in continuing provocation after the patient is removed from the challenge chamber. Occupational materials such as grain or wood dust[31] are best tested by the patient tipping the material from one receptacle to another as illustrated in Figure 3.III.6. Small amounts (10 to 1000 mg) of materials such as antibiotics or the complex salts of platinum which are highly allergenic and which exist in a fine powder form are best mixed with a vehicle such as lactose (250 g) previously dried overnight at 105 °C and the patient instructed to create a dust in the atmosphere of the challenge chamber[32,33]. Vapours from soldering fluxes can readily be tested by asking the subject to repeat the soldering manoeuvre in the challenge chamber.

One of the problems with these techniques as with common inhalant allergens has been the lack of knowledge of the dose of material inhaled by the patient. Whenever possible measurements of the concentration of the occupational material produced in the challenge chamber should be made and compared with that found at work. This has proved possible with bronchial provocation tests with toluene diisocyanate (TDI). A known concentration of TDI can be produced in the challenge chamber by passing air at known flow rates over TDI in a gas washing bottle (Figure 3.III.7). The flow of air is adjusted until a steady state concentration of TDI is reached at the required level as measured by a Universal Instruments Model 7000 TDI Monitor[34].

Information from such comparative studies has shown that sensitized individuals may develop asthma on contact with levels very much lower than the threshold limit value (TLV) set as a standard for occupational safety.

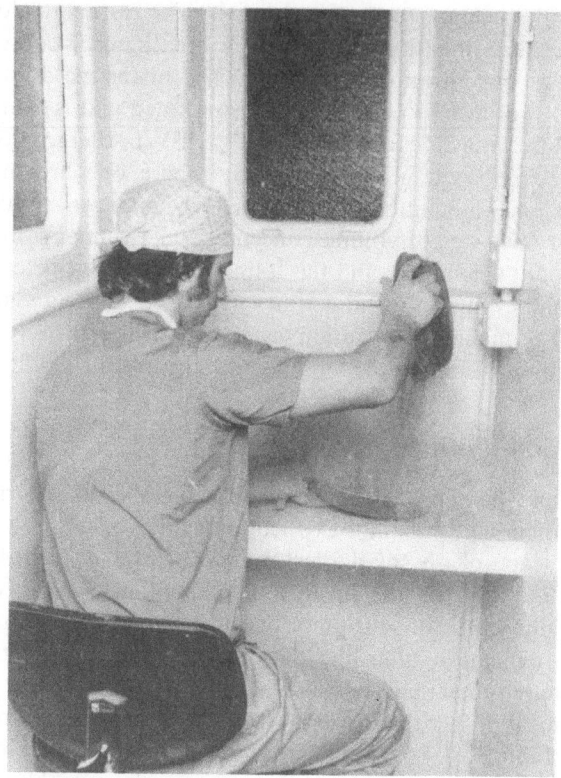

Figure 3.III.6   An 'occupational type' of bronchial provocation test with the dust of western red cedar

Dose and exposure times

The initial concentration for bronchial provocation testing with allergens should be assessed by skin prick testing and the concentration provoking a skin reaction with a weal diameter of less than 3 mm should be used[23]. It is difficult to be sure of the appropriate initial concentration of methacholine or histamine since the dose at which individuals react varies greatly. For this reason it is best to start at low concentrations such as 0.15 mg/ml of methacholine and 0.03 mg/ml of histamine. Whatever the technique used for bronchial provocation testing, the concentration of allergen, histamine or methacholine should be increased two- to five-fold if initial tests are negative. The tests should be repeated at 10 minute intervals for allergen and every 5 minutes for histamine or methacholine if cumulative dose–response curves are required. If the history suggests that the bronchial provocation test might result in late asthmatic reactions or extrinsic allergic bronchio-alveolitis then only one test should be performed on a particular day and increasing concentrations given on subsequent days. It may not be possible to use skin tests to assess the starting concentration for bronchial provocation testing

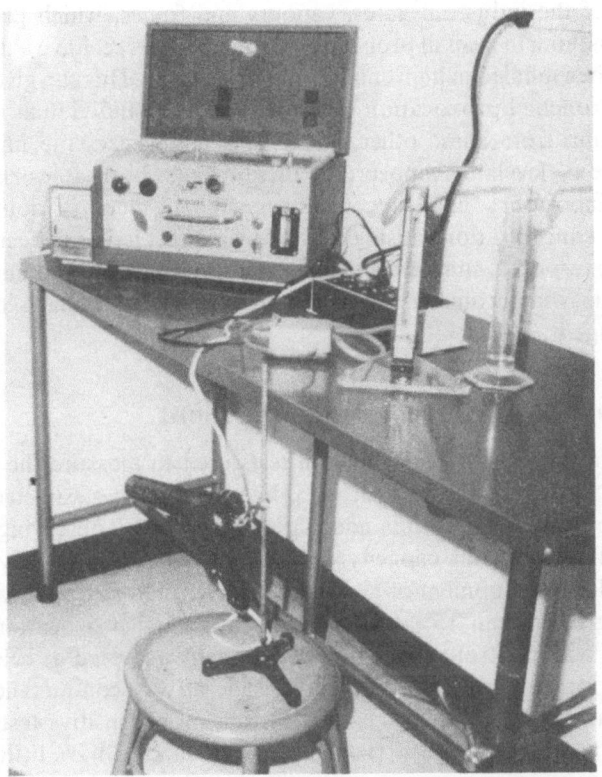

Figure 3.III.7   The apparatus required for an 'occupational type' of bronchial provocation test with toluene di-isocyanate (TDI)

with many agents causing occupational asthma or extrinsic allergic bronchio-alveolitis either because Type I allergic reactions are not involved in the pathogenesis or appropriate solutions cannot be prepared. In these circumstances it is necessary to gauge the initial dose from careful knowledge of the patient's history and work conditions. In general it is essential to start with extremely low doses to avoid untoward reactions. Where measurements have been made at work, it is possible to begin bronchial provocation testing with these agents at lower concentrations. Experience suggests that the occupational type of bronchial provocation test should be continued for 15 to 30 minutes. However, care is required since a single inhalation of epoxy resin fumes has been shown to lead to marked changes in respiratory function[35].

It is difficult to know what the top concentration of the allergen should be for bronchial provocation testing. In one study bronchial provocation tests with pollen allergens at a concentration of 10 000 protein nitrogen units gave rise to a positive test in patients with allergic rhinitis who had never previously wheezed[13].

Many of the industrial gases, vapours and fumes, which produce occupational asthma in a small proportion of the work force, have a direct irritant activity when inhaled in high enough concentrations. This can give rise to false positive bronchial provocation tests particularly in individuals who already have asthma from some other cause. This emphasizes the importance of knowledge of levels of exposure to these agents, both at work and in the hospital laboratory challenge chamber. When there is doubt about a particular concentration causing asthma by a direct irritant effect rather than an allergic response, similar bronchial provocation tests should be performed on patients with bronchial hyper-reactivity whose asthma is caused by a different agent.

Measurement of the respiratory reactions

The appropriate respiratory function tests used to measure the response to bronchial provocation tests depend in part on the expected outcome. Asthmatic reactions are often adequately followed by observing changes in FEV_1 and forced vital capacity (FVC) or in peak expiratory flow rates (PEFR). The development of an obstructive ventilatory defect, with a fall in FEV_1 of greater than 15% following the bronchial provocation test when compared with control values, is conventionally accepted as evidence of an asthmatic reaction. Measurement of specific airway conductance and flow rates at various lung volumes can be used as more sensitive tests of airflow obstruction. In general these tests have been found to have little advantage over spirometric measurements in identifying asthmatic reactions to bronchial provocation tests although they have been found to show greater proportional changes from the pre-test values[36]. In a study of a group of patients with occupational asthma due to western red cedar, immediate falls in flow rates at low lung volumes were seen in some patients following bronchial provocation tests with extracts of the wood dust, which were not accompanied by changes in the FEV_1[37]. Studies using bronchial provocation tests with methacholine on patients with allergic rhinitis but no asthma showed that significant change in specific airway conductance (SG_{AW}) occurred while the falls in FEV_1 did not come into the asthmatic range. This information could be interpreted as showing that the FEV_1 is an insensitive test of the response of the airways of patients with allergic rhinitis to methacholine: alternatively it could be considered a more specific test[38]. Although measurement of specific airways' conductance may be a more sensitive test in asthmatic subjects, the differences between SG_{AW} and FEV_1 are slight and the advantage of this sensitivity may be offset both by the simplicity of the FEV_1 measurements and its greater specificity. When the respiratory reaction provoked by a bronchial provocation test involves the peripheral gas exchanging part of the lung as in extrinsic allergic bronchio-alveolitis, carbon monoxide gas transfer should be measured and expressed both as transfer factor (DL_{CO}) and transfer coefficient (K_{CO}). Where possible total lung capacity (TLC) and residual volume (RV) should also be measured to help in determination of the site of reaction.

Respiratory function should be measured 30 minutes before and immediately before the bronchial provocation test. When there is a long exposure time during the bronchial provocation test, as with many occupational dusts, the patient should perform a peak expiratory flow manoeuvre during the test to identify any severe respiratory reaction. If this occurs the bronchial provocation test should be stopped. Measurements should be made every 5 minutes after the test for an hour and then hourly for the rest of the day. It is essential that bronchial provocation tests are conducted in the early morning to identify late reactions. Respiratory function tests should also be measured during the evening and if necessary during the night, particularly if the patient is woken by respiratory symptoms. Carbon monoxide gas transfer and lung volumes should be measured immediately before the test and then every 4 hours until the values have returned to pre-test levels.

Bronchial provocation tests with occupational agents in particular have shown that a single exposure to the provoking agent may give rise to attacks of

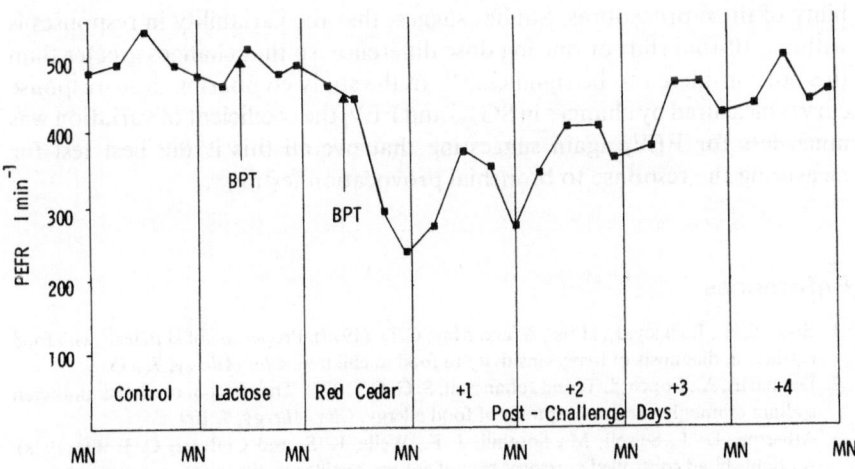

Figure 3.III.8 Recurrent asthma following a bronchial provocation test with western red cedar. PEFR = Peak expiratory flow rate in litres per minute; MN = midnight; BPT = bronchial provocation test

asthma which persist for many days or even weeks[39]. An example of a recurrent nocturnal asthmatic reaction following a bronchial provocation test with western red cedar is shown in Figure 3.III.8: this clearly indicates the importance of control days particularly with regard to late respiratory reactions. It is obviously essential to make sure that the patient's respiratory function is remaining steady throughout both day and night before performing the bronchial provocation test and to follow the reaction carefully over several days. Bronchial provocation tests performed when the patient already has recurrent nocturnal asthma may give rise to a falsely positive test and the reaction can be attributed to the wrong agent.

Reproducibility

Problems may arise when comparisons are made in the same subject during bronchial provocation tests on several occasions. Tests should be compared only when they have been performed with similar baseline function. There is an exponential relationship between the radius of a tube and its resistance to flow so that patients with pre-existing airflow obstruction will have a greater increase in airway resistance for a given reduction in airway calibre[40]. Further, there is some evidence that non-specific bronchial hyper-reactivity may increase in patients following inhalation of allergen which has led to late asthmatic reactions in particular. This may result in subsequent bronchial provocation tests with the same quantity of allergen giving rise to a more marked effect on airflow obstruction[41]. The increasing attention to dose-response curves following both allergen inhalation and the inhalation of histamine or methacholine has made it necessary to consider the reproducibility of these procedures. Studies suggest that the variability in responses is within a 10-fold shift or one log dose difference, so that changes greater than this are considered to be significant[42]. In the study comparing dose–response curves measured by changes in SG_{AW} and FEV_1 the coefficient of variation was much less for FEV_1 again suggesting that overall this is the best test for measuring the response to bronchial provocation testing[38].

References

1. Bock, S. A., Buckley, J., Holst, A. and May, C. D. (1977). Proper use of skin tests with food extracts in diagnosis of hypersensitivity to food in children. *Clin. Allergy*, **7**, 375
2. Dannaeus, A., Foucard, T. and Johansson, S. G. O. (1977). The effect of orally administered sodium cromoglycate on symptoms of food allergy. *Clin. Allergy*, **7**, 109
3. Atherton, D. J., Sewell, M., Soothill, J. F., Wells, R. S. and Chilvers, C. E. D. (1978). A double blind controlled crossover trial of antigen avoidance diet in atopic eczema. *Lancet*, **1**, 401
4. Huggins, K. G. and Brostoff, J. (1975). IgE antibodies in allergic rhinitis patients with negative skin tests. *Lancet*, **2**, 148

5. Taylor, G. and Shivalkar, P. R. (1971). Changes in nasal airways resistance on antigenic challenge in allergic rhinitis. *Clin. Allergy*, **1**, 63

6. Mygind, N. and Thomsen, J. (1975). I.C.I. 74, 917: A new antiallergic drug administered by pressurized aerosol. *Acta Allergologica (Kbh)*, **30**, 298

7. Britton, M. G., Empey, D. W., John, G. C., McDonnell, K. A. and Hughes, D. T. D. (1978). Histamine challenge and anterior nasal rhinometry: Their use in the assessment of pseudophedrine and triprolidine as nasal decongestants in subjects with hay fever. *Br. J. Clin. Pharmacol.*, **6**, 51

8. Phillips, M. J., Ollier, S. and Davies, R. J. (1980). Anterior rhinometry in the evaluation of the effects of ketotifen, clemastine, cromoglycate and placebo in nasal allergen provocation. *Respiration.* (In press)

9. Holopainen, E., Tarkiainen, E. and Malmberg, H. (1976). Nasal challenge. *Rhinology*, **14**, 181

10. Lowell, F. C. and Schiller, I. W. (1947). Reduction in the vital capacity of asthmatic subjects following exposure to aerosolised pollen extracts. *Science*, **105**, 312

11. Aas, K. (1970). Bronchial provocation tests in asthma. *Arch. Dis. Children*, **45**, 221

12. Aas, K. (1975). *Bronchial Provocation Tests*, p. 42. (Springfield, Illinois: Charles C. Thomas)

13. Townley, R. G., Dennis, M. and Itkin. I. H. (1965). Comparative action of acetyl beta methylcholine, histamine and pollen antigens in subjects with hay fever and patients with bronchial asthma. *J. Allergy*, **36**, 121

14. Pepys, J., Davies, R. J., Breslin, A. B. X., Hendrick, D. J. and Hutchcroft, B. J. (1974). The effects of inhaled beclomethasone dipropionate (Becotide) and sodium cromoglycate on asthmatic reactions to provocation tests. *Clin. Allergy*, **4**, 13

15. Muittari, A., Ahonen, A., Kellomaki, L., Kuusisto, P., Lehtinen, J. and Veneskoski, T. (1978). The effect of ICI 74917 on asthma and bronchial provocation tests. *Clin. Allergy*, **8**, 281

16. Rosenthal, R. R. (1979). Inhalation challenge procedures, indications and techniques: The emerging role of broncho provocation. *J. Allergy Clin. Immunol.*, **64**, 561

17. Pepys, J. and Hutchcroft, B. J. (1975). Bronchial provocation tests in the aetiological diagnosis and analysis of asthma. *Am. Rev. Resp. Dis.*, **112**, 829

18. Newman-Taylor, A. J. and Davies, R. J. (1980). Inhalation challenge testing. In Weill, H. and Turner-Warwick, M. (eds.) *Occupational Lung Diseases.* (New York: Marcel Dekker Inc.) (In press)

19. Townley, R. G., Buttra, A. K., Nair, N. M., Brodky, F. D., Watt, G. D. and Burk, K. M. (1979). Inhalation challenge studies. *J. Allergy Clin. Immunol.*, **64**, 569

20. Bruce, C. A., Rosenthal, R. R., Lichtenstein, L. M. and Norman, P. S. (1975). Quantitative inhalation bronchial challenge in ragweed hay fever patients: A comparison with ragweed allergic asthmatics. *J. Allergy Clin. Immunol.*, **56**, 331

21. Hargreave, F. E. and Pepys, J. (1972). Allergic respiratory reactions in bird fanciers provoked by allergen inhalation provocation tests. *J. Allergy Clin. Immunol.*, **50**, 157

22. Rosenberg, G. L., Rosenthal, R. R. and Norman, P. S. (1975). Inhalational challenge with ragweed pollen in ragweed sensitive asthmatics. *J. Allergy Clin. Immunol.*, **55**, 2

23. Davies, R. J. (1974). Bronchial provocation tests with common allergens, vapours and fumes. In Brent. L. and Holborow. E. J. (eds.) *Progress in Immunology.* 2. Vol. 4. p. 349. (Amsterdam and Oxford: North Holland Publishing Co.)

24. Sherwood Burge, P., O'Brien, I. M. and Harries, M. G. (1979). Peak flow rate recordings in the diagnosis of occupational asthma due to colophony. *Thorax*, **34**, 208

25. Reed, C. E., Bhansali, P. V., Irvin, C. and Polcyn, R. E. (1979). Site of deposition of aerosols delivered by two methods using a dosimeter. *J. Allergy Clin. Immunol.*, **63**, 164

26. Dolovich, M., Obminski, G., Cockcroft, R. W., Hargreave, F. E. and Newhouse, M. T. (1979). Standardisation of inhalation tests: Influence of method of aerosol generation and inhalation. *J. Allergy Clin. Immunol.*, **63**, 165

27. Cockcroft, D. W., Killian, D. N., Mellon, J. J. A. and Hargreave, F. E. (1977). Bronchial reactivity to inhaled histamine: a method and clinical survey. *Clin. Allergy*, **7**, 235

28. Dolovich, M. B., Sanchis, J. A., Rossman, C. and Newhouse, M. T. (1977). Aerosol penetrants, a sensitive index of peripheral airways obstruction. *J. Appl. Physiol.*, **40**, 268

29. Chai, H., Farr, S., Froehlich, L. A., Mathison, D. A., McLean, J. A., Rosenthal, R. R., Sheffer, R. A. L., Spector, S. L. and Townley, R. G. (1975). Standardisation of bronchial inhalation challenge procedures. *J. Allergy Clin. Immunol.*, **56**, 323

30. Beaupré, A. and Malo, J. L. (1979). Comparison of histamine bronchial challenges with the Wright nebuliser and the dosimeter. *Clin. Allergy*, **9**, 575

31. Pickering, C. A. C., Batten, J. C. and Pepys, J. (1972). Asthma due to inhaled wood dusts, western red cedar and iroko. *Clin. Allergy*, **2**, 213

32. Davies, R. J., Hendrick, D. F. and Pepys, J. (1974). Asthma due to inhaled chemical agents: ampicillin, benzyl penicillin and 6-amino penicillanic acid and related substrates. *Clin. Allergy*, **4**, 227

33. Pickering, C. A. C. (1972). Inhalation tests with chemical allergens, complex salts of platinum. *Proc. R. Soc. Med.*, **65**, 272

34. Karr, R. M., Davies, R. J., Butcher, B. T., Lehrer, S. B., Wilson, M. R. Dharmarajan, V. and Salvaggio, J. E. (1978). Occupational asthma. *J. Allergy Clin. Immunol.*, **61**, 54

35. Fawcett, I. W., Newman-Taylor, A. J. and Pepys, J. (1971). Asthma due to inhaled chemical agents – epoxy resin systems containing phthalic anhydride, trimellitic anhydride and triethylene tetramine. *Clin. Allergy*, **7**, 1

36. Haydu, S. P., Empey, D. and Hughes, D. T. D. (1974). Inhalation challenge tests in asthma: an assessment of spirometry, maximum expiratory flow rates and plethysmography in measuring the responses. *Clin. Allergy*. **4**. 371

37. Chan-Yeung, M. (1973). Maximal expiratory flow and airway resistance during induced bronchoconstriction in patients with asthma due to western red cedar (*Thuja plicata*). *Am. Rev. Resp. Dis.*, **108**, 1103

38. Fish, J. E. and Kelly, J. F. (1979). Measurements of responsiveness in broncho provocation testing. *J. Allergy Clin. Immunol.*, **64**, 592

39. Newman-Taylor, A. J., Davies, R. J., Hendrick, D. J. and Pepys, J. (1979). Recurrent nocturnal asthmatic reactions to bronchial provocation tests. *Clin. Allergy*, **9**, 213

40. Benson, M. K. (1978). Bronchial responsiveness of inhaled histamine and isoprenaline in patients with airway obstruction. *Thorax*, **33**, 211

41. Cockcroft, D. W., Ruffin, R. E., Dolovich, J. and Hargreave, F. E. (1977). Allergen-induced increase in non-allergic bronchial reactivity. *Clin. Allergy*, **7**, 503

42. Rosenthal, R. R., Norman, P. S., Summer, W. R. and Permutt, E. S. Role of the parasympathetic system in antigen induced bronchospasm. *J. Appl. Physiol.*, **42**, 600

3
Diagnostic Tests

PART IV:
Laboratory Techniques in Immediate Hypersensitivity

T. A. E. PLATTS-MILLS

INTRODUCTION

Prior to 1921 direct skin testing with allergens was the only test that was available for diagnosing immediate hypersensitivity. When passive transfer testing was introduced by Prausnitz and Küstner (P–K testing) this test was widely used to confirm the presence of reagins in sera from allergic persons[1]. Subsequently it became clear that these sera also contained heat stable non-reaginic antibodies which could inhibit P–K testing[2,3]. Modern laboratory techniques relevant to immediate hypersensitivity are largely directed to the measurement of reagins and 'blocking' antibodies. Since it became clear that skin-sensitizing activity in the P–K test is mediated exclusively by IgE antibodies, *in vitro* measurements of IgE antibodies have replaced P–K testing[4,5]. In addition, it became clear that measurements of total serum IgE could give considerable diagnostic help in immediate hypersensitivity[6]. The first *in vitro* technique for measuring 'blocking' antibodies was inhibition of antigen-induced histamine release from peripheral blood leukocytes[7]. However, it has become clear that 'blocking' activity in serum is attributable to IgG antibodies[8] while blocking activity in nasal secretions is attributable to both IgG and IgA antibodies[9]. Thus *in vitro* techniques for measuring class-specific antibodies have largely replaced methods for assessing inhibition of histamine release. Finally, techniques used for assessing or standardizing allergen preparations will be briefly considered because the quality of allergen extracts is essential for all methods of detecting specific sensitivity either *in vivo* or *in vitro*. The following discussion is not a laboratory manual but is designed to outline some of the procedures which are in use and to indicate some of the problems. In addition, those techniques which may be of routine diagnostic use will be distinguished from those which are research techniques.

TECHNIQUES FOR MEASURING TOTAL SERUM IgE

Measurement of total serum IgE has become a routine clinical test. Results for total IgE are expressed in international units defined by WHO standard sera. In general, all assays should use a local serum substandardized from the WHO standard. The unit of IgE is considered to represent 2.4 ng IgE[10]. Total IgE levels are generally less than 5 units at birth and rise over 10 years[11].

While it is clear that normal ranges are essential for IgE levels this is not a simple matter. Since up to 15% of the population will develop inhalant allergy, any normal range should specify whether allergic (or skin test positive) patients were excluded[12, 13]. The relationship between total IgE and allergy is not very close, and many highly allergic patients have total IgE < 100 units/ml, while some individuals with total > 3000 units/ml have no allergic symptoms. On the other hand the finding of high (> 500 units) or low (< 50 units) serum IgE may be clinically useful in many different situations. Certainly in any report on allergic patients measurement of total serum IgE is an essential part of defining the patient group.

Double antibody inhibition radioimmunoassay (RIA)

The RIA for IgE in serum is a direct modification of the assays used routinely for measuring hormone levels[14, 15]. The technique was developed by Gleich *et al.*[6] and has become the reference technique for measuring IgE levels (Figure 3.IV.1A). The main advantage of the assay is that inhibition occurs in the fluid phase and therefore the chances of non-specific inhibition are minimized. The RIA for IgE has proved very suitable for measuring IgE in secretions[16, 17]. In addition, the RIA has been modified[16] so that it is capable of measuring down to 0.1 ng of IgE/ml. For laboratories experienced with RIA the assay is not difficult, and requires only very small quantities of pure IgE and monospecific rabbit anti-IgE.

Radioimmunosorbent technique (RIST)

RIST is a solid phase competitive technique which was the first commercially available assay for IgE levels[18] (Figure 3.IV.1B). The competition occurs for anti-IgE on the surface of particles of sepharose or bromacetylcellulose. Unfortunately minor degrees of inhibition can occur with a variety of abnormal sera or secretions and this non-specific inhibition has given rise to erroneous results. Indeed it now appears likely that RIST is not accurate below 100 units/ml[19, 20]. A particularly glaring example of non-specific inhibition was the apparent presence of high levels of IgE in human breast milk[21]. However, erroneous results have also been obtained showing high levels of IgE in patients with cancer when the levels were normal. The RIST technique also showed apparently normal levels of IgE in sera from patients with common variable hypogammaglobulinaemia[22], when the levels are in fact very low by RIA, by paper RIST, or as detected by skin testing with anti-IgE[12, 23]. Thus although RIST may distinguish between low and high IgE levels it becomes totally inaccurate below 50 units/ml and is not applicable to measurements of IgE in secretions.

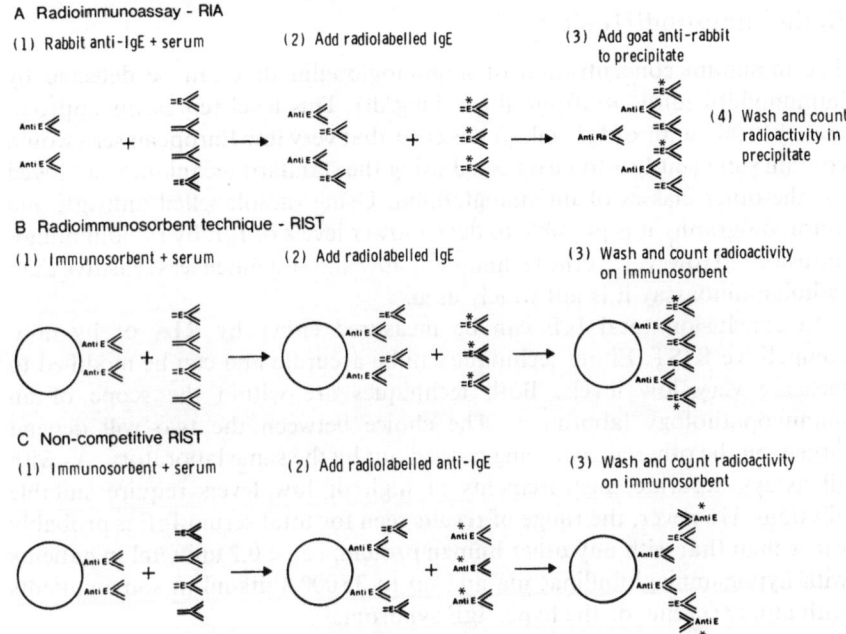

Figure 3.IV.1 Techniques for measuring total serum IgE

Non-competitive RIST

This modification of the RIST avoids many of the problems because it does not depend on inhibition (Figure 3.IV.1C). Although this technique is often called paper RIST or PRIST, essentially the same particle linked to anti-IgE can be used and is reacted with unknown or standard IgE in the same way[24]. However, the final stage of the assay uses radiolabelled rabbit anti-IgE instead of IgE. The important difference is that if 20% of the anti-IgE on the particle is blocked non-specifically (e.g. by mucus) it will not affect results. Furthermore, using the non-competitive RIST the radioactive counts are directly related to the IgE present. This makes the technique more sensitive at low levels. Correspondingly, the non-competitive RIST can be modified to measure very low levels of IgE (down to 1.0 ng/ml). The non-competitive RIST is applicable to nasal secretions[25]. However, because the technique involves a solid phase there is always the possibility of non-specific binding that could interfere with the results, so that results under new conditions should be related to the results of RIA. At a practical level the advantages of the non-competitive RIST are that the same radiolabelled anti-IgE can be used for the radioallergosorbent test (RAST). In addition the technique is relatively easy on reagents and does not require a second antibody.

Radioimmunodiffusion

The minimum concentration of immunoglobulin that can be detected by immunodiffusion is $\simeq 10\,\mu g/ml$ (or $1\,mg/dl$). This level represents approximately 10 000 units of IgE/ml, so it is clear that very few European sera would contain sufficient IgE to be detected using the standard techniques employed for the other classes of immunoglobulin. Using radiolabelled anti-IgE and autoradiography it is possible to detect lower levels of IgE by radioimmuno-diffusion[26]. However, as the technique is slow and still much less sensitive than radioimmunoassay it is not widely used.

In conclusion total IgE can be measured either by RIA or by non-competitive RIST. Either technique can be accurate and can be modified to measure very low levels. Both techniques are within the scope of an immunopathology laboratory. The choice between the two will depend largely on the other assays being carried out by the same laboratory. As with all assays accurate measurements of high or low levels require suitable dilutions. However, the range of results seen for total serum IgE is probably wider than that with any other human protein, i.e. < 0.2 units/ml in patients with hypogammaglobulinaemia and up to 35 000 units/ml in some patients with atopic eczema or the hyper-IgE syndrome[27].

TECHNIQUES FOR MEASURING SPECIFIC IgE AND IgG ANTIBODIES

The original work on IgE demonstrated that IgE antibodies could bind radiolabelled allergens either on immunodiffusion plates or in the fluid phase[4]. Although radioimmunoelectrophoresis is a very reliable technique for demonstrating the presence of IgE antibodies[28], it proved very difficult to establish a quantitative technique for measuring IgE binding activity with the allergen 'free'[29]. In 1968 Wide et al. introduced the radioallergosorbent technique where the allergen is bound to a particle[5]. This technique has been used very extensively both for research and as an adjunct to clinical diagnosis. In some parts of the world RAST has replaced skin testing as the primary method for diagnosing allergic diseases. However, there is no evidence that any in vitro technique is superior to skin testing. Although RAST results may correlate quite well with skin tests they are generally less sensitive[30]. Indeed, the in vitro techniques are less sensitive than P–K testing[31]. Although P–K testing or passive sensitization of basophils *in vitro* is not simple[32], it should still be regarded as the final arbiter of IgE antibodies, since these techniques demonstrate the biological activity as well as the ability to bind allergens.

Recently antigen binding assays for IgE antibodies have been modified by using IgE myeloma serum as a source of carrier protein[31,33-35]. Antigen binding techniques generally require large quantities of monospecific antisera and purified allergens, so that it is most unlikely that these assays will become routine. None the less they appear to have major advantages over RAST for a variety of research purposes.

The radioallergosorbent technique (RAST)

RAST is very simple to carry out and is not very demanding on reagents (Figure 3.IV.2). The allergen on the discs need not be purified and although the anti-IgE used for radiolabelling should be specifically purified only very small quantities are required. On the other hand, the quality of RAST

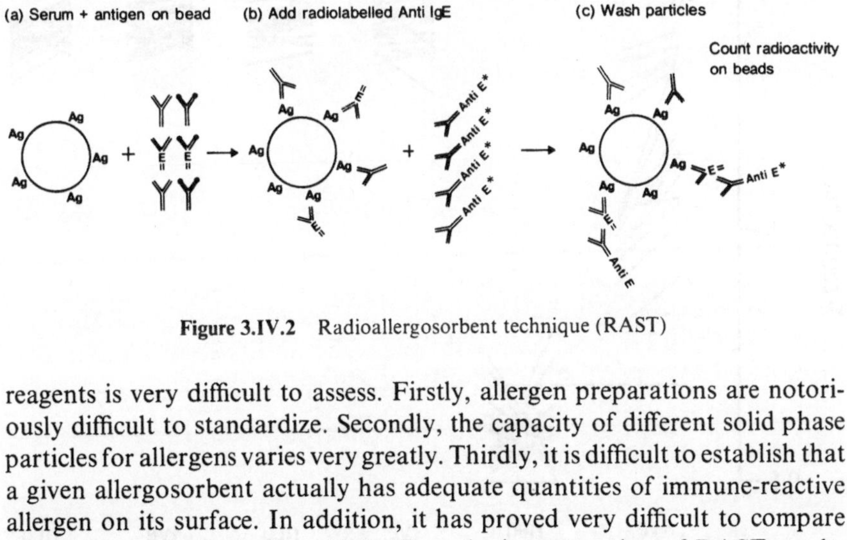

Figure 3.IV.2 Radioallergosorbent technique (RAST)

reagents is very difficult to assess. Firstly, allergen preparations are notoriously difficult to standardize. Secondly, the capacity of different solid phase particles for allergens varies very greatly. Thirdly, it is difficult to establish that a given allergosorbent actually has adequate quantities of immune-reactive allergen on its surface. In addition, it has proved very difficult to compare different preparations of anti-IgE. Thus the interpretation of RAST results depends on how carefully the assay is carried out, and it is impossible to assess results without knowing the details of the assay and the actual binding levels observed. Because RAST is so widely used some of the problems will be discussed in detail.

Negative background in RAST

The negative background for RAST is dependent on the quantity of human IgE that binds non-specifically to the beads. This non-specific binding is directly related to the total serum IgE so that with sera containing greater than 1000 units total IgE/ml the background will rise slightly and with sera above 5000 units/ml the increasing background may well become a serious problem. However, the problem of negative background is more difficult because it will vary from one sorbent to another and also from one allergen to another[36]. Thus the negative background for each allergosorbent preparation should be known. This background problem becomes very severe when interpreting RAST results on sera from patients with atopic eczema. Many of these sera are reported to have a weakly positive RAST for food allergens, but the total IgE levels may be very high[36]. In applying RAST to fluids other than serum the background variations also have to be considered. It has been suggested that apparent positive RAST results in nasal secretions reflected higher levels of total IgE in the secretions[37]. If background binding on RAST beads represents a percentage of the total immunoglobulin present, it is not surprising that

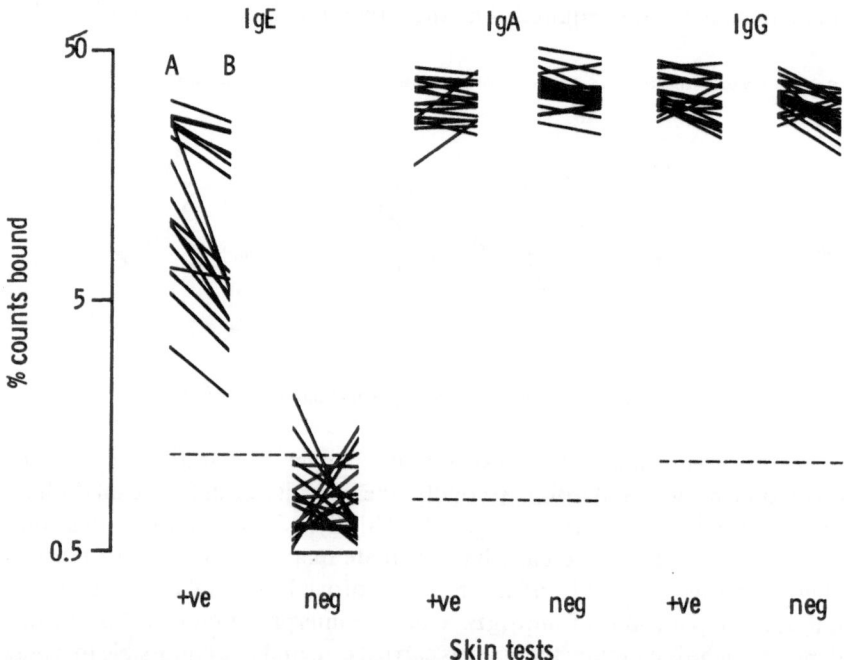

Figure 3.IV.3   The results for RAST assay for IgE, IgA and IgG antibodies to *Dermatophagoides pteronyssinus*. Sera from 17 skin test positive and 17 skin test negative individuals were assayed at two dilutions 1/6 (A) and 1/12 (B). *D. pteronyssinus* extract was linked to cyanogen-bromide-activated cellulose discs; after incubation with serum the discs were incubated with ^{125}I-labelled anti-IgE, anti-IgA or anti-IgG. Only for IgE was there a consistent relationship between the two dilutions of allergic sera and only for IgE was the negative serum background low enough for the assay to be useful. Comparable results using an antigen binding assay show clear differences for each class[35]. The background binding using bovine serum albumin instead of human serum is also shown (– – – – –)

other classes of immunoglobulin usually give very high background binding[38] (Figure 3.IV.3). Indeed, in most laboratories it has not proved possible to adapt RAST directly for other classes of immunoglobulins.

Inhibition of RAST by IgG antibodies

Sera from allergic patients who have not received desensitizing injections generally contain detectable but low levels of IgG antibody. Most of these sera will contain between two and six times more IgG binding activity for an allergen than IgE binding activity[31]. However, following desensitizing injections the IgG antibody in serum selectively rises so that it may be 50 times higher than IgE antibody[17,35,39]. Under these circumstances an apparent fall in RAST result may occur which is in fact due to IgG antibodies blocking allergen on the discs[33,40]. This problem can usually be overcome by diluting the sera[41]. However, with some sera dilution is not possible because the IgE antibody levels are too low. It is obvious that the degree of inhibition caused by IgG antibody will depend on whether the allergen on the sorbent is in excess. Using sepharose or microfine cellulose beads, the allergen is often present in large excess. However, with cellulose discs the quantity of allergen may only be sufficient to bind a proportion of antibodies[40]. Under these circumstances any increase in the ratio of IgG antibody:IgE antibody would inhibit IgE binding.

Ideally RAST is carried out using a high capacity sorbent and high quality or purified allergen, under conditions where all the specific antibody in a sample will be absorbed. Using at least two dilutions of each serum sample and referring the results to a standard curve for the same allergen, it is possible to give accurate quantitative results. In addition the background activity is measured using negative sera with a range of total IgE levels, so that a clear distinction between positive and negative results can be made.

At the other extreme RAST is often carried out using low capacity discs linked to a poor extract. The sera are assayed at one dilution without knowing total IgE levels or the background for the allergen being used. In addition the results for many different allergens are related to a single standard and expressed as percentage counts bound. Under these circumstances all the weakly positive and negative results become confused, while no effective distinction is obtained between positive and strongly positive sera. Thus RAST can easily be reduced to a method which does little more than identify strongly positive sera.

Antigen binding radioimmunoassay (or radioimmunoprecipitation)

Serum from patients with inhalant allergies does not contain precipitins against allergens. In order to measure non-IgE antibodies their ability to bind allergens has to be assessed. This can be done by determining their ability to 'block' P–K or direct skin tests *in vivo*[2,3], or histamine release *in vitro*[7]. However, binding activity can be assessed more easily by using radiolabelled allergens. Initially, ammonium sulphate was used to precipitate the globulin fraction of sera[42]. Subsequently it became clear that different classes could be precipitated using class-specific antisera[43,44], not only for IgG and IgA but also for IgE[31,33–35]. Antigen binding techniques can be modified to give estimates of total antigen binding activity. However, full saturation requires very high concentrations of antigens, e.g. 100 µg/ml[43]. Using 1 µg of antigen E

Serum sample

+

Allergen * (Radiolabelled with ^{125} Iodine)

+

Carrier Protein if necessary (e. g. IgE myeloma serum)

- 4 hours -

Goat anti-IgG (or anti-IgA or anti-IgE)

- Overnight to precipitate -

Wash, precipitate and count Radioactivity

Counts directly related to the quantity of specific IgG (or IgA or IgE) antibody in the serum.

Figure 3.IV.4   Antigen binding radioimmunoassay

per assay Yunginger and Gleich measured serum IgG antibodies in the sera of patients who had been treated with desensitizing injections[45]. In order to detect the levels of IgG antibody found in the serum of untreated patients or in nasal secretions much lower quantities of radiolabelled allergen have been used[9,31,41]. The problem is that the negative background in antigen binding assays is directly related to the quantity of allergen added[31]. Thus antigen binding assays generally represent a compromise between sensitivity (i.e. low allergen concentrations) and full saturation of all antibodies. However, it has been shown by several groups that the avidity of different classes of antiallergen antibodies is comparable[31,33]. Thus by using low concentrations of allergen the relationship between different classes is accurately reflected. In addition *in vivo* exposure to allergens is probably at very low concentrations (< 10 ng/ml), so antibodies measured in the presence of low concentrations may reflect the biologically relevant antibodies.

A simple outline of an antigen binding assay is shown in Figure 3.IV.4. For measuring IgE antibodies the assay requires large quantities of anti-IgE and IgE myeloma serum. In addition, only purified (or partially purified) allergens can be radiolabelled satisfactorily. Despite these disadvantages, there are considerable advantages in an assay which can measure IgG, IgA and IgE antibodies in parallel and which is equally applicable to secretions or serum. There are several ways in which antigen binding assays for IgE antibodies have direct advantages over RAST. Firstly, the quantity of IgE in the serum sample does not alter the background. This is particularly important for measuring IgE antibodies in sera from patients with atopic eczema[46]. Secondly, these assays require very little purified allergen; thus an antigen binding assay may be the easiest way to measure IgE antibodies against a purified allergen which is only available in small quantities (e.g. the minor ragweed allergen Ra3)[47].

The main application for antigen binding assays has been to measure the production of IgG antibodies following desensitizing injections[17, 41, 45, 48, 49]. It is possible that these assays will become part of the routine assessment of desensitization for bee venom allergy[50]. For inhalant allergies it is not clear that serum IgG or blocking antibodies have any direct relationship to clinical improvement. Some studies have found a relationship between blocking antibodies and response[51, 52] but generally the relationship has been poor or non-existent. Even measuring IgG and IgE antibodies in parallel it has not been possible to relate clinical improvement to any aspect of serum antibody levels[39, 48]. At present it seems very unlikely that routine measurements of IgG antibody to inhalant allergens would give useful clinical information.

Solid phase techniques for measuring IgG antibodies

Direct modification of RAST to classes other than IgE has proved very difficult, primarily because RAST background for each class represents a percentage of the total immunoglobulin present. Since IgG and IgA antibodies to allergens rarely represent more than 0.2% of the total IgG or IgA, any background binding over 0.1% will make the RAST assay useless. This problem is illustrated in Figure 3.IV.3, which shows the results of IgG, IgA and IgE RAST, using a *Dermatophagoides pteronyssinus* allergosorbent. Only for the IgE RAST is there a significant difference between allergic sera and the negative sera. This is because the percentage of anti-IgA or anti-IgG counts bound with negative sera is too high. The control without serum is very low for all three classes, i.e. $< 0.1\%$ counts bound.

Alternative modifications of solid phase techniques have used immunosorbent to bind IgG or IgA followed by fluid phase radiolabelled allergen. The binding of IgG can be achieved by using Staph A coated sepharose, while

IgA can be bound using anti-IgA or sepharose[25]. These techniques can be very simple to carry out. However, it is difficult to know what proportion of the IgG or IgA is bound to the discs, and to exclude non-specific binding of other classes. In addition because each of these solid phase techniques is different and uses a different radiolabel it is not possible to directly relate results for different classes. More recently Delespesse *et al.* have introduced the idea of using radiolabelled Staph A to replace anti-IgG in the IgG RAST[53]. This technique clearly has some of the problems of IgG RAST. However, the reagents and technique are so simple that it may prove to have a role in measuring the IgG antibody response following desensitizing injections. The problems of a solid phase technique for IgG antibodies have clearly not yet been resolved. However, the practical advantages are very great and further modifications may produce an assay that is sufficiently simple to be of clinical use.

Conclusions concerning antibody measurements

For routine diagnostic use, skin tests are the first choice, while RAST has a limited role where skin testing is difficult or undesirable. For research purposes RAST can give accurate and sensitive measurements of IgE antibody, but the technique is often abused. For measurements of IgG antibody, antigen binding techniques are preferred. For comparing different classes or for measurements on secretions, antigen binding assays for IgG, IgA and IgE antibodies are the most satisfactory techniques.

ALLERGEN STANDARDIZATION

Allergen extracts depend entirely on the quality of the allergen source used to prepare them. In assessing an allergen extract it has been traditional to measure protein nitrogen content (or PNU) (1 PNU = 0.01 μg protein N). Using 'good' preparations of allergen and a short duration of aqueous extraction, PNU may well give a reasonable guide to the 'allergenic' activity of an extract. However, using special techniques designed to increase protein extraction, PNU may bear very little relationship to allergen content[54]. Largely because of these discrepancies there has been an increasing demand to standardize allergen extracts on the basis of their allergenic activity. When a 'major' allergen is available in purified form, it seems logical to use assays of this protein to standardize extracts. This procedure has already been adopted for standardization of ragweed pollen extracts (using antigen E content[54]), for grass pollen extracts (using Rye I)[55], and for bee venom (using phospholipase A content). However, for the majority of allergens no purified protein is available. Clearly, skin testing a large group of allergic persons is the most convincing way of establishing the quality/strength of an allergen extract. This technique has been recommended by some authorities[56]. The problem with skin testing is firstly that it represents a large amount of work and secondly that it is very difficult to compare a group of patients from one country to another. In addition, for some allergens it would be very difficult to find a suitable group of patients. It might of course be argued that if patients are difficult to find, the reagent need not remain available. In this respect it seems worth distinguishing between diagnostic extracts and desensitizing extracts. Desensitizing injections carry far greater hazards than prick testing. Furthermore, the diagnostic value of skin testing is obvious for many allergies in which there is no evidence that desensitization is beneficial. Thus there is a good case for insisting that desensitizing extracts should be standardized and probably that the number of extracts available should be reduced. On the other hand, some of the reasons for demanding that desensitizing extracts should be controlled do not apply to diagnostic extracts.

In vitro techniques for standardization

A variety of techniques have been suggested to standardize allergen extracts in vitro, where the major allergen has not been purified. These include RAST inhibition, direct RAST and crossed radioimmunoelectrophoresis (CRIE). RAST inhibition is carried out by incubating allergosorbent beads with a standard human serum pool in the presence of serial dilutions of allergen extract. The allergen extract is in effect being compared with the allergen extract on the RAST bead[57]. RAST inhibition is a simple technique which certainly offers a satisfactory way for an individual laboratory to maintain the consistency of the allergen extracts they produce[58].

Crossed radioimmunoelectrophoresis (CRIE) is a beautiful technique which allows direct identification of multiple proteins in an extract (by the Laurell technique) followed by an autoradiographic demonstration of which proteins bind IgE antibodies[59]. CRIE may well represent the best way of assessing allergen extracts in a technically excellent central laboratory, as has been established in Denmark. However, for general purposes CRIE may well be too difficult to carry out and interpret. This would certainly be so if standardization is to depend primarily on the individual companies that produce allergen extracts. There might thus be a case for moving allergen standardization into the hands of a central laboratory and also for encouraging a reduction in the number of companies producing allergen extracts.

Analytical isoelectric focusing has been proposed as a method of assessing allergen extracts. However, the technique gives no evidence whether the individual bands seen have allergenic activity. Furthermore, many allergens, particularly *Cladosporium*[60] and *Dermatophagoides pteronyssinus*[61], have multiple isoallergens (see also reference 62). These isoallergens are antigenically and allergenically identical but have different isoelectric points. Thus different allergen extracts may have a different distribution of isoallergens while having very similar allergen content. At present it seems unlikely that analytical isoelectric focusing represents a useful technique in assessing allergen extracts.

An interesting feature of the techniques for assessing allergen extracts is that, in general, they would give no indication about the presence of contaminating allergens. Most reagents or pharmaceutical products are standardized by their quantity of active material and also their contamination with other substances. Indeed, since allergen extracts include multiple proteins it would be extremely difficult to exclude contamination with other allergens. This aspect of allergen quality will continue to depend on the quality of material used for making extracts. Any realistic view of allergen standardization would suggest that standardizing a large number of allergen extracts would nevertheless be very difficult. On the other hand the important allergens could, and indeed must, be standardized in the future, using some combination of skin tests, PNU, RAST inhibition and assays of major allergen content.

References

1. Coca, A. F. and Grove, E. F. (1925). Studies on hypersensitiveness. XIII. A study of the atopic reagins. *J. Immunol.*, **10**, 445
2. Cooke, R., Barnard, J., Hebald, S. and Stull, A. (1935). Serological evidence on immunity with co-existing sensitization in a type of human allergy, hay fever. *J. Exp. Med.*, **62**, 733
3. Loveless, M. H. (1940). Immunological studies of pollinosis. I. The presence of two antibodies related to the same pollen-antigen in the serum of treated hay fever patients. *J. Immunol.*, **38**, 1925
4. Ishizaka, K., Ishizaka, T. and Hornbrook, M. M. (1967). Allergen binding activity of γE, γG and γA, antibodies in sera from atopic patients: *in vitro* measurements of reaginic antibody. *J. Immunol.*, **98**, 490
5. Wide, L., Bennich, H. and Johansson, S. G. O. (1967). Diagnosis of allergy by an *in vitro* test for allergen antibodies. *Lancet*, **2**, 1105
6. Gleich, G. J., Averback, A. K. and Svedlund, H. A. (1971). Measurement of IgE in normal and allergic serum by radioimmunoassay. *J. Lab. Clin. Med.*, **77**, 690
7. Lichtenstein, L. M., Norman, P. S., Osler, A. G. and Winkenwerder, W. L. (1966). *In vitro* studies of human ragweed allergy: changes in cellular and humoral activity associated with specific desensitization. *J. Clin. Invest.*, **45**, 1126
8. Lichtenstein, L. M., Holtzman, N. A. and Burnett, L. S. (1968). A quantitative *in vitro* study of the chromatographic distribution and immunoglobulin characteristics of human blocking antibody. *J. Immunol.*, **101**, 317
9. Platts-Mills, T. A. E., von Maur, R. K., Ishizaka, K., Norman, P. S. and Lichtenstein, L. M. (1976). IgA and IgG anti-ragweed antibodies in nasal secretions. Quantitative measurements of antibodies and correlation with inhibition of histamine release. *J. Clin. Invest.*, **57**, 1041
10. Bazarel, M. G. and Hamburger, R. H. (1972). Standardization and stability of immunoglobulin E. *J. Allergy Clin. Immunol.*, **49**, 189
11. Orgel, H. A., Hamburger, R. N., Bazaral, M., Gorrin, H., Groshong, T., Lenoir, M., Miller, J. R. and Wallace, W. W. (1975). Development of IgE and allergy in infancy. *J. Allergy and Clin. Immunol.*, **56**, 296

12. Waldman, T. A., Strober, W., Polmar, S. M. and Terry, W. D. (1972). IgE levels and metabolism in immune deficiency diseases. In Ishizaka, K. and Drayton, D. H. (eds.) *The Biological Role of the Immunoglobulin E Systems*, pp. 247–258. (Washington D.C.: USPHS)

13. Nye, L., Merrett, T. G., Landon, J. and White, R. J. (1975). A detailed investigation of circulating IgE in a normal population. *Clin. Allergy*, **5**, 13

14. Addison, G. M. and Hales, C. N. (1975). Radioactive immunoassay. In *Clinical Aspects of Immunology*, 3rd Edn. (Oxford: Blackwell)

15. Tomioka, H. and Ishizaka, K. (1971). Mechanisms of passive sensitization II. Presence of receptors for IgE on monkey mast cells. *J. Immunol.*, **107**, 971

16. Nakajima, S., Gillespie, D. N. and Gleich, G. J. (1975). Differences between IgA and IgE as secretory proteins. *Clin. Exp. Immunol.*, **21**, 306

17. Platts-Mills, T. A. E. (1979). Local production of IgG, IgA and IgE antibodies in grass pollen hay fever. *J. Immunol.*, **122**, 2218

18. Wide, L. (1971). Solid-phase antigen–antibody systems. In Kirkham, K. E. and Hunter, W. M. (eds.) *Radioimmunoassay Methods*, pp. 405–412. (Edinburgh: E. and S. Livingstone)

19. Polmar, S. H., Waldmann, T. A. and Terry, W. D. (1973). A comparison of three radioimmunoassay techniques for the measurement of serum IgE. *J. Immunol.*, **110**, 1253

20. Johansson, S. G. O., Bergland, A. and Kjellman, N. I. M. (1976). Comparison of IgE values as determined by different solid phase radioimmunoassay methods. *Clin. Allergy*, **6**, 91

21. Underdown, B. J., Knight, A. and Papsin, F. R. (1976). The relative paucity of IgE in human milk. *J. Immunol.*, **116**, 1435

22. McLaughlan, P., Stanworth, D. R., Webster, A. D. B. and Asherson, G. L. (1974). Serum IgE in immunodeficiency disorders. *Clin. Exp. Immunol.*, **16**, 375

23. Stites, D. P., Ishizaka, K. and Fudenberg, H. H. (1971). Serum IgE levels in patients and family members with various immune deficiency states. *Clin. Res.*, **19**, 452

24. Ceska, M. and Lundquist, U. (1972). A new and simple radioimmunoassay method for the determination of IgE. *Immunochemistry*, **9**, 1021

25. Johansson, S. G. O., Deuschl, H. and Zetterström, O. (1979). Use of glutaraldehyde-modified Timothy grass pollen extract in nasal hyposensitization treatment of hay fever. *Int. Arch. Allergy Appl. Immunol.*, **60**, 447

26. Rowe, D. S. (1971). Measurements of concentrations of human serum immunoglobulins. *Clin. Exp. Immunol.*, **9**, 695

27. Buckley, R. H., Wray, B. B. and Belmaker, E. Z. (1972). Hyperimmunoglobulinemia E and undue susceptibility to infection. *Pediatrics*, **49**, 59

28. Tse, K. S., Wicher, K. and Arbesman, C. E. (1973). Effect of immunotherapy on the appearance of antibodies to ragweed in external secretions. *J. Allergy Clin. Immunol.*, **51**, 208

29. Zeiss, C. R., Pruzansky, J. J., Patterson, R. and Roberts, M. (1973). A solid phase radioimmunoassay for the quantitation of human reaginic antibody against ragweed antigen E. *J. Immunol.*, **110**, 414

30. Norman, P. S., Lichtenstein, L. M. and Ishizaka, K. (1973). Diagnostic tests in ragweed hay fever. *J. Allergy Clin. Immunol.*, **52**, 210

31. Platts-Mills, T. A. E., Snajdr, M. J., Ishizaka, K. and Frankland, A. W. (1978). Measurement of IgE antibody by an antigen binding assay: correlation with PK activity and IgG and IgA antibodies to allergens. *J. Immunol.*, **120**, 1201

32. Levy, D. A. and Osler, A. G. (1966). Studies on the mechanisms of hypersensitivity phenomena. XIV. Passive sensitization *in vitro* of human leukocytes to ragweed pollen antigen. *J. Immunol.*, **97**, 203

33. Pauli, B., Jacob, G. L., Yunginger, J. W. and Gleich, G. J. (1978). Comparison of binding of IgE and IgG antibodies to honey bee venom phospholipase-A. *J. Immunol.*, **120**, 1917

34. Zeiss, C. R., Pruzansky, J. J., Levitz, D. and Wang, J. (1978). The quantitation of IgE antibody specific for ragweed antigen E (AgE) from the basophil surface in patients with ragweed pollenosis. *Immunology*, **35**, 237

35. Chapman, M. D. and Platts-Mills, T. A. E. (1978). Measurement of IgG, IgA and IgE antibodies to *Dermatophagoides pteronyssinus* by antigen-binding assay, using a partially purified fraction of mite extract (F_4P_1). *Clin. Exp. Immunol.*, **34**, 126

36. Aas, K. (1978). The diagnosis of hypersensitivity to ingested foods: Reliability of skin prick testing and the radioallergosorbent test with different materials. *Clin. Allergy*, **8**, 39

37. Mygind, N. and Weeke, B. (1975). Local IgE antibodies in nasal secretions. *Lancet*, **2**, 502

38. Soothill, J. F. (1976). Some intrinsic and extrinsic factors predisposing to allergy. *Proc. R. Soc. Med.*, **69**, 439

39. Chapman, M. D., Platts-Mills, T. A. E., Gabriel, M., Ng, H. K., Allan, W. G. L., Hill, L. E. and Nunn, A. J. (1980). The antibody response following prolonged hyposensitization with *D. pteronyssinus* extract. *Int. Arch. Allergy Appl. Immunol.*, **61**, 431

40. Lynch, N. R., Durand, P., Newcomb, R. W., Chai, H. and Bigley, J. (1975). Influence of IgG antibody and glycopeptide allergens on the correlation between the radioallergosorbent test (RAST) and skin testing or bronchial challenge with *Alternaria*. *Clin. Exp. Immunol.*, **22**, 35

41. Lichtenstein, L. M., Ishizaka, K., Norman, P. S., Sobotka, A. K. and Hill, B. M. (1973). IgE measurements in ragweed hay fever. Relationship to clinical severity and the results of immunotherapy. *J. Clin. Invest.*, **52**, 472

42. Farr, R. S. (1958). A quantitative immunochemical measure of the primary interaction between I* BSA and antibody. *J. Infect. Dis.*, **103**, 239

43. Osler, A. G., Mulligan, J. J. and Rodriguez, E. (1966). Weight estimates of rabbit anti-human serum albumin based on antigen-binding and precipitin analyses: specific haemagglutinating activities of 7S and 19S components. *J. Immunol.*, **96**, 334

44. Newcomb, R. W., Ishizaka, K. and de Vald, B. L. (1969). Human IgG and IgA diphtheria antitoxins in serum, nasal fluids and saliva. *J. Immunol.*, **103**, 215

45. Yunginger, J. W. and Gleich, G. J. (1973). Seasonal changes in IgE antibodies and their relationship to IgG antibodies during immunotherapy for ragweed hay fever. *J. Clin. Invest.*, **52**. 1268

46. Chapman, M. D., Platts-Mills, T. A. E., Fuenmajor, M. and Champion, R. H. (1980). IgE antibodies to inhalant allergens in patients with atopic eczema: measurement by antigen binding assay. (Manuscript in preparation)

47. Platts-Mills, T. A. E., Chapman, M. D. and Marsh, D. G. (1980). Human IgE and IgG antibody responses to the 'minor' ragweed allergen Ra3: correlation with skin tests and comparison with other allergens. (Manuscript in preparation)

48. Gleich, G. J., Jacob, G. L., Yunginger, J. W. and Henderson, L. L. (1977). Measurement of absolute levels of IgE antibodies in patients with ragweed hay fever: effect of immunotherapy on seasonal changes and relationship to IgG antibodies. *J. Allergy Clin. Immunol.*, **60**, 188

49. Sobotka, A. K., Valentine, M. D., Ishizaka, K. and Lichtenstein, L. M. (1976). Measurement of IgG-blocking antibodies: development and application of a radioimmunoassay. *J. Immunol.*, **117**, 84

50. Hunt, K. J., Valentine, M. D., Sobotka, A. K., Benton, A. W., Amodio, F. J. and Lichtenstein, L. M. (1978). A controlled trial of immunotherapy in insect hypersensitivity. *N. Engl. J. Med.*, **249**, 157

51. Lichtenstein, L. M., Norman, P. S. and Winkenwerder, W. L. (1968). Clinical and *in vitro* studies on the role of immunotherapy in ragweed hay fever. *Am. J. Med.*, **44**, 514

52. Starr, M. S. and Weinstock, M. (1970). Studies in pollen allergy. III. The relationship between blocking antibody levels and symptomatic relief following hyposensitization with allpyral in hay fever patients. *Int. Arch. Allergy*, **38**, 514

53. Delespesse, G., Debisschop, M. J. and Flament, J. (1979). Measurement of IgG antibodies to house dust mite and grass pollen by a solid-phase radioimmunoassay. *Clin. Allergy*, **9**, 503

54. Baer, H., Godfrey, H., Maloney, C. J., Norman, P. S. and Lichtenstein, L. M. (1970). The potency and antigen E content of commercially prepared ragweed extracts. *J. Allergy*, **45**, 347

55. Baer, H., Maloney, C. J., Norman, P. S. and Marsh, D. G. (1974). The potency and group I antigen content of six commercially prepared grass pollen extracts. *J. Allergy Clin. Immunol.*, **54**, 157

56. Aas, K. and Belin. L. (1972). Standardization of diagnostic work in allergy. *Acta Allergy (Kbh)*, **27**, 439

57. Tovey, E. and Vandenberg, R. (1979). Mite allergen content in commercial extracts and bed dust determined by radioallergosorbent tests. *Clin. Allergy*, **9**, 253

58. Gleich, G. J., Larson, J. B., Jones, R. T. and Baer, H. (1974). Measurement of the potency of allergen extracts by their inhibitory capacities in the radioallergosorbent test. *J. Allergy Clin. Immunol.*, **53**, 158

59. Lowenstein, H., Marcussen, B. and Weeke, B. (1976). Identification of allergens in extract of horse hair and dandruff by means of crossed radioimmunoelectrophoresis. *Int. Arch. Allergy Appl. Immunol.*, **51**, 38

60. Aukrust, L. (1979). Crossed radioimmunoelectrophoretic studies of distinct allergens in two extracts of *Cladosporium herbarum*. *Int. Arch. Allergy Appl. Immunol.*, **58**, 371

61. Chapman, M. D. and Platts-Mills, T. A. E. (1980). Purification and properties of the major allergen from *Dermatophagoides pteronyssinus*-Antigen P_1. *J. Immunol.* (In press, August 1980)

62. Marsh, D. G. (1975). Allergens and the genetics of allergy. In Sela, M. (ed.) *The Antigens*, Vol. III, pp. 271–359. (New York: Academic Press)

4
Allergy in Infancy and Childhood

PART I:
Genetic Aspects

M. W. TURNER

INTRODUCTION

The heritability of allergic diseases has been recognized for more than a century[1] but the first serious investigation of the subject was that by Cooke and Van der Veer[2] in 1916. In a study of 594 allergic individuals they found 48% with a positive family history compared to only 14% of 76 non-allergic persons. This and later reports[3,4] indicate that between one-half and three-quarters of all allergic patients have a positive family history. A more recent study[5] of 1598 Australian school children aged between 6 and 17 years produced somewhat lower frequencies. When neither parent was affected by allergic illness only 7% of the offspring had developed rhinitis at the time of the investigation; when one parent alone (of either sex) had an allergic history, 15–17% of the children suffered from hay fever and when both parents gave a positive history, 30% of the children were found to have hay fever. These frequencies are clearly lower than other reports but many of the children under study were still very young and could be expected to develop symptoms in due course. Nevertheless, the cumulative genetic effect observed when a bilateral family history is present suggests that genetic factors loom large in the aetiology of allergic illness although the mode of inheritance is certainly complex. The allergic diseases (restricted in this review to the classic triad of allergic rhinitis, asthma and atopic eczema) are not themselves inherited as specific diseases. For example, a parent with hay fever may have a child who will develop infantile eczema but at no stage manifest symptoms of respiratory allergy. Thus the atopic inherits a general predisposition to develop hyper-sensitivity to common environmental antigens but the particular clinical manifestations are determined by other factors which may be genetic or environmental or both. Such a multifactorial pathogenesis for atopy, in which both polygenic and environmental factors are equally important, is now generally accepted.

There is at present no evidence to suggest that different genetic factors operate in childhood atopy as opposed to disease of adult onset and this brief review will draw on illustrative material from both the paediatric and adult age groups. Emphasis will be given to those genetic aspects which have attracted most attention in the last decade, namely the genetic control of serum IgE levels, the association between atopic disease and histocompati-bility (HLA) antigens and the associated question of possible allergen-specific *Ir* genes.

GENETIC CONTROL OF SERUM IgE LEVELS

Unselected population studies

It was clear from the early studies of Johansson *et al.*[6] that the distribution of serum IgE levels (called IgND at that stage) spanned a wide range and was apparently multimodal. This multimodality has been repeatedly confirmed[7, 8, 9] and evidence has been presented for low, intermediate and high groups within the observed distribution[8, 9]. In both of these latter (independent) studies the distribution of IgE levels was claimed to follow the Hardy–Weinberg law describing segregation of two alleles at a single locus. The IgE distribution frequency is heavily skewed towards low levels and a putative allele for low levels would have, it is suggested, a frequency[8, 9] of about 0.75.

Family studies

Other authors have attempted to delineate the mode of inheritance of serum IgE levels by family studies. Gerrard and co-workers[10] determined serum IgE levels in 80 unselected families, dividing the levels at 150 units/ml, into 'low' and 'high' categories for the purpose of analysis. The authors concluded that a genetic effect was apparent and that their results were consistent with the presence of two dominant genes controlling low IgE levels. The absence of one or other such gene would permit high levels of IgE.

Marsh and co-workers[11, 12] have also studied the genetics of total IgE levels in 30 families with at least one member clinically allergic to grass or ragweed pollen allergens. For these analyses a cut-off point of 95 units/ml was selected for separating putative low and high basal IgE phenotypes. This value was selected because only 21% of the non-allergic subjects had IgE levels above and only 22% of allergic subjects had IgE levels below this level. At this point the sum of the percentages of allergic and non-allergic subjects with IgE levels atypical of the respective group was minimized.

The authors believe that their results point to a single Mendelian gene R/r playing a major role in the determination of an individual's IgE level. It is suggested that the 'high IgE phenotype' is inherited as a recessive trait and corresponds to the rr genotype. The 'low IgE phenotype' corresponds to the RR and Rr genotypes and in this respect this theory is different from other hypotheses[9, 13] since here the heterozygote is presumed to have low IgE levels. The gene product of the dominant R allele may, it is suggested, exert its effect in one of the following possible ways. It may regulate the rate of biosynthesis of IgE or the secretion of IgE from plasma cells. It may exert control at the level of T-cell regulation or on the differentiation of B cells into IgE-producing plasma cells. Finally it may act by degrading or binding circulating IgE. While suggesting that this is a major regulatory locus for IgE the authors concede that further alleles, possibly determining very high and very low IgE levels, are also possible. Finally, their studies failed to establish any link between the hypothetical IgE regulator locus and the Gm or HLA systems.

Twin studies

Since environmental factors are a major influence on the serum IgE level, the study of such levels in twins might be expected to be particularly valuable. Bazaral et al.[13] studied IgE levels in middle-aged male monozygous twins (54 pairs) and dizygous twins (39 pairs). As a necessary prerequisite to the main aim of this study the variance in IgE level in a single individual over a period of time was estimated in 23 individuals by taking a second serum sample after an interval of 6.5 to 63 months. The authors found that the mean intrapair variance for the IgE levels of the same individuals at different times was only 3% of the variance of the population from which the sample was drawn. Thus the authors concluded that the short-term fluctuations in the serum IgE level of a single individual relative to the range of population values are sufficiently small to allow analysis of genetic effects on IgE levels. Serum IgE levels in monozygotic twins were very similar and usually not much more different than pairs of levels determined in a single individual at different times. In contrast, levels measured in dizygotic twins were often very different from each other. The genetic effects on basal serum IgE levels were found to be large in children and considerable in adults, thus confirming the suggestion that a significant proportion of the variance of serum IgE is indeed genetic.

ASSOCIATIONS BETWEEN ATOPIC DISEASE AND HLA

The human major histocompatibility complex (or MHC) is commonly known as the HLA (or human leukocyte antigen) system. The complex includes genes which determine serologically defined leukocyte antigens (e.g. HLA-A, -B and -C) and antigens which lead to a thymus-derived lymphocyte response as shown by their ability to stimulate in mixed lymphocyte culture (HLA-D). A series of antigens which are detected serologically appear to be similar if not identical to the D antigens and these are known as DR (D related) antigens. Many investigators believe these to be the human equivalent of the so-called immune associated (Ia) antigens described in the mouse. Work on the MHC of mice, rats and guinea-pigs has revealed the existence of many genes which appear to control specifically immune responses to a variety of antigens. These are known as the *Ir* genes and their existence in the human genome has been widely assumed although formal proof has not been forthcoming.

Following the reported associations between certain antigens in the mouse MHC and susceptibility to leukaemogenic viruses[14] there has been much interest in searching for similar associations in man between possession of certain HLA antigens and susceptibility to various diseases. The literature in this field is by now extensive and even within the narrower context of atopic disease is already considerable. As is often the case with rapidly developing areas of research, many of the early studies which did much to stimulate subsequent interest have themselves been criticized for various deficiencies. In several instances the clinical criteria used to define patients were inadequately described and apparently contradictory results were reported from different centres. With more precise definition of the clinical subgroups encountered under the descriptive umbrella 'atopy' it became clear that many of the associations could themselves be restated more precisely. For example, one of the first published reports was of an association between the HLA haplotype A1, B8 and serious childhood asthma[15]. The same antigens were also found to be increased in a prospective study of infants who had developed reaginic disease (positive skin tests and/or eczema) in the first year of life[16] but the latter appeared to be in sharp contrast with a brief report by Krain and Terasaki[17] that the antigens A3 and A9 were increased in 45 adults with atopic dermatitis. Prompted by these apparent contradictions a study was undertaken in the author's laboratory with the aim of delineating HLA antigen associations with any one of four atopic subgroups[18]. These subgroups were themselves derived from two polar groups of patients. These consisted of, firstly, 40 patients who had presented initially with infantile eczema at a mean age of 7 months. By the time the patients were studied (mean age 8.2 years) 28 had additionally developed asthma and/or hay fever and 12 had suffered only from eczema. The second polar group consisted of 40 patients who had presented with allergic rhinitis and a positive skin test to grass pollen at a mean age of 13.6 years. When these patients were investigated their mean age was 23.7 years and 19 of the 40 had gone on to develop asthma in addition to their hay fever whereas 21 had suffered only from allergic rhinitis. None of these 40, however, had ever suffered from eczema. No significant association of any single HLA antigen was observed with any of the four patient subgroups but the presumed haplotype HLA-A1, B8 was found to be significantly increased in patients with eczema complicated by asthma and/or hay fever and A3, B7 occurred frequently among patients presenting with hay fever and then developing asthma (see Figure 4.I.1). These results support the reports of an

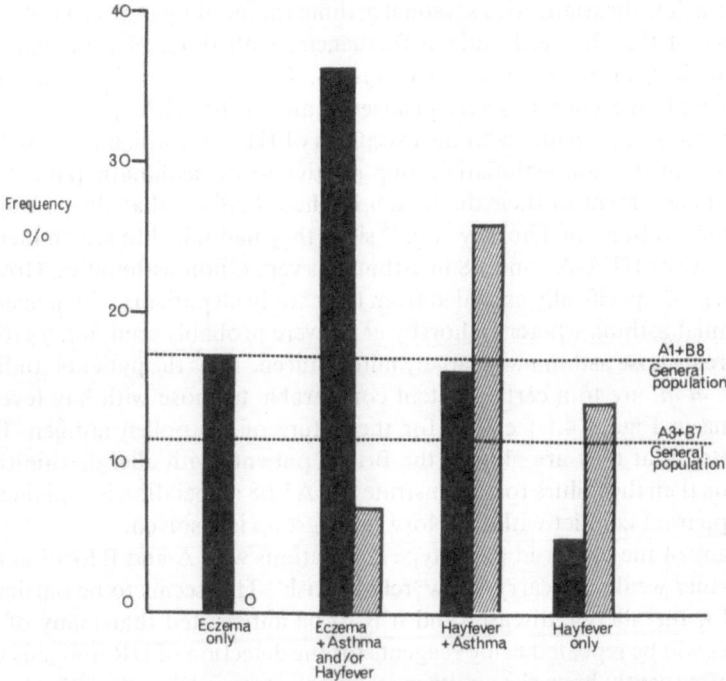

Figure 4.I.1 Frequencies of the HLA antigen combination A1 + B8 (solid columns) and A3 + B7 (hatched columns) in atopic patients classified by clinical manifestations. The general population frequencies for these antigens are indicated by the horizontal lines. (Reproduced from Turner *et al.*[18] with the permission of the publishers)

increase of the presumed haplotype A1, B8 in some series[15,16] and provide a possible explanation of why it was not detected by Krain and Terasaki[17] since it is possible that many of their patients had uncomplicated eczema. Considerable, though not significant, differences in the frequency of A3, B12 and BW35 were observed in this study and each of these antigens has previously been reported to be elevated in atopic dermatitis[17,19]. Again, patient selection may have had an important bearing on the results obtained by different groups.

The haplotype A1, B8 has been associated with many diseases (e.g. coeliac disease[20], dermatitis herpetiformis[21], chronic active hepatitis[22] and myasthenia gravis[23]) and we believe it to be a marker of hyper-reactivity or of a particular type of reactivity of the immune response of an antigen non-specific type. Considerable support for this view comes from Eddleston's observation that higher antibody titres to several antigenically distinct viruses were found in individuals with the presumed haplotype A1, B8 than in those with either A1 or B8 antigens alone[24]. In an independent study of clinically defined allergic subgroups, Bruce et al.[25] tissue-typed a population of 41 North American Caucasians with seasonal asthma (induced by ragweed pollen) and compared the observed antigen frequencies with those of a matched non-asthmatic (but ragweed-sensitive) group. Chi-square analysis showed no significant difference in the frequencies of any of the HLA specificities in the two groups of patients, with the exception of HLA-B5 which appeared to be elevated in the non-asthmatic group relative to the asthmatic patients. The authors comment in their discussion of these findings that their results are contrary to those of Thorsby et al.[15] since they had failed to see an increased incidence of HLA-A1 and B8 in asthmatics versus non-asthmatics. However, Bruce et al. specifically excluded from their study all patients with a history of perennial asthma whereas Thorsby et al. were probably studying a group of children whose asthma was largely mite induced. Thus the patients studied by Bruce et al. are to a certain extent comparable to those with hay fever and asthma in Figure 4.I.1 except for the nature of the pollen antigen. If it is accepted that they are akin to the British patients with allergic rhinitis and asthma then the failure to demonstrate any A1 B8 association is explained and the apparent conflict with the Norwegian group is resolved.

Many of the observed tissue type associations with A and B locus antigens are rather weak and carry a low 'relative risk'. This seems to be particularly true for the allergic diseases and it is to be anticipated that many of these studies will be repeated using reagents for the detection of DR antigens which not infrequently have shown stronger disease associations than the A and B locus antigens. Such results will be awaited with considerable interest but already there is some evidence of such associations in the field of allergy. Rachelefsky et al.[26] have tested B lymphocyte specificities in 30 families with at least one member having extrinsic asthma (presumably either perennial or seasonal). Reagents for the detection of five 'group' antigens were used and 88% of 30 asthma patients were found to have the B lymphocyte Group 2 antigen compared with 24% of 109 control subjects. Such studies require confirmation and further evaluation in terms of clinical subgroups but progress in this area is still relatively slow since the reagents are not generally available and interlaboratory disagreement exists over certain specificities.

Morris et al.[43] have recently studied 103 adult asthmatic patients and failed to find any association with seven defined DR antigens.

An interaction between atopic disease, tissue type and vulnerability to steroid-responsive nephrotic syndrome (SRNS) has been reported by Thomson et al.[27] and is, perhaps, a good example of the complex interactions which are probably extremely common in the field of allergy. These authors showed that atopic symptoms were more common in children with steroid-responsive nephrotic syndrome than in matched controls and that HLA-B12 was more common in children with SRNS than in adult controls. Atopic symptoms (particularly hay fever), positive prick tests with grass pollen antigens and a higher mean serum concentration of IgE antibody to Timothy grass pollen were more common in nephrotic children with HLA-B12 than in those without HLA-B12.

There have been several hypotheses to account for the observed associations between certain tissue types and vulnerability to different diseases. The 'molecular mimicry' hypothesis[14] suggests that the HLA antigen associating with a particular disease is antigenically cross-reactive with the causative agent. Another theory suggests that HLA antigens act as receptors and are capable of binding viruses or pathologically important molecules. The localization of structural genes for the complement components C2, C4 and Factor B to the MHC locus of chromosome 6 provides another explanation for some of the observed associations. However, tissue-type associations with immunopathology are most often interpreted in terms of the antigen specific *Ir* gene hypothesis of Benacerraf and McDevitt[28, 29] which postulates that individual antigens are specifically recognized by the products of individual dominant immune response genes located in the genome in close relationship with the MHC. This theory envisages a class of molecules distinct from immunoglobulins but capable of interacting specifically with antigen and composed partially or totally of gene products of the MHC. Their function, it has been suggested, is to interact with appropriate cell receptors on T cells, B cells and macrophages and to control the differentiation of immunocompetent cells in immune responses. There is, however, no direct evidence for the existence of *Ir* genes in man but the best circumstantial evidence is probably from the allergic diseases and these data are briefly reviewed in the next section.

ALLERGEN SPECIFIC *Ir* GENES?

In 1973 Marsh and co-workers[30] were able to show a highly significant association between an allergic individual's ability to develop marked skin sensitivity to allergen Ra5 (following exposure to ragweed pollen) and the possession of the HLA antigen B7 or one of an immunologically related group of antigens called B7 'Creg'. Since skin sensitivity to particular antigens is generally believed to correlate well with the ability to synthesize specific IgE antibody after inhalation of immunogenically limiting doses of antigen the authors suggested that they had in effect demonstrated an association between a specific immune response and the HLA system. However, as these authors discussed in a later paper[31], their family studies[11] had suggested that genetic determination of total IgE level was of overriding importance in determining *specific* IgE-mediated skin sensitivity to highly purified allergens and it seemed likely that this would mask any anticipated effect of HLA-linked *Ir* genes. Subsequent work from this laboratory has suggested how the apparent conflict in these two pieces of work may be reconciled[32]. It was discovered that a significant association existed between IgE-mediated sensitivity to rye grass Group I allergen and the possession of HLA-B8 especially at low total serum

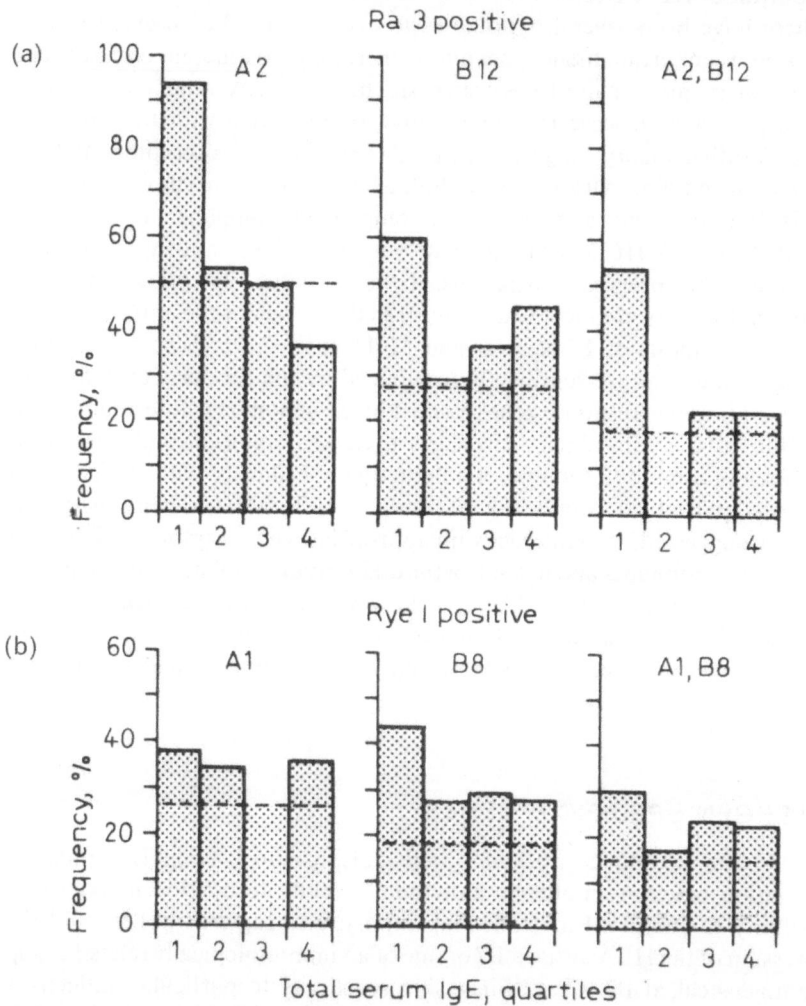

Figure 4.I.2   (a) Distribution frequencies of HLA-A2, B12 and the A2, B12 phenotype in Ra3 responders ($n = 76$) subdivided according to IgE quartiles in a total Ra3 study group of 126 allergic Caucasian subjects. Quartile divisions were at 127, 202 and 430 U ml^{-1}.

(b) Distribution frequencies of HLA-A1, B8 and the A1, B8 phenotype in Rye I responders ($n = 136$) subdivided according to IgE quartiles in the overall Rye I study group of 214 allergic Caucasian subjects. Quartile divisions were at 112, 203 and 400 U ml^{-1}. (Reproduced from Marsh *et al.*[31] with permission and excluding intermediate responders)

IgE levels. For a relatively complex allergen such as rye grass Group I, both the antigenic exposure and the overall capacity to synthesize IgE need to be highly limiting, in order to see the *strongest* associations between a specific IgE response and a particular HLA type. A similar study of the relationship between total serum IgE, Ra3 responsiveness and HLA-A2 frequency was even more interesting. Figure 4.I.2 shows in diagrammatic form the data for both Ra3 and rye Group I sensitive individuals. The overall populations in both studies were divided into quartiles based on total serum IgE levels and the respective HLA frequencies calculated for each of the quartiles. For both allergens the association between the most frequently observed HLA specificities was much more pronounced in the subgroup having genetically limiting low serum IgE levels.

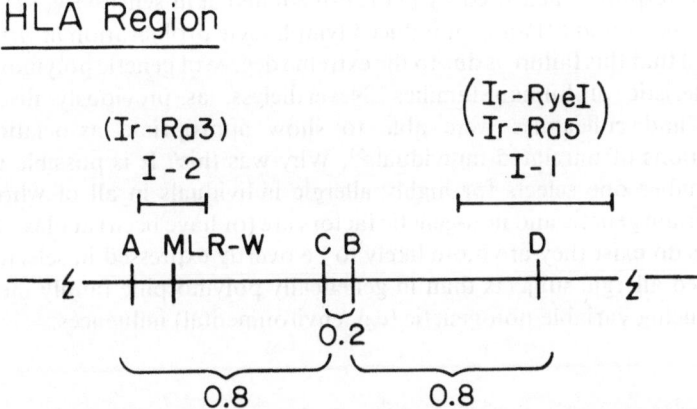

Figure 4.I.3   Gene map of the HLA region showing possible locations of hypothetical immune response subregions. The region I-1 contains the postulated Ir–Rye I and Ir–Ra5 loci and I-2 the postulated Ir–Ra3 locus. Note that these I regions are postulated to encompass the MLR regions D and MLR-W respectively. The map distances given are in centimorgans. (Reproduced from Marsh *et al.*[31] with permission)

Although alternative interpretations of these data are possible, the authors have hypothesized that certain *Ir* locus alleles controlling responsiveness to Ra3 and Rye I are in linkage disequilibrium with the alleles HLA-A2 and B8 respectively. The close association between A2 and Ra3 responsiveness and between B8 and Rye I responsiveness in people with low IgE phenotypes has provided further support for this suggestion which was originally based on population studies[11]. The authors have suggested that an 'Ir–Ra3' locus exists in the MHC and maps more closely to the A than to the B locus. Conversely an 'Ir–Rye I' locus maps more closely to the B than to the A locus (see Figure 4.I.3). Furthermore, since the association between B8 and Rye I responsiveness is weaker than that between A2 and Ra3 responsiveness it is suggested that the distance between the B and Ir–Rye I loci is greater than that between A and Ir–Ra3 and that these genes map in the chromosomal regions involved in the mixed lymphocyte response, i.e. MLR-W and D respectively.

Marsh and colleagues are the first to admit that their study provides working hypotheses which will be useful for future investigations but do not yet prove the existence of *Ir* genes in man. Appropriate family studies should provide such data and there have been three publications claiming 'linkage' between familial HLA haplotypes and IgE-mediated skin sensitivity to antigen E of ragweed pollen[33-35]. The Baltimore group subsequently studied 76 members of 13 large families and sought evidence of associations between familial HLA haplotypes and immune responses to four different pollen antigens (ragweed antigen E, Ra3, Ra5 and rye grass Group I)[36]. The authors found no evidence of association between specific HLA haplotype and specific immune response measured by (1) IgE-mediated skin sensitivity, (2) serum IgG antibody and (3) antigen-induced lymphocyte proliferation *in vitro*. It is assumed that this failure is due to the extreme degree of genetic polymorphism characteristic of human families. Nevertheless, as previously discussed, Marsh and colleagues were able to show appropriate associations in populations of unrelated individuals[31]. Why was this? It is possible that in such studies one selects for highly allergic individuals in all of whom the appropriate genetic and non-genetic factors are (or have been) at play. Thus if *Ir* genes do exist they are more likely to be overtly expressed in selected and unrelated allergic subjects than in genetically polymorphic family members experiencing variable non-genetic (e.g. environmental) influences.

CONCLUSIONS

It appears probable that at least three independent genetic systems operate in the acquisition of allergic illnesses. There is one (clearly critical) gene which predisposes certain individuals to develop one or more of the atopic diseases but we have practically no information on its chromosomal location or on the mechanism of action of its translated products(s). A second genetic system controls total serum IgE levels and is not linked to either the HLA or Gm systems. Thirdly there is a measure of HLA-linked genetic influence. This may operate by determining which particular atopic syndrome becomes manifest or it may represent a group of genes controlling specific IgE and IgG responses to allergens.

The basic defect in atopic disease is still the subject of much speculation and aspects of this controversy are discussed elsewhere in this volume. The association of immunodeficiency with allergic disease in infancy and childhood has been stressed[16,37] and may represent a cause and effect situation whereby there is failure to eliminate antigen by one mechanism (by an antibody/complement/phagocyte defect) which then permits sensitization of the IgE system. However, another interpretation can be placed upon these findings and several authors have argued that a deficiency of either specific or non-specific suppressor T cells might preferentially result in an increased formation of IgE antibodies and the development of clinical allergy[38-40]. Indeed, Strannegård and Strannegård[39] have suggested that there is a basic, genetically determined defect in some or all of the T lymphocytes of the atopic which makes them more vulnerable to the inhibitory action of cyclic AMP. An increased sensitivity to cyclic AMP may result in decreased T-cell numbers (reported in the newborns of parents with a family history of atopic disease[39, 41]) and an impaired balance between helper and suppressor T cells. Since IgE production is known to be particularly dependent on T-cell regulation the end stage of the lymphocyte defect is seen as excessive production of this immunoglobulin and atopic disease.

Progress in understanding the genetics of atopic disease was slow between 1916, when Cooke and Van der Veer[2] published their results and 1968 when Johansson et al.[6] studied the distribution of IgE levels in an atopic population. Most of what we know today has been learned in the past decade largely as a result of progress in the field of immunology, associated firstly with the characterization of IgE reaginic antibody and more recently with the elucidation of the mechanisms involved in lymphocyte differentiation and regulation. These advances have given convenient 'handles' such as serum IgE and HLA antigens which in turn have been exploited to provide genetic information. Although further knowledge of the basic atopic defect and its heritability may point, at some future date, towards effective preventative strategies it will be necessary in the short term to rely mainly on the manipulation of the environment (e.g. avoidance of cow's milk in early infancy[42]) for successful prevention of these diseases.

References

1. Wyman, M. (1872). In *Autumnal Catarrh* (Hayfever). (Cambridge: Hurd & Houghton)
2. Cooke, R. A. and Van der Veer, A. (1916). Human sensitization. *J. Immunol.*, 1, 201
3. Ratner, B. and Silberman, D. E. (1952). Allergy – its distribution and the hereditary concept. *Ann. Allergy*, 9, 1
4. Van Arsdel, P. P. and Motulsky, A. G. (1959). Frequency and heritability of asthma and allergic rhinitis in college students. *Acta Genet.*, 9, 101
5. Turner, K. J., Rosman, D. L. and O'Mahony, J. (1974). Prevalence and familial association of atopic disease and its relationship to serum IgE levels in 1061 school children and their families. *Int. Arch. Allergy Appl. Immunol.*, 47, 650
6. Johansson, S. G. O., Bennich, H. and Wide, L. (1968). A new class of immunoglobulin in human serum. *Immunology*, 14, 265
7. Spitz, E., Gelfand, E. W., Sheffer, A. L. and Austen, K. F. (1972). Serum IgE in clinical immunology and allergy. *J. Allergy Clin. Immunol.*, 49, 337
8. Bazaral, M., Orgel, H. A. and Hamburger, R. N. (1971). IgE levels in normal infants and mothers and an inheritance hypothesis. *J. Immunol.*, 107, 794

9. Oprée, W., Krause, H. and Stockberg, H. (1972). Genetic aspects of serum IgE levels in atopic families. *Acta Allergol.*, **27**, 247

10. Gerrard, J. W., Horne, S., Vickers, P., MacKenzie, J. W. A., Goluboff, N., Garson, J. Z. and Maningas, C. S. (1974). Serum IgE levels in parents and children. *J. Pediatr.*, **85**, 660

11. Marsh, D. G., Bias, Wilma B. and Ishizaka, K. (1974). Genetic control of basal serum immunoglobulin E level and its effect on specific reaginic sensitivity. *Proc. Natl. Acad. Sci. USA*, **71**, 3588

12. Marsh, D. G. (1976). Allergy: A model for studying the genetics of the human immune response. In Johansson, Strandberg and Uvnas (eds.) *Molecular and Biological Aspects of the Acute Allergic Reaction*. Nobel Symposium No. 33, pp. 23–57. (New York: Plenum Press)

13. Bazaral, M., Orgel, H. A. and Hamburger, R. N. (1974). Genetics of IgE and allergy: serum IgE levels in twins. *J. Allergy Clin. Immunol.*, **54**, 288

14. Snell, G. D. (1968). The H-2 locus of the mouse: observations and speculations concerning its comparative genetics and its polymorphism. *Folia. Biol. (Praha)*, **14**, 335

15. Thorsby, E., Engeset, A. and Lie, S. O. (1971). HL-A antigens and susceptibility to diseases. A study of patients with acute lymphoblastic leukemia, Hodgkin's disease and childhood asthma. *Tissue Antigens*, **1**, 147

16. Soothill, J. F., Stokes, C. R., Turner, M. W., Norman, A. P. and Taylor, B. (1976). Predisposing factors and the development of reaginic allergy in infancy. *Clin. Allergy*, **6**, 305

17. Krain, L. S. and Terasaki, P. (1973). HL-A types in atopic dermatitis. *Lancet*, **1**, 1059

18. Turner, M. W., Brostoff, J., Wells, R. S., Stokes, C. R. and Soothill, J. F. (1977). HLA in eczema and hay fever. *Clin. Exp. Immunol.*, **27**, 43

19. Desmons, F., Delmas-Marsalet, Y., Goudemand, J. and Defrenne, C. (1976). HL-A antigens and atopic dermatitis. *Allergol. Immunopath.*, **4**, 29

20. McNeish, A. S., Nelson, R. and Mackintosh, P. (1973). HL-A1 and 8 in childhood coeliac disease. *Lancet*, **1**, 668

21. Gebhard, R. L., Katz, S. I., Marks, J., Shuster, S., Trapani, R. J., Rogentine, G. N. and Strober, W. (1973). HL-A antigen type and small-intestinal disease in dermatitis herpetiformis. *Lancet*, **2**, 760

22. Mackay, I. R. and Morris, P. J. (1972). Association of auto-immune active chronic hepatitis with HL-A1, 8. *Lancet*, **2**, 793

23. Pirskanen, R., Tulikairen, A. and Hokkaren, E. (1972). Histo-compatibility (HL-A) antigens associated with myasthenia gravis. *Ann. Clin. Res.*, **4**, 304

24. Eddleston, A. L. (1977). Genetically determined immune hyperreactivity in human liver disease. *Proc. R. Soc. Med.*, **70**, 525

25. Bruce, C. A., Bias, Wilma B., Norman, P. S., Lichtenstein, L. M. and Marsh, D. G. (1976). Studies of HLA antigen frequencies, IgE levels, and specific allergic sensitivities in patients having ragweed hayfever, with and without asthma. *Clin. Exp. Immunol.*, **25**, 67

26. Rachelefsky, G., Terasaki, P. I., Park, M. S., Katz, R., Siegel, S. and Saito, S. (1976). Strong association between B-lymphocyte group-2 specificity and asthma. *Lancet*, **2**, 1042

27. Thomson, P. D., Barratt, T. M., Stokes, C. R., Turner, M. W. and Soothill, J. F. (1976). HLA-antigens and atopic features in steroid responsive nephrotic syndrome of childhood. *Lancet*, **2**, 765

28. Benacerraf, B. and McDevitt, H. O. (1972). Histocompatibility-linked immune response genes. *Science*, **175**, 273

29. McDevitt, H. O. and Landy, M. (1972). *Genetic Control of Immune Responsiveness*. (New York: Academic Press)

30. Marsh, D. G., Bias, Wilma B., Hsu, Susan H. and Goodfriend, L. (1973). Association of the HL-A7 cross reacting group with a specific reaginic antibody response in allergic man. *Science*, **179**, 691

31. Marsh, D. G., Chase, G. A., Goodfriend, L. and Bias, Wilma B. (1977). 'Mapping' of postulated Ir genes within HLA by studies in allergic populations. *Monogr. Allergy*, **11**, 106

32. Marsh, D. G. and Bias, Wilma B. (1976). Atopic allergy: a model for studying the genetics of immune response in man. In Bergsma, D. and Schimke, R. N. (eds), *Growth Problems and Clinical Advances*. Proc. Birth Defects Conference, Kansas City, 1975, pp. 223–237 (National Foundation March of Dimes Original Article Series, Vol. XII, No. 6)

33. Levine, B. B., Stember, R. H. and Fotino, M. (1972). Ragweed hayfever: genetic control and linkage to HL-A haplotypes. *Science*, **178**, 1201

34. Blumenthal, M. N., Amos, D. B., Noreen, H., Mendell, N. R. and Yunis, E. J. (1974). Genetic mapping of Ir locus in man: linkage to second locus of HL-A. *Science*, **184**, 1301

35. Buckley, C. E., Dorsey, F. C., Corley, R. B., Ralph, W. B., Woodbury, M. A. and Amos, D. B. (1973). HL-A linked human immune response genes. *Proc. Natl. Acad. Sci. USA*, **70**, 2157

36. Black, P. L., Marsh, D. G., Jarrett, E., Delespesse, G. J. and Bias, W. B. (1976). Family studies of association between HLA and specific immune responses to highly purified pollen allergens. *Immunogenetics*, **3**, 349

37. Turner, M. W., Mowbray, J. F., Harvey, B. A. M., Brostoff, J., Wells, R. S. and Soothill, J. F. (1978). Defective yeast opsonization and C2 deficiency in atopic patients. *Clin. Exp. Immunol.*, **34**, 253

38. Strannegård, I.-L., Lindholm, L. and Strannegård, Ö. (1976). Studies of T lymphocytes in atopic children. *Int. Arch. Allergy Appl. Immunol.*, **50**, 684

39. Strannegård, Ö. and Strannegård, I-L. (1978). T lymphocyte numbers and function in human IgE-mediated allergy. *Immunol. Rev.*, **41**, 149

40. Jarrett, E. E. E. (1977). Activation of IgE regulatory mechanisms by transmucosal absorption of antigen. *Lancet*, **2**, 223

41. Juto, P. and Strannegård, Ö. (1979). T lymphocytes and blood eosinophils in early infancy in relation to heredity for allergy and type of feeding. *J. Allergy Clin. Immunol.*, **64**, 38

42. Matthew, D. J., Taylor, B., Norman, A. P., Turner, M. W. and Soothill, J. F. (1977). Prevention of eczema. *Lancet*, **1**, 321

43. Morris, M. J., Faux, J. A., Ting, A., Morris, P. J. and Lane, D. J. (1980). HLA-A, B and C and HLA-DR antigens in intrinsic and allergic asthma. *Clin. Allergy*, **10**, 173

4
Allergy in Infancy and Childhood
PART II:
Other Aspects

J. F. PRICE

Allergy is an important cause of acute and chronic illness in childhood. At least 200 000 children in the United Kingdom will have asthma during the school years[1]. The United States National Health Survey, 1959–61, showed that asthma, hay fever and other allergies accounted for one-third of all chronic conditions in children under 17 years of age. Prevalence rates were 25.8 per 1000 for asthma, 24.5 per 1000 for hay fever, and 24 per 1000 for 'other allergies'. These figures indicate that at least five million children in the United States suffer from some chronic allergic condition, and over one-and-a-half million have asthma, which was responsible for more school absence than any other single chronic condition. Of total days lost from school 23% were due to this disease[2].

IMMUNODEFICIENCY AND ATOPY

Atopy, a term conceived 50 years ago[3], is used to describe the tendency of individuals to synthesize IgE antibody after contact with otherwise innocuous environmental antigens. Heat-labile antibodies in the serum of allergic subjects were capable of conferring prolonged sensitization and were called 'reagins'[4]. Most reaginic antibody is IgE; divalent molecules of this immunoglobulin are attached to basophils and mast cells, and the bridging of these molecules by antigen triggers the release of histamine and other vasoactive substances[5,6]. This results in immediate or Type I hypersensitivity reactions. Such reactions can be elicited in the skin of 95% of asthmatic children over the age of 5[7].

The causative antigens, where known, are usually common in the environment of the population at large; so host factor variation must underlie the state of atopy. This variation is partly genetic. A high incidence of positive skin tests in the relatives of atopic patients, and clustering of asthma, eczema and hay fever in families is well recognized. Concordance for asthma is greater in monozygotic than dizygotic twins. However, the concordance rate is low even in monozygotic pairs (less than 20%)[8,9] so environmental influence must also be important. Negro children born in England have the same prevalence of asthma as European children born in England, but the prevalence is much lower in negro children born in the West Indies[10]. Also asthma is rare in Gambian children in villages but common in the children living in the larger towns[11]. The observation that environmental factors can influence the state of atopy has clear therapeutic implications.

Genetically predisposed children (with allergic parents) often develop skin sensitivity to inhalant antigens during infancy, and sensitization may be particularly liable to occur in early life[12]. If this is so one would expect allergy to seasonal antigens to vary with the month of birth. More boys (but not girls) with pollen allergy were found to have been born in the spring, but the same trend was seen with non-seasonal antigens (animal epithelia)[13]. The results of a study of asthmatic children are more convincing[14]. Of those that were sensitive to *Dermatophagoides pteronyssinus*, the largest number were born between October and December, the smallest number in April to June. These periods correspond to the highest and lowest frequencies of live mites in house dust[15]. In contrast, the distribution of month of birth in the children who were not *Dermatophagoides*-sensitive followed general population trends. Susceptibility to sensitization is certainly not confined to infancy. Atopic children give an increasing number of positive skin reactions throughout childhood[7]. Adults who are brought up in a country where pollen counts are low may develop hay fever when they emigrate to the United Kingdom, and industrial exposure to castor bean antigens can also initiate IgE-mediated allergy[16].

There is a relationship between immunodeficiency and atopy. Allergy is common in the Wiskott–Aldridge syndrome and X-linked agammaglobulinaemia. In one study IgA deficiency was 35 times more frequent that expected in 'atopic' adults[17], though the definition of atopy was a very broad one. Atopy is common but these immunodeficiency states are rare. Perhaps common minor or transient defects of the immune system (close to or within the normal range) cause failure of proper exclusion and elimination of antigen. If this were so allergy could result from chronic overstimulation of normal (but potentially damaging) systems, by excess contact with antigen. Of course this hypothesis assumes that mechanisms exist in non-allergic subjects which reduce antigen entry. If there are such mechanisms they are unlikely to be antigen specific.

Transient low levels of serum IgA (at 3 months) in infants of allergic parents were found to be associated with the development of eczema and immediate hypersensitivity[18]. This is strong evidence for the aetiological role of immunodeficiency. However, another group were unable to detect any immunoglobulin deficiency in infants similarly selected[19]. A defect of yeast opsonization is found in 5% of the general population, but in a quarter of infants with unexplained frequent infection, many of these infants have eczema and other allergies[20]. Of atopics (children with eczema and adults with hay fever) 27% showed defective yeast opsonization[21], which appears to be a functional deficiency of the alternative pathway of complement[22]. Patients with another complement abnormality, low C2, frequently have allergies[23], and C2 deficiency was found in 18% of this same atopic group[21]. The two defects were mutually exclusive. There is no direct evidence that these two complement defects are causative in atopy, but they are probably familial and the fact that they occur independently in atopic subjects indicates that the low levels are not the result of *in vivo* consumption.

The mechanism of a failure to exclude antigen in IgA deficiency and defective yeast opsonization might be an indirect one through *Escherichia coli* endotoxin. IgA prevents the attachment of *E. coli* to gut mucosal cells[24]. The sera of patients with defective yeast opsonization fix complement poorly with endotoxin[22]. In both cases deficiency could result in abnormal persistence of endotoxin, which might then act as an adjuvant for ingested antigen and so lead to an IgE response. The means by which C2 deficiency could cause defective antigen handling at mucosal surfaces is not clear.

A failure to exclude antigen may also operate in other situations. Children with cystic fibrosis (CF) have a high prevalence of positive skin prick tests to inhalant antigens[25] and frequently have symptoms suggesting respiratory allergy[26], although the range of antigens to which they are sensitized differs from that seen in asthmatics. A mucosal defect is likely in these children but there is disagreement whether the defect is primary or secondary to chronic infection. The incidence of atopy in the parents (heterozygotes) of CF children is disputed[27, 28].

Once antigens have entered, their mode of elimination may also be important. Soothill and Steward observed in mice a variation in antibody affinity to protein antigens administered in saline[29], and this variation was later shown to be related to capacity for elimination of antigen[30]. Antibody affinity in mice closely correlates with clearance of polyvinyl pyrolidone (PVP) which is a test of macrophage function[31]. In man there is a range of PVP clearance similar to that seen in mice, but it remains to be seen whether low affinity antibody production or defects of macrophage function predispose to the development of reaginic allergy in humans.

CHILDHOOD ECZEMA

Childhood eczema usually occurs in atopic children: 20% subsequently develop asthma and 45% hay fever[32]; most give positive immediate skin reactions[33] and have high levels of serum IgE[34, 35]. There is about a 50% incidence of eczema in the infants of allergic parents[19, 36]. The overall incidence is not known precisely, but eczema is more common before the age of 2 years and only about a third have symptoms which persist to adulthood[37]. The problems of eczema are also discussed in Chapter 6.

Pathology

The epidermis shows hyperplasia and acanthosis. There is intra- and intercellular oedema (spongiosis) with flattening of the rete ridges. Keratinocytes are enlarged, and the cytoplasmic tonofibrils which make keratin are aggregated into irregular runs. The impression is of rapid cell proliferation which is outpacing keratinization.

The corium is infiltrated with lymphocytes, monocytes, eosinophils and basophils. There is vascular dilatation and oedema[38].

Pathogenesis

Allergic factors

In most children with eczema, IgE immunoglobulin and IgE antibodies to common environmental antigens are increased[34, 35]. Skin biopsies taken from adults with atopic eczema contain abnormally high levels of IgE[39] and increased numbers of IgE-producing B lymphocytes[40] and IgE-staining mast cells[41]. However, it is uncertain whether this increased IgE synthesis is the cause of eczema or simply reflects the frequent association of eczema with respiratory allergy[42, 43]. Intradermal injection of food or inhalant antigens induces a weal and flare response rather than the skin lesions of atopic dermatitis. In a proportion of children with eczema IgE levels are normal and prick skin tests negative[44], and typical atopic dermatitis can occur in patients with agammaglobulinaemia and absent weal and flare responses[45].

Most of the evidence that IgE-mediated reactions are involved in the pathogenesis of eczema comes from studies in adults (who are a highly selected group, as many children with eczema lose their symptoms). Patients with extensive skin involvement show the highest IgE levels[46, 47]. Resolution of the disease either spontaneously or after long-term treatment with steroids is associated with a fall in IgE[48]. When IgE is measured repeatedly over several years, the level roughly parallels the state of the skin in individual patients[49]. A study of 116 adult patients showed serum IgE levels closely correlated with severity of eczema and this relationship was independent of coexisting asthma and hay fever[50]. Some patients with eczema have evidence of impaired cell-mediated immunity, and it has therefore been postulated that a deficiency of IgE suppressor T cells might be the reason for the rise in IgE immunoglobulin[51,52].

In 1936, Grube and Sandford found eczema to be seven times more common in artificially fed than exclusively breast-fed infants[53]. In 1943 their conclusions were disputed by Edgren[37] and the role of hypersensitivity to cow's milk and other ingested food antigens in the aetiology of infantile eczema is still controversial. A recent prospective study of 49 infants of atopic parents showed a significantly lower incidence of eczema in those who were breast-fed and given an antigen avoidance regime (3/20), as compared with a control group who received artificial feeds (9/19). A possible mechanism might be that, in its effect upon sensitizing antigens, *E. coli* endotoxin acts as an adjuvant, and a protective effect of breast feeding might then result from inhibition of *E. coli* in the colon. However, in this study there was inconclusive evidence that immediate hypersensitivity to cow's milk antigens was greater in the artificially fed babies[54]. A second approach to investigating the role of food antigens is to examine the effects of elimination diets in established eczema. In 1954 Keston[55] reported a beneficial effect from a strict antigen avoidance diet in two-thirds of eczematous children under 3 years. Other authors have expressed the opposite view[56] and unfortunately hardly any controlled trials have been done. Two recent studies have indicated an improvement in eczema with elimination diets. In the first, 19 out of 20 infants showed subjective clinical improvement during a 6-week diet period. The trial was not controlled but there was concurrent reduction in eosinophilia and serum IgE[57]. The second study was a double-blind controlled trial of cow's milk and egg antigen avoidance in 20 children aged between 2 and 8 years. Fourteen children responded better to the elimination diet than to the control diet, while only one was better during the control period. There was no correlation between positive prick skin tests to milk and egg and response to the avoidance diet[58]. These studies suggest that dietary antigens in milk (and perhaps egg, wheat, fish, etc.) play a part in the development of eczema and influence its severity, but they do not clarify the role of IgE-mediated reactions in its pathogenesis.

Non-allergic factors

Itching and scratching are an important feature of childhood eczema. Itch is due to direct stimulation of nerve endings and is not affected by acetylcholine or catecholamines[59]. Simple tests have been devised to test itch threshold, such as stroking the forehead with a cotton wisp. One study has shown that atopic children have a heightened response to this test which is maximal at 1 year and declines by 4 years. This timing would correspond to the period of spontaneous remission in many children[60]. Often simply preventing scratching by bandaging without any other treatment will result in marked improvement in eczema, and there have been cases of eczema and paraplegia where the eczema has cleared below the spinal cord lesion.

The skin of eczematous children shows a number of abnormal physiological responses to non-allergic stimuli.

(1) White dermatographism; a white line response to pressure (in contrast to the normal red line)[61, 62].

(2) Delayed blanch; a spreading white reaction 5–30 minutes after intradermal injection of acetylcholine, methacholine[63] and nicotinic acid esters[64]. Seventy per cent of adults[65] and children[66] with eczema show this response. The blanching may be due to extreme vasodilatation and subsequent oedema[67].

(3) A lower digital temperature than normal, more marked constriction and slow dilatation in response to lowering and raising environment temperature[68].

Some have proposed that in eczematous patients there is an imbalance of autonomic control. β-Adrenergic blockade normally increases sweat output but has no such effect in patients with eczema. β-Adrenergic agonists stimulate deoxyribonucleic acid (DNA) synthesis in normal epidermal cells but not in cells cultured from the eczematous skin[69]. In some ways the relationship of non-allergic to allergic factors in the aetiology of childhood eczema is analogous to the situation in the lungs of children with asthma. Hyper-reactivity is an integral part of the disease and appears to exert an effect which is to some extent independent of immunological reactions.

Clinical features

The lesions frequently appear in the first 3 months of life. Sometimes the onset is related to the introduction of cow's milk, wheat or eggs. Such infants develop urticaria, colic, and a diffuse erythematous flush followed by typical eczema. More usually this association with the introduction of specific foods is less obvious; first papules and then vesicles appear over small areas of the cheeks and napkin area. They spread to the scalp, trunk and extremities and are accompanied by intense pruritis. The babies make incessant efforts to scratch the affected areas and the skin becomes weepy, crusted and infected. Small infants with eczema are susceptible to serious infection such as staphylococcal pneumonia. In a few the whole body becomes bright red (atopic erythroderma), secondary infection is common and there may be generalized lymphadenopathy.

The eczema tends to improve during the first 3 to 5 years of life and in many children clears completely. When the eczema persists the flexures, extremities and scalp, especially behind the ears, are the areas most frequently involved. The lesions vary in appearance; they may be dry and scaling or moist and weeping, but they always itch. The hands and feet often feel abnormally cold.

Children with severe eczema have a characteristic facial appearance. The skin is pale, there is an extra skin fold under the eyes (Dennie line or Morgan fold) and part of the eyebrows may be lost as a result of continuous scratching. Gradually the eczematous skin becomes hyperpigmented and shows lichenification; there is papular thickening with accentuation of normal surface lines. Exacerbations sometimes occur at times of emotional stress or after excessive sweating. The disease may be milder during the summer months when the child wears less clothing and the skin is exposed to sunshine.

Atopic eczema must be differentiated from other disorders of infancy and childhood in which erythema, oedema and exudative scaling and crusting skin lesions occur. These are listed in Table 4.II.1. Usually the association with other disorders, the family history, eosinophilia and high serum IgE make the diagnosis straightforward. Identical skin lesions are seen in two primary immunodeficiency diseases – sex-linked (Bruton's) agammaglobulinaemia and the Wiskott–Aldridge syndrome, a sex-linked recessive disorder characterized by thrombocytopaenia, eczema, and recurrent infections.

The most common complication of eczema is secondary bacterial infection, often with *Staphylococcus aureus* or the β-haemolytic *Streptococcus*. A generalized vesicular eruption with high pyrexia and severe systemic illness may result from infection with herpes simplex (Kaposi's varicelliform eruption). This latter condition is uncommon, but it is advisable that children with eczema are kept away from adults who have 'cold sores'. Eczema vaccinatum used to be seen after vaccination or exposure of an eczematous child to a recently vaccinated individual but is now very rare. Cataracts occur in 5–10% of adults with eczema but are hardly ever seen in childhood.

Table 4.II.1 Diseases causing skin lesions which may resemble atopic eczema

Seborrhoeic dermatitis
Scabies
Primary irritant dermatitis
Contact dermatitis
Ichthyosis
Phenylketonuria
Acrodermatitis enteropathica
Histiocytosis X (Letterer–Siwe)
Wiskott–Aldrich syndrome
X-linked agammaglobulinaemia

Treatment

General measures are aimed at reducing the damage done by itching, scratching and further itching. Extremes of temperature and humidity are best avoided, and exposure to sunlight and salt water is sometimes helpful. Cotton clothing should be worn in preference to wool. Bathing should be kept to a minimum and soap should not be used. Simple emulsifying ointments must be applied after bathing to keep the skin moist. Cetaphil, a non-lipid lotion containing cetyl alcohol, is a useful non-drying cleansing agent. The fingernails should always be kept short. In infants and toddlers scratching can be prevented with cotton stockings and mittens.

All children with eczema tend to scratch during the night and may do considerable damage to their skin while asleep. Some have very disturbed sleep and their schooling suffers as a result. Antihistamines with some sedative properties, promethazine, trimeprazine or diphenhydramine may be useful. If daytime drowsiness is a problem, clemastine is a suitable alternative with negligible sedative effect.

Exacerbations require topical therapy. Coal tar ointments (3–5%) and occlusive dressings are safe and often very effective. Unfortunately they are messy and if the lesions are extensive hospital admission may be necessary for their proper application. They have become less widely used since the introduction of topical steroids. A preparation of 0.5–1% hydrocortisone is suitable for use in children as a cream for weeping lesions or an ointment if the skin is dry. The more potent fluorine-containing topical steroids should be avoided as far as possible. Although they may be dramatically effective, the eczema often rebounds when they are withdrawn. In addition they may be absorbed in sufficient quantity to cause adrenal suppression, and their long-term use may result in damage to the epidermis. There have been reports of benefit from the use of corn starch/oatmeal baths (Aveeno). Systemic antibiotics (e.g. erythromycin) are an important part of treatment because secondary infection is so common. Topical antibiotics are of little value, and some like neomycin are liable to cause skin sensitization. It is preferable to use a mild topical antiseptic and give antibiotics systemically.

Breast feeding and antigen avoidance measures during the first months of life may prevent eczema developing, and the children of atopic parents are a clearly identified 'at risk' group. There is evidence that antigen avoidance diets, especially those which exclude cow's milk and egg, may be beneficial in established eczema. More extensive elimination diets are difficult to administer and if applied rigorously in infants can result in malnutrition. At present there is no way of identifying the children most likely to respond to an elimination diet.

It is important to give consideration to the unwanted side-effects of any treatment used for what is, in most children, a self-limiting disease.

RESPIRATORY ALLERGY

Diagnosis in children

Sometimes a specific allergy can be identified as a cause of asthma or rhinitis from the history, for example when symptoms develop only at a particular time of year or after contact with certain animals. It is more usual for symptoms to be perennial and the history difficult to interpret. Two main *in vitro* tests have been devised for the diagnosis of immediate (Type I) hypersensitivity, the measurement of IgE antibodies in serum, and the assay of histamine released from sensitized leukocytes. The alternative approach, antigen provocation, has been applied to three organs, the skin, nose and lung. In practice the diagnosis is often made from a combination of the history and one or more of these tests.

The precision of any allergy test depends on the purity and standardization of the antigen used. Unfortunately many antigen extracts are crude protein mixtures which contain non-specific irritant substances. Standardization by measurement of protein nitrogen content is unreliable when the active constituent forms only a small proportion of the total protein.

The interpretation of tests for immediate hypersensitivity is especially difficult in children. Serum IgE levels[70] and immediate skin reactions[7] increase throughout childhood and the size of response which is clinically significant may vary with age.

All allergy tests cause children some degree of discomfort and should only be done when specific immunotherapy, allergen avoidance or hyposensitization is proposed and the history is not clear-cut.

In vitro *tests*

IgE antibody measurement – The method most readily available is the radio-allergosorbent test (RAST), a modified antiglobulin reaction. A positive RAST to pollens, dust, house mite, and some moulds and animal danders agrees well with the history and results of provocation tests. In Scandinavian children with allergy to codfish the offending antigen has been identified and highly purified; the correlation for RAST, history and skin prick tests in these children is virtually 100%[71]. Discrepancies between RAST and *in vitro* tests may be due to poor quality of the allergen extracts, and the value of IgE antibody measurement will increase as individual antigens are defined more precisely. RAST has the advantage that it is not influenced by the patient's drug therapy and may be particularly useful in infants and young children when skin tests are unreliable and nasal or bronchial provocation tests impossible. The main disadvantages are that the tests are expensive, require special laboratory facilities and the results are not available immediately.

Leukocyte histamine release – The release of histamine from isolated leukocytes when challenged with allergen has been carefully assessed in patients with ragweed-sensitive allergic rhinitis. The test is reproducible and correlates well with clinical symptoms[62, 73]. The disadvantages of this test as a means of allergy diagnosis in children are that it requires a relatively large blood sample, is time consuming, and a limited number of allergens can be tested.

Provocation tests

Skin tests – Skin tests are the easiest to perform and therefore the most widely used diagnostic tests for allergy in children. They can be done by the scratch, prick or intracutaneous method. The scratch test is the least sensitive and the response is difficult to measure accurately. The intracutaneous technique is very sensitive and may be useful where the only extracts available contain low concentrations of allergen. However, intracutaneous injections are more likely to produce immunologically non-specific reactions and may be dangerous in very sensitive children. For the common inhaled antigens intracutaneous testing appears to have little advantage over prick testing. When intracutaneous and prick skin tests were compared with bronchial provocation in asthmatic children, a positive bronchial reaction did not occur if the response to intracutaneous testing was less than 5 mm. If the prick test response was less than a 5 mm weal, then a large intracutaneous reaction only marginally increased the likelihood of a positive bronchial test[74]. The results of carefully performed prick tests in adults correlate well with history, IgE antibody, nasal and bronchial provocation[75, 76]. However, Aas concluded from studies on 534 asthmatic children that if judged by bronchial reactivity, a diagnosis of house dust allergy based on history and skin testing would be incorrect in about a third of cases[77]. He found similar discrepancies between cutaneous and bronchial testing with animal danders, wool and pollens[78].

Skin tests of course only demonstrate cutaneous sensitivity and there is no universal agreement about the size of skin response which can be taken to indicate respiratory allergy. Of randomly selected school children 34% gave a 3 mm or greater weal response to prick testing with house dust mite or grass pollen but only about 17% had symptoms of respiratory allergy[79]. A study of asthmatic children in Denver showed that if the skin weal was less than 5 mm, only 15% of tests with dust and 19% with pollens were also positive on bronchial provocation. However, in children over 5 years, a weal response of greater than 5 mm (or one which is comparable to a positive control with 0.1 mg/ml histamine) and a strongly suggestive history, gives a high probability of a positive bronchial provocation test to the same antigen[74, 78, 80]. The advantages of skin tests are that several antigens can be tested at the same time, the results are immediately available, and they cause minimal upset to the child.

Nasal tests – Nasal provocation testing is an attractive prospect because the nasal mucosa is easily available, the response gives more direct evidence of respiratory allergy and the tests are safe. However, there are inherent difficulties in administering antigens to the nose in a quantitative way and making objective reproducible measurements of the response. The simplest method is to spray particles of antigen into the nose, or preferably to apply antigen to one nostril and then to compare the appearance of the nasal mucosa with that on the other side. If the child has acute rhinitis at the time the test is done then a non-specific response is highly likely, so it is important to use adequate controls. A positive response is shown by sneezing, rhinorrhoea and nasal obstruction. Several investigators have tried to make the test more precise by measuring changes in nasal airway calibre. The most promising of these techniques involves the simultaneous measurement of nasal airflow and the pressure drop across the nose by posterior rhinomanometry. Reproducible measurements of 'nasal resistance' in both adults and children have been reported[81-83]. Nasal provocation tests with pollens and house dust mite correlate well with skin tests and RAST[84]; however, the degree of reactivity in the different organs varies considerably[82]. It has not been established that nasal provocation tests have any advantage over skin tests as a means of diagnosis in allergic children.

Bronchial tests – Bronchial provocation testing is the most direct way to detect a specific allergy in asthma. Aas concluded from his experience of performing over 20 000 inhalation challenges in asthmatic children, that bronchial provocation tests were necessary for precise allergy diagnosis[85]. However, others argue that the administration of single doses of soluble antigen creates a highly artificial situation which does not reflect the events following natural exposure. Some of the nebulized antigen is swallowed, the amount inhaled may vary considerably, and administration of high concentrations of antigen can induce immunologically specific but clinically insignificant responses[86]. Antigen inhalation challenge tests are hazardous if done in centres which do not specialize in the technique.

The degree of bronchial obstruction which develops 10–20 minutes after antigen challenge does not always correlate with severity of symptoms. Aas noted that some children developed prolonged airflow obstruction which was resistant to symptomatic treatment. Another group observed two distinct patterns of response to bronchial provocation. Of 54 asthmatic children with a positive reaction to house dust 25 gave a reaction within half an hour of the test, and 29 gave a late reaction 8 to 13 hours after provocation. Some of those who showed an immediate reaction also showed a late reaction[87]. Warner found 31 of 45 children with positive bronchial provocation tests to the house dust mite (*Dermatophagoides pteronyssinus*) had late reactions. In contrast to the previous study no late reactions were seen without preceding immediate ones. The children with dual (immediate and late) bronchial reactions had more frequent attacks of asthma than those with immediate reactions only[80]. Dual reactions have also been observed in asthmatic children after bronchial provocation with Timothy pollen and cat fur[83] (see Figures 4.II.1 and 4.II.2).

In some ways the late reaction more closely resembles a severe asthma attack than the immediate one, but the mechanism is not clear. The time of onset would suggest an antigen–antibody complex and complement-mediated reaction (Type 3). However, late reactions to common inhaled antigens such as house dust differ from those seen in some forms of adult asthma, avian

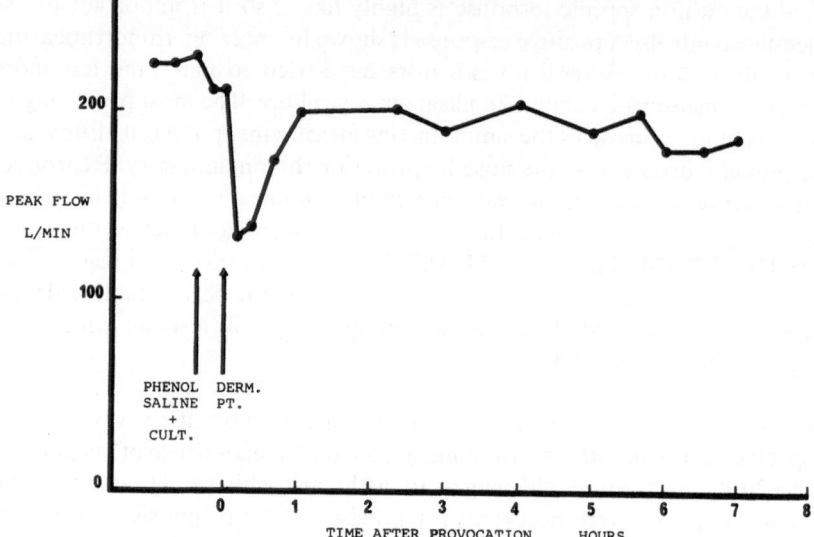

Figure 4.II.1   An immediate bronchial reaction, in a child with perennial asthma, to inhalation of a solution containing *Dermatophagoides pteronyssinus*. The bronchial challenge was preceded by inhalation of the control solution: mite culture medium in phenol saline

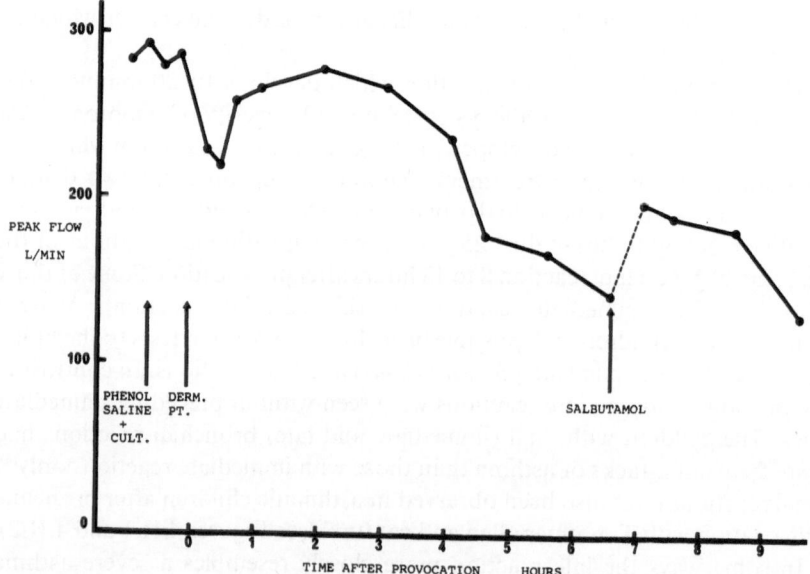

Figure 4.II.2   A dual (immediate and late) reaction to bronchial provocation with *Dermatophagoides pteronyssinus* in a child with perennial asthma. The late reaction though more slowly developing is ultimately more severe than the immediate one and is only partially reversed by a bronchodilator

allergy or bronchopulmonary aspergillosis, in that fever, leukocytosis, crepitations and pulmonary infiltrations are absent[88]. It may be that the reaction is localized to the bronchi rather than the alveoli. The observation that late bronchial reactions to pollens occurred in adult asthmatic patients with large immediate reactions and high serum IgE antibody led some to suggest that late bronchial reactions were IgE dependent[89]. Others have proposed that late reactions might result from the absorption of antigen through the gastrointestinal tract, reaching the lungs via the bloodstream[90]. Loss of late reactions is associated with improvement in asthma after hyposensitization to *Dermatophagoides*, and this emphasizes their clinical importance[91].

In summary, the bronchial provocation test is specific for allergy diagnosis and may be valuable in the assessment of the response to therapy. In experienced hands the test is safe but the high incidence of late bronchial reactions means that children should be admitted to hospital overnight. The test should only be used in special centres where specific allergy diagnosis cannot be established by other means and the outcome will influence treatment.

Childhood asthma

Asthma is a complex disorder with a broad spectrum of clinical features. It is characterized by recurrent and reversible obstruction of the lower airways causing symptoms of dyspnoea and wheezing, but there is no adequate definition in terms of pathology or pathogenesis. There may be several disease entities operating through a final common pathway (limited by the reactive properties of the bronchi) or there may be a common basic disorder, attacks of asthma being precipitated by a variety of trigger mechanisms. In children epidemiological studies favour the latter; they show that most asthmatic children share two major abnormalities, bronchial hyper-reactivity and the state of atopy.

Epidemiology

Estimates of prevalence range from 1.8 to 4.8% in the United Kingdom, 4.9 to 12.1% in the United States of America and 4.6 to 11% in Australia. Very low prevalence rates (0.8 to 1.4%) are reported from Scandinavia. These figures may represent real differences but are subject to a number of variables, such as the definition of asthma, the methods of patient sampling, and the types of questionnaire used.

The primary variable in epidemiological studies of children is whether wheezing with a respiratory infection constitutes asthma. The relationship of 'wheezy bronchitis' to asthma has been clarified as a result of a prospective long-term epidemiological study in Melbourne. The children diagnosed as having wheezy bronchitis could not be distinguished immunologically or physiologically from those with asthma[92]. When such children are included in the asthmatic population the prevalence rate increases to between 10 and 19%. Childhood asthma is more common in boys than girls with a ratio of 2 to 1, and boys tend to have more severe symptoms. After puberty this sex difference disappears. About 80% of asthmatic children develop symptoms before the age of 5 and about a third before 2 years of age. The majority with mild recurrent wheezing at the age of 7 will have lost their symptoms by the time they are 14, but the more severe the child's symptoms, the less likely they are to lose their asthma[93].

The morbidity from asthma is considerable. The disease is responsible for more school absence than any other single chronic condition. Fortunately, the mortality is low, although about 40 children in the United Kingdom and about 100 children in the United States die of asthma each year. There was a dramatic increase in asthma deaths in England and Wales between 1960 and 1966. This increase was particularly evident in 10- to 14-year-olds and was attributed to the increased use of aerosol bronchodilators. The death rate has now declined but has not fallen below the levels in the 1950s. More recent reports suggest that children under the age of 3 are particularly at risk of respiratory failure and death[94,95].

Pathology

Our knowledge is limited to the autopsy findings in the small group of asthmatics who have died or have had lung biopsy performed. The pathological changes are constant and largely independent of the patient's age. The lungs are overinflated and incompressible. Many of the bronchi are blocked with thick plugs of mucus which contain epithelial cells, eosinophils, lymphocytes, polymorphs and sometimes Charcot–Leyden crystals. The smooth muscle which surrounds the small bronchi is hypertrophied as are the mucous glands and goblet cells in the mucosal wall. The mucosa is infiltrated with eosinophils, lymphocytes, mast cells and polymorphs and there is thickening of the basement membrane of the bronchi. The alveoli are overdistended but the elastic tissue is normally intact in children; the emphysema often seen in older patients dying of asthma is not usually evident. In young children there is often enlargement of the hilar lymph nodes. We do not know to what extent these observed changes are primary or whether they are secondary to severe asthma and its treatment.

Pathogenesis

Bronchial hyper-reactivity – It has been known for over 30 years that a variety of non-allergic stimuli will provoke airways obstruction in asthmatic subjects[96]. This can be shown experimentally by their response to the inhalation of methacholine or histamine or by the effects of exercise. With repeated testing, 90% of asthmatic children develop abnormal bronchoconstriction during a standardized exercise test. Patients with a past history of wheezy bronchitis behave similarly[97]. Kernig and Godfrey found abnormal bronchial lability after exercise in first degree relatives of asthmatic children and suggested a genetic influence[98]. Increased irritability of the airways in response to non-antigenic stimuli could be due to partial β-adrenergic blockade[99], adenylcyclase deficiency[100], an over-responsive cholinergic system[101], or a combination of these three.

Atopy – Whereas in adults 'intrinsic' asthma occurs in association, not with atopy, but with autoallergic phenomena and certain tissue types[102], in childhood this form of asthma is rare. Most asthmatic children give immediate skin reactions and have high levels of IgE antibody to common inhaled antigens. The number of positive skin tests and their size tends to increase throughout childhood[7]. It is not precisely clear why asthmatic children show this highly familial tendency, but there may be an analogy with the situation in experimental animals, in which the IgE response is influenced by the balance of helper and suppressor T lymphocytes[103] and by the mode of presentation of antigen[104].

Immediate reactions in the skin are not, however, invariably associated with symptoms of asthma or hay fever[79]. Davis found a high incidence of positive skin tests in the non-wheezy sisters of asthmatic boys. Although atopy is a major characteristic of asthmatic children, it may not therefore be the only determinant of the capacity to wheeze[105]. The high incidence of late reactions after bronchial provocation with common antigens in children with perennial asthma suggests that other allergic mechanisms could be involved[80,83].

The house dust mite – Atopy indicates a wide ranging susceptibility and is antigen non-specific; most asthmatic children react on skin testing to more than one antigen. It is difficult to establish the relative importance of individual allergies, but there is some evidence that allergy to the house dust mite (*Dermatophagoides pteronyssinus*) is a major cause of perennial wheezing.

Exposure to dust has long been recognized as a cause of asthma[106], but it was not until 1964 that the progliphid mites were identified as important antigens in dust[107]. There are 15 species, the commonest being *Dermatophagoides pteronyssinus*, the European house mite, and *Dermatophagoides farinae*, the North American house mite. They live off keratin shed from the skin, and high counts are found in domestic mattresses and furniture upholstery. Children's soft toys are often inhabited by mites, but counts on cots and prams are lower, and mites are virtually absent from hospital ward mattresses[108].

More than 80% of asthmatic children over the age of 5 give an immediate skin reaction to *Dermatophagoides* (about 60% have positive reactions to other common inhaled antigens like grass pollens, animal danders and moulds)[7]. A similar proportion give an immediate reaction on nasal provocation and IgE antibodies can be detected in about 60%[108]. Of 85 children with moderately severe perennial wheezing 69 gave a positive bronchial reaction to provocation with house mite[14].

Mite sensitivity develops early in life – by the age of 2 half of an unselected group of asthmatics had a positive skin reaction to *Dermatophagoides*[108]. A relationship has been demonstrated between the seasonal variation in mite counts and severity of symptoms. A group of Dutch children had most wheezing in autumn and early winter when mite counts were highest, and the converse was found for both symptoms (recorded by diary card score) and mite counts in mid-summer[109]. One might expect that measures taken to eradicate the house mite from the bedroom would result in clinical improvement. This was the finding in a small uncontrolled study but there was no associated fall in IgE antibody[110]. Hyposensitization to *Dermatophagoides pteronyssinus* has been shown to give benefit in mite-sensitive children with perennial asthma, although many of the patients gave positive immediate reactions to other antigens[91].

When asthmatic children with a positive skin or bronchial reaction to mite are compared with those without mite allergy, there are certain differences. Mite-sensitive asthma is characterized by an earlier age of onset of wheezing. Nocturnal symptoms are common, and this might be expected as mites inhabit mattress dust and bedding. Finally, children with mite sensitivity are more likely to have been born in autumn and early winter when mite counts are high and so might have been sensitized during a susceptible period in early infancy[14].

Clinical features

In the early stages, particularly in infants and toddlers, the clinical patterns of asthma vary considerably. Many babies present with loud wheezing and tachypnoea but remain well, active, and gain weight. A small group – often with eczema and a strong family history of atopy – develop serious attacks which can lead to respiratory failure. These children are likely to have severe asthma persisting into adulthood. Some have wheezing associated with recurrent acute lower respiratory tract infections. Respiratory viruses are usually responsible and the children show the characteristic bronchial lability and immediate hypersensitivity of asthma. Fifty per cent of infants with proven respiratory syncytial virus bronchiolitis go on to have further attacks of wheezing and it may be that bronchiolitis is the reaction of potential asthmatics to infection with this virus (rather than rhinitis or mild bronchitis)[111].

Once asthma is established the patterns of illness will depend on the precipitating causes (Table 4.II.2), and the frequency, duration and severity of attacks. About three-quarters of asthmatic children have acute episodes of wheezing which vary in severity but nevertheless allow lung function to return to normal between attacks. In such cases viral respiratory infection often seems to be responsible for precipitating wheezing. The prognosis for these children is good and most of them cease to wheeze before the age of 14. A second group, about one-quarter of children with asthma, have more frequent and sometimes prolonged wheezing triggered by infective, allergic, emotional or physical stimuli. The majority have evidence of small airways

Table 4.II.2   Factors which may precipitate wheezing in asthmatic children

Antigen + IgE
Viral respiratory infection
Exercise
Laughing
Coughing
Emotion
Chemical irritants
Changes in air temperature

obstruction in between episodes of wheezing, but many of this group also improve in later childhood. Finally, a third small group, 1–2% of the asthma population, have severe and continuing wheezing throughout childhood. Four out of five are boys, their symptoms usually start before the age of 2 and many also have eczema and rhinitis. They may be small in stature, with chest deformity, and all have abnormal pulmonary function between attacks. Most continue to wheeze in adult life.

Treatment

Pharmacological – When the attachment of antigen leads to bridging of IgE molecules on the surface of mast cells, this is followed by the release of histamine which induces not only bronchoconstriction (directly or reflexly via the vagus) but also mucosal oedema and hypersecretion of mucus. Several other chemical mediators, such as slow reacting substance (SRS-A), serotonin, kinins and eosinophil chemotactic factor (ECF) have also been implicated. Three types of drug are used to block the sequence of events which leads to airways obstruction – bronchodilators, sodium cromoglycate and corticosteroids. A simple scheme of the sites of action of these drugs is shown in Figure 4.II.3. Intermittent bronchodilator therapy is usually sufficient for acute episodic asthma, though bronchodilators have little effect in infants[112]. Those children with more frequent attacks should be given regular cromoglycate or theophylline therapy and a sympathomimetic used for acute attacks. An inhaled corticosteroid should be given if control is still not achieved, and as steroids act in part by sensitizing beta receptors it is appropriate to give a sympathomimetic drug at the same time. Although systemic steroids are important in the treatment of acute severe asthma it is rarely necessary to use them for long-term treatment in children.

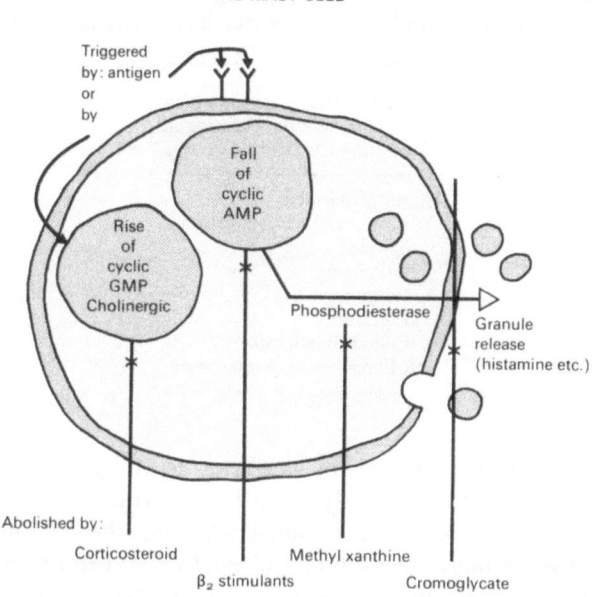

Figure 4.II.3   A schematic representation of the sites of action of drugs used to block antigen-induced airways obstruction

Immunological – Immunological treatment consists of antigen avoidance and hyposensitization therapy. As with eczema, there is evidence that breast feeding during infancy prevents or delays the development of asthma[113]. In established asthma, house dust and dust mite avoidance measures may improve symptoms and should be carried out where possible. The most important area is the child's bedroom. Upholstered furniture, feather pillows or quilts, woollen rugs and soft toys should be removed, and the bed mattress should be cleaned and then enclosed in a plastic cover. Other beds in the room should be treated similarly. The room should be carefully damp dusted, the bed vacuum-cleaned weekly and curtains washed frequently. Linoleum or vinyl covered flooring is preferable to carpeting, as it is easier to keep dust free. Dust should be removed from upholstered furniture in other rooms in the house. Families with an asthmatic child should be discouraged from keeping pet animals.

Controlled trials have shown that hyposensitization to house dust[114] and house dust mite[91], if continued for at least a year, results in clinical improvement in carefully selected asthmatic children. This form of treatment is painful and has potential adverse effects, so should be reserved for those children with proven allergy who cannot be adequately controlled with drug therapy. The evidence of beneficial effect from pollen hyposensitization is inconclusive and there are no controlled trials with other inhalant antigens.

Allergic rhinitis

Pathogenesis

In addition to functioning as an olfactory organ, the nose warms, moisturizes and filters the inspired air and has an important role in defence against airborne hazards. Among these hazards are antigens which can provoke reagin-mediated allergic reactions. The mechanism of allergic rhinitis is better understood than that of eczema and asthma. Sensitization probably occurs when small amounts of antigen are inhaled and absorbed over a period of time, leading to the synthesis of IgE antibody in atopic subjects. Subsequently, when particles are deposited in the nose, the soluble antigen which is eluted combines with IgE on mast cells in the lumen or the submucosa. Vasoactive substances are released which provoke itching, rhinorrhoea, mucosal oedema and the accumulation of eosinophils.

Allergic rhinitis can be seasonal or perennial. The antigens responsible for seasonal symptoms are contained in the windborne pollens of grasses, trees and weeds. In the United Kingdom the most important pollens are those of *Phleum pratense* (Timothy), *Dactylis glomerata* (cocksfoot) and *Lolium perenne* (rye). Grass and weed pollen grains are very light and are carried for miles by the wind. Because tree pollens are heavier they tend to cause symptoms in more localized areas. Pollen grains from plants that are insect pollinated are rarely responsible for allergic rhinitis.

The antigens thought to be important in children with perennial rhinitis are those in household dust, and in Europe the major component is *Dermatophagoides pteronyssinus*. Outdoor earth or road dust does not usually cause nasal allergy. Some children become sensitized to feathers and the epithelia of household pets. Food antigens are very unlikely to be responsible for allergic rhinitis.

Clinical features

Seasonal allergic rhinitis is estimated to occur in 5–9% of children and is quite rare under the age of 5. It is still not clear whether allergic rhinitis predisposes to asthma. Many patients with only nasal symptoms have abnormal bronchial lability[115], but epidemiological studies suggest that relatively few of them develop asthma. One such investigation showed that after 4 years the incidence of asthma in patients who had previously suffered from allergic rhinitis was 1% in males and 3% in females[116]. The exact incidence of perennial rhinitis is not known but it has been claimed that 10% of the population in Great Britain are affected[117] and over 30% develop symptoms before the age of 10[118]. Most children with perennial asthma also have rhinitis.

The symptoms are sneezing, rhinorrhoea, nasal obstruction and itching of nose, palate and pharynx. Many children also have a conjunctivitis. The nasal mucosa looks pale, bluish and oedematous. Children with nasal allergy often develop characteristic mannerisms, nose wrinkling and repeated upward rubbing of the nose with the hand (allergic salute). The latter may cause a horizontal skin crease to appear on the dorsum of the nose near the tip. Some have dark rings under the eyes (allergic shiners) which are attributed to venous stasis from impaired blood flow through the swollen nasal mucosa. Perennial rhinitis in small children must be differentiated from unilateral choanal atresia, foreign body, recurrent upper respiratory tract infection and nasal polyps (found in 20% of children with cystic fibrosis). Vasomotor rhinitis, a non-allergic condition which is possibly due to an imbalance of autonomic control, tends to cause nasal obstruction with relatively little itching, sneezing or rhinorrhoea.

Unlike eczema and asthma, the prognosis for spontaneous resolution of allergic rhinitis is relatively poor. A prospective study showed that less than 10% of children with allergic rhinitis had become symptom free after 5 years[119], and a 20-year follow-up of nearly 700 children found that 80% still had rhinitis[120].

The relationship of allergy and secretory otitis media is controversial (see Chapter 9, Part I). Otitis media frequently complicates allergic rhinitis, but only about a quarter of children with chronic secretory otitis media have evidence of immediate hypersensitivity[121].

Treatment

Antigen avoidance measures for perennial rhinitis are the same as those described for children with asthma. Hyposensitization therapy is discussed in Chapter 8.

The drugs used in treatment are antihistamines, sympathomimetics, sodium cromoglycate, and topical corticosteroids. Antihistamines (promethazine, chlorpheniramine, clemastine) may control itching and sneezing, but often fail to relieve obstruction and cause drowsiness. Sympathomimetic agents with mainly alpha-receptor activity (ephedrine, phenylephrine) vasoconstrict the nasal mucosa and help relieve obstruction, but their prolonged use (more than a week) may cause severe persistent nasal congestion (*Rhinitis medicamentosa*). Sodium cromoglycate, though somewhat less effective in the treatment of allergic rhinitis than in asthma, has been shown to improve seasonal and perennial symptoms. Finally, when topical corticosteroid (beclomethazone) is administered by pressurized aerosol it often produces marked improvement, which can be maintained with a very small dose. As yet no serious side-effects have been observed from beclomethazone given in this way.

References

1. Court, D. and Jackson, A. (1975). *Paediatrics in the Seventies*. (Oxford: Oxford University Press)
2. Schiffer, C. G. and Hunt, E. P. (1963). *Illness Among Children*. Children's Bureau Publication No. 405 Washington DC, United States, Department of Health Education and Welfare
3. Coca, A. F. and Cooke, R. A. (1923). On the classification of the phenomena of hypersensitiveness. *J. Immunol.*, **8**, 163
4. Coca, A. F. and Grove, E. (1925). Studies in hypersensitiveness. XIII. A study of atopic reagins. *J. Immunol.*, **10**, 445
5. Ishizaka, K., Ishizaka, T. and Hornbrook, M. M. (1966). Physico-chemical properties of reaginic antibody IV. Presence of a unique immunoglobulin as a carrier of reaginic activity. *J. Immunol.*, **97**, 75
6. Ishizaka, T., Soto, C. S. and Ishizaka, K. (1973). Mechanisms of passive sensitisation: 3. Number of IgE molecules and their receptor sites on human basophil granulocytes. *J. Immunol.*, **111**, 500
7. Smith, M. J. (1973). Skin tests and atopic allergy in children. *Clin. Allergy*, **3**, 269
8. Spaich, D. and Ostertag, M. (1936). Untersuchungen über allergische Erkrankungen bei Zwillingen. *Zeitschr. f. Menschl. Vererb. Konstitutionslehre*, **19**, 731
9. Edfors-Lubs, M. L. (1971). Allergy in 7000 twin pairs. *Acta Allergol.*, **26**, 249
10. Smith, J. M., Harding, L. K. and Cumming, G. (1971). The changing prevalence of asthma in school children. *Clin. Allergy*, **1**, 57
11. Godfrey, R. C. (1975). Asthma and IgE levels in rural and urban communities of the Gambia. *Clin. Allergy*, **5**, 201
12. Soothill, J. F. (1976). Some intrinsic and extrinsic factors predisposing to allergy. *Proc. R. Soc. Med.*, **69**, 439
13. Bjorksten, F. and Suoniemi, I. (1976). Dependence of immediate hypersensitivity on the monnth of birth. *Clin. Allergy*, **6**, 165
14. Warner, J. O. and Price, J. F. (1978). House dust mite sensitivity in childhood asthma. *Arch. Dis. Child.*, **53**, 710
15. Blythe, M. E. (1976). Some aspects of the ecological study of the house dust mites. *Br. J. Dis. Chest*, **70**, 3
16. Ordman, D. (1955). An outbreak of bronchial asthma in South Africa affecting more than 200 persons caused by castor bean dust from an oil processing factory. *Int. Arch. Allergy*, **7**, 10
17. Kaufman, H. S. and Hobbs, J. R. (1970). Immunoglobulin deficiencies in an atopic population. *Lancet*, **2**, 1061
18. Taylor, B., Norman, A. P., Orgel, H. A., Stokes, C. R., Turner, M. W. and Soothill, J. F. (1973). Transient IgA deficiency and pathogenesis of infantile atopy. *Lancet*, **2**, 111
19. Kaufman, H. S. and Frick, O. L. (1976). Immunological development in infants of allergic parents. *Clin. Allergy*, **6**, 321
20. Soothill, J. F. and Harvey, B. A. (1976). Defective opsonisation: a common immunity deficiency. *Arch. Dis. Child.*, **51**, 91
21. Turner, M. W., Mowbray, J. F., Harvey, B. A. M., Brostoff, J., Wells, R. S. and Soothill, J. F. (1978). Defective yeast opsonisation and C2 deficiency in atopic patients. *Clin. Exp. Immunol.*, **34**, 253

22. Soothill, J. F. and Harvey, B. A. M. (1977). A defect of the alternative pathway of complement. *Clin. Exp. Immunol.*, **27**, 30

23. Mowbray, J. F. (1976). Association of heterozygous C2 deficiency with both disease and HLA. In *HLA and Disease*, p. 204. (Paris: Editions Inserm)

24. Hanson, L. A. (1976). *Esch. coli* infections in childhood: significance of bacterial virulence and immune defence. *Arch. Dis. Child.*, **51**, 737

25. Warren, C. P. W., Tai, E., Batten, J. C., Hutchcroft, B. J. and Pepys, J. (1975). Cystic fibrosis – immunological reactions to *A. fumigatus* and common allergens. *Clin. Allergy*, **5**, 1

26. Warner, J. O., Taylor, B. W., Norman, A. P. and Soothill, J. F. (1976). Association of cystic fibrosis with allergy. *Arch. Dis. Child.*, **51**, 507

27. Warner, J. O., Norman, A. P. and Soothill, J. F. (1976). Cystic fibrosis heterozygosity in the pathogenesis of allergy. *Lancet*, **1**, 990

28. Silverman, M., Hobbs, F. D. R., Gordon, I. R. S. and Carswell, F. (1978). Cystic fibrosis, atopy and airways lability. *Arch. Dis. Child.*, **53**, 873

29. Soothill, J. F. and Steward, M. W. (1971). The immunopathological significance of the heterogeneity of antibody affinity. *Clin. Exp. Immunol.*, **9**, 193

30. Alpers, J. H., Steward, M. W. and Soothill, J. F. (1972). Differences in immune elimination in inbred mice. The role of low affinity antibody. *Clin. Exp. Immunol.*, **12**, 121

31. Morgan, A. G. and Soothill, J. F. (1975). Relationship between macrophage clearance of PVP and affinity of anti-protein antibody response in inbred mouse strains. *Nature (London)*, **254**, 711

32. Stifler, W. C. (1965). A 21 year follow up of infantile eczema. *J. Pediatr.*, **66**, 166

33. Meara, R. H. (1955). Skin reactions in atopic eczema. *Br. J. Dermatol.*, **67**, 60

34. Berg, T. and Johansson, S. G. O. (1969). IgE concentrations in children with atopic diseases. *Int. Arch. Allergy Appl. Immunol.*, **36**, 219

35. Church, J., Kleban, D. and Bellanti, J. (1976). Serum immunoglobulin E concentrations and radioallergosorbent tests in children with atopic dermatitis. *Pediatr. Res.*, **10**, 97

36. Soothill, J. F., Stokes, C. R., Turner, M. W. and Norman, A. P. (1976). Predisposing factors and the development of reaginic allergy in infancy. *Clin. Allergy*, **6**, 305

37. Edgren, G. (1943). Prognose und erblichkeitsmomente bei ekzima infantum. *Acta Pediatr.*, **30** (Suppl. 2), 1

38. Prose, P. H. (1965). Pathologic changes in eczema. *J. Pediatr.*, **66**, 178

39. Jansen, C. T., Haapalahti, J. and Hopsu-Haver, V. K. (1973). Immunoglobulin E in the human atopic skin. *Arch für Dermatol. Forsch.*, **246**, 299

40. Cormane, R. H., Husz, S. and Hamerlinck, F. (1974). Immunoglobulin – and complement-bearing lymphocytes in allergic contact dermatitis and atopic dermatitis (eczema). *Br. J. Dermatol.*, **90**, 597

41. Anan, S. (1976). Cellules porteuses d'immunoglobulins au niveau de la peau. *Rev. Française d'Allergie*, **16**, 65

42. Ohman, S. and Johansson, S. G. O. (1974). Immunoglobulins in atopic dermatitis. *Acta Dermatovenereol. (Stockholm)*, **54**, 193

43. Johnson, E. E., Irons, J. S., Patterson, R. and Roberts, M. (1974). Serum IgE concentrations in atopic dermatitis. *J. Allergy Clin. Immunol.*, **54**, 94

44. Price, J. F., Cogswell, J. J., Joseph, M. C. and Cochrane, G. M. (1976). Exercise-induced bronchoconstriction, skin sensitivity and serum IgE in children with eczema. *Arch. Dis. Child.*, **51**, 912

45. Peterson, R. D. A., Page, A. R. and Good, R. A. (1962). Wheal and erythema allergy in patients with agammaglobulinaemia. *J. Allergy*, **33**, 406

46. Clendenning, W. E., Clack, W. E., Ogawa, M. and Ishizaka, K. (1973). Serum IgE studies in atopic dermatitis. *J. Invest. Dermatol.*, **61**, 233

47. Stone, St. P., Gleich, G. J. and Muller, S. A. (1976). Atopic dermatitis and IgE. *Arch. Dermatol.*, **112**, 1254

48. Johansson, S. G. O. and Fuhlin, L. (1970). Immunoglobulin E in 'healed' atopic dermatitis and after treatment with corticosteroids and azathioprine. *Br. J. Dermatol.*, **82**, 10

49. Wuthrich, B. (1975). *Zur Immunopathologie der Neurodermitis constitutionalis*, p. 47. (Bern, Stuttgart, Weir: Hans Huber)

50. Wuthrich, B. (1978). Serum IgE in atopic dermatitis. *Clin. Allergy*, **8**, 241

51. Schopf, E. and Boehringer, D. (1974). IgE and cell-mediated immunity in atopic dermatitis. *J. Dermatol.*, **1**, 133

52. McGeady, S. J. and Buckley, R. H. (1974). Studies of cell-mediated immune function in atopic eczema. *J. Allergy Clin. Immunol.*, **53**, 72

53. Grube, S. and Sandford. H. (1936). The influence of breast and artificial feeding on infantile eczema. *J. Pediatr.*. **89**. 223

54. Matthew, D. J., Taylor, B., Norman, A. P., Turner, M. W. and Soothill, J. F. (1977). Prevention of eczema. *Lancet*, **1**, 321

55. Keston, B. M. (1954). Allergic eczema. *N.Y. State J. Med.*, **54**, 244

56. Norins, A. (1971). *Atopic Dermatitis*. Symposium on pediatric dermatology. In Jacobs, A. H. (ed.) *The Pediatric Clinics of North America*, p. 801. (Philadelphia: W. B. Saunders Company Ltd.)

57. Juto, P., Engberg, S. and Winberg, J. (1978). Treatment of infantile atopic dermatitis with a strict elimination diet. *Clin. Allergy*, **8**, 493

58. Atherton, D. J., Sewell, M., Soothill, J. F. and Wells, R. S. (1978). A double-blind controlled crossover trial of an antigen-avoidance diet in atopic eczema. *Lancet*, **1**, 401

59. Arthur, R. P. and Shelley, W. B. (1959). The peripheral mechanism of itch in man. In Wolstenholme, G. E. W. and O'Connor, Maeve (eds.) *Pain and Itch: Nervous Mechanisms*, pp. 84–95. Ciba Foundation Study Group No. 1. (Boston. Little. Brown and Co.)

60. Kepecs, J. G., Robin, Milton and Munro Clare (1960). Tickle in atopic dermatitis: interference with the organisation of a patterned response. *Arch. Gen. Psychiatry*, **3**, 243

61. Ebbecke, U. (1917). Die hokale vasomotorische reaktion (L.V.R.) der Haut und der inneren organe. *Arch. Ges. Physiol.*, **169**, 1

62. Whitfield, A. (1938). On the white reaction (white line) in dermatology. *Br. J. Dermatol.*, **50**, 71

63. Lobitz, W. C. and Campbell, C. J. (1953). Physiologic studies in atopic dermatitis (disseminated neurodermatitis). 1. The local cutaneous response to intradermally injected acetylcholine and epinephrine. A.M.A. *Arch. Dermatol. Syphilol.*. **67**, 575

64. Callaway, J. L. (1956). Dermatological research: an office procedure. *J. Invest. Dermatol.*, **27**, 215

65. West, J. R., Johnson, L. A. and Winkelman, R. K. (1962). Delayed blanch phenomenon in atopic individuals. *Arch. Dermatol.*, **85**, 227

66. Winkelman, R. K. (1966). Non-allergic factors in atopic dermatitis. *J. Allergy*, **37**, 29

67. Ramsay, C. (1969). Vascular changes accompanying white dermatographism and delayed blanch in atopic dermatitis. *Br. J. Dermatol.*, **81**, 37

68. Weber, R. G., Roth, G. M. and Kierland, R. R. (1955). Further contributions to the vascular physiology of atopic dermatitis. *J. Invest. Dermatol.*, **24**, 19

69. Carr. R. and Reed, C. E. (1973). Effect of catecholamines on D.N.A. synthesis in epidermis from normal subjects and patients with atopic eczema. *J. Allergy Clin. Immunol.*. **51**, 255

70. Berg, T. and Johansson, S. G. O. (1969). Immunoglobulin levels during childhood with special regard to IgE. *Acta Paediatr. Scand.*, **58**, 513

71. Aas, K. and Lundkvist, U. (1973). The radioallergosorbent test with a purified allergen from codfish. *Clin. Allergy*, **3**, 255

72. Lichtenstein, L. M. and Osler, A. G. (1964). Studies on the mechanism of hypersensitivity phenomena. 9. Histamine release from human leukocytes by ragweed pollen antigen. *J. Exp. Med.*. **120**. 507

73. Lichtenstein, L. M., Norman, P. S., Osler, A. G. *et al.* (1966). *In vitro* studies of human ragweed allergy. Changes in cellular and humoral activity associated with specific desensitisation. *J. Clin. Invest.*, **45**, 1126

74. Cavanaugh, M. J., Bronsky, E. A. and Buckley, J. M. (1977). Clinical value of bronchial provocation testing in childhood asthma. *J. Allergy Clin. Immunol.*, **59**, 41

75. Bryant. D. H., Burns, M. W. and Lazarus, L. (1975). The correlation between skin tests. bronchial provocation tests and serum levels of IgE specific for common allergens in patients with asthma. *Clin. Allergy*, **5**, 145

76. Pepys, J., Roth, A. and Carroll, K. B. (1975). RAST, skin and nasal tests and the history in grass pollen allergy. *Clin. Allergy*, **5**, 431

77. Aas, K. (1969). Allergic asthma in childhood. *Arch. Dis. Child.*, **44**, 1

78. Aas, K. (1970). Bronchial provocation tests in asthma. *Arch. Dis. Child.*, **45**, 221

79. Godfrey, R. C. and Griffiths, M. (1976). The prevalence of immediate positive skin tests to *Dermatophagoides pteronyssinus* and grass pollen in schoolchildren. *Clin. Allergy*, **6**, 79

80. Warner, J. O. (1976). Significance of late reactions after bronchial challenge with house dust mite. *Arch. Dis. Child.*, **51**, 905

81. Solomon, W. R., McLean, J. A., Cookingham, M. D., Ahronheim, G. and DeMuth, G. R. (1965). Measurement of nasal airway resistance. *J. Allergy*, **36**, 62

82. Taylor, G. and Shivalkar, P. R. (1971). Changes in nasal airways resistance on antigenic challenge in allergic rhinitis. *Clin. Allergy*, **1**, 63

83. Price, J. F., Hey, E. N., Levinsky, R. J. and Soothill, J. F. (1978). Factors underlying the immediate and dual responses to antigen challenge in childhood asthma. *Arch. Dis. Child.*, **53**, 835

84. Stenius, B., Wide, L., Seymour, W. M., Holford-Stevens, V. and Pepys, J. (1971). Clinical significance of specific IgE to common allergens 1. Relationship of specific IgE against *Dermatophagoides* spp. and grass pollen to skin and nasal test and history. *Clin. Allergy*, **1**, 37

85. Aas, K. (1975). *The Bronchial Provocation Test.* (Springfield: Charles C. Thomas)

86. Spector, S. L. and Farr, R. S. (1974). Bronchial inhalation procedures in asthmatics. *Med. Clin. N. Am.*, **58**, 71

87. Van Lookeren Campagne, J. G., Knol, K. and De Vries, K. (1969). House dust provocation in children. *Scand. J. Resp. Dis.*, **50**, 76

88. Booij-Noord, H., de Vries, K., Slunter, H. J. and Orie, N. G. M. (1972). Late bronchial obstructive reaction to experimental inhalation of house dust extract. *Clin. Allergy*, **2**, 43

89. Robertson, D. G., Kemgan, A. T., Hargreave, F. E., Chalmers, R. and Dolovitch, J. (1974). Late asthmatic responses induced by ragweed pollen antigen. *J. Allergy Clin. Immunol.*, **54**, 244

90. Wilson, A. F., Novey, H. S., Berke, R. A. and Surprenant, E. J. (1973). Deposition of inhaled pollen and pollen extract in human airways. *N. Engl. J. Med.*, **288**, 1056

91. Warner, J. O., Price, J. F., Soothill, J. F. and Hey, E. N. (1978). Controlled trial of hyposensitisation to *Dermatophagoides pteronyssinus* in children with asthma. *Lancet*, **2**, 912

92. Williams, H. E. and McNichol, K. N. (1969). Prevalence, natural history and relationship of wheezy bronchitis and asthma in children. An epidemiological study. *Br. Med. J.*, **4**, 321

93. McNichol, K. N. and Williams, H. E. (1973). Spectrum of asthma in childhood 1. Clinical and physiological components. *Br. Med. J.*, **4**, 7

94. Buranakal, B., Washington, J., Hillman, B., Mancuso, J. and Sly, R. M. (1974). Causes of death during acute asthma in children. *Am. J. Dis. Child.*, **128**, 343

95. Simons, F. E. R., Person, W. E. and Bierman, C. W. (1977). Respiratory failure in childhood status asthmaticus. *Am. J. Dis. Child.*, **131**, 1097

96. Curry, J. J. (1946). The action of histamine on the respiratory tract in normal and asthmatic subjects. *J. Clin. Invest.*, **25**, 785

97. Godfrey, S. (1974). *Exercise Testing in Children.* (London: W. B. Saunders Company Ltd.)

98. Kernig, P. and Godfrey, S. (1973). Prevalence of exercise-induced bronchial lability in families of children with asthma. *Arch. Dis. Child.*, **48**, 513

99. Szentivanyi, A. (1968). The β-adrenergic theory of atopic abnormality in bronchial asthma. *J. Allergy*, **42**, 203

100. Sutherland, E. W. and Robinson, G. A. (1966). The role of cyclic 3,5-AMP in response to catecholamines and other hormones. *Pharmacol. Rev.*, **18**, 145

101. Nadel, J. A. (1968). Mechanism of airways response to inhaled substances. *Arch. Environ. Health*, **16**, 171

102. Brostoff, J., Mowbray, J. F., Kapoor, A., Hollowell, S. J., Rudolf, M. and Saunders, K. B. (1976). 80% of patients with intrinsic asthma are homozygous for HLA W6. *Lancet*, **2**, 872

103. Tada, T., Okumura, K. and Tariguchi, M. (1973). Reagin-mediated hypersensitivity. In Goodfriend, L. (ed.) *Mechanisms in Allergy*, p. 43. (New York: Marcel Dekker)

104. Jarrett, E. E. E., Haig, D. M., McDougall, W. and McNulty, E. (1976). Rat IgE production. II. Primary and booster reaginic antibody responses following intradermal or oral immunisation. *Immunology*, **30**, 671

105. Davis, J. B. (1976). Asthma and wheezy bronchitis in children. Skin test reactivity in cases, their parents and siblings. A controlled population study of sex differences. *Clin. Allergy*, **6**, 329

106. Van Helmont, J. B. (1662). *Physick Refined.* (London: Lodwick Lloyd)

107. Voorhorst, R., Spieksma-Boezeman, M. I. A. and Spieksma, F. T. M. (1964). Is a mite (*Dermatophagoides* sp.) the producer of the house dust allergen? *Allergie und Asthma Forsch.*, **10**, 329

108. Sarsfield, J. K. (1974). Role of house dust mites in childhood asthma. *Arch. Dis. Child.*, **49**, 711

109. Van Bronswijk, J. E. M. H. and Sinha, R. N. (1971). Proglyphid mites (*Acari*) and house dust allergy. *J. Allergy*, **47**, 31

110. Sarsfield, J. K., Gowland, G., Toy, R. and Norman, A. L. E. (1974). Mite-sensitive asthma of childhood. Trial of avoidance measures. *Arch. Dis. Child.*, **49**, 716

111. Rooney, J. C. and Williams, H. E. (1971). The relationship between proven bronchiolitis and subsequent wheezing. *J. Pediatr.*, **79**, 744

112. Lenney, W. and Milner, A. D. (1978). At what age do bronchodilators work? *Arch. Dis. Child.*, **53**, 532

113. Chandra, R. K. (1979). Prospective studies of the effect of breast feeding on incidence of infection and allergy. *Acta Paediatr. Scand.*, **68**, 691

114. Aas, K. (1971). Hyposensitisation in house dust allergy asthma. *Acta Paediatr. Scand.*, **60**, 264

115. Fairshter, R. D., Chiu, J. T., Wilson, A. F. and Novey, H. S. (1977). Large airway constriction in allergic rhinitis. *J. Allergy Clin. Immunol.*, **59**, 243

116. Broder, I., Higgins, M. W., Matthews, K. P. *et al.* (1974). Epidemiology of asthma and allergic rhinitis in a total community. Tecumseh, Michigan IV. Natural History. *J. Allergy Clin. Immunol.*, **54**, 100

117. McAllen, M. K. and Langman, M. J. S. (1969). A controlled trial of dexamethazone snuff in chronic perennial rhinitis. *Lancet*, **1**, 968

118. Viner, A. S. and Jackman, N. (1976). Retrospective study of 1271 patients diagnosed as perennial rhinitis. *Clin. Allergy*, **6**, 251

119. Smith, J. M. (1971). A five year prospective study of rural children with asthma and hay fever. *J. Allergy*, **47**, 23

120. Rackeman, F. and Edwards, M. (1952). Asthma in children, a follow up study of 688 patients after an interval of 20 years. *N. Engl. J. Med.*, **246**, 858

121. Reisman, R. E. and Bernstein, J. (1975). Allergy and secretory otitis media: clinical and immunologic studies. *Pediatr. Clin. N. Am.*, **22**, 251

5
Gastrointestinal Reactions

M. H. LESSOF and P. D. BUISSERET

INTRODUCTION

The respiratory and gastrointestinal tracts are two major routes for antigen entry into the body; in view of the heavy and continuous antigenic load to which these two systems are exposed it is remarkable that they are not in a permanent state of immune uproar. The immunological differences between the two systems are as great as the anatomical differences. Once antigenic material has reached the alveolus the situation is the same as though it had been injected intravenously; the major specific (i.e. immune) and non-specific (i.e. humoral and mechanical) defences will by then have been circumvented. In the gut of the intact individual, however, this extraordinary vulnerability never occurs. The gut lumen remains at all times the *milieu exterieur* despite the intimacy with which it is applied to the *milieu interieur*[1]. Nevertheless in the alimentary tract the barrier separating the two *milieux* is only one cell thick.

There is an immediate and obvious paradox in the apparent unresponsiveness of the body to the endless traffic of food antigens passing through the bowel, as compared with the rapid response to oral immunization with viral or bacterial pathogens. The ingestion of a boiled egg does not irrevocably sensitize the normal individual to ovalbumin, whereas the ingestion of live attenuated polio virus on a sugar lump can confer lifelong immunity to poliomyelitis. Evidently a course is successfully steered between the Scylla of non-responsiveness with the resultant vulnerability to ingested pathogens and the Charybdis of total responsiveness with immunological upheavals whenever foreign material is ingested[2]. The dangers will evidently lie either in repeated gastrointestinal infections or in inappropriate immune responses (i.e. allergies) to what should be innocuous foods. The immune system of the gastrointestinal tract is uniquely tuned and organized to avoid both dangers in normal circumstances.

IMMUNE RESPONSES IN THE GASTROINTESTINAL TRACT

The major lymphoid tissue of the intestines is located in the Peyer's patches, aggregations of highly specialized cells situated in clumps from the duodenum to the caecum. The patches vary in size from a few millimetres to several centimetres across and are of heterogeneous shape and number. They are situated predominantly in the gut wall opposite that to which the mesentery, with its blood vessels and lymphatics, is attached[3]. Provision is made for the closely regulated entry of antigenic material from the lumen, its presentation to B lymphocytes and the subsequent production of specific antibody for secretion into the gut lumen. That the antibody is principally IgA, with its limited biological capabilities, is an important reason why serious immunological overreaction does not occur in the gut. This is so principally because IgA does not fix complement by the classical pathway[4], nor does it opsonize antigen for subsequent phagocytosis[5]. Even though IgA can activate the alternative complement pathway *in vitro*, its ability to do so is limited[6] and in any case it is not certain that the necessary complement components are present in the intestinal secretions or that they can function there[7].

While IgA is a relatively minor constituent of the immunoglobulin content of the serum, it is the major immunoglobulin of most secretions[8] including tears, saliva, colostrum and milk, the mucus of the respiratory tract (excluding the alveolus) and the gastrointestinal tract. It is synthesized by plasma cells which face the external environment[9, 10].

The sequence of events when antigenic material enters the gut is sum-

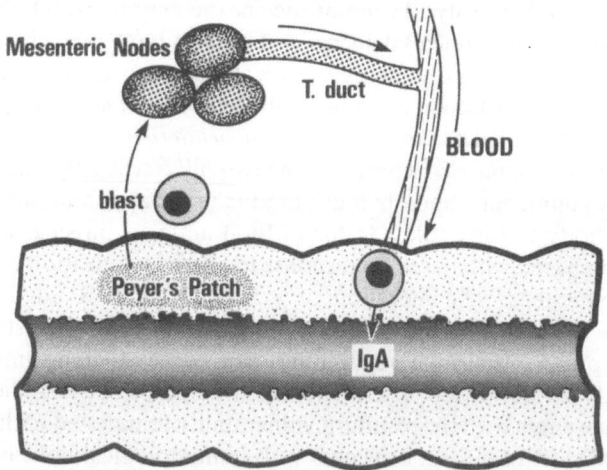

Figure 5.1 Sequence of events following oral immunization. Sensitization occurs in the Peyer's patch. IgA-precursors migrate via the mesenteric lymphatics and thoracic duct to the systemic circulation and then selectively home back to the intestinal lamina propria where IgA is synthesized. During lactation these cells also home to the acini of the mammary glands. (Modified from Lamm, 1976)[5]

marized in Figure 5.1. Following penetration of the outer epithelial cell layer of the intestinal mucosa, antigen is presented to B lymphocytes within the Peyer's patch. However, immediate transformation into an antibody-secreting plasma cell does not occur. Following sensitization the Peyer's patch B lymphocytes migrate to the mesenteric lymph nodes, where they begin the process of differentiation into plasmablasts. From the mesenteric nodes the plasmablasts pass via the thoracic duct into the systemic circulation. They then exhibit the remarkable property of selective homing back to the intestinal lamina propria from whence they originated, and upon their return they complete their transformation into actively secreting IgA plasma cells. These steps will now be considered in detail.

PENETRATION OF THE INTESTINAL EPITHELIUM BY ANTIGEN

Peyer's patches lack an afferent lymphatic, so that antigen must enter them by some different route. After measuring the clearance rate of different sized molecules from the blood of perfused rabbit intestine, Loehry and his colleagues[11, 12] suggested a hypothetical 'pore' size of 8–12 Å which allows water and other small molecular weight solutes to diffuse passively. The existence of such pores conflicts however with the demonstrable tight junctions which are present between epithelial cells, and this incongruity has not been resolved. Secondly, material is pinocytosed by villous epithelial cells, transported through the cell cytoplasm and exocytosed into the lamina propria, for removal by way of the villous microvasculature and lacteals to the portal vein tributaries and to the intestinal lymphatics. This route of entry is probably the major one involved in the absorption of nutritional material[13]. In ungulates and many other lower mammals very large molecules achieve entry in this way during the neonatal period. The newborn ungulate is born agammaglobulinaemic and absorbs large quantities of intact IgG (mol. wt. 160 000) from maternal colostrum and milk. At the end of the first 24 hours of life the newborn foal has a serum IgG equal to or even greater than that of its mother[14, 15]. At this stage the epithelial cells of the small intestine, which have a life span of only about 24 hours, are replaced by fresh cells which, though morphologically similar, do not have the capacity for such avid absorption of macromolecules of this size. This phenomenon of 'closure' is seen in many mammals including rodents[16], ruminants[17] and pigs[18], but it does not appear to occur in humans. The human neonate is born with a serum IgG acquired *in utero*, by transplacental diffusion from and in equal concentration to the serum of its mother. Unlike the species mentioned above, the feeding or withholding of maternal colostrum does not affect the serum immunoglobulin concentration of human newborns[19], suggesting that there is no transient hyperpermeable state, and abrupt perinatal changes in permeability of the intestines to macromolecules do not normally occur.

There also exists a specific route of entry for macromolecules for presentation to B lymphocytes. In 1974 Owen and Jones[20] studied the morphology of Peyer's patches with the transmission and scanning electron microscopes, and they described a cell always found in association with the lymphoid follicles. Unlike the adjacent epithelial cells, they had no microvilli and were often recessed below the level of the surrounding cells (Figure 5.2).

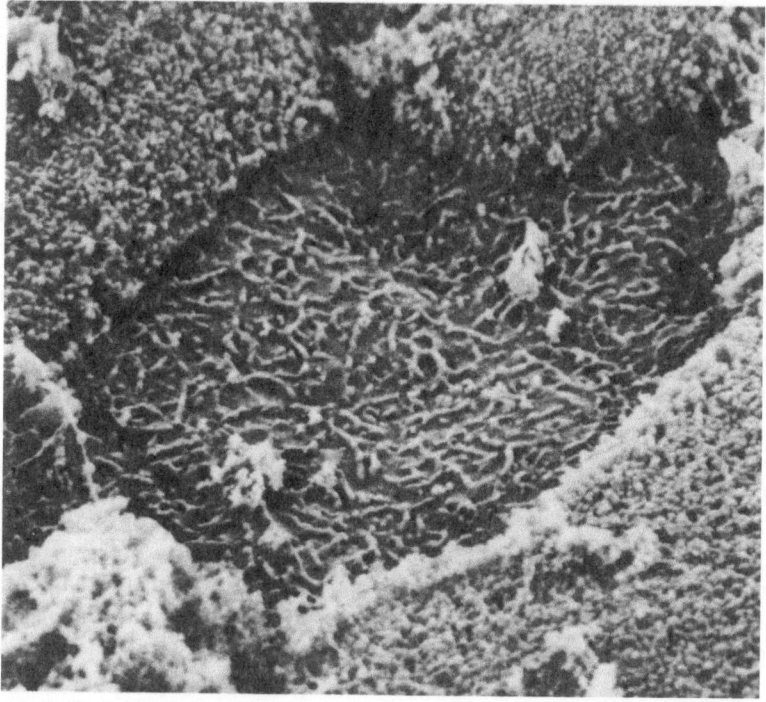

Figure 5.2 Scanning electron micrograph of the surface of a human M cell. Microfolds converge, diverge and end abruptly. Mucus obscures the bottom left-hand corner. The M-cell surface appears recessed below the level of the adjacent columnar epithelial cells and, unlike them, the M cell has no surface microvilli. (× 4500) (From Owen, 1974[20]. Reproduced by permission of the author and Messrs. William & Wilkins Co., Baltimore)

Under the scanning electron microscope the surface of these cells appeared wrinkled or thrown into folds. They were called therefore 'microfold cells' abbreviated shortly afterwards to 'M cells'. Their extraordinary morphology reflects both their pinocytotic capability and their close functional relationship with the lymphocytes of Peyer's patches. The nucleus of the M cell is situated quite deeply in the epithelial cell monolayer; the overlying cytoplasm is highly attenuated and forms a network of filaments or strands. Lymphocytes migrate into the interstices of these cytoplasmic strands or 'microfolds' and, so to speak, peer into the gut lumen through this cytoplasmic lace curtain. Using horseradish peroxidase Owen subsequently showed[21] that luminal material initially adheres to the surface of the M cell and is then avidly pinocytosed. Within 1 hour this material is transported through the M-cell cytoplasm and exocytosed into the extracellular space wherein lies the waiting lymphocyte. The lymphocyte pinocytoses the material, migrates out of the M-cell net, and is replaced by a fresh lymphocyte (Figure 5.3). Although M cells appear to fulfil the function of a macrophage in presenting material to lymphocytes, the available evidence suggests that they are derived from the intestinal columnar epithelial cells (Owen, personal communication). The lymphocytes which lodge temporarily alongside are T lymphocytes. In all mammalian species so far studied, M cells are found throughout the gut, wherever Peyer's patch lymphoid follicles exist, including the appendix[20,21,21a]. They are peculiar to the intestines and are not found in any other mucous membrane, including the tracheo-bronchial tree[22].

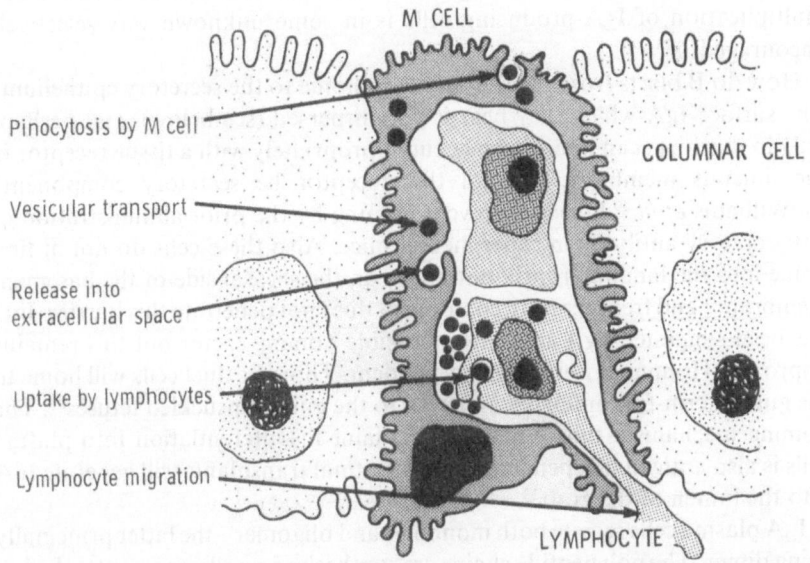

Figure 5.3 Schematic diagram showing the sequential uptake of antigen by an M cell, transport of antigen through the M-cell cytoplasm into the 'extracellular space' where it is pinocytosed by a T lymphocyte and removed for subsequent presentation to IgA precursor cells within the Peyer's patch. (Modified from Owen, 1977)[21]

Following passage through the M cell and uptake by T lymphocytes, antigen is presented to B lymphocytes within the Peyer's patch. Peyer's patches possess very few plasma cells, and little antibody is secreted there. The majority of cells present are B blasts, and of these 85% bear surface IgA. Transformation does not occur within the Peyer's patch and intracellular IgA is infrequently observed at these sites, contrasting markedly with the situation in the draining mesenteric nodes and thoracic duct[23]. It is not known where the preponderant B lymphocytes of Peyer's patches arise. The rate of mitosis in Peyer's patch tissue is incompatible with this being a central source of B cells, and it does not appear to be a mammalian bursa-equivalent as was first thought[24]. The IgA blasts seem undoubtedly to have been derived originally from IgM-bearing precursors. Indeed, phylogenetically the oldest immuno-globulin-producing cell produces IgM. At some point during B-cell matur-ation switching occurs, which induces a cell bearing surface IgM to produce either IgM, IgG or IgA[25]. The switching pathway does not appear to be IgM → IgG → IgA, but IgG and IgA are switched independently from each other. IgA-bearing cells thus represent a terminal differentiation event[26]. Cells committed ultimately to produce IgA localize in mucous membranes, especially those of the gut and respiratory tract. Cells not yet committed to an immunoglobulin class when they reach these sites are also induced to differentiate into IgA-producing cells. Thus the subsequent division and multiplication of IgA-producing cells is in some unknown way selectively encouraged[27, 28].

How do B blasts from the thoracic duct home to the secretory epithelium? The surface IgA which they bear is polydispersed (see below), and perhaps only in this form can interaction occur appropriately with a tissue receptor in the mucous membrane[5]. Could this receptor be secretory component? McWilliams et al.[29] failed to prevent homing by the prior administration of antisecretory antibody in experimental mice. Also these cells do not at first home into the lamina propria but arrive on the serosal side of the basement membrane; and free secretory component does not penetrate this barrier. IgD has been suggested by Lamm[5] as a possible homing factor but this remains unproven. Homing is not antigen dependent. Thoracic duct cells will home to the gut of germ-free animals[30] and even to the gut of unsuckled fetuses[31]. The homing mechanism thus remains unexplained. Differentiation into plasma cells is also antigen independent; fetal intestinal transplants will generate IgA into the lumen of the graft[32].

IgA plasma cells secrete both monomer and oligomer – the latter principally being dimer. The polypeptide chains are synthesized on ribosomes attached to the membranes of the endoplasmic reticulum. Bonding of the H and L chains takes place within the cisternae before the assembled molecule is secreted by the Golgi apparatus. Polydispersion occurs extracellularly, very close to the moment of secretion[33], and its extent is dependent on the amount of J chain present. The J chains are synthesized by the same plasma cells and are divalent[34]. IgA which remains monomeric and is not bound to other IgA molecules by J chain is the source of IgA in the serum. It has no observed function and is cleared by the liver rapidly and excreted in the bile[35].

Dimeric IgA exists in two forms: IgA_1 and IgA_2, depending on the configuration of the covalent bonds between the H and L chains (Figure 5.4)[36, 37]. In vitro, IgA_2 is more resistant to enzymic proteolysis than IgA_1 and is present in secretions in the proportions of $IgA_1 : IgA_2 \simeq 2.5 : 1$, twice the proportion of IgA_2 monomer found in the serum. This selective increase in the proportion of IgA_2 in secretions may be regarded therefore as a molecular evolutionary advance.

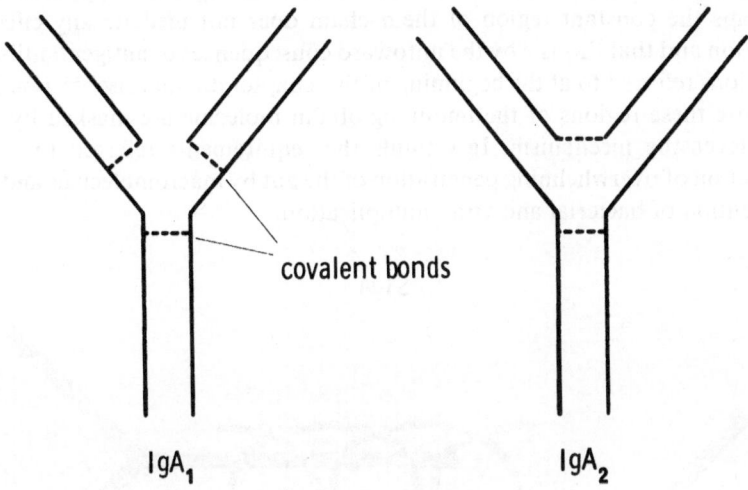

Figure 5.4 The two subclasses of IgA differ in respect of the arrangement of covalent bonds between the heavy and light chains. This, together with differences in the amino acid sequences at the hinge region of the H chain renders IgA_2 considerably more resistant to proteolysis than IgA_1. (Modified from Grey et al., 1968)[36]

Following the secretion by the plasma cell and polydispersion, IgA dimer couples with secretory component, which is a small molecular weight protein synthesized by the epithelial cells of the gut lumen. Secretory component (SC) is produced only by secretory epithelial cells and by no others[34, 38], and binds with IgA dimer. Binding occurs on the plasma membrane of the epithelial cell[39] where SC acts as a receptor for the newly synthesized dimer. Once binding has occurred the compound is pinocytosed by the epithelial cell and is transported to the luminal surface where it is exocytosed into the lumen. Secretory component confers considerable resistance to proteolysis of IgA both by the intracellular enzymes during transit through the epithelial cell and also by the intraluminal gut proteases. Thus the finished product of the plasma cell is 'secretory IgA' (SIgA) – two molecules of IgA bound together by one molecule of J chain and one molecule of SC (Figure 5.5). SIgA has unique properties, some of which have been referred to. It is a protein, and to be effective in the proteolytic atmosphere of the gut lumen it must resist enzymic digestion. This it achieves principally by being bound to SC and partly by the bonding configuration of its H and L chains. It is not cytophilic and does not fix complement by the classical pathway, although it may be able to activate the alternative complement pathway[6, 7]. It does not act as an opsonin[5]. It binds at its variable regions to ingested antigens, and as these complexes are not absorbed[40, 41], the ingress of foreign macromolecules is hampered. It also binds to bacterial and viral antigens and prevents their adhesion to the epithelial plasma membrane[42], an essential prelude to endocytosis and to bacterial or viral multiplication[43]. It has reasonably been suggested that perhaps the constant region of the α-chain does not mediate any effector function and that this is why the untoward consequences of antigen/antibody reactions referred to at the beginning of this chapter do not arise[5, 44], possibly because these regions of the immunoglobulin molecule are masked by SC. Whatever the mechanism, IgA fulfils the requirements referred to – the inhibition of overwhelming penetration of the gut by macromolecules and the prevention of bacterial and viral multiplication.

SIgA

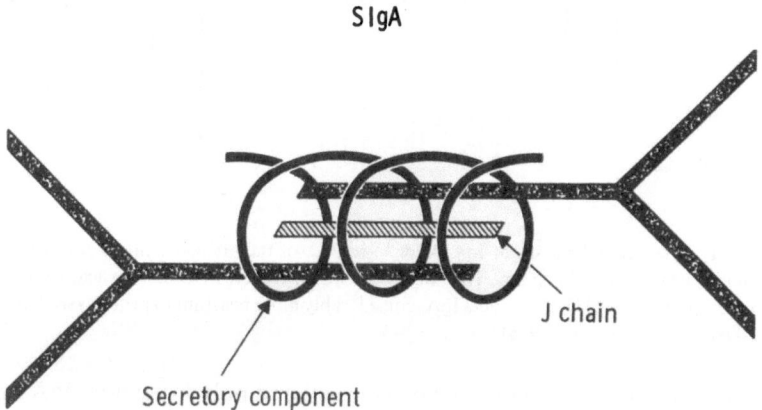

Secretory component

J chain

Figure 5.5 Diagrammatic representation of a molecule of secretory IgA (SIgA). Two molecules of IgA are bound by one molecule of J chain and one molecule of secretory component (SC). (Modified from Heremans, 1969)[198]

IgA-producing cells lack an immunological memory[45, 46] and in contrast to IgM producers[47] are the most thymus dependent of the B-cell family. Their dependency is directed towards the proliferation of plasma cells and the promotion of antibody secretion[48, 49], and in this way the relationship between T and M cells forms an essential link in the sensitization of IgA plasma cell precursors[21]. Nude mice are severely deficient in IgA, and the administration of T cells repairs the IgA deficit[50]. In man, thymic dysfunction is often associated with diminished IgA production[51, 52], despite the fact that such patients have normal numbers of IgA-bearing peripheral blood lymphocytes which are capable of synthesizing and secreting IgA in response to mitogens *in vitro*. The raised levels of IgM often found in these patients may represent a compensatory mechanism. They may, on the other hand, indicate a failure of T cells to initiate switching from IgM-bearing precursors.

IgA present in serum might be regarded as an 'overspill', a way of clearing non-functioning IgA monomer. It does not contribute to secretory IgA (SIgA), which is secreted entirely locally[53]. The evidence for this comes from several sources. In infants, SIgA is found in the tears and saliva before IgA appears in the serum[54,55]. Dysenteric stools contain antibody to *Shigella* before it is detectable in the serum[56]. If polio virus is administered parenterally as Salk vaccine, no anti-polio virus antibody appears in the secretions and the serum response is predominantly IgG. If polio virus is given orally, on the other hand, large amounts of SIgA directed against polio virus are found in the secretions of the nasopharynx and intestines together with an IgG response in the serum.

A lack of IgA is the commonest of immune deficiencies and is found in one in 700 individuals[57]. Many such individuals are in normal good health but there is nevertheless an increased incidence of recurrent sinopulmonary infections and gastrointestinal infections[58]. There is also an increased incidence of antibodies to foods[60,61] and an increase in reticulin antibodies and other autoimmune phenomena, perhaps because ingested antigens stimulate the production of circulating antibody which cross-reacts with autoantigens.

IMMUNE TOLERANCE

Apart from the protective factors which operate at the level of the gastrointestinal mucosa there exists a separate mechanism to prevent inappropriate immune responses to ingested and absorbed macromolecules. If a hapten such as dinitrochlorobenzene or picryl chloride is injected intracutaneously a local, cell-mediated immune reaction results. If an experimental animal is first given the hapten orally and it is subsequently injected intracutaneously, there is no immune response to the injection[62-64]. If the portal vein is anastomosed to the inferior vena cava, bypassing the liver, this tolerance by prior feedings of the hapten is abolished and full cutaneous sensitivity is maintained[65,66]. The mechanism whereby oral feeding induces tolerance and the precise role played by the liver is not yet known, though this phenomenon is likely to be crucially important in the normal immunological functioning of the digestive system and in the pathogenesis of gastrointestinal allergies.

PATHOGENESIS OF FOOD ALLERGIES

We should now consider how the foregoing relates to the development of food allergies. Occasionally food intolerance may develop *de novo* in an otherwise healthy and immune-intact adult. How this arises is unknown, though some individuals will report that the allergy was preceded by a severe infection, usually gastroenteritis. In neonates and small children gastroenteritis may

sufficiently damage the intestinal epithelium to cause a transient disaccharidase deficiency and also to allow the temporary ingress of whole milk proteins
and lead to cow's milk sensitization[67]. This may be one mechanism whereby a
previously healthy adult becomes sensitized to food proteins, especially since
jejunal biopsy of milk-allergic infants shows a deranged epithelium across
which macromolecules may more readily pass[68, 69].

Rarely, adult women may note the onset of catastrophic food allergies
which commence during the last trimester of a pregnancy or shortly after
delivery. How the two events may relate is unclear. Immune responses during
pregnancy are altered and it is possible that α-fetoprotein may be one factor
responsible for this. Murgita and Tomasi[70, 71] showed that α-fetoprotein has a
powerful suppressive effect on both T and B lymphocytes. Of the B series,
those most thymus dependent (i.e. IgA plasma cell precursors) are those most
sensitive to the suppressive activity of α-fetoprotein.

In the majority of patients with food allergy the allergic state develops in
infancy or childhood and a number of factors are known to operate, both
genetic and environmental[72, 73]. An infant born to an atopic parent is more
likely to develop food allergy than an infant without this familial trait. Infants
fed at their mother's breast and not given formula feeds derived from cow's
milk are less likely to develop subsequent milk allergy whether there is a
genetic predisposition or not (Table 5.1). This raises questions about the

Table 5.1 Relation between breast feeding and
bottle feeding and atopy in parents in 72 milk-
allergic children (Buisseret, 1978)[73]

	Bottle fed	Breast fed
Parental atopy	43	19
No parental atopy	10	0

relevance of breast feeding to the subsequent development of food allergy.
Amman and Stiehm[19] showed that the concentration of IgA in colostrum and
breast milk is very high and greatly exceeds that of the other major immunoglobulin classes (Figure 5.6). The IgA in these secretions is synthesized
by the plasma cells of the mammary acini and has the full configuration of
secretory IgA. The IgA plasma cell precursors arising in the Peyer's patches of
the intestine home not only to the intestinal lamina propria as described above
but, during lactation only, also home to the secretory acini of the mammary
tissues. It will be recalled that these cells are sensitized specifically to gut-
derived antigens. When they home to lactating breast tissue the resulting SIgA
produced in colostrum and milk is specifically directed against gut-derived
antigen[74–76]. When the neonate suckles at the maternal breast the SIgA
contained in the colostrum and milk is neither digested nor absorbed[19] but
remains intact within the neonatal gut and can ultimately be recovered intact

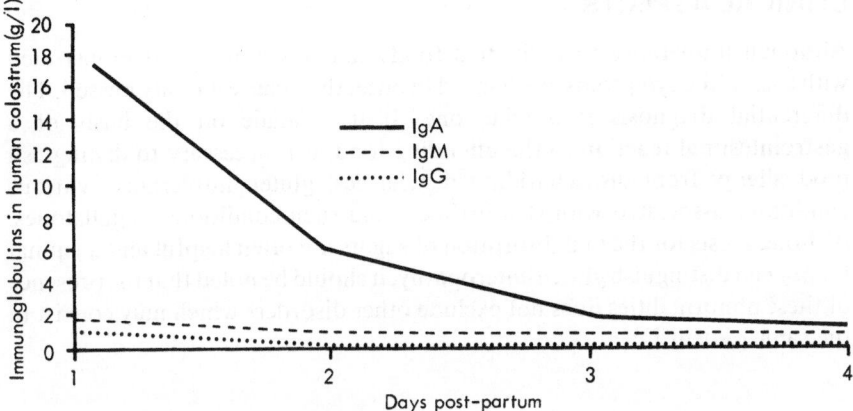

Figure 5.6   Concentrations of IgA. IgG and IgM in human colostrum and milk (Modified from Amman and Stiehm. 1966)[19]

in the neonatal faeces. During the passage of this colostral and milk SIgA through the infant gut, the luminal epithelial surface is thus protected not only from bacterial and viral adherence but also from the incursion of food antigens. Thus the infant denied colostrum and milk is exposed to foreign bovine milk proteins at a time when the child is unable to produce its own IgA necessary to lessen the risk of sensitization. Once lactation is fully established, the human neonate receives about 1.5 grams/day of SIgA by this route[77].

It has been shown that non-breast-fed infants absorb intact bovine milk proteins. Delire and his colleagues[78] found that 96% of infants who were fed cow's milk 'formula' had circulating immune complexes to bovine proteins, as compared to 8% of breast-fed infants. The bovine proteins were complexed with transplacentally derived maternal IgG. Gunther *et al.*[79] found that the titre of bovine milk protein antibodies of bottle-fed infants was much higher than in those who had been breast fed. The relevance of these findings in clinical allergy will be discussed below.

In general, where tests are employed which are based on the agglutination of protein-coated particles, the presence of circulating antibodies to food proteins correlates only weakly with the presence or absence of allergy to that food. Almost 100% of neonates, for example, have circulating antibodies to bovine milk proteins, albeit mostly in fairly low titres[79]. The incidence of bovine milk allergy. while largely conjectural, is unlikely to exceed 10% of all newborns and is probably less. In general, the presence of IgE antibodies to food proteins, whether demonstrated by skin tests or by the radioallergo-sorbent test (RAST), correlates reasonably well with allergy to a number of specific foods. On the other hand, unequivocal allergy to bovine milk may exist in spite of a negative skin test[73] or RAST to that food. The problems of diagnosis in these cases will be discussed below.

CLINICAL ASPECTS

Although intolerance to individual foods can sometimes be demonstrated with ease, if the symptoms are delayed in onset their cause is easily missed. The differential diagnosis is a wide one. If it is made on the basis of a gastrointestinal reaction to the offending food, it is necessary to distinguish food allergy from disaccharidase deficiencies, gluten intolerance, various conditions associated with steatorrhoea, and such conditions as gallstones. Although tests for the malabsorption of sugars are often helpful and a jejunal biopsy can distinguish gluten enteropathy, it should be noted that the presence of these abnormalities does not exclude other disorders which may coexist in the same patient[80].

Food allergy and milk intolerance in childhood

As noted above, exposure to an ingested antigen can stimulate the production of secretory IgA antibody at the mucous surfaces, and a normal sequel to this is the development of a specific tolerance to the same antigen if it is later injected[81, 82]. When absorbed proteins *fail* to induce systemic tolerance this can be advantageous to the host if the protein is bacterial but highly damaging when the antigen concerned is a regularly ingested food such as cow's milk.

There are at least 20 proteins present in milk, but casein, α-lactalbumen, β-lactoglobulin and bovine serum albumen are responsible for most of the reactions that are observed. Reactions against single allergens are exceptional and two or more proteins are usually involved[83].

If, as Parish and his colleagues[84] suggest, experimental results can be extrapolated to man, the most extreme forms of hypersensitivity to milk may lead to cot deaths when small quantities of cow's milk are aspirated. In the more general experience, however, cow's milk intolerance is a cause of gastrointestinal symptoms and of asthma, eczema and rhinorrhoea in some cases. It is not clear what mechanisms determine whether a child is protected or susceptible. One suggestion that has been made is that a transient IgA deficiency predisposes to the development of cow's milk allergy[85, 86] but if true, this factor could operate in various ways – for example by modifying the intestinal flora or increasing the susceptibility to gastroenteritis[87]. This in turn, by causing mucosal damage, could allow an increased absorption of macromolecules and so stimulate the development of all types of antibody to foods. The effect of breast feeding on intestinal infection is also complex. In poor communities, for the baby to be fully protected against infective enteritis, breast milk has to be given alone, i.e. without additional cow's milk[88].

Changes in milk protein absorption cannot entirely explain the immunological effects that are seen in selective IgA deficiency. In the most severe form of this deficiency, circulating precipitins to cow's milk are often present[59]; but these antibodies are largely directed against bovine IgM[89], which is by no means the most common sensitizing protein in milk. The presence of this unexpected type of antibody suggests a defect in immune regulation. In support of this view, there is another state of partial immune deficiency – the much less common Wiskott–Aldrich syndrome – in which precisely the same type of milk antibodies are found.

Whatever the mechanism, the beneficial effect of antigen avoidance during the susceptible period of early life has been demonstrated by controlled trial studies, especially in babies with a family history of allergic disease[90]. In one such study it was suggested that an appropriate allergen-avoidance regime should include both breast feeding and measures against the house dust mite. In another study, breast feeding for a period of 6 months appeared to nullify any hereditary risks of food allergy (of whatever type) or of eczema[91]. Since this cannot be explained solely by the avoidance of cow's milk, it is possible that human milk has some kind of protective effect – for example, by coating the mucosa with SIgA. However, it is now well documented that breast feeding does not provide a complete protection against sensitization to cow's milk or to other foods contained in the milk of the lactating mother[92–94].

Pathological studies

When children intolerant to cow's milk are challenged with milk and then subjected to a jejunal biopsy within 24 hours, the changes which are seen range from a minor infiltrate of the villi with a variety of cells, including eosinophils, to villous atrophy that can be as pronounced as in coeliac disease[95, 96]. The evidence suggests an immediate hypersensitivity reaction, and Shiner[95] has suggested that this is followed by an Arthus type of reaction and a cellular delayed hypersensitivity response. In the lamina propria, an increase in immunocytes is seen, with cells which contain largely IgA and IgM but also IgE. Precipitating antibodies to dietary proteins are detectable in the blood but, as in gluten enteropathy, are probably only indirectly connected with the disease. By contrast with coeliac disease, antireticulin antibodies cannot usually be found[97]. The gut changes disappear on withdrawal of the offending food and reappear on rechallenge, with an increase in plasma cells and eosinophils and, in the more severe cases, the development of oedema, haemorrhage or fat necrosis. This is associated[98] with a rise in IgA and IgM in the intestinal secretions and an activation of serum complement.

As in many other immunological disorders, it is likely that more than one mechanism is involved. Circulating IgG antibodies to milk proteins are found, but they also occur frequently in other bowel disorders – notably in ulcerative colitis[99]. This suggests that they represent a secondary reaction to absorption of milk proteins, which is particularly likely to occur if the bowel wall is damaged or ulcerated. IgG antibodies of the 'short term sensitizing' type have been claimed to be of aetiological importance in some cases[100] and IgG or IgE, complexed with antigen, have also been suspected of being responsible for a number of late symptoms. In addition, it is possible that some of the clinical reactions which occur at a distance from the site of protein absorption are the 'metastatic' effects of mediators which are initially liberated in the gut[101].

Clinical studies

Intolerance to cow's milk can develop within days of its introduction into an infant's diet, but exceptionally it can also afflict the breast-fed infant whose mother drinks milk[93]. There are many additional cases in which cow's milk intolerance develops secondarily as a sequel to infective enteritis[102, 103], apparently as a result of damage to the small bowel mucosa and a consequent depletion of mucosal sugar-splitting enzymes[104]. The mechanism is not necessarily immunological but is a cause of prolonged diarrhoea even after the infection has cleared. By increasing the permeability of the mucosa to foreign protein in young infants, it may also provide a further predisposing factor for the development of a true allergy to cow's milk and other foods.

In a study carried out by Iyngkaran et al.[103], 23 infants with infective enteritis were subjected to jejunal biopsy before and after cow's milk challenge. No fewer than 18 infants developed histological changes in the mucosa after cow's milk, and in 17 of these the level of three mucosal disaccharidases – lactase, sucrase and maltase – were much reduced. Ten of these infants developed diarrhoea after cow's milk, usually with the presence of reducing sugar in the stools. In view of these findings, there is a good case for excluding cow's milk protein and lactose in those cases where an infant, while recovering from infective enteritis appears to develop a secondary sugar or milk intolerance.

Cow's milk intolerance is often transient[80, 83]. However, it may persist and even extend to other foods, one after another, including soya flour and other milk substitutes. This accords with Iyngkaran's suggestion that mucosal damage, by leading to increased mucosal permeability, allows the absorption of potentially antigenic food proteins in substantial amounts. Whereas the response to small quantities of absorbed proteins, in the experimental situation, is to induce tolerance[105], it is possible that there are factors which can modify this response, such as the actual amount of protein that is absorbed or the question of whether the absorption route which this protein follows is the physiological pathway outlined earlier.

Symptoms

The 'immediate' symptoms of milk allergy, occurring within an hour, include a full-blown anaphylactic reaction, with vomiting, diarrhoea, hypotension and bronchospasm in the most severe cases. Each of these symptoms can occur alone, as may swelling of the lips and mouth, abdominal pain, and bloating or rhinorrhoea. 'Late' symptoms also occur after an interval of more than an hour. In some cases repeated challenges are necessary over days or weeks before asthma, eczema, or some of the more insidious gastrointestinal reactions develop.

Gross intestinal bleeding is an occasional symptom[106], with diarrhoea stools in which blood is intermingled. Proctoscopy shows a friable intestinal mucosa which bleeds easily. Wilson *et al.*[107] reported that the cow's milk sensitive infant can also develop iron deficiency anaemia as a result of occult intestinal bleeding, but large quantities of milk are probably required to produce such effects. Intestinal absorption of fat is impaired in some milk sensitive children with or without eosinophilia[108, 80] and, occasionally, gluten enteropathy and milk intolerance coexist. Growth retardation and psychological disturbances may also be prominent features in some cases[73].

Waldmann and his colleagues[109] described six children who had diarrhoea, vomiting, hypoproteinaemia, anaemia and eosinophilia, together with such other symptoms as rhinorrhoea, bronchial asthma, and eczema. The feeding of milk was capable of increasing both the symptoms and the protein loss in some cases, with improvement after the introduction of a milk-free diet. Mucosal biopsies were normal except for an eosinophilic infiltration of the lamina propria in three patients.

Diagnosis and management

As noted above, postinfective disorders of the bowel may give rise to deficiencies of sugar splitting enzymes and either mimic cow's milk allergy or coexist with it. Tests for the malabsorption of sugars may be useful in such cases[110]. Diagnostic tests for the presence of milk allergy are less helpful, however, since skin tests and radioallergosorbent tests for specific foods are seldom positive at this age. Challenge tests remain the most useful way of establishing a diagnosis of milk intolerance with certainty before initiating a long-term milk exclusion diet, with all the problems which that involves. At least two dietary elimination periods and at least one challenge are required[83], and in these circumstances there are considerable advantages in the procedure advocated by Walker-Smith and Phillips[111]. Small intestinal biopsy is carried out at diagnosis, repeated some time after withdrawal of the offending protein, and followed at once by a challenge test. If symptoms develop, a further biopsy is carried out. The same procedure has been used in transient gluten intolerance[112] and in soya protein intolerance[113].

The withdrawal of milk from the diet is essential in severe cases, but cautious reintroduction after 6 months or more has often demonstrated the transient nature of the condition. The prophylactic use of oral disodium cromoglycate is discussed below.

Food allergies in adults

In the adult a substantial minority of patients with asthma also have a history of specific food intolerance. On the other hand, gastrointestinal symptoms suggestive of food intolerance can be due to a variety of causes, which include disaccharidase deficiency, gluten enteropathy, cystic fibrosis and galactos-aemia, and such indirect causes as gallstones, psychiatric illness, low-grade intestinal infections, and the pharmacological effects of histamine or other natural ingredients of certain foods. When these causes are excluded and a gastrointestinal allergy is suspected, both food and non-food substances still need to be considered. Drugs or antibiotics may be involved, as in patients who react to traces of penicillin in the milk of penicillin-treated cows. In addition, reactions occur to food additives such as monosodium glutamate[114], colouring agents such as tartrazine, and preservatives such as benzoic acid[115]. Some of the foods to be implicated are listed in Table 5.2, but the list could

Table 5.2 Foods causing symptoms of intolerance in 100 patients (Lessof *et al.*, 1980)[121]

Milk	46	Artificial colours	7
Eggs	40	Pork/bacon	7
Nuts/peanuts	22	Chicken	6
Fish/shellfish	22	Tomato	6
Wheat/flour	9	Soft fruits	6
Chocolate	8	Cheese (not milk)	6

Also: yeast (3), banana, beef, cucumber, onion, pine-apple, sweetcorn, tea/coffee (2 each), apple, celery, cream, ginger, marmite, peas, potato, quails, soya, sultanas (1 each)

be considerably longer. Despite some variations, most reports emphasize milk, egg, fish, wheat, and many give a prominent place to chocolate and soft fruit[116]. The importance of wheat intolerance in some reported series may have derived from the inclusion of patients with gluten enteropathy, but it is clear that cases of non-gluten wheat intolerance also occur[117].

Apart from the more dramatic symptoms such as vomiting, diarrhoea or abdominal pain, gastrointestinal effects are similar to those seen in children and include abdominal distension, constipation, and various symptoms associated with malabsorption or protein-losing enteropathy. Exceptionally, a haemorrhagic proctitis can occur[118]. Allergic symptoms also develop outside the intestinal tract which are nevertheless food induced or 'alimentary'. The smell of food can provoke rhinitis or asthma; local contact can provoke angioedema of the face or mouth; and a considerable time after the food has been ingested, symptoms ranging from headache to bronchial asthma, urticaria and eczema are seen. In the most severe cases acute anaphylactic reactions and shock occur within minutes of contact with the offending substance.

A number of other gastrointestinal syndromes are known to be associated with allergic causes (Table 5.3), including the milk-induced gastrointestinal bleeding[107] which has been referred to above. Eosinophilic gastroenteritis is another uncommon syndrome characterized by diffuse eosinophilic infiltration of the pyloric region, associated with peripheral blood eosinophilia in the absence of intestinal parasites or vasculitis, neoplasm or other recognized causes. On jejunal biopsy, it is sometimes associated with blunting of the villi and submucosal oedema[119]. The diagnosis can be confirmed if the patient responds to a provocative challenge with suspected foods[120]; but this response

Table 5.3   Gastrointestinal allergy syndromes

---

1. Food-related gastrointestinal symptoms (vomiting, diarrhoea, pains, bloating, constipation)

2. Secondary syndromes (steatorrhoea and 'coeliac-like' syndromes, protein losing enteropathy, blood loss and iron deficiency anaemia, eosinophilic gastroenteritis)

3. Remote effects (anaphylaxis, rhinorrhoea, serous otitis media, asthma, eczema, urticaria, angioedema)

---

is by no means invariable. However, evidence of food allergy is worth pursuing since the response to dietary restriction or to an intravenous or elemental diet can be dramatic[119]. Yet another syndrome needs consideration. It is not uncommon for milk intolerance to develop as a secondary effect in ulcerative colitis or haemorrhagic proctitis, possibly as a further result of defects of sugar splitting enzymes.

Diagnosis

The problem of diagnosis depends partly on the difficulty in distinguishing food allergy from food fads and anxiety states. When reactions occur after a delay of an hour or more, there may be little to suggest, either to patient or doctor, that foods are responsible. This is especially so in conditions such as milk-induced eczema in which occasional small amounts of the offending food are often well tolerated. It may require repeated challenges with substantial quantities of the offending food before a cumulative effect is seen and an eczematous reaction occurs, which often takes a considerable time to subside. The practice of excluding the suspect food and then giving a single food challenge, repeated after an interval, may not therefore reproduce the patient's symptoms. Furthermore, there are serious defects in the practice of giving a 'blind' challenge through a nasogastric tube, since a patient whose reaction is triggered by an oral or nasal stimulus will give a false negative reaction in this type of test. Where it is thought desirable to introduce a 'blind' element, it is preferable to give prophylactic capsules which cannot be identified by the patient, followed by an open challenge (or challenges) with the appropriate food. The capsules may contain salicylate[121], cromoglycate, or placebo.

In seeking diagnostic confirmation, skin prick tests and radioallergosorbent tests are both useful, provided that satisfactory test extracts are available. Most patients with egg, fish or nut intolerance give positive skin reactions, especially when their symptoms are of the immediate variety. However, it is only a minority of patients with milk intolerance who have positive tests, even when the alternative diagnosis of disaccharidase deficiency appears to have been excluded (see Table 5.4). In patients with negative IgE tests, the question

Table 5.4   Diagnostic tests in 100 cases of specific food intolerance (after Lessof et al., 1980)[121]

Food	No. of patients	Positive skin tests	Positive RAST	Total patients with +ve tests*	% of patients with positive tests
Milk	46	12	3	14 (1)	30
Egg	40	23	19	30 (12)	75
Nuts	22	10	14	16 (8)	73
Fish	22	16	8	17 (7)	77

* Number in brackets had both positive skin tests and RAST

therefore arises whether tests for other types of antibody – such as precipitating, or short-term sensitizing, IgG antibodies – may provide diagnostic help. As yet such tests have not been able to discriminate reliably between symptomatic patients and healthy controls[121]. Another approach to the problem has been that of Haddad et al. [122], who have noted that patients who have negative skin tests with raw milk may nevertheless have specific IgE in their serum which reacts with milk digests. Although this work awaits confirmation, there are other instances in which foods may be allergenic in one form but not in another. For example, allergic reactions may be seen with raw apple but not after cooking[123] and some patients may be allergic to boiled fish, others to fresh fish[124].

In the difficult case, for example in cases of suspected milk allergy where prolonged dietary restriction is envisaged, jejunal biopsy may be undertaken on an appropriately restricted diet, followed by a challenge with the suspect food. If symptoms then develop, the biopsy can be repeated[68].

Remote manifestations of food allergy

Manifestations outside the intestinal tract are common in cases of food intolerance. Asthma or eczema was noted in 64 out of 100 of our own food intolerant patients and all but seven of the remainder had symptoms that extended beyond the gut, including urticaria or angioedema in 22 and rhinorrhoea (with or without gastrointestinal symptoms) in seven. The serum IgE levels in these patients are represented in Figure 5.7 which also shows the incidence of positive confirmatory tests to the specific foods involved – either skin prick tests or RAST.

Many of our patients with asthma or eczema were themselves aware that they had more than one type of allergy. With this in mind, we used the RAST method to look for IgE antibodies to three common inhaled allergens in their serum. An associated allergy to grass pollen, dust mite or cat was thus diagnosed in 49 out of 64 patients with asthma or eczema, including all 16

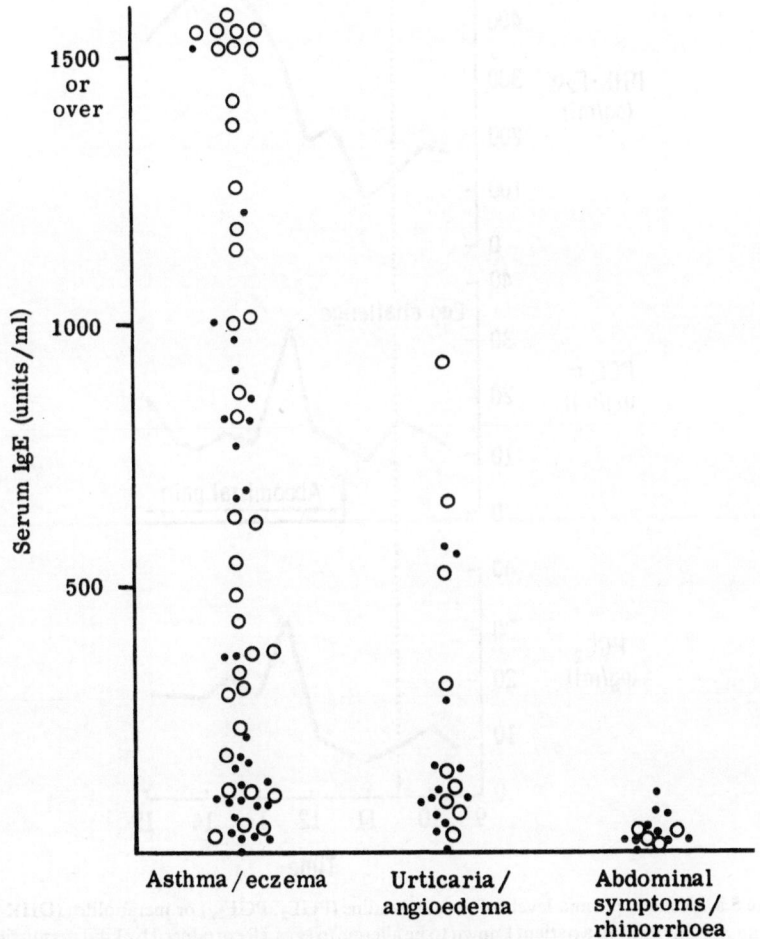

Figure 5.7   Serum IgE levels in 100 patients with food intolerance

Column 1: Patients with asthma or eczema (including those with other symptoms).

Column 2: Patients with urticaria or angioedema, *excluding* patients in column 1.

Column 3: Patients with abdominal symptoms or rhinorrhoea, excluding those in columns 1 and 2.

(○) Patients with positive food allergy tests.

(●) Patients with negative food allergy tests

patients with an IgE level of over 1000 units/ml. A point of interest, however, was the presence of a subgroup with 'low-IgE asthma' and negative tests. This subgroup included five patients who had milk intolerance, IgE levels below 40 units/ml, negative skin tests and RAST, and no evidence of IgG antibodies.

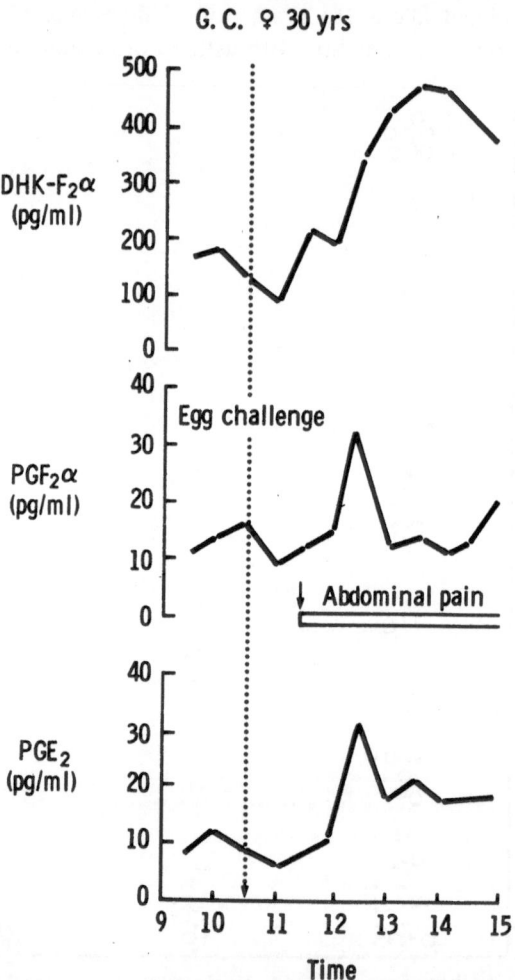

Figure 5.8 Venous plasma levels of prostaglandins (PGE$_2$, PGF$_{2\alpha}$) or metabolites (DHK-F$_{2\alpha}$) after an egg challenge in a patient known to be allergic to eggs. (Reproduced by kind permission of Dr L. J. F. Youlten)

They nevertheless had asthmatic reactions, which sometimes developed an hour or more after drinking milk. This long-recognized form of 'alimentary asthma' appears to differ from asthma which is initiated by inhaled allergens or initiated reflexly after hyperventilation. It is presumably triggered by the systemic route after absorption of milk proteins from the gut and may indicate the transmitted effect of mediators which are first liberated in the gastro-intestinal tract. In keeping with this is the evidence that venous blood levels of prostaglandins rise after a food challenge in allergic subjects (Figure 5.8)[118] and raised plasma levels of histamine have been reported in food-induced and other types of urticaria[125]. Slow reacting substance (SRS-A), which is released from mast cells during allergic reactions, could also play a part through its constricting effect on the peripheral airways[126]. This theoretical concept needs further investigation.

Other explanations are possible for the systemic symptoms which are so common in food allergy. These include the possibility that immune complexes may trigger these symptoms, and such complexes could contain either IgG or IgE[127]. This could not easily explain the asthmatic attacks of patients who have no detectable IgG or IgE food antibodies, but whatever the explanation, if the mechanism of alimentary asthma differs from that of asthma caused by inhaled allergens, the therapeutic approach may need to be reconsidered. It is known, for example, that some asthmatic patients improve when they take aspirin[128]. If prostaglandin studies can identify aspirin-responsive patients or if it is confirmed that histamine measurements are abnormal in food-induced urticaria or in patients who have food-induced headaches, this may have considerable therapeutic implications.

Management of food allergy

The recognition of offending food allergens is the cornerstone of treatment, yet when several foods are involved, their elimination from the diet is by no means simple. In infancy, in cases in which cow's milk is the sole offending food the use of vegetable protein milks or protein hydrolysates is of value, as is goat's milk on occasions – though each of these may sometimes lead to renewed allergic reactions, directed against the milk substitute itself. More refined elemental diets are reserved for the exceptionally severe case.

In the older infant, once milk substitutes have been introduced, simple foods are added every few days, in order to assess which ones may be administered on a long-term basis and which should be excluded. The occasional ingestion of small amounts of the offending food is usually well tolerated. Spontaneous remission is common in milk intolerance[83] especially in those cases which follow gastroenteritis[103]. For this reason, a further milk challenge every 6 months or so should help to determine whether a strict diet, with all its nutritional and psychological problems, needs to be continued. There is as yet no controlled trial evidence that sublingual or other forms of 'hyposensitization' produce a higher rate of remissions than is seen spontaneously.

The prophylactic use of oral disodium cromoglycate[129], now appears to provide a relatively simple approach to those cases where there are multiple food allergies or where there is a need to avoid a complex and restricted diet[130, 131]. Symptoms which may remit with this treatment include some which are not usually acknowledged as being attributable to food reactions, such as fever, polyarthritis, joint pains, lassitude, irritability and headache. This supports the view[73], that in food-intolerant subjects unusual symptoms should not be dismissed as psychogenic without careful enquiry.

Disodium cromoglycate tends to reduce rather than abolish the more severe reactions[132]; and it is not entirely without its adverse effects. Although few reactions are seen in healthy subjects, headache, rhinorrhoea and urticaria have occurred sufficiently often in a double blind trial[130] to suggest that subjects who react adversely to foods may also be unduly sensitive to chemicals such as cromoglycate.

An intriguing observation is that oral cromoglycate can also benefit a coexisting allergic rhinitis. There is, however, no evidence that this is a direct effect of this treatment. It is the common experience of patients who have allergic reactions to more than one allergen – for example to animal fur and grass pollen – that exacerbations of one type of allergy may lower the threshold for reacting to an unrelated allergen. It seems probable that the reverse is also true and that measures which improve allergic reactions of one type may make the patient less likely to react to a second stimulus.

Occasionally, patients who complain mainly of diarrhoea or abdominal pain may be unwilling or unable to avoid the offending food and derive no benefit from oral cromoglycate. In such cases prostaglandin synthetase-inhibiting drugs may be effective in preventing the untoward reactions and allow an unrestricted diet to be followed while the patient remains on low-dose maintenance treatment with either aspirin or indomethacin[118].

The methods of treatment discussed so far have concerned the less extreme types of reaction. When anaphylaxis occurs, this still requires the immediate injection of adrenaline[133] or the use of comparable preparations in pressurized aerosol form, containing adrenaline or isoprenaline. Oral or injected anti-histamines also have a useful place, and it is possible that the H_2 receptor antagonist cimetidine will in some circumstances potentiate the effect of conventional antihistamine drugs[134].

GLUTEN ENTEROPATHY

The difficulty in identifying patients with an intolerance to specific foods is well seen in coeliac disease and in the adult type of gluten enteropathy. Gluten intolerance, and its indirect consequences, can continue for many years, totally unrecognized despite its association with malabsorption, aphthous ulceration and anaemia or, in children, with short stature and poor growth. By the time adult life is reached, there is also atrophy of the spleen and other lymphatic tissue in up to 50% of cases. Indeed, the presence of Howell–Jolly bodies in the peripheral blood film may suggest the diagnosis in previously unsuspected cases.

A jejunal biopsy demonstrates villous atrophy of the small bowel mucosa, with basement membrane thickening and infiltration of the submucosa by lymphocytes, eosinophils and plasma cells[135–137]. A similar sensitivity to gluten can be found in approximately 60% of patients with dermatitis herpetiformis, a condition in which there is a recurrent, itching vesicular rash[138]. The gastrointestinal symptoms are usually milder in dermatitis herpetiformis than in coeliac disease. As in coeliac disease they respond to a gluten-free diet, though the skin eruption responds more slowly and may take several months to clear[139, 140].

Quite apart from dermatitis herpetiformis, the other disorders that have been reported in patients with gluten enteropathy often have features suggesting an immunological basis. Asthma, eczema and hay fever have been noted in 10 (29%) of 35 patients with gluten enteropathy but only in 5% of controls[141]. Diabetes mellitus, thyroid disease, liver disease, glomerulonephritis, and ulcerative colitis are also more common than expected[142, 143]. The association which has perhaps aroused the greatest interest of all has been with diffuse interstitial lung disease[144, 145]. Since avian precipitins may be present in such cases, Berrill and his colleagues[146] reviewed 16 patients who had been diagnosed as having bird fancier's lung. All had a history of recent exposure to birds and had avian precipitins in their blood. Eight had features of malabsorption, and of these, five proved to have jejunal villous atrophy. The response of these patients to a gluten-free diet suggested a true gluten enteropathy, and the question then arose whether sensitization to avian antigens might occur in such cases because of absorption through an abnormal intestinal mucosa. Once again, the 'leaky gut' syndrome could explain a number of secondary effects. The leakage of proteins could provide the means by which these patients become sensitized to the subsequent inhalation of avian antigen. In support of this view, nine out of 26 patients with coeliac disease have been reported as having avian antibodies but were found to differ from patients with bird fancier's lung by possessing a different type of antibody. They were found to have precipitins that react with a component of hen egg yolk – but not with the antigens (present in bird droppings) to which bird fanciers produce their reaction[147].

In gluten enteropathy other immunological abnormalities may also be found on investigation. Antinuclear antibodies, parietal cell and antithyroid antibodies are found in a significant number of patients[148, 149] and up to 50% have antireticulin antibodies. The antireticulin antibodies increase after a gluten challenge and can often be absorbed out by gluten, indicating a cross-reaction between the two substances. There also appear to be abnormalities affecting entire classes of immunoglobulins. IgA and IgM levels are increased in the jejunal secretions and contain antibodies with a specificity for gluten[150, 151]. Serum IgM levels may be low but rise on a gluten-free diet[152]; and in 2% of patients there is an isolated IgA deficiency, which persists after treatment[153], suggesting that this is independent of gluten enteropathy or may even predispose to it.

Pathologically, apart from the villous atrophy of the small bowel, there is evidence on immunofluorescence studies of an increase in the number of IgM- and IgG-containing cells in the mucosa and a decrease of cells containing IgA[154]. In both coeliac disease and dermatitis herpetiformis there is deposition of IgA and occasionally complement around the basement membrane of the small bowel mucosa[155]. In dermatitis herpetiformis, deposits of IgA and complement have also been demonstrated in the dermal papillae of skin even in the uninvolved areas[156] and although their specificity is unknown, circulating immune complexes are found in the blood[157].

Pathogenesis

Most of these findings have been interpreted as indicating a primary abnormality in the immune response to gluten. The resulting mucosal damage persists indefinitely unless a gluten-free diet is maintained[158]. Because of the multiplicity of autoantibodies and because of the immune complex test results, it has been suggested that tissue damage in the gut and skin are probably mediated by circulating immune complexes, formed between gluten and the corresponding antibody. If so, an Arthus-like reaction could account for some of the histological changes. The skin reactions to gluten subfractions that have been reported[159] could also represent a response to gluten.

An alternative explanation is possible. Autoantibodies, including antibodies to reticulin, could arise in a secondary response to the tissue damage which affects the small bowel mucosa. Strober and his colleagues[151] postulated that the initial cause of this type of damage might be a toxic effect of gluten peptides on susceptible mucosal cells. Mucosal cell susceptibility could, in this case, be due to a genetically determined enzyme deficiency. This is reminiscent of other non-immunological food reactions – for instance, the haemolytic anaemia induced by fava beans in cases of glucose-6-phosphate dehydrogenase deficiency.

The two theories concerning the aetiology of gluten enteropathy are not mutually exclusive. Many of the immunological findings could result from the leakage of antigenic material across the gut due to some other cause. Associated allergies are common, but the same is true of other conditions with bowel wall damage, such as ulcerative colitis[160]. The finding of antibody to gluten and other foods could also be due to increased absorption and is reminiscent of the findings in Crohn's disease[161]. Furthermore, in gluten enteropathy, the titre of these antibodies falls as the patient improves on a gluten-free diet[162, 163].

A genetic component in the pathogenesis of gluten-sensitive enteropathy has been suggested by the finding of HLA-B8 in approximately 80% of patients with this condition[164]. Despite the suggestion that this may be linked to the influence of an immune-response (*Ir*) gene, genetic linkages cannot be explained on so simple a basis. The well-known links between inflammatory disorders of connective tissue and HLA-B27 show a clear predilection for those disorders involving the sacroiliac joints and other synovial or uveal tissue. Reported links with HLA-B8, on the other hand, are predominantly with disorders of the gastrointestinal tract and endocrine organs.

INFLAMMATORY BOWEL DISEASE

Although Crohn's disease frequently involves the small intestine, can involve the upper gastrointestinal tract, and has other striking differences from ulcerative colitis, the two diseases have much in common and probably have both a clinical and a pathological relationship to one another. This view is supported by the occurrence of both diseases in close relatives and by their similar age, sex and geographical distribution[165].

Ulcerative colitis, which involves the mucosa and submucosa of the rectum and colon, varies in severity from the very mild case of proctitis to the fulminating case. It resembles Crohn's disease in having a number of extraintestinal manifestations such as erythema nodosum, uveitis, arthritis and liver disease. Diarrhoea, blood in the stools and abdominal pain remain the most common clinical features, together with the effects of blood and protein loss from the ulcerated bowel surface, fever, secondary infection and the further complications caused by anaemia and electrolyte disturbances. The mucosa is diffusely but superficially infiltrated with a variety of inflammatory cells, often with a striking eosinophilia. Crypt abscesses are common.

Crohn's disease, in contrast, involves a more deep ulceration, with fissures and fistula formation. Characteristically, thickening of the bowel wall reduces the lumen considerably. In acute Crohn's disease the mucosa is haemorrhagic, and even in the less acute forms it is oedematous and thickened in a patchy 'cobblestone' pattern. Inflammation extends to the serous surface, and the mesentery, lymphatics and mesenteric lymph nodes are all involved. Histologically, a lymphocytic and plasma cell infiltration in the bowel wall are sometimes associated with granuloma formation both in the bowel and draining lymph nodes. This has led to the speculation[166] that a defective clearing of macrophage-ingested material determines the granulomatous response that is so typical of the Crohn's lesion.

The associated extraintestinal manifestations in both conditions suggest that immunological reactions play an important part. In addition to those listed above, erythema multiforme, urticaria, sacroiliitis and spondylitis, pyoderma gangrenosa and thyoma have all been noted.

There is no evidence of any abnormality of serum or secretory immuno-globulins in these patients or of a defect in humoral or cellular immunity[167]. IgA- and IgG-containing cells are present in the rectal submucosa in increased numbers. Deposits of the C3 component of complement have also been noted, together with local antibodies to anaerobic bacteria[168], which have been variously thought to form immune complexes, leading to an Arthus reaction in the mucosa, or else to cross-react with colon antigens and cause tissue damage in that way. A number of circulating autoantibodies (including antibodies to colon) have been demonstrated by a variety of techniques; but they bear no relationship to the severity or stage of activity of the disease and persist long after total colectomy[169].

Aetiology and secondary phenomena

The evidence for a transmissible agent in either ulcerative colitis[170, 171] or Crohn's disease[172, 173] is still contentious. The increased risk of ulcerative colitis in infants who are weaned early[174] could be explained either by an increased risk of infective gastroenteritis or by early exposure to other antigenic stimuli. In Crohn's disease there is a significantly increased incidence of gastroenteritis in the first 6 months of life, regardless of the type of feeding[175].

From the immunological point of view, the complications which affect the skin, eyes, joints and liver may represent a response either to an infection or to tissue damage and breakdown caused in some other way. The difficulty in distinguishing between primary changes and those which are secondary to tissue damage is nowhere more clearly seen than in the association between inflammatory bowel disease and allergies to milk and other foods which have been reported[176]. Patients have significantly fewer reactions on a milk-free diet[177] and relapse may occur when milk is reintroduced. However, it has not been established whether a deficiency of sugar-splitting enzymes or some other non-immunological cause of milk intolerance may have played a part. Neither IgG nor IgE antibodies to milk protein appear to correlate with the patient's clinical condition[100, 178]. Any increase in circulating antibodies to milk protein could, in these circumstances, represent merely a reaction to an increased absorption of milk as part of a 'leaky gut' syndrome.

An increased incidence of asthma, rhinitis and eczema[160, 179] could also be explained as a secondary effect in inflammatory bowel disease. On the other hand, the reported high incidence of familial allergy may reflect the conscientiousness with which a questionnaire is completed by patients who are concerned about a serious illness. This finding therefore requires confirmation. Evidence of Type I allergy in inflammatory bowel disease, apart from this, is indirect and circumstantial – an increased number of circulating basophils and of mast cells in the lamina propria[180]; a response to cromo-glycate, especially in patients who have a high tissue eosinophil count[181]; an increased number of IgE-containing cells in the rectum in idiopathic proctitis[182]. None of these is seen in Crohn's disease, and all could be secondary effects, due to a damaged bowel wall.

Management

The traditional problems of inflammatory bowel disease include not only the management of the local bowel disorder, but also the problems of anaemia, electrolyte disturbance, tissue breakdown, fever, secondary infections, fistula formation, and all the secondary complications listed above.

Whereas the effect of corticosteroids may be mainly anti-inflammatory, the reported effectiveness of oral and rectal disodium cromoglycate (DSCG) in haemorrhagic proctitis[181] suggested the possibility that antiallergic measures may have a place. Those patients who responded to DSCG had significantly more eosinophils in their rectal biopsies than those who failed to respond which, it was argued, supported the hypothesis that an allergic reaction is important in this condition. However, when DSCG and sulphasalazine were compared in their ability to prevent relapse in 120 patients with ulcerative colitis[183], sulphasalazine proved to be greatly superior.

The part played by sulphasalazine itself may be non-specific. It is cleaved by bacteria in the colon to release 5-aminosalicylic acid[184], and it has been suggested that the prostaglandin synthetase inhibiting effect of this substance may explain its action, in a syndrome in which there is known to be an excessive production of prostaglandins[185]. Khan and his colleagues[186] therefore gave retention enemas of sulphasalazine and its individual components, 5-aminosalicylic acid and sulphapyridine, to a total of 62 patients. In controlled trial conditions they were able to produce evidence that 5-aminosalicylic acid is as effective as the parent compound in controlling both the clinical and the histological changes of active ulcerative colitis.

Other approaches have been made to the immunological management of these disorders. Thalidomide was tried (successfully) in one case[187] because of its known suppressive effects on immune complexes. Claims have also been made for the effectiveness of levamisole in Crohn's disease, but these claims have not been substantiated[188].

WORMS AND PARASITES

The immune defences of the gastrointestinal tract are capable in most circumstances of distinguishing between food, drink and the potentially damaging agents of disease. These reactions are not always entirely protective, however. Many of the clinical problems of allergy arise when vigorous reactions are directed against swallowed dusts and pollens, protozoa, helminths, viruses and bacteria, chemical substances and even the damaged constituents of the body's own cells. Allergic reactions to parasites and infective agents do have a considerable protective value[189]; yet the disability caused by the immunological response itself may be considerable. This is not only because of the immediate type of reaction within and outside the gut. Parasite-induced reactions involving IgE also extend to some types of eosinophilic response, as in certain cases of tropical eosinophilia which are associated with reaginic antibodies to human filarial parasites[190].

Parasite antigens are a potent stimulus for the synthesis of antiparasite antibodies of the IgE class, and there may be associated clinical features, such as urticaria[191]. It is, however, a curious observation that the allergic manifestations of early schistosomiasis, such as urticaria and asthma, may be suppressed later in the disease[192]. It is possible that this suppression occurs at a time when the total IgE has risen out of all proportion to the IgE antibody directed specifically against schistosomal antigens. The possible mechanism of this suppression will be discussed below. The sensitivity of gut-orientated IgE reactions is such that very high IgE levels are common in districts where parasitic infestations are endemic. The effect that this may have on other immunological reactions is of interest, since there is evidence that parasitic infection can potentiate the IgE response to an unrelated antigen, provided that it is simultaneously administered[193]. However, it appears that an allergic reaction to parasites may also confer a degree of protection against the subsequent development of other allergic manifestations. The evidence is as yet inconclusive, but asthma and hay fever are uncommon in communities in which the population is heavily parasitized[194].

There is now some experimental evidence about the way this protection may operate. This evidence is derived from passive skin sensitization studies. In this technique, passive sensitization is achieved by injecting, into the skin, serum which contains IgE antibody. This antibody becomes attached to mast cells, and successful sensitization is demonstrated when a later injection of the appropriate antigen leads to a weal and flare reaction. It is not possible to sensitize the skin in this way, however, if all the mast cell IgE-binding sites are already occupied, as in IgE myeloma[195]. This suggests that any cause of a high IgE level may protect against other IgE-mediated reactions. In keeping with this is the fact that passive skin sensitization is hard to produce in parasitized people who have high levels of circulating IgE[196]. But this may be an oversimplification. When the mast cells in human lung fragments are exposed to high-IgE serum from West African subjects, subsequent mast cell sensitization by other types of IgE antibodies can be blocked[197]. The time sequence is critical, and the high-IgE serum cannot displace IgE antibodies which have already become attached.

The biological implications of these findings deserve further consideration. Continuing IgE stimulation by parasite infection may indeed carry a partial protection against the development of other allergies. In communities in which naturally occurring, parasitic antigens are removed from the environment by improved hygiene and environmental measures, it is theoretically possible that a dramatically increased susceptibility to inhalant and food allergens may then emerge for the first time.

References

1. Lachmann, P. J. (1977). *Immunology of the Gut*. Ciba Foundation Symposium. No. 46. pp. 1–3. (Amsterdam: Excerpta Medica)
2. Poston. R. (1979). Nutrition and immunity. In Jarrett. R. J. (ed.) *Nutrition and Disease*. pp. 173–215. (London: Croom Helm)
3. Bockman, D. E. and Cooper, M. D. (1973). Pinocytosis by epithelium associated with lymphoid follicles in the Bursa of Fabricius and Peyer's patches. An electron microscope study. *Am. J. Anat.*, **136**, 455
4. Götze. O. and Müller-Eberhard, H. J. (1971). The C3 activator system: an alternate pathway of complement activation. *J. Exp. Med.*, **134**, 905
5. Lamm, M. E. (1976). Cellular aspects of immunoglobulin A. *Adv. Immunol.*, **2**, 223
6. Colten, H. R. and Bienenstock, J. (1974). Lack of C3 activation through classical or alternate pathways by human secretory IgA anti-blood group A antibody. *Adv. Exp. Med. Biol.*, **45**, 305
7. Ballow, M., Faye Fang, Good, R. A. and Day, N. K. (1974). Developmental aspects of complement components in the newborn. *Clin. Exp. Immunol.*, **18**, 257
8. Chodirkar, W. B. and Tomasi, T. B. (1963). Gamma globulins: quantitative relationships in human serum and non-vascular fluids. *Science*, **142**, 1080
9. Tomasi, T., Tan, E., Solomon, A. and Prendergast, R. (1965). Characteristics of an immune system common to certain external secretions. *J. Exp. Med.*, **121**, 101
10. Rubin. W., Fauci, A. S., Sleisenger, M. H. and Jeffries, G. H. (1965). Immunofluorescent studies in adult celiac disease. *J. Clin. Invest.*, **44**, 475
11. Loehry, C. A., Axon, A. T. R., Hilton, P. J., Hider, R. C. and Creamer, B. (1970). Permeability of the small intestine to substances of different molecular weight. *Gut*, **11**, 466
12. Loehry, C. A., Kingham, J. and Baker, J. (1973). Small intestinal permeability in animals and man. *Gut*, **14**, 683
13. Walker, W. A. and Isselbacher, K. J. (1974). Uptake and transport of macro molecules by the intestine: possible role in clinical disorders. *Gastroenterology*, **67**, 531
14. Jeffcott, L. B. (1973). The mechanism of transfer of maternal immunity to the foal. In *Proceedings of the 3rd International Conference on Equine Infectious Diseases, Paris, 1972*, pp. 419–435. (Basel: Karger)
15. Jeffcott, L. B. (1974). Studies on passive immunity in the foal. I. γ-globulin and antibody variations associated with the maternal transfer of immunity and the onset of active immunity. *J. Comp. Pathol.*, **84**, 93
16. Clarke, R. M. and Hardy, R. N. (1969). Use of [^{125}I]polyvinyl pyrrolidone K.60 in the quantitative assessment of the uptake of macromolecular substances by the intestine of the young rat. *J. Physiol.*, **204**, 113
17. Porter, P. (1970). Intestinal absorption of colostral IgA anti-*E. coli* antibodies by the neonatal piglet and calf. In Brambell, F. W. R. (ed.) *The Transmission of Passive Immunity from Mother to Young*, pp. 397–404. (Amsterdam and London: North Holland)
18. Hardy, R. N. (1969). The absorption of polyvinyl pyrrolidone by the newborn pig intestine. *J. Physiol.*, **204**, 633
19. Amman, A. J. and Stiehm, E. R. (1966). Immunoglobulin levels in colostrum and breast milk and serum from formula and breast-fed newborns. *Proc. Soc. Exp. Biol. Med.*, **122**, 1098

20. Owen, R. L. and Jones, A. L. (1974). Epithelial cell specialisation within human Peyer's patches: an ultrastructural study of intestinal lymphoid follicles. *Gastroenterology*, **66**, 189

21. Owen, R. L. (1977). Sequential uptake of horseradish peroxidase by lymphoid follicle epithelium of Peyer's patches in the normal, unobstructed mouse intestine: an ultra-structural study. *Gastroenterology*, **72**, 440

21a. Owen, R. L. and Nemanic, P. (1978). Antigen processing structures of the mammalian intestinal tract: an SEM study of lymphoepithelial organs. *Scanning Electron Microsc.*, **2**, 1978

22. Bienenstock, J. and Johnston, N. (1976). A morphologic study of rabbit bronchial lymphoid aggregates and lymphoepithelium. *J. Lab. Invest.*, **35**, 343

23. Guy-Grand, D., Griscelli, C. and Vassalli, P. (1974). The gut associated lymphoid system: nature and properties of the large dividing cells. *Eur. J. Immunol.*, **4**, 435

24. Friedberg, S. H. and Weissman, I. L. (1974). Lymphoid tissue architecture: II. *J. Immunol.*, **113**, 1477

25. Goldblum, R. M., Ahlstedt, S., Carlsson, B. *et al.* (1975). Antibody-forming cells in human colostrum after oral immunisation. *Nature (London)*, **257**, 797

26. Manning, D. D. and Jutila, J. W. (1974). Immunosuppression of congenitally athymic (nude) mice with heterologous anti-immunoglobulin heavy-chain antisera. *Cell. Immunol.*, **14**, 453

27. Gowans, J. L. and Knight, E. J. (1964). The route of recirculation of lymphocytes in the rat. *Proc. R. Soc. Series B*, **159**, 257

28. Hall, J. G., Parry, D. M. and Smith, M. E. (1972). The distribution and differentiation of lymph-borne immunoblasts after intravenous injection into syngeneic recipients. *Cell. Tissue. Kinet.*, **5**, 269

29. McWilliams, M., Phillips-Quagliata, J. M. and Lamm, M. E. (1975). Characteristics of mesenteric lymph node cells homing to gut-associated lymphoid tissue in syngeneic mice. *J. Immunol.*, **115**, 54

30. Griscelli, C., Vassalli, P. and McLuskey, R. T. (1969). The distribution of large, dividing lymph node cells in syngeneic recipient rats after intravenous injection. *J. Exp. Med.*, **130**, 1427

31. Halstead, T. E. and Hall, J. G. (1972). The homing of lymph-borne immunoblasts to the small gut of neonatal rats. *Transplantation*, **14**, 339

32. Ferguson, A. (1974). Secretion of IgA into 'antigen-free' isografts of mouse small intestine. *Clin. Exp. Immunol.*, **17**, 691

33. Buxbaum, J. N., Zolla, S., Scharff, M. D. *et al.* (1974). The synthesis and assembly of immunoglobulins by malignant human plasmacytes. *Eur. J. Immunol.*, **4**, 367

34. Brandtzaeg, P. (1974). Presence of J chain in human immunocytes containing various immunoglobulin classes. *Nature (London)*, **252**, 418

35. Orlans, E., Peppard, J., Reynolds, J. and Hall, J. (1978). Rapid active transport of immunoglobulin A from blood to bile. *J. Exp. Med.*, **147**, 568

36. Grey, H. M., Abel, C. A., Yount, W. J. and Kunkel, H. A. (1968). A subclass of human γ-A globulins (γ-A$_2$) which lacks the disulfide bonds linking heavy and light chains. *J. Exp. Med.*, **128**, 1223

37. Plaut, A. G., Wistar, R. and Capra, J. D. (1974). Differential susceptibility of human IgA immunoglobulins to streptococcal IgA protease. *J. Clin. Invest.*, **54**, 1295

38. Poger, M. E. and Lamm, M. E. (1974). Localisation of free and bound secretory component in human intestinal epithelial cells. *J. Exp. Med.*, **139**, 629

39. Brandtzaeg, P. (1978). Further evidence for role of secretory component and J chain in the glandular transport of IgA. *Adv. Exp. Med. Biol.*, **107**, 219

40. Walker, W. A., Isselbacher, K. J. and Bloch, K. J. (1972). Intestinal uptake of macro molecules: effect of oral immunization. *Science*, **177**, 608

41. André, C., Lambert, R., Bazin, H. *et al.* (1974). Interference of oral immunization with the intestinal absorption of heterologous albumin. *Eur. J. Immunol.*, **4**, 701
42. Williams, R. C. and Gibbons, R. J. (1972). Inhibition of bacterial adherence by secretory immunoglobulin A: a mechanism of antigen disposal. *Science*, **177**, 697
43. Kallenins, G. and Winberg, J. (1978). Bacterial adherence to periurethral epithelial cells in girls prone to urinary tract infections. *Lancet*, **2**, 540
44. Stokes, C. R., Taylor, B. and Turner, M. W. (1974). Association of house dust and grass pollen allergies with specific IgA antibody deficiency. *Lancet*, **2**, 485
45. Ogra, P. L. and Karzon, D. T. (1968). Poliovirus antibody response in serum and nasal secretions following intranasal inoculation with inactivated poliovaccine. *J. Immunol.*, **102**, 15
46. Clough, J. D., Zaccari, J. and Strober, W. (1970). Rabbit IgA, IgM and IgG antihapten responses assayed by C1a fixation and transfer. *J. Immunol.*, **105**, 687
47. Kojima, S. and Ovary, Z. (1975). Effect of *Nippostrongylus brasiliensis* infection of antihapten IgE antibody responses in the mouse. *Cell. Immunol.*, **15**, 274
48. Katz, D. H. and Benacerraf, B. (1972). The regulatory influence of activated T cells on B cell response to antigen. *Adv. Immunol.*, **15**, 1
49. Mond, J. J., Caporale, L. H. and Thorbecke, G. J. (1974). Kinetics of B cell memory development during a thymus 'independent' immune response. *Cell. Immunol.*, **10**, 105
50. Pritchard, H., Riddaway, J. and Micklem, H. S. (1973). Immune responses in congenitally thymus-less mice. *Clin. Exp. Immunol.*, **13**, 125
51. Eidelman, S. and Davis, S. D. (1968). Immunoglobulin content of intestinal mucosal plasma cells in ataxia telangiectasia. *Lancet*, **1**, 884
52. McFarlin, D. E., Strober, W. and Waldmann, T. A. (1972). Ataxia-telangiectasia. *Medicine (Baltimore)*, **51**, 281
53. O'Daly, J. A., Craig, S. W. and Cebra, J. J. (1971). Localization of b markers, α-chain and s.c. of s. IgA in epithelial cells lining Lieberkühn's crypts. *J. Immunol.*, **106**, 286
54. Haworth, J. C. and Dilling, L. (1966). Concentration of γ-A globulin in serum, saliva and nasopharyngeal secretions of infants and children. *J. Lab. Clin. Med.*, **67**, 922
55. McKay, E. M. and Thom, H. (1969). Observation on neonatal tears. *J. Pediatr.*, **75**, 1245
56. Davies, A. (1922). An investigation into the serological properties of dysentery stools. *Lancet*, **2**, 1009
57. Cassidy, J. T., Oldham, G. and Platts-Mills, T. A. E. (1979). Functional assessment of a B cell defect in patients with selective IgA deficiency. *Clin. Exp. Immunol.*, **35**, 296
58. Gerrard, J. W. (1974). Breast feeding: second thoughts. *Pediatrics*, **4**, 757
59. Buckley, R. H. and Dees, S. C. (1969). Correlations of milk precipitins with IgA deficiency. *N. Engl. J. Med.*, **281**, 465
60. Huntley, C., Robbins, J., Lyerly, A. and Buckley, R. (1971). Characterisation of precipitating antibodies to ruminant serum and milk proteins in humans with selective IgA deficiency. *N. Engl. J. Med.*, **284**, 7
61. Butler, J. E. and Oskvig, R. (1974). Cancer, autoimmunity and IgA deficiency related by a common antigen–antibody system. *Nature (London)*, **249**, 830
62. Sulzberger, M. B. (1929). Hypersensitiveness to arsphenamine in guinea-pigs. *Arch. Derm. Syph.*, **20**, 669
63. Chase, M. W. (1946). Inhibition of experimental drug allergy by prior feeding of the sensitizing agent. *Proc. Soc. Exp. Biol. Med.*, **61**, 257
64. Asherson, G. L., Zembala, M., Perera, M., Mayhew, B. and Thomas, W. R. (1977). Production of immunity and unresponsiveness in the mouse by feeding contact sensitizing agents and the role of suppressor cells in the Peyer's patches, mesenteric lymph nodes and other lymphoid tissue. *Cell. Immunol.*, **33**, 145
65. Cantor, H. M. and Dumont, A. E. (1967). Hepatic suppression of sensitization of antigens absorbed into the portal system. *Nature*, **215**, 744

66. Triger, D. R., Cynamon, M. H. and Wright, R. (1973). Studies on hepatic uptake of antigen: I. Comparison of inferior vena cava and portal vein routes of immunization. *Immunology*, **25**, 941

67. Harrison, M., Kilby, A., Walker-Smith, J. A., France, N. E. and Wood, C. B. S. (1976). Cow's milk protein intolerance: a possible association with gastroenteritis, lactose intolerance and IgA deficiency. *Br. Med. J.*, **1**, 1501

68. Walker-Smith, J. A. (1978). Gastrointestinal allergy. *Practitioner*, **220**, 562

69. Iyngkaran, N., Robinson, J. J., Prathar, K., Sumithran, E. and Yadav, M. (1978). Cow's milk protein sensitive enteropathy. Combined clinical and biological criteria for diagnosis. *Arch. Dis. Child.*, **53**, 20

70. Murgita, R. A. and Tomasi, T. B. (1975a). Suppression of the immune response by α-fetoprotein: I. *J. Exp. Med.*, **141**, 269

71. Murgita, R. A. and Tomasi, T. B. (1975b). Suppression of the immune response by α-fetoprotein: II. *J. Exp. Med.*, **141**, 440

72. Freier, S. (1974). *Clinical Immunology – Allergy in Paediatric Medicine*, p. 107. (Oxford: Blackwell)

73. Buisseret, P. (1978). Common manifestations of cow's milk allergy in children. *Lancet*, **1**, 304

74. Bienenstock, J., McDermott, M., Befus, D. and O'Neill, M. (1978). A common mucosal immunologic system involving the bronchus, breast and bowel. *Adv. Exp. Med. Biol.*, **107**, 53

75. Mestecky, J., McGhee, J. R., Michalek, S. M., Arnold, R. R., Crago, S. S. and Babb, J. L. (1978). Concept of the local and common mucosal immune response. *Adv. Exp. Med. Biol.*, **107**, 185

76. Lamm, M. E., Weisz-Carrington, P., Estela-Roux, M., McWilliams, M. and Phillips-Quagliata, J. M. (1978). Development of the IgA system in the mammary gland. *Adv. Exp. Med. Biol.*, **107**, 35

77. McLelland, D. B. L., McGrath, J. and Samson, R. R. (1978). Antimicrobial factors in human milk. *Acta Paediatr. Scand.* (Suppl.), **271**, 3

78. Delire, M., Cambiaso, C. L. and Masson, P. L. (1978). Circulating immune complexes in infants fed on cow's milk. *Nature (London)*, **272**, 632

79. Gunther, M., Aschaffenburg, R., Matthews, R. H., Parish, W. E. and Coombs, R. R. A. (1960). The level of antibodies to the proteins of cow's milk in the serum of normal human infants. *Immunology*, **3**, 296

80. Kuitunen, P., Visakorpi, J. K., Savilahti, E. and Pelkonen, P. (1975). Malabsorption syndrome with cow's milk intolerance. Clinical findings and course in 54 cases. *Arch. Dis. Child.*, **50**, 351

81. Pomeranz, J. R. (1970). Immunologic unresponsiveness following a single feeding of picryl chloride. *J. Immunol.*, **104**, 1486

82. Thomas, H. C. and Parrott, D. M. V. (1974). The induction of tolerance to a soluble protein antigen by oral administration. *Immunology*, **27**, 631

83. Goldman, A. S. and Heiner, D. C. (1977). Clinical aspects of food sensitivity. Diagnosis and management of cow's milk sensitivity. *Pediatr. Clin. N. Am.*, **24**, 133

84. Parish, W. E., Barrett, A. M., Coombs, R. R. A., Gunther, M. and Camps, F. E. (1960). Hypersensitivity to milk and sudden death in infancy. *Lancet*, **2**, 1106

85. Taylor, B., Norman, A. P., Orgel, H. A., Stokes, C. R., Turner, M. W. and Soothill, J. F. (1973). Transient IgA deficiency and pathogenesis of infantile atopy. *Lancet*, **2**, 111

86. Soothill, J. F., Stokes, C. R., Turner. M. W., Norman, A. P. and Taylor, B. (1976). Predisposing factors and the development of reaginic allergy in infancy. *Clin. Allergy*, **6**, 305

87. Grulee, C. G., Sanford, H. N. and Herron, P. (1934). Breast and artificial feeding. *J. Am. Med. Assoc.*, **103**, 735

88. Gerrard, J. W. (1974). Breast feeding: second thought. *Pediatrics*, **54**, 757

89. Barrett, D. J., Bertani, L., Wara, D. W. and Amman, A. J. (1979). Milk precipitins in selective IgA deficiency. *Ann. Allergy.* **42.** 73

90. Matthew, D. J., Taylor, B., Norman, A. P., Turner, M. W. and Soothill, J. F. (1977). Prevention of eczema. *Lancet*, **1**, 321

91. Saarinen, U. M., Kajosaari, M., Backman, A. and Siimes, M. A. (1979). Prolonged breast-feeding as prophylaxis for atopic diseases. *Lancet*, **2**, 163

92. Shannon, W. R. (1921). Demonstration of food proteins in human breast milk by anaphylactic experiments on guinea-pigs. *Am. J. Dis. Child.*, **22**, 223

93. Jakobsson, I. and Windberg, T. (1978). Cow's milk as a cause of infantile colic in breast-fed infants. *Lancet*, **2**, 437

94. Gerrard, J. W. (1979). Allergy in breast fed babies to ingredients in breast milk. *Ann. Allergy*, **42**, 69

95. Shiner, M., Ballard, J. and Smith, M. E. (1975). The small-intestinal mucosa in cow's milk allergy. *Lancet*, **1**, 136

96. Withrington, R. and Challacombe, D. N. (1979). Eosinophil counts in duodenal tissue in cow's milk allergy. *Lancet*, **1**, 675

97. Essen, R. von, Savilahti, E. and Pelkonen, P. (1972). Reticulin antibody in children with malabsorption. *Lancet*, **1**, 1157

98. Matthews, T. S., and Soothill, J. F. (1970). Complement activation after milk feeding in children with cow's milk allergy. *Lancet*, **2**, 893

99. Wright, R. and Truelove, S. C. (1965). Circulating antibodies to dietary proteins in ulcerative colitis. *Br. Med. J.*, **2**, 142

100. Parish, W. E. (1970). Short-term anaphylactic IgG antibodies in human sera. *Lancet*, **2**, 591

101. Lessof, M. H., Buisseret, P. D., Merrett, J., Merrett, T. G. and Wraith, D. G. (1980). Assessing the value of skin prick tests. *Clin. Allergy*, **10**, 115

102. Harrison, M., Kilby, A., Walker-Smith, J. A., France, N. E. and Wood, C. B. S. (1976). Cow's milk protein intolerance: a possible association with gastroenteritis, lactose intolerance, and IgA deficiency. *Br. Med. J.*, **1**, 1501

103. Iyngkaran, N., Davis, K., Robinson, M. J., Boey, C. G., Sumithran, E., Yadav, M., Laun, S. K. and Duthucheary, S. D. (1979). Cow's milk protein-sensitive enteropathy. *Arch. Dis. Child.*, **54**, 39

104. Barnes, G. L. and Townley, R. R. W. (1973). Duodenal mucosal damage in 31 infants with gastroenteritis. *Arch. Dis. Child.*, **48**, 343

105. André, C., Vaerman, J. P., Heremans, J. F. (1978). Oral immunization of rats with human serum albumin: interference with intestinal absorption and tolerogenic effect. In Hemmings, W. A. (ed.) *Antigen Absorption by the Gut*, pp. 65–71. (Lancaster: MTP Press)

106. Rubin, M. I. (1940). Allergic intestinal bleeding in newborn: clinical syndrome. *Am. J. Med. Sci.*, **200**, 385

107. Wilson, J. F., Heiner, D. C. and Lahey, M. E. (1964). Milk-induced gastrointestinal bleeding in infants with hypochromic microcytic anaemia. *J. Am. Med. Assoc.*, **189**, 568

108. Davidson, M., Burnstine, R. C. and Kugher, M. M. *et al.* (1965). Malabsorption defect induced by ingestion of β-lactoglobulin. *J. Pediatr.*, **66**, 545

109. Waldmann, T. A., Wochner, R. D., Laster, L. and Gordon, R. S. (1967). Allergic gastro-enteropathy; a cause of excessive gastrointestinal protein loss. *N. Engl. J. Med.*, **276**, 761

110. Editorial (1978). Sugar malabsorption in childhood. *Lancet*, **2**, 1292

111. Walker-Smith, J. and Phillips, A. (1979). The pathology of gastrointestinal allergy. *Proceedings of the Mast Cell International Symposium. Davos.* pp. 629–37

112. Walker-Smith, J. A. (1970). Transient gluten intolerance. *Arch. Dis. Child.*, **45**, 523

113. Ament, M. D. and Rubin, C. E. (1972). Soy protein – another cause of flat intestinal lesion. *Gastroenterology*, **62**, 227

114. Kwok, R. H. M. (1968). Chinese restaurant syndrome. *N. Engl. J. Med.*, **278**, 796

115. Lockey, S. D. (1972). Sensitizing properties of food additives and other commercial products. *Ann. Allergy*, **30**, 638
116. Speer, F. (1973). Management of food allergy. In Speer, F. and Dockhorn, R. J. (eds.) *Immunology in Children*, pp. 397–402. (Springfield, Ill.: C. C. Thomas)
117. Dahl, R. (1979). Wheat sensitive–but not coeliac. *Lancet*, **1**, 43
118. Buisseret, P. D., Youlten, L. J. F., Heinzelmann, D. I. and Lessof, M. H. (1978). Prostaglandin-synthesis inhibitors in prophylaxis of food intolerance. *Lancet*, **1**, 906
119. Nelson, T. L., Klein, G. L. and Galant, S. P. (1979). Severe eosinophilic gastroenteritis successfully treated with an elemental diet. *J. Allergy Clin. Immunol.*, **63**, 198
120. Caldwell, J. H., Tennenbaum, J. I. and Bronstein, H. A. (1975). Serum IgE in eosinophilic gastroenteritis. Response to intestinal challenge in 2 cases. *N. Engl. J. Med.*, **292**, 1388
121. Lessof, M. H., Wraith, D. G., Merrett, T. G., Merrett, J. and Buisseret, P. D. (1980). Food allergy and intolerance in 100 patients – local and systemic effects. *Q. J. Med.*, **49**, 259
122. Haddad, Z. H., Verma, S. and Kalra, V. (1979). IgE antibodies to peptic and peptic-tryptic digests of beta-lactoglobulin: significance in food hypersensitivity. *J. Allergy Clin. Immunol.*, **63**, 198
123. Kennedy, P. (1978). Acute reactions to apple eating. *Br. Med. J.*, **2**, 1501
124. Bluemink, E. (1970). Food allergy: the chemical nature of the substances eliciting symptoms. *World Rev. Nutr. Dietet.*, **12**, 505
125. Harries, M. G., O'Brien, I. M. and Burge, P. S. (1979). Histamine release in experimentally induced asthma and urticaria. *Proceedings of the Mast Cell International Symposium, Davos.*, 193–8
126. Lewis, R. A. (1979). SRS-A – its role in the inflammatory process. *Proceedings of the Mast Cell International Symposium, Davos.*, 97–100
127. Brostoff, J., Carini, C. and Wraith, D. G. (1979). IgE complexes produced by allergen challenge and the effect of sodium cromoglycate. *Proceedings of the Mast Cell International Symposium, Davos.*, 380–93
128. Kordansky, D., Adkinson, N. F., Norman, P. S. and Rosenthal, R. R. (1978). Asthma improved by non-steroidal anti-inflammatory drugs. *Ann. Intern. Med.*, **88**, 508
129. Freier, S. and Berger, R. (1973). Disodium cromoglycate in gastrointestinal protein intolerance. *Lancet*, **1**, 913
130. Vaz, G. A., Tan, L. K. T. and Gerrard, J. W. (1978). Oral cromoglycate in treatment of adverse reactions to foods. *Lancet*, **1**, 1066
131. Wraith, D. G., Young, G. V. W. and Lee, T. H. (1979). The management of food allergy with diet and Nalcrom. *Proceedings of the Mast Cell International Symposium, Davos.*, 443–6
132. Gerrard, J. W. (1979). Oral cromoglycate: its value in the treatment of adverse reactions to foods. *Ann. Allergy*, **42**, 135
133. American Academy of Pediatrics Committee on Drugs: Anaphylaxis (1973). *Paediatrics*, **51**, 136
134. Hutchcroft, B. J., Moore, E. G. and Orange, R. P. (1979). The effects of H_1 and H_2 receptor antagonism on the response of monkey skin to intradermal histamine, reverse-type anaphylaxis, and passive cutaneous anaphylaxis. *J. Allergy Clin. Immunol.*, **63**, 376
135. Holmes, G. K. T., Asquith, O., Stokes, P. L. and Cooke, W. T. (1974). Cellular infiltrate of jejunal biopsies in adult coeliac disease in relation to gluten withdrawal. *Gut*, **15**, 278
136. Shiner, M. (1973). Ultrastructural changes suggestive of immune reactions in the jejunal mucosa in childhood coeliac disease after gluten challenge. *Gut*, **14**, 1
137. Shiner, M. and Shmerling, D. H. (1972). The immunopathology of coeliac disease. *Digestion*, **5**, 69
138. Marks, J., Shuster, S. and Watson, A. J. (1966). Small bowel changes in dermatitis herpetiformis. *Lancet*, **2**, 1280
139. Weinstein, W. M., Brow, J. R., Parker, F. and Rubin, C. E. (1971). The small intestinal

mucosa in dermatitis herpetiformis. II. Relationship of the small intestinal lesion to gluten. *Gastroenterology*, **60**, 362

140. Fry, L., Seah, P. P., Riches, D. J. and Hoffbrand, A. V. (1973). Clearance of skin lesions in dermatitis herpetiformis after gluten withdrawal. *Lancet*, **1**, 288

141. Hodgson, H. J. F., Davies, R. J., Gent, A. E. and Hodson, M. E. (1976). Atopic disorders and adult coeliac disease. *Lancet*, **1**, 115

142. Scott, B. B. and Losowsky, M. S. (1975). Coeliac disease: a cause of various associated diseases? *Lancet*, **2**, 956

143. Cooper, B. T., Holmes, G. K. T. and Cooke, W. T. (1978). Coeliac disease and immunological disorders. *Br. Med. J.*, **1**, 537

144. Hood, J. and Mason, A. M. S. (1970). Diffuse pulmonary disease with transfer defect occurring with coeliac disease. *Lancet*, **1**, 445

145. Lancaster-Smith, M. J., Benson, M. K. and Strickland, I. D. (1971). Coeliac disease and diffuse interstitial lung disease. *Lancet*, **1**, 473

146. Berrill, W. T., Eade, O. E., Fitzpatrick, P. F., Hyde, I., MacLeod, W. M. and Wright, R. (1975). Bird-fancier's lung and jejunal villous atrophy. *Lancet*, **2**, 1006

147. Faux, J. A., Hendrick, D. J. and Anand, B. S. (1978). Precipitins to different avian serum antigens in bird fancier's lung and coeliac disease. *Clin. Allergy*, **8**, 101

148. Dingle, P. R., Ferguson, A., Horn, D. B., Tubman, J. and Hall, R. (1966). The incidence of thyroglobulin antibodies and thyroid enlargement in a general practice in north-east England. *Clin. Exp. Immunol.*, **I**, 277

149. MacCuish, A. C., Barnes, E. W., Irvine, W. J. and Duncan, L. J. P. (1974). Antibodies to pancreatic islet cells in insulin-dependent diabetes with coexisting autoimmune disease. *Lancet*, **2**, 1529

150. McClelland, D. B. L., Barnetson, R. S. T. C., Parkin, D. M., Warwick, R. R. G., Heading, R. C. and Shearman, D. J. C. (1972). Small-intestinal immunoglobulin levels in dermatitis herpetiformis. *Lancet*, **2**, 1108

151. Strober, W., Falchuk, Z. M., Rogentine, G. N., Nelson, D. L. and Klaeveman, H. L. (1975). The pathogenesis of gluten-sensitive enteropathy. *Ann. Intern. Med.*, **83**, 242

152. Brown, D. L., Cooper, A. G. and Hepner, G. W. (1969). IgM metabolism in coeliac disease. *Lancet*, **1**, 858

153. Mawhinney, H. and Tomkin, G. H. (1971). Gluten enteropathy associated with selective IgA deficiency. *Lancet*, **2**, 121

154. Gasbanini, G., Miglio, F., Serra, M. A. and Bernardi, M. (1974). Immunological studies of the jejunal mucosa in normal subjects and adult coeliac disease patients. *Digestion*, **10**, 122

155. Shiner, M. and Ballard, J. (1972). Antigen–antibody reactions in jejunal mucosa in childhood coeliac disease after gluten challenge. *Lancet*, **1**, 1202

156. Seah, P. P., Fry, L., Stewart, J. S., Chapman, B. L., Hoffbrand, A. V. and Holborow, E. J. (1972). Immunoglobulins in the skin in d. herpetiformis and coeliac disease. *Lancet*, **1**, 611

157. Mowbray, J. F., Hoffbrand, A. V., Holborow, E. J., Seah, P. P. and Fry, L. (1973). Circulating immune complexes in dermatitis herpetiformis. *Lancet*, **2**, 400

158. McCrae, W. M., Eastwood, M. A., Martin, M. R. and Sircus, W. (1975). Neglected coeliac disease. *Lancet*, **1**, 187

159. Anand, B. S., Truelove, S. C. and Offord, R. E. (1977). Skin test for coeliac disease using a subfraction of gluten. *Lancet*, **1**, 118

160. Roberts, D. L., Rhodes, J., Heatley, R. V. and Newcombe, R. G. (1978). Atopic features of ulcerative colitis. *Lancet*, **1**, 1262

161. Ratnaike, R. N. and Wangel, A. G. (1977). Immunological abnormalities in coeliac disease and response to dietary restriction. I. Immunoglobulins, antibody and complement. *Aust. N.Z. J. Med.*, **7**, 349

162. Alarcon-Segovia, D., Herskovic, T., Wakelin, K. G., Green, P. A. and Scudamore, H. H. (1964). Presence of circulating antibodies to gluten and milk fractions in patients with non-tropical sprue. *Am. J. Med.*, **36**, 485

163. Ferguson, A. and Carswell, F. (1972). Precipitans to dietary proteins in serum and upper intestinal secretions of coeliac children. *Br. Med. J.*, **I**, 75

164. Gibhard, R. L., Falchuk, Z. M., Katz, S. I., Sessions, C., Rogentine, G. N. and Strober, W. (1974). Dermatitis herpetiformis: immunologic concomitants of small intestine disease and relationship to histocompatibility antigen HL-A8. *J. Clin. Invest.*, **54**, 98

165. Wright, R. (1977). *Immunology of Gastrointestinal and Liver Disease*, p. 132. (London: Edward Arnold)

166. Ward, M. (1977). The pathogenesis of Crohn's disease. *Lancet*, **2**, 903

167. Skinner, J. M. and Whitehead, R. (1974). A morphological assessment of immunoreactivity in colonic Crohn's disease and ulcerative colitis. *J. Clin. Pathol.*, **27**, 202

168. Monteiro, E., Fossey, J., Shiner, M., Drasar, B. S. and Allison, A. C. (1971). Antibacterial antibodies in rectal and colonic mucosa in ulcerative colitis. *Lancet*, **1**, 249

169. Watson, D. W. (1974). Ulcerative colitis autoimmune epiphenomena and colonic cancer. *Cancer*, **34**, 867

170. Farmer, G. W., Vincent, M. M., Fuccillo, D. A., Horta-Barbosa, L., Ritman, S., Sever, J. L. and Gitnick, G. L. (1973). Viral investigations in ulcerative colitis and regional enteritis. *Gastroenterology*, **65**, 8

171. Rosen, P., Armstrong, D. and Rice, N. (1973). Gastrointestinal cytomegalovirus infection. *Arch. Intern. Med.*, **132**, 274

172. Mitchell, D. N. and Rees, R. J. W. (1970). Agent transmissible from Crohn's disease tissue. *Lancet*, **2**, 168

173. Aronson, M. D., Phillips, C. A., Beeken, W. L. and Forsyth, B. (1975). Isolation and characterization of a viral agent from intestinal tissue of patients with Crohn's disease and other intestinal disorders. *Prog. Med. Virol.*, **21**, 165

174. Acheson, H. D. and Truelove, S. C. (1961). Early weaning in aetiology of ulcerative colitis. A study of feeding in infancy and in controls. *Br. Med. J.*, **2**, 929

175. Whorwell, P. J., Holdstock, G., Whorwell, G. M. and Wright, R. (1979). Bottle feeding, early gastroenteritis, and inflammatory bowel disease. *Br. Med. J.*, **I**, 382

176. Andresen, A. F. R. (1953). Allergic manifestations in the gastrointestinal tract. *Gastroenterology*, **23**, 20

177. Wright, R. and Truelove, S. C. (1965). A controlled therapeutic trial of various diets in ulcerative colitis. *Br. Med. J.*, **2**, 138

178. Jewell, D. P. and Truelove, S. C. (1972). Circulating antibodies to cow's milk proteins in ulcerative colitis. *Gut*, **13**, 796

179. Pugh, S. M., Rhodes, J., Mayberry, J. F., Roberts, D. L., Heatley, R. V. and Newcombe, R. G. (1979). Atopic disease in ulcerative colitis and Crohn's disease. *Clin. Allergy*, **9**, 221

180. Lloyd, G., Green, F. H. Y., Fox, H., Mani, V. and Turnberg, L. A. (1975). Mast cells and immunoglobulin E in inflammatory bowel disease. *Gut*, **16**, 861

181. Heatley, R. V., Calcraft, B. J., Rhodes, J., Owen, E. and Evans, B. V. C. (1975). Disodium cromoglycate in the treatment of chronic proctitis. *Gut*, **16**, 559

182. Heatley, R. V., Rhodes, J., Calcraft, B. J., Whitehead, R. H., Fifield, R. and Newcombe, R. G. (1975). Immunoglobulin E in rectal mucosa of patients with proctitis. *Lancet*, **2**, 1010

183. Willoughby, C. P., Heyworth, M. F., Piris, J. and Truelove, S. C. (1979). Comparison of disodium cromoglycate and sulphasalazine as maintenance therapy for ulcerative colitis. *Lancet*, **1**, 119

184. Gould, S. R. (1975). Prostaglandins, ulcerative colitis, and sulphasalazine. *Lancet*, **2**, 988

185. Gould, S. R., Brash, A. R. and Connolly, M. E. (1977). Increased prostaglandin production in ulcerative colitis. *Lancet*, **2**, 98

186. Khan, A. K. A., Piris, J. and Truelove, S. C. (1977). An experiment to determine the active therapeutic moiety of sulphasalazine. *Lancet*, **2**, 892

187. Waters, M. F. R., Laing, A. B. G., Ambikapathy, A. and Lennard Jones, J. E. (1979). Treatment of ulcerative colitis with thalidomide. *Br. Med. J.*, **I**, 792

188. Swarbrick, E. T. and O'Donoghue, D. P. (1979). Levamisole in Crohn's disease. *Lancet*, **1**, 392

189. Ferguson, A. and Jarrett, E. E. E. (1975). Hypersensitivity reactions in the small intestine. I. Thymus dependence of experimental 'partial villous atrophy'. *Gut*, **16**, 114

190. Ottesen, E. A., Neva, F. A., Paranjape, R. S., Tripathy, S. P., Thiruvengadam, K. V. and Beaven, M. A. (1979). Specific allergic sensitisation to filarial antigens in tropical eosinophilia syndrome. *Lancet*, **1**, 1158

191. Habte-Gabr, E., Tirunch, M. and Hailu, M. (1977). Chronic urticaria: its relationship to parasitic infestation and response to anthelminthic drugs. *Ethiopian Med. J.*, **15**, 9

192. Weltman, J. K. and Senft, A. W. (1979). Modulation of the allergic response in schistosomiasis by non-specific IgE. *J. Allergy Clin. Immunol.*, **63**, 176 (abstract)

193. Jarrett, E. E. E. and Stewart, D. C. (1972). Potentiation of rat reaginic (IgE) antibody by helminth infection. *Immunology*. **23**. 749

194. Godfrey, R. C. (1975). Asthma and IgE levels in rural and urban communities of the Gambia. *Clin. Allergy*, **5**, 201

195. Ogawa, M., McIntyre, R., Ishizaka, K., Ishizaka, T., Terry, W. D. and Waldmann, T. A. (1971). Biologic properties of *E. myeloma* proteins. *Am. J. Med.*, **51**. 193

196. Bazaral, M., Orgel, H. A. and Hamburger, R. N. (1973). The influence of serum IgE levels of selected recipients, including patients with allergy, helminthiasis and tuberculosis, on the apparent P-K titre of a reaginic serum. *Clin. Exp. Immunol.*, **14**, 117

197. Godfrey, R. C. and Gradidge, C. F. (1976). Allergic sensitisation of human lung fragments prevented by saturation of IgE binding sites. *Nature (London)*, **259**, 484

198. Heremans, J. F. (1969). In Dayton, D. H. (ed.) *The Secretory Immunologic System*, pp. 309-324. US Dept. of Health, Education and Welfare, Public Health Service, National Institute of Health, Bethesda, Maryland

6
Allergy and the Skin

M. G. C. DAHL

INTRODUCTION

The skin has a limited number of ways in which it can react to pathological stimuli. In this respect it does not differ from other organs. The unique accessibility of the skin has enabled its pathological responses to be studied visually in minute detail both macroscopically and histologically. This minute visual assessment of skin pathology has in the past led to a multiplicity of descriptive diagnoses, terms and eponyms which have proved confusing to non-dermatologists and dermatologists alike. This descriptive approach has proved comparatively unhelpful at any but the most superficial clinical level, since it has generally provided little information about pathophysiology.

The development of immunology over the last two decades has enabled a new set of normal and abnormal physiological mechanisms to be examined in the context of skin diseases. Disordered immunity has been clearly demonstrated in many of these. However, it must be remembered that the effector mechanisms which are activated by immune reactions and which result in the different reaction patterns which are recognized as diseases, may also be activated in other ways or may themselves be intrinsically abnormal. Thus the final pattern of response – which we may refer to as a specific disease at the purely clinical level – may be initiated in a variety of different ways, some of which may properly be regarded as allergic and others not. The common patterns of disease which are most frequently considered as 'allergic' by general physicians, allergists and dermatologists, are urticaria, cutaneous vasculitis and eczema. It is with these three conditions that this discussion is concerned.

URTICARIA

Urticaria is a physical sign rather than a disease. It may be produced by different mechanisms – some undoubtedly immune – others apparently not. In many patients it is the only feature of their illness although in some it occurs as part of a more generalized disease such as systemic lupus erythematosus[1].

Mechanisms of urticaria

Urticarial lesions are the result of a sudden localized accumulation of fluid in the dermis. The term angioedema is used for more diffuse oedematous reactions additionally involving deeper tissues. Urticaria and angioedema commonly coexist. The oedema fluid is derived from plasma as a result of a sudden increase in local vascular permeability. It is the multiplicity of the factors which may affect vascular permeability and the complexity of their interrelationships which make the understanding of the mechanisms underlying urticarial reactions so difficult.

Many naturally occurring substances increase vascular permeability and produce urticarial reactions when injected intradermally. Such agents include histamine, serotonin, kinins, prostaglandins and anaphylotoxins, i.e. C3a and C5a resulting from complement activation. Theoretically any stimulus which results in local liberation of such vasoactive substances may result in urticaria. Events which directly or indirectly increase their rates of production or decrease their rates of degradation are also likely to cause or exacerbate urticarial reactions. Inflammatory changes in dermal blood vessels (vasculitis) also increase vascular permeability and in some circumstances produce urticarial lesions.

Mast cells in the perivascular dermis are one source of vasoactive mediators. Liberation of mast cell mediators occurs in some types of urticaria, but it seems that mast cell involvement is not invariable. Following both immune and non-immune stimulation, mast cells release histamine, serotinin and slow-reacting substance of anaphylaxis (SRS-A) all of which increase local vascular permeability[2]. Eosinophil, neutrophil and platelet chemotactic factors are also produced and are almost certainly involved in the development of the cellular infiltrate which follows. These cells, particularly eosinophils, probably play a part in limiting the reaction by inactivating primary mediators[3, 4] including histamine and SRS-A.

Acute urticaria in atopics

Allergic reactions involving antigen-specific IgE bound to dermal mast cells are central to some types of urticaria. Urticaria is common in atopic subjects and a history of previous urticarial attacks was obtained in 23% of patients attending hospital with hay fever and in 36% of adults with atopic eczema[5]. Characteristically the urticarial attacks in these patients are brief (2–3 days) and the patient is often aware of the cause of the reaction. Immediate urticarial weal and flare reactions are produced by skin prick testing with the appropriate antigen. The reactions can be passively transferred to normal recipients with serum and antigen-specific IgE can be detected in serum by RAST. The reactions can normally be suppressed with H1 antihistamines. This evidence therefore implicates allergic stimulation of the mast cell by way of antigen-specific IgE and it is this form of urticaria that is most clearly allergic in aetiology. The clinical pattern exhibited by such patients depends largely on the route by which the allergen gains access to the body. Skin thickness is a critical factor in determining whether antigen is able to penetrate. Direct penetration through intact skin may occur, usually in areas of thin skin adjacent to mucous membranes. Contact urticaria to egg protein or to animal urine (in animal house technicians) are examples.

Mucous membranes themselves are frequently involved giving rise to conjunctivitis and periorbital oedema with airborne allergens such as grass pollens and to swelling of the lips and tongue following contact with food allergens. Generalized urticarial eruptions of this type may also result from antigen absorption and distribution to the skin via the bloodstream following ingestion, injection or occasionally inhalation of allergen. Not all examples of urticaria due to IgE-mediated allergic reactions are brief and self-limiting. An unusual example of chronic urticaria of 17 years' duration in which an allergic IgE/mast cell mechanism was well documented has been reported due to radiographic contrast material retained in the subarachnoid space[6]. Nevertheless this mechanism is rarely demonstrated in chronic urticaria and allergic urticaria of this type is characteristically short-lived. Many patients do not seek hospital or specialist dermatologist advice and for this reason the prevalence of this type of urticaria in some series is much lower than its probable occurrence in the general population.

Chronic idiopathic urticaria

The majority of patients who develop prolonged continuous or frequently repeated episodes of urticaria are not atopic. In most studies serum IgE levels have been normal[7-9] although in a proportion of individuals elevated levels have sometimes been reported[10]. In general such patients differ from atopic individuals with acute urticaria in the following ways.

(1) The disease is chronic (by definition).
(2) A causative allergen is seldom apparent.
(3) Serum IgE levels are usually normal.
(4) The response to H1 antihistamines is often poor.

Clinical differences in the lesions between acute atopic urticaria and chronic idiopathic urticaria have been poorly documented. The author's clinical impressions suggest that urticarial lesions in atopics characteristically consist of a pink or slightly blanched weal surrounded by a bright red flare whereas in chronic urticaria the weal is frequently a more dusky red with little surrounding flare. The lesions of chronic idiopathic urticaria tend to be comparatively less itchy. Such clinical differences are difficult to quantify but deserve further study by quantitative methods.

Evidence of complement activation has been found in some patients with chronic urticarial skin lesions. Low serum levels of early classical pathway complement components have been reported[11, 12]. Complement activation by immune complexes or an intrinsic defect in the control of the complement system[12] has been postulated. In other patients without evidence of immune complex formation low levels of C1, C1q, C1s, properdin factor B and C3 were found in the presence of normal C4 and C2 levels. These observations suggested activation of complement by the C1-bypass pathway[14]. The majority of these patients had unusual disease with involvement of other organs including arthritis and renal disease. It is pertinent to question to what extent these complement abnormalities can be extended to the majority of chronic urticaria patients with disease limited to the skin.

In one investigation[10], complement abnormalities (low CH50 and some-times low C3 levels) were found in eight of 48 patients. In another study[15] of 150 patients with chronic urticaria and angioedema, abnormalities of C1 subcomponents were found in about 40% of cases. Immunofluorescence studies of the skin for the presence of immunoglobulin and complement have occasionally been reported as negative in chronic urticaria[12]. However, the author has noted deposition of C3 in papillary vessels of lesional skin in several chronic urticaria patients without histological evidence of necrotizing vasculitis. These various observations do suggest that complement activation may be more important in the common non-vasculitic type of chronic urticaria than previously recognized. However it seems that the changes may be subtle and comparatively rarely reflected by abnormal levels of the major complement components in serum. This is clearly an area of investigation which requires extension.

The histological changes in the skin in chronic urticaria are usually non-specific and consist mainly of a perivascular infiltrate of mononuclear cells and polymorphs. Occasionally there are frank changes of necrotizing vasculitis which were originally associated with hypocomplementaemia[11]. Nevertheless it appears that patients with hypocomplementaemic urticaria do not always show the histological changes of necrotizing vasculitis[12] and that vasculitic urticaria may also be associated with normal complement levels[16]. Both the histological findings and the presence of immunoreactants detected by immunofluorescence may be critically dependent on the age of the lesions. This factor is frequently unknown when spontaneous lesions are studied. If complement activation is responsible for the development of the clinical lesion and of the cellular infiltrate it might be anticipated that complement deposition would be present in early lesions (and absent later) whereas the most florid histological changes might be found at a later stage. Little consideration has hitherto been given to the possible dynamics of the lesion when studying the skin by histological techniques.

Lesions of necrotizing vasculitis can be induced by intradermal injection of histamine which is thought to localize immune complexes in the resulting area of increased vascular permeability[17, 18]. Lesions can also be induced by this method in some patients with non-vasculitic chronic urticaria. The author has used this technique in several such patients and has been able to demonstrate by immunofluorescence early deposition of C3 in the walls of dermal blood vessels. A similar study of spontaneous lesions was usually negative. This technique should prove useful in further studies of the dynamic aspects of such lesions.

Studies of suction blisters in the skin of chronic urticaria patients have shown that blister fluid levels of histamine are usually higher than in controls[19]. In some patients the levels were particularly high in blisters raised over urticarial weals whereas in other patients levels were also high in clinically normal skin. Such studies provide evidence for the involvement of histamine in the reaction but its precise role and importance is unclear. Blood leukocytes (basophils) from patients with chronic urticaria have been found to contain normal total amounts of histamine and after treatment with compound 48/80 or calcium ionophore release histamine in quantities comparable to normal individuals. However when passively sensitized with IgE and then challenged with anti-IgE, histamine release was diminished[20, 21]. These observations suggest a defect specifically in the immune mechanism of histamine release from mast cells. It is not known whether this defect is a primary or secondary phenomenon and at present its significance is unclear.

Inherited or acquired deficiencies of the inhibitors of vasoactive mediators could theoretically contribute to the development of urticarial reactions[22]. C1 esterase inhibitor deficiency in hereditary angioedema is an example which is considered separately (see: hereditary angioedema, page 186). Deficiencies of other protease inhibitors might have similar consequences since unrestrained protease activity would allow accumulation of C1 esterase, plasmin, kallikrein etc., resulting in excessive activation of the complement, fibrinolytic and kallikrein systems respectively with consequent accumulation of vasoactive mediators. Low plasma levels of α_1-antitrypsin and antichymotrypsin activity have been found in some chronic urticaria patients, particularly those with prominent angioedema[23]. Excessive oedematous reactions to intradermal kallikrein were also found in some patients[22, 23] but such reactions did not correlate with low plasma protease activity[23]. The importance of these biochemical abnormalities is at present unclear, particularly since it is not known whether the observed abnormalities are primary or secondary to the disease process itself.

The possible mechanisms which may be involved in chronic urticaria may be summarized as follows:

(1) IgE mediated immune reactions involving skin mast cells (probably uncommon).

(2) Complement activation, either by immune mechanisms or due to intrinsic defects of the complement system.

(3) Vasculitis – possibly induced by immune complexes and complement activation or by other unknown mechanisms.

(4) Defective control mechanisms of vasoactive mediators.

No comprehensive study has yet attempted to look at all these possible mechanisms in patients with chronic urticaria. Moreover many of the investigative techniques which have been used are not readily available to clinicians in general. In these circumstances the satisfactory classification and understanding of chronic urticaria patients at the clinical level remains very difficult.

Physical urticarias

Urticaria may be provoked by a variety of physical stimuli including exposure to cold, heat, light, pressure and vibration. Such patients are particularly suitable for study since their reactions can be induced in a reproducible fashion. Cold-induced urticaria has been the most extensively investigated and it might be anticipated that this superficially homogeneous group would show uniform findings. This is not the case.

In some patients with cold urticaria the reaction can be passively transferred with serum to normal recipients[24, 25]. Following induction of lesions in one limb by immersion in cold water, raised levels of mast cell mediators have been detected in effluent blood including histamine[25–27], eosinophil chemotactic factor[26] and a neutrophil chemotactic factor[28]. Mast cell degranulation has been observed[29] and a mechanism involving IgE and mast cells seems probable in these patients[25].

In other patients with cold urticaria passive transfer has been achieved with IgM[30]. Cold urticaria may also be associated with cryoglobulinaemia and in such patients passive transfer studies were positive with IgG and IgG–IgM cryoglobulin[31–33]. In a family with dominantly inherited cold urticaria extensive studies of immunoglobulin, complement and mast cell mediators failed to show any abnormality[34]. In the less common heat urticaria evidence for mediation by histamine[35, 36] has been found in some patients while in another patient there was evidence of complement activation with normal plasma histamine levels[37]. Urticaria induced by light also seems to be heterogeneous in its pathogenesis[38].

Dermographism

Immediate or simple dermographism is common. Patients are usually young adults who present with pruritus but are otherwise fit. Linear wealing develops within 2–3 minutes of scratching normal skin with a bluntly pointed instrument or finger nail. A similar reaction can be elicited in some asymptomatic individuals and it has been suggested that there are two types – one physiological and asymptomatic, the other pathological and symptomatic[39]. Passive transfer has been achieved in some patients[40, 41] with a heat-labile serum factor suggesting involvement of IgE[40]. Raised blood histamine levels have been noted[42] after extensive induction of lesions and patients usually respond well to H1 antihistamines[39]. After induction of lesions the affected sites are refractory to further stimuli for several hours[43]. The available evidence implicates IgE and mast cells although mast cell degranulation is alleged not to occur[44].

The cause of immediate dermographism is seldom apparent. However it has been noted to follow insect bites[45], scabies infestation and treatment with penicillin[46]. In a diabetic patient studied by the author severe dermographism was associated with insulin allergy. Dermographic wealing has been noted to persist for several days at the sites of positive immediate prick tests. These observations suggest the involvement of exogenous allergens in some cases of dermographism.

Cholinergic urticaria

Cholinergic urticaria is a distinctive condition in which small urticarial weals develop after stimuli such as exercise, emotional stress and generalized heat, e.g. taking a hot bath. Young adults are usually affected and the weals, which occur particularly on the upper trunk, are characteristically small and surrounded by a prominent flare. Itching is the only symptom and attacks subside after 15–30 minutes. The clinical features may be incomplete consisting of erythema without wealing or even pruritus only. Many mildly affected individuals do not seek medical attention but occasionally the condition can be severe and disabling. Systemic symptoms[47], including wheezing[48], have occasionally been described during attacks.

Cholinergic urticaria is mediated through sympathetic cholinergic nerve fibres which innervate sweat glands in the skin[49]. It appears that urticaria develops as an abnormal response to liberation of acetyl choline. Histamine appears to be involved since wealing is reduced by H1 antihistamine treatment or by pretreatment with histamine liberating agents[49, 50]. Urticarial weals with satellite lesions can be induced by intradermal injection of methacholine[51] and other agents which induce sufficient axon reflex[48], but these tests are positive only in severely affected individuals and the diagnosis should be made clinically on the basis of morphology and distribution of the rash and its association with stress, heat and exercise[52]. Exogenous causes for cholinergic urticaria have not been defined.

Treatment

Since the clinician is frequently unable to find a cause for the urticaria or to elucidate its mechanism, treatment has often to be pragmatic and empirical. H1 antihistamines are of value in suppressing acute urticaria in atopics and other treatment is seldom required. In such cases the cause can often be established and further episodes prevented by its avoidance. The effect of H1 antihistamines in patients with chronic idiopathic urticaria is variable and frequently unsatisfactory[5]. Combination of H1 with H2 antihistamines such as cimetidine has not been beneficial[53]. Terbutaline, a β_2-adrenergic stimulant has been reported to benefit some patients[54].

The author has occasionally found dapsone apparently effective in controlling chronic idiopathic urticaria. One such patient had hypocomplementaemia and vasculitic urticaria. The mode of action of dapsone is not known but further studies of this drug in urticaria may be worth while. Systemic corticosteroids usually suppress chronic urticaria but the long-term side-effects are usually unacceptable.

Some patients are aware that their lesions are exacerbated by aspirin ingestion[5, 55]. The mechanism is unclear but avoidance of aspirin in its many forms is important for such patients. Certain azo-dyes, particularly tartrazine, also exacerbate some patients with chronic urticaria[56, 57]. Good results have been claimed for the use of diets free of such dyes[57] but the author's experience has been disappointing.

The management of physical urticaria consists primarily of avoiding the physical agent responsible. The empirical use of antihistamines and sometimes systemic corticosteroids may be helpful. Dermographism usually responds well to H1 antihistamines. Anticholinergic drugs such as Pro-Banthine have been recommended for the treatment of cholinergic urticaria. However the author, in common with others[58], has found this drug completely ineffective. Several affected patients have responded quite well to a combination of H1 and H2 antihistamines. Hydroxyzine has also been recommended for this condition[59].

HEREDITARY ANGIOEDEMA

Angioedema commonly occurs in association with urticaria and its causes must be considered with the many causes of urticaria. As in patients with urticaria, a cause of angioedema is frequently not established although the report of α_1-antitrypsin deficiency in angioedema[23] has already been discussed. However a small proportion of patients with angioedema lack C1 esterase inhibitor activity[60]. In these patients the clinical pattern is rather distinctive and the condition is often familial.

Lesions of this hereditary angioedema recur at irregular intervals. Attacks often arise spontaneously but have sometimes been attributed to stress and may certainly be provoked by trauma. Dental extraction is a particularly important provoking factor since lesions in the region of the mouth and tongue may produce respiratory obstructions. Subcutaneous oedema develops over the course of a few hours and persists for 2–3 days. It may be extensive, perhaps involving an entire limb. The lesions are not itchy but may be rather sore. Involvement of intestinal mucosa may produce abdominal colic with signs of intestinal obstruction. Laryngeal involvement[61] producing asphyxia is the major cause of the considerable mortality which may be as high as 30%.

Details of the complement system have been most recently reviewed by Gigli[62]. C1 esterase is the activated form of C1. It is normally generated to some extent spontaneously and particularly by the participation of C1 in antigen–antibody reactions and by the action of plasmin on C1. Patients who lack the C1 esterase inhibitor therefore have excess circulating C1 esterase activity. The substrates for C1 esterase are C4 and C2 which are split into C4a, C4b and C2a respectively. Levels of both C4 and C2 are therefore low during attacks and C4 levels are also reduced during asymptomatic periods. This provides a useful screening test for the disease. The combination of C4b and C2a produces the enzyme C3 convertase which is responsible for activation of C3 and the continuing complement activation cascade. In the process of formation of C2a, a kinin-like substance, C2-kinin is also produced and it is this C2-kinin which is thought to be the mediator of the disease process[63].

Production of C2-kinin appears also to be dependent on Hageman factor, a protein which is itself involved both in coagulation and in the plasma bradykinin-forming system. The C1 esterase inhibitor also acts as a controlling mechanism on several enzymes in this system and excessive C1 esterase activity leads to increased plasmin production from plasminogen. As has already been mentioned plasmin itself produces C1 esterase from C1. This mechanism therefore further contributes to excessive C1 esterase activity.

Diagnosis of hereditary angioedema depends on the demonstration of reduced activity of the C1 esterase inhibitor in the serum. A low absolute level, which is the usual abnormality, can be detected by a quantitative immunochemical method. However, in a minority of affected families this quantitative method gives normal results but the protein is functionally inactive[64]. In such patients the defect can only be confirmed using a chemical esterolytic assay[65]. Low levels of C4 in the presence of normal quantities of the inhibitor detected immunochemically should raise the suspicion of a functional defect and lead to further investigation. Measurement of C4 is also a useful screening test since the levels are low even between attacks and C4 levels are usually normal in other forms of angioedema.

The administration of the C1 esterase inhibitor, either in fresh frozen plasma[66] or in partially purified form[67], has been useful in terminating acute attacks. Such treatment is however impractical for routine prophylaxis. Inhibitors of plasmin such as ε-aminocaproic acid and tranexamic acid have been effective when given prophylactically[68–71] and the successful use of tranexamic acid in pregnancy has been described[72]. However the side-effects of these drugs, including renal failure[73] and myositis[74, 75] have been significant and have stimulated other therapeutic approaches. Androgens have a prophylactic effect in hereditary angioedema[76] but their use has also been limited by long-term side-effects. However danazol, an inhibitor of pituitary gonadotrophin, has little androgenic effect[77] and has been successfully used in prophylactic treatment[78, 79]. Its effect appears to be to increase functionally active C1 esterase inhibitor in both the quantitatively and functionally deficient forms of the disease and C4 levels may return to normal[78, 80]. One reasonable therapeutic approach has been to use danazol for men and postmenopausal women and to reserve tranexamic acid for premenopausal women[72]. Nevertheless some caution is needed in the prolonged use of danazol since its long-term side-effects are as yet largely unknown and there is preliminary evidence of altered cholesterol metabolism[81].

CUTANEOUS VASCULITIS

A diagnosis of cutaneous vasculitis rests ultimately on the histological demonstration of an inflammatory process involving skin blood vessels and producing damage to the wall of those vessels. Microscopically such damage consists of endothelial swelling and necrosis, infiltration of the vessel wall with inflammatory cells and leakage of red cells into the perivascular space. In severe cases there may be complete disruption of the vessel wall. Other features include thrombotic vascular occlusion, deposition of fibrinoid material and necrosis of adjacent tissues. The diversity of clinical lesions seen in vasculitis is initially confusing but can be more easily understood if one considers the following variable factors.

(1) Damage to the vessel wall may be mild or severe.
(2) Different sizes of vessels may be involved.
(3) Vessels at different depths within the skin may be involved.

Severe damage to a vessel may lead to rupture and the predominating sign of purpura. These purpuric lesions are almost always palpable, a feature which distinguishes them from other types of purpura. Milder vessel damage may result predominantly in increased vascular permeability leading to local oedema and urticarial lesions (see: chronic idiopathic urticaria, page 181). Nodular lesions usually result from the involvement of larger vessels deeper in the dermis or in the subcutaneous fat with prominent cellular infiltration and oedema. Necrosis, ulceration and ultimately scarring result mainly from ischaemia. Haemorrhagic bullae are often an initial sign of superficial necrosis and pustular lesions occur when the inflammatory cell exudate is intense.

The inflammatory cell type is variable. Neutrophils predominate in some cases, a mixture of neutrophils and mononuclear cells occur in others, while some show a predominantly mononuclear or granulomatous histology. In patients with a neutrophil infiltrate, small nuclear fragments (nuclear dust) which are derived from disintegrating neutrophil polymorphs (leukocytoclasis) are present in the infiltrate. The histology of the cellular infiltrate may alter with the age of the lesion.

Classification of vasculitis

No system of classification of cutaneous vasculitis is entirely satisfactory. There is at present insufficient understanding of either the causes or the pathological mechanisms to allow a comprehensive aetiological or mechanistic classification. Certain patterns of cutaneous vasculitis, for example Henoch–Schönlein syndrome and erythema nodosum, are clinically well defined, but many other patterns of disease do not fit so easily into a purely descriptive classification. Classifications have been made on the basis of the type and size of blood vessels which are involved[82]; on the histological features of the inflammatory cells; and on the basis of a bewildering mixture of clinical, histological and other pathological features[83]. Immune complexes have been implicated in the pathogenesis of some types of vasculitis (see below) and a classification has been proposed on the basis of the physico-chemical properties of these immune complexes[84]. Unfortunately current investigational methods detect circulating immune complexes in only a minority of patients. Each classification has some merit, but all have serious deficiencies.

The classification suggested in Table 6.1 is modified from that recently proposed by Shuster[85]. It is unsatisfactory in that it is based on a mixture of clinical and histological features, but it nevertheless serves as a useful

Table 6.1 Classification of cutaneous vasculitis (Modified from Shuster, 1978)[85]

Clinico-pathological category	Name	Type of inflammatory infiltrate
Leukocytoclastic vasculitis	Henoch–Schönlein syndrome allergic vasculitis urticarial vasculitis erythema multiforme	predominantly polymorph or mixed polymorph and mononuclear leukocytoclasis
Nodular vasculitis	erythema nodosum erythema induratum	polymorph and mononuclear or mononuclear and granulomatous
Granulomatous vasculitis	polyarteritis nodosa allergic granulomatosis Wegener's granulomatosis	granulomatous

framework for discussion in the light of current ignorance. It is necessarily didactic and oversimplified.

Leukocytoclastic vasculitis[86]

Lesions show a predilection for the lower limbs, lower trunk and forearms. Involvement of the upper trunk or face is uncommon. Mild lesions are often symptomless but nodules and ulceration may be painful. Dependent oedema is common due to increased vascular permeability. Non-specific systemic symptoms include general malaise, myalgia and fever. Vessels of other organs are frequently involved leading to nephritis, arthritis, gastrointestinal haemorrhage, radiological pulmonary shadowing and pleural effusion and various neurological changes. Renal failure is the commonest fatal complication.

Allergic vasculitis is perhaps the best general term to apply to the majority of patients with the leukocytoclastic type of vasculitis. The condition may be transient and self-limiting, acute fulminating and fatal, or chronic with a significant mortality from renal failure and morbidity from skin lesions, arthritis and neurological disease.

Henoch–Schönlein syndrome is a type of leukocytoclastic vasculitis affecting both children[87] and adults[88]. Occasionally it is preceded by a respiratory tract infection. Purpura, arthralgia, renal involvement (proteinuria) and gastrointestinal involvement (abdominal pain and gastrointestinal haemorrhage) are the commonest clinical findings. Apart from historical reasons there seems little merit in retaining the eponym since the disease cannot be clearly distinguished from other types of leukocytoclastic vasculitis[86].

Urticarial vasculitis (synonyms: urticarial angiitis, vasculitic urticaria) is a useful clinical term to describe a condition which appears similar to chronic idiopathic urticaria. However, unlike ordinary urticaria the lesions tend to last longer, that is for 1–3 days compared with a few hours, and very close inspection may reveal subtle evidence of purpura. Biopsy reveals leukocytoclastic vasculitis[1, 11, 89] compared to the non-specific perivascular infiltrate without microscopic vessel damage which is found in chronic urticaria. Interestingly, hypocomplementaemia is common in this group of patients[11, 89] whereas serum complement levels are often normal in other types of allergic vasculitis[86].

Erythema multiforme[90] is a condition which is clinically more distinctive than the other types of leukocytoclastic vasculitis. Its name implies polymorphic features but these are no more so than in other types of vasculitis. It is an acute self-limiting condition usually running a course of 1–3 weeks but with a tendency to recur in some patients. Lesions most characteristically occur on the palms and backs of the hands, elbows, buttocks and knees. There may be prominent involvement of mucous membranes of the eye, mouth and urogenital tract (Stevens–Johnson syndrome). Acute generalized skin involvement with erythema and necrosis and sloughing of the epidermis (adult type of toxic epidermal necrolysis) appears to be an uncommon variant of erythema multiforme. Erythematous macules and urticarial plaques with purpura are the commonest clinical type of lesion but there may also be papules, vesicles and bullae. Peripheral extension with central clearing gives rise to the characteristic target or iris lesions but these are by no means always present. Kidneys, joints and sometimes other internal organs may be involved. Histologically the infiltrate is more mononuclear than in the preceding types of leukocytoclastic vasculitis but nevertheless endothelial damage, polymorph infiltration and leukocytoclasis are found in early lesions[91].

Nodular vasculitis

Erythema nodosum[92] is clinically a well-circumscribed type of vasculitis which is generally familiar to physicians in specialties other than dermatology. Lesions characteristically occur on the anterior aspect of the lower legs, but less commonly involve the thighs and upper arms. Clinically deep tender nodules develop which may initially exhibit little visible change. Over the course of days or weeks the nodules enlarge to form irregular red indurated plaques of varying size. Individual lesions tend to resolve without scarring over a course of 2–6 weeks and often exhibit bruise-like discoloration in the later stages. Joint involvement is common but renal disease less so.

The vessels involved are mainly located in subcutaneous fat[93]. In early lesions small vessels and medium-sized venules show endothelial proliferation and mural invasion with polymorphs and mononuclear cells. Red cell extravasation occurs commonly[94] but without thrombosis. Mononuclear cells and giant cell granulomata predominate in older lesions. Vessels within the dermis usually show less florid changes.

Lesions of *erythema induratum*[95] occur characteristically on the sides and backs of the lower legs. Women are almost exclusively affected. The lesions start as deep, slightly tender nodules of dusky purple coloration. They enlarge slowly and may ulcerate, sometimes persisting for several weeks and ultimately healing with scarring. Systemic signs and symptoms are usually absent.

Both arteries and veins in the subcutaneous fat are involved in the inflammatory process. The inflammatory infiltrate is intense and consists of mononuclear and plasma cells with granuloma formation. There is endothelial proliferation and mural invasion with inflammatory cells and fibrosis[96]. These features together with thrombosis frequently produce vascular obliteration with infarction.

Granulomatous vasculitis

Polyarteritis nodosa, allergic granulomatosis and *Wegener's granulomatosis* are all types of granulomatous vasculitis which are considerably less common than the previously considered types of vasculitis. In polyarteritis nodosa and allergic granulomatosis small and medium-sized arteries are involved. Renal and cardiac involvement with polymyositis and peripheral neuritis are the commonest features of polyarteritis nodosa[97]. A benign form involves only the skin[98, 99]. Pulmonary involvement predominates in allergic granulomatosis[100] with asthma, pulmonary infiltration and eosinophilia. Cutaneous nodules may develop. In both polyarteritis nodosa and allergic granulomatosis there is granulomatous destruction of arterial walls but in allergic granulomatosis there are also numerous granulomata present which are not directly related to vessels[100]. In Wegener's granulomatosis there is granulomatous vasculitis involving particularly the upper and lower respiratory tract and the kidney. Both arteries and veins are involved histologically. A variety of skin lesions occur in a minority of patients and include petechial haemorrhages, papulonecrotic lesions and ulcers. Renal failure is the commonest cause of death in all these types of granulomatous vasculitis.

Pathogenic mechanisms

The histological similarity of leukocytoclastic vasculitis to the experimental Arthus reaction has long suggested an immune pathogenesis for this type of vasculitis. There is now considerable evidence to implicate the involvement of circulating immune complexes. Similar mechanisms may operate in nodular and granulomatous types of vasculitis but the evidence for this is at present tenuous.

Evidence of circulating immune complexes can be found in some patients with vasculitis. The demonstration of cryoglobulin[101] provides the most direct evidence but not all complexes are cold-precipitable and their detection may depend on more indirect methods. Anticomplementary activity in serum[102] and low serum levels of early complement components[11, 103, 104] are features suggestive of the presence of complement-binding immune complexes. C1q-binding activity is perhaps the most widely used test for inferring the presence of immune complexes and high binding activity has been found in some patients[105]. Nevertheless evidence suggestive of circulating immune complexes is only obtainable in a proportion of patients using currently available methods.

Many studies have demonstrated by immunofluorescence the presence of immunoglobulin and complement components in affected lesional blood vessels[106]. The presence of similar deposits in normal perilesional skin[107] has been used as an argument that the localization of complexes in vessels precedes and perhaps initiates the vasculitis. Experimental evidence indicates that immune complexes can be induced to localize in vascular endothelium by increasing vascular permeability. Advantage has been taken of this to induce vasculitic lesions by the local injection of histamine into the skin of patients with cutaneous vasculitis. In areas of histamine-induced wealing early accumulation of neutrophils as well as deposition of immunoglobulin and complement components has been noted[17,18]. Amorphous and occasionally crystalloid deposition of putative immune complexes beneath the vascular endothelium has been observed by electron microscopy[17]. Early events in histamine-induced lesions have also been studied by immunoelectron microscopy. Localization of C3, IgM and IgG between endothelial cells and pericytes has been demonstrated by this technique[108].

So far there has been little published evidence that experimental localization of complexes by these techniques actually leads to the development of lesions. However the author's observations in patients with urticarial vasculitis indicate that a variety of vasodilating stimuli including intradermal injection of histamine, blunt trauma, and in some cases even saline injection or the trauma of venepuncture may be followed after a few hours by the development of typical urticarial vasculitis lesions.

The tissue damage which occurs in vasculitis is thought to result mainly from complement activation induced by the immune complexes. Among the results of complement activation are formation of anaphylotoxin which releases histamine and formation of the C5a complex which is chemotactic for polymorphs. Polymorphs which have engulfed complexes release lysosomal proteolytic enzymes which may not only destroy the cells producing leukocytoclasis but also damage adjacent structures. The relationship of the complement system to Hageman factor and the kinin system has already been mentioned (see: hereditary angioedema, page 186). Both immune complexes and Hageman factor activate the proteolytic enzyme kallikrein and Hageman factor also promotes thrombus formation. It follows that the degree of damage resulting from immune complex deposition is likely to be dependent on several independently variable factors including (1) the concentration of complexes, (2) the ability of complexes to activate complement, (3) the availability of polymorphs, and (4) the availability of the effector enzyme systems, e.g. kallikrein, Hageman factor etc. The effector systems mentioned above, i.e. the accumulation of polymorphs and the activation of proteolytic enzyme systems, require time for their development and clinical lesions do not develop for 2–6 hours after complex deposition.

Factors which are involved in the formation and removal of complexes and in the repair of vasculitic damage may be expected to influence the duration of clinical disease. Continuing disease may result from the continuing presence of immune complexes in the plasma either because of their persistent formation or because of impaired clearance by the reticuloendothelial system[109]. Local clearance of complexes from the lesions as well as the repair of tissue damage, for example by fibrinolysis[110] may also be expected to influence the severity and duration of lesions.

The physico-chemical properties of the immune complexes themselves are also important in determining the clinical features of the disease which is produced[101]. IgM complexes may be so large as to increase blood viscosity and lead to a frank hyperviscosity syndrome[111]. The relative amounts of antigen and antibody in complexes may also affect a variety of properties including the histological type of inflammation which is produced. Soluble complexes produced in antigen excess typically produce leukocytoclastic vasculitis similar to the experimental Arthus reaction. However the experimental injection of less soluble complexes formed at equivalence of antigen and antibody results in the production of granulomata[112]. So far this interesting experimental observation has not been applied to the study of granulomatous vasculitis in man.

Aetiology

A large number of agents have been incriminated in the initiation of vasculitis. These include infectious agents, injection of foreign protein and drugs. Vasculitis is also a feature of some 'autoimmune' diseases including particularly systemic lupus erythematosus, chronic active hepatitis, rheumatoid disease and ulcerative colitis. The evidence incriminating these factors consists mainly of guilt by association. Removal or treatment of the causative agent leads in some cases to clearance of the vasculitis but such evidence is suggestive rather than proof of causation. However the circumstantial clinical evidence is extremely strong in the case of certain infectious agents and drugs. Virus infections, particularly herpes simplex and orf, are frequently associated with erythema multiforme as are drug reactions, for which sulphonamides are at present mainly responsible. Streptococcal infection has been particularly implicated in the causation of erythema nodosum and there is an association between this condition as well as erythema induratum with tuberculous infection. Nevertheless further evidence of causation is required.

Such evidence might include the following: (1) demonstration of the alleged causative antigen in circulating immune complexes, (2) demonstration of the antigen as well as antibody fixed in the vessels of the lesions, and (3) evidence that injection of the antigen–antibody complexes induces tissue damage analogous to that of vasculitis. Evidence satisfying the first two criteria has been obtained in vasculitis associated with hepatitis B antigenaemia[113]. Considerable experimental evidence of this type has also been produced to implicate streptococcal infection in the causation of vasculitis[114–117]. Antigen, apparently derived from a variety of other infectious agents, has been detected in the vasculitic lesions of other patients. Vasculitic skin lesions have been induced in primates by the injection of complexes composed of streptococcal antigen and human streptococcal antibody[114]. Thus there is limited experimental evidence to support the view that immune reactions initiated by exogenous agents may in some circumstances lead to the development of vasculitis by the mechanisms previously suggested.

Treatment

In many patients an acute episode of cutaneous vasculitis is brief and self-limiting. Symptoms may be minimal and in such a situation no specific treatment is required. This type of vasculitis is commonly seen following acute infections and in adverse drug reactions. In cases in which an infectious cause is suspected this should be treated when possible and drugs which may have been responsible should be withdrawn. Immunosuppressive treatment with systemic corticosteroids and more general supportive measures are required in more severe reactions or when signification involvement of internal organs is present.

The management of more chronic types of vasculitis poses greater problems. Efforts should be made to find possible causative factors such as occult infection or neoplasia which may be amenable to treatment. In the absence of such factors the hazards of long-term immunosuppressive treatment with systemic corticosteroids and drugs such as azathioprine have to be weighed against the severity of the disease. Immunosuppressive treatment is not invariably effective.

Other forms of treatment may influence other aspects of the effector and repair systems which operate in vasculitis. Dapsone is occasionally effective[118-120] and recent evidence suggests that this drug may inhibit polymorph function[121]. Fibrin deposition is prominent in vasculitic lesions and fibrinolysis is required for its removal and repair. Fibrinolytic activity is reduced in the blood[122, 123] and in the skin[110] of some patients with cutaneous vasculitis and beneficial effects have been claimed for the use of drugs which enhance fibrinolytic activity[124]. The author's limited experience of this form of treatment has been disappointing.

If circulating immune complexes play a central role in the pathogenesis of vasculitis it would be logical to remove them by plasmaphoresis. This technique has been successfully used to treat some patients with severe and resistant disease. There is evidence of defective clearance of complexes from the circulation by the reticuloendothelial system in patients with systemic lupus erythematosus and cutaneous vasculitis[109]. It is not clear whether this is a primary defect or the result of overloading of the reticuloendothelial system. Plasmaphoresis in such patients produced not only clinical improvement and a fall in circulating immune complex levels but also improved reticuloendothelial function. A combination of immunosuppressive drugs and intermittent plasmaphoresis may be justified in some severely affected patients.

ECZEMA

The term eczema is usually considered synonymous with dermatitis. However the latter term is also used in other contexts, for example dermatitis artefacta, perioral dermatitis and dermatitis herpetiformis. Eczema implies specific clinical and particularly histological features and for this reason it is preferred by the author. The clinical features of eczema include redness, scaling, vesiculation, exudation and crusting. Itching is often severe and excoriation encourages secondary bacterial infection. Not all these features are necessarily present. Histological changes are found in both the epidermis and dermis. Epidermal changes are the most characteristic and consist of intercellular oedema (spongiosis) and vacuolation of keratinocytes which break down to form intraepidermal vesicles. Dermal blood vessels and lymphatics are dilated and there is oedema with an inflammatory infiltrate composed mainly of mononuclear cells which may also be present in the epidermal vesicles. Hyperkeratosis and parakeratosis are variable features.

Although the eczemas have the above features in common they present varied clinical patterns. Allergic contact eczema often exhibits a characteristic distribution determined by the circumstances of allergen exposure. It is the type of eczema which has been most extensively studied since the causes can be verified by patch testing and it can be readily induced in man and experimental animals. Atopic eczema is also well delineated with its association with immediate hypersensitivity and allergic respiratory disease and a rather characteristic distribution pattern and clinical course. Other less clearly defined patterns of endogenous eczema are common especially in adults. They have less specific features although the distribution is frequently symmetrical and may involve sites such as the scalp, trunk and lower legs. This distribution does not suggest involvement of a contact allergen and patch tests are negative. No association with atopy has been clearly established. Little is known of the aetiology or mechanism of these types of eczema. Irritant and toxic agents are also able to induce eczematous reactions in which immunological or allergic mechanisms may not be involved.

Atopic eczema

Although this condition often starts in early childhood the term infantile eczema is a misnomer. In patients with a childhood onset there is certainly a tendency to spontaneous improvement, but there is an understandable tendency for this aspect to be overemphasized by clinicians. Several studies have indicated that childhood atopic eczema persists into adult life in 30–80% of patients[125–129]. Clinically identical patterns of eczema, often associated with asthma or rhinitis, may appear for the first time in adult life.

At the onset, especially in childhood, the rash is frequently rather diffuse involving particularly the face, trunk and extensor surfaces of the limbs. When the napkin area is involved the depths of the skin folds in the groin are characteristically spared and this is a useful sign in distinguishing it from an infective intertrigo, especially candidosis. At this early stage redness and fine scaling predominate, often without macroscopic vesiculation or much secondary bacterial infection. As the condition becomes more chronic, the characteristic involvement of flexures tends to develop with thickening and scaling (lichenification) of the epidermis which tends to fissure especially around the joints. At this stage vesiculation (especially on the palms and soles), weeping, crusting and secondary bacterial infection (usually staphylococcal) are common features.

A personal or family history of allergic rhinitis or asthma is common, but by no means invariable. Some useful diagnostic criteria have recently been suggested[130]. Their use should certainly help to ensure greater uniformity in clinical research but their rigid clinical application would probably exclude many patients with mild forms of the disease. A clear distinction between atopic eczema, seborrhoeic dermatitis, irritant napkin dermatitis and infective flexural intertrigo is often very difficult in early infancy.

Immunological factors

There are abnormalities of both humoral and cell-mediated immunity in patients with atopic eczema. IgA deficiency is more common in atopics than in normal controls[131]. Transient IgA deficiency at the age of 3 months has been associated with an increased risk of developing atopic disease in the first year of life[132]. This finding led to the hypothesis that a transient defect of IgA-mediated intestinal humoral immunity could lead to excessive absorption of antigens in neonatal life and to inappropriate development of IgE antibody responses with consequent atopic disease. While such a hypothesis is an attractive one, another study[133] has failed to confirm the basic premise of transient neonatal IgA deficiency in atopic disease. Moreover the workers who originally reported this observation were themselves unable to confirm it in a more recent study[134].

The most obvious abnormality of humoral immunity in atopic eczema is the presence of high levels of serum IgE[135]. Immediate weal and flare prick test reactions to allergens involved in allergic respiratory disease are frequently found[136,137] and many patients have coexisting allergic respiratory disease such as allergic rhinitis and asthma. Serum IgE levels tend to be highest in those patients with both eczema and allergic respiratory disease[138] and IgE levels show some correlation with the severity of skin disease[137-141]. The proportion of B lymphocytes bearing surface IgE is increased in the blood of patients with atopic eczema[142,143]. Such evidence has led some investigators to implicate IgE in the pathogenic mechanism of atopic eczema in addition to its established role in allergic respiratory disease.

A number of other observations cast doubt on a primary role for IgE in atopic eczema. These may be summarized as follows.

(1) IgE levels are only moderately raised in patients with pure atopic eczema (without respiratory disease) and in some the levels are normal[144].

(2) Serial measurements of serum IgE in individual patients do not correlate with changes in severity of the eczema[145, 146].

(3) Eczema is not induced by skin testing with common respiratory allergens which produce typical IgE-mediated immediate hypersensitivity reactions in the skin.

(4) Exacerbation of IgE-mediated allergic respiratory disease is not usually associated with simultaneous exacerbation of atopic eczema in patients with both conditions.

While such observations do not exclude the possibility that IgE is involved in the mechanism of eczema its role at present remains unclear. Serum levels of IgG4 have also been found to be elevated in atopic eczema[147]. However, further studies to examine a possible role for this immunoglobulin are still awaited.

Several lines of evidence indicate defective cell-mediated immunity in patients with atopic eczema. Such individuals are particularly susceptible to infectious diseases including disseminated vaccinia (eczema vaccinatum), herpes simplex (eczema herpeticum), warts[148], molluscum contagiosum[149, 150] and chronic dermatophyte infection[151]. Cell-mediated immune mechanisms are thought to be involved in the normal control of all these conditions.

Cell-mediated hypersensitivity is the predominant mechanism of allergic contact eczema. Patients with atopic eczema are less susceptible than non-atopics to sensitization with experimental contact allergens such as dinitro-chlorobenzene[152] or to naturally occurring poison ivy[153]. These findings suggest a defect in the afferent pathway for the induction of cell-mediated hypersensitivity.

Previously established delayed skin test reactivity to tuberculin is diminished during exacerbation of atopic eczema[154]. This observation suggests an additional defect in the efferent limb of delayed cell-mediated hypersensitivity reactions. Further evidence of an efferent pathway defect comes from the recent observation that delayed skin test reactions to streptokinase–streptodornase and candidin are frequently negative in patients with atopic eczema despite normal *in vitro* lymphocyte transformation to these antigens[155].

A review of 40 studies indicates that circulating T-lymphocyte numbers are reduced in atopic eczema[156]. The mononuclear cells in the eczematous skin are predominantly T lymphocytes[157] and the presence of extensive eczema could itself lead to diminished circulating T-cells because of redistribution in the skin. *In vitro*, lymphocytes with T-cell characteristics can be induced by incubation with thymosin[158]. Normal individuals have significantly fewer thymosin-inducible T-cells than patients with atopic eczema. The numbers of thymosin-inducible T-cells correlate with IgE levels[158] and it has been suggested that these cells represent immature T-suppressor cells whose functional deficiency leads to inadequate suppression of IgE responses[158].

In malignant lymphomas[159] and various immunodeficiency diseases[160] it has been shown that *in vitro* lymphocyte stimulation with the T-cell mitogen concanavalin A fails to lead to the production of leukocyte migration inhibitor factor (LMIF). This inhibition of LMIF production correlates with decreased cell-mediated immunity. A highly significant depression of LMIF production has been found in lymphocytes from patients with atopic eczema following *in vitro* stimulation with concanavalin A, phytohaemagglutinin and tuberculin[161]. These observations provide further evidence for a defect of cell-mediated immunity in atopic eczema.

Eczema, indistinguishable from atopic eczema also occurs in primary immunodeficiency diseases of which the Wiskott–Aldrich syndrome[162,163] is an example. Raised IgE levels and depressed cell-mediated immunity are also characteristic of this condition. This constant feature of an inverse relationship between IgE levels and cell-mediated immunity in primary immunodeficiencies and in atopy has suggested that these two aspects of the immune system may be interdependent. Some confirmation of such an interrelationship comes from animal experiments[164] in which T-cell depletion was followed by increased IgE production.

It has not been clear whether the observed defects in cell-mediated immune mechanisms are primary or secondary phenomena. The direct relationship of tuberculin skin test reactivity with the severity of the eczema[154] is compatible either with a primary defect affecting both processes or with a depression of reactivity secondary to the eczema. None of the numerous other abnormalities related to cell-mediated immune mechanisms has been studied sequentially in a similar way. However the interesting recent finding[165] of depressed T-lymphocyte numbers in healthy 1-month-old children born to atopic parents (especially asthmatic fathers) suggests a primary defect of cellular immunity. If confirmed, this observation may link the common type of atopic eczema with that which occurs less commonly in major immunodeficiency diseases.

Management

The treatment of atopic eczema is unsatisfactory. Corticosteroids suppress the condition and used topically these are the most successful agents currently available. Systemic corticosteroids are seldom justified. The action of corticosteroids is suppressive rather than curative and their regular long-term topical use leads to atrophy of both the epidermis and dermis. The main clinical result of this atrophy are telangiectasia, shear purpura (ecchymosis), striae and fragile skin. Significant systemic absorption occurs but is seldom of clinical importance except in young children in whom the use of potent topical steroid may result in a Cushingoid appearance, hirsuties and even retardation of growth. Absorption of topical corticosteroid is enhanced by the presence of extensive eczema and by the use of polythene occlusion.

Bland emollients may provide some symptomatic relief of itching especially in patients with ichthyosis which frequently coexists with atopic eczema. Emollients also help to reduce fissuring by increasing the elasticity of the abnormal keratin. Oral antihistamines may help to diminish irritation, but are often disappointingly ineffective.

Bacteria, especially *Staphylococcus aureus*, are present in enormous numbers on the skin of patients with atopic eczema, particularly in the lesions[166]. Although many patients do not have overt evidence of infection, recurrent skin sepsis is a major feature in some. This aspect of the disease is frequently neglected. Both topical and systemic antibiotics dramatically decrease the numbers of *Staphylococcus aureus* in diseased skin[166] and systemic cloxacillin alone significantly increased the rate of healing of eczema compared with placebo[167]. The author's usual preference is for oral flucloxacillin in prolonged courses of at least 1 month or in some cases on a long-term basis. Antiseptic soaks of potassium permanganate are very useful for infected eczema of the hands and feet. Although bacteria are considered as secondary invaders in the eczematous skin of atopics a more primary role has been suggested for bacteria in some types of eczema (see: bacterial allergy in eczema, page 205). A possible role for bacterial allergy in atopic eczema deserves further study.

Measures designed to enhance the depressed cell-mediated immunity have not so far been successful. Levamisole has been without benefit[168, 169] and the use of thymosin[158] is still only theoretical.

The hypothesis that transient neonatal immunodeficiency predisposes to atopy[132] has stimulated attempts to enhance natural immunity and to avoid exposure to allergens in the neonatal period. It has been suggested that breast-feeding achieves this goal both by avoiding exposure to allergens in cows' milk or artificial milk formulae and also by providing secretory IgA in breast milk[134]. Available data on the effect of breast-feeding is conflicting, some studies suggesting that it protects against the development of atopic eczema[134, 170] and others that it does not[171, 172]. Although the encouragement of breast-feeding may be desirable for a variety of reasons its widespread encouragement as a means of preventing atopic eczema should still be regarded as controversial.

In children with established atopic eczema significant improvement occurred with an egg- and milk-free diet[173]. These allergens were arbitrarily chosen for exclusion because they are common dietary causes of immediate type hypersensitivity reactions in atopic patients. This interesting study appears to have been carefully performed in a double-blind way but has not yet been confirmed. However, in spite of the improvement, in none of the patients did the eczema clear completely. A further common clinical observation casts doubt on a major role for a dietary causation of atopic eczema. Admission to hospital almost invariably produces rapid and dramatic improvement in atopic eczema even though the patients continue on a normal diet. The reasons for this phenomenon are not clear but dietary factors have to be discounted.

Allergic contact eczema

There are no clinical features which clearly distinguish eczema due to external allergens from other types. However the pattern and distribution of the rash often suggests the diagnosis and this may be reinforced by a history of exposure to a known contact allergen. However the routine use of patch tests with a standard battery of the most common contact sensitizers will reveal many unsuspected cases of allergic contact dermatitis. Identification and elimination of a contact allergen offers an opportunity to cure the condition – an opportunity which is not at present available in any other form of eczema. Failure to detect contact allergy accounts for a significant number of patients with persistent eczema labelled as endogenous. It is important to remember that all types of eczema may be complicated by the development of allergy to topically applied drugs. Identification of such problems depends on a high index of suspicion and on the widespread use of routine standard patch testing in patients with chronic eczema of all types.

The number of potential contact allergens is enormous and the circumstances under which they may be encountered is infinitely greater. Fortunately, however, a small number of allergens accounts for the great majority of cases. These allergens include metallic ions, especially chromate, nickel and cobalt; antioxidants and accelerators used in the manufacture of rubber; topically applied therapeutic agents and a variety of miscellaneous substances. Such substances can be conveniently tested by using a standard battery of about two dozen contact allergens for routine patch testing. Such standard batteries are now in widespread use. Their composition tends to be similar but is modified when necessary to take into account allergens which may be locally important.

Other standard allergen batteries are useful for testing patients with particular patterns of eczema, for example suspected allergy to shoes (rubber chemicals, leather tanning agents, glues, etc.) or for investigating patients from particular occupations, for example dentists or nurses (acrylic monomers, local anaesthetics, drugs etc.).

Much clinical research in human contact dermatitis has revolved around the identification of potential contact allergens. Such work is of great clinical importance. A specialist in contact dermatitis necessarily requires a wide knowledge of industrial chemistry and manufacturing processes ranging from heavy engineering to the manufacture of clothing and cosmetics. Fortunately much of this encyclopaedic information is available in standard reference texts[174,175].

It is essential to bear in mind that a positive patch test is only an indication of previous sensitization to the allergen. Its relevance to a particular episode of eczema depends on other circumstantial evidence of exposure to the relevant agent and clinical improvement after its elimination. Sensitivity to multiple allergens is common and this can considerably complicate identification of the cause of an episode of eczema.

Aetiological factors

In order to cause eczema, a contact allergen must necessarily penetrate intact skin. Such agents are therefore usually of small molecular weight and act as haptens. Conjugation with protein in the skin is thought to produce the complete antigen. Allergens conjugated with various proteins including albumin[176], skin proteins[176,177], erythrocytes[178] and leukocytes[178] will induce lymphocyte transformation in sensitized human subjects. It is not clear whether *in vivo* the carrier protein is specific. However there is increasing evidence that the epidermal Langerhans cell (see below) is specifically involved in transferring antigen recognition to lymphocytes.

Much work in animals over the last 40 years has established that cell-mediated hypersensitivity mechanisms are of central importance in allergic contact eczema. The most important evidence in favour of this can be summarized as follows.

(1) The inflammatory cells found in allergic contact eczema are mononuclear cells of the lymphocyte series.

(2) Allergic contact sensitivity can be passively transferred to non-sensitized animals by the injection of lymphoid cell suspensions from sensitized animals, but not by the injection of serum[179].

(3) During the induction of contact sensitivity histological changes occur in the draining lymph nodes which are typical of cell-mediated hypersensitivity reactions[180]. These changes consist of T lymphocyte proliferation in the paracortical areas. Similar changes are seen in skin allograft rejection.

(4) Lymphocyte transformation can be achieved *in vitro* in some cases of human allergic contact eczema using protein conjugates of the causative agent as antigen[176–178].

Although cell-mediated hypersensitivity reactions are clearly of paramount importance in allergic contact hypersensitivity the possible role of antibody in human allergic eczema has received little study. An increased number of circulating lymphocytes bearing surface IgD has been reported in patients with allergic contact eczema[142] and this observation has been confirmed by others[143]. IgD-bearing lymphocytes appeared in a patient experimentally sensitized with DNCB[143]. These observations have raised speculation of a role for IgD in human allergic contact dermatitis but as yet further data are not available.

Perhaps the most interesting new facet of allergic contact hypersensitivity to emerge in recent years is the role played by the Langerhans cell[181]. First described in 1868 by Paul Langerhans, it is only in the last decade that the electron microscope has allowed systematic study of this cell. Langerhans cells were originally found in the epidermis but have also been identified in thymus[182] and lymph nodes[183]. Indistinguishable cells occur in large numbers in the lesions of histocytosis X[184]. Langerhans cells can be identified electron microscopically by their specific intracytoplasmic granules and by the absence of structural features and organelles typical of epidermal keratinocytes or melanocytes. In common with some other immunologically active cells, Langerhans cells express Ia antigens[185, 186] and bear Fc and C3 receptors[187]. They appear to be derived from bone marrow[188].

The work of Silberberg and her colleagues has done much to establish a role for Langerhans cells in allergic contact eczema. It was noted that in human allergic contact hypersensitivity reactions to a variety of allergens, close apposition of mononuclear cells to epidermal Langerhans cells invariably occurred[189]. This apposition was not found in non-reactive patch tests to various allergens, in irritant dermatitis reactions or in a variety of other dermatoses. A similar association of the two cell types was found in guinea-pigs sensitized either actively or passively to DNCB[190, 191]. Langerhans cells are also found in the dermis in both human and guinea-pig allergic contact hypersensitivity reactions and have occasionally been identified in dermal lymphatics in guinea-pig reactions[191].

Langerhans cells are phagocytic and will engulf foreign material such as ferritin[192]. However they are much less active in this respect than keratinocytes and it appears unlikely that the cell has a primary phagocytic role. It has however been demonstrated that a variety of soluble small molecular weight substances, all of them contact allergens, have a special affinity for the Langerhans cell[193]. This observation has led to the hypothesis that the Langerhans cell acts as an allergen trap which absorbs haptens as they traverse the epidermis and converts them to complete antigens. The close association between Langerhans and mononuclear cells in allergic contact dermatitis reactions suggests that they are involved in transferring antigen recognition to T lymphocytes[194].

Management

The management of allergic contact eczema can be considered under the headings of prevention and treatment. Preventive measures in allergic industrial dermatitis depend on the use of protective clothing, automated manufacturing processes and improved ventilation. Substitution of a non-allergenic or less allergenic chemical may also be possible in some circumstances. Unfortunately financial considerations often oppose those of safety. Many industrial manual workers are unable to work satisfactorily while wearing protective gloves. In these circumstances the use of barrier cream may afford some protection. Minor cuts and abrasions on the hands inevitably result in increased skin penetration by allergens and patients quite frequently note that eczema started initially around such an injury. Measures designed to minimize trauma such as filtration of swarf from cutting oils, education of employees and closer medical supervision of employees can all reduce such problems.

Topical agents used in the treatment of skin disease are among the most frequent causes of allergic contact dermatitis. Some of the commonest culprits are topical antibiotics – particularly neomycin, framycetin and sodium fusidate. The indiscriminate use of ointments containing these substances for trivial skin infections and often non-infective conditions must be condemned. Creams which have an aqueous phase will support the growth of bacteria and require the addition of preservatives some of which are sensitizers. Parabens (esters of p-aminobenzoic acid) and ethylenediamine are among the most important of these. Ointments, which are generally free of preservatives, are usually preferable to creams. However lanolin, a constituent of some ointment bases, is an important sensitizer and is still used in some preparations. A particular difficulty facing general practitioners and dermatologists is that the minor ingredients (preservatives, wetting agents, emulsifiers, etc.) of topical drug formulations are not stated on their containers. Although manufacturers are invariably helpful in providing this information when approached on an individual basis it is not generally available. It is therefore very difficult to know which other topical drug formulations contain the substance to which the patient may have already been shown to be allergic. Approaches to the pharmaceutical industry have not so far resolved this problem.

In animals it has been clearly demonstrated that the ability to develop contact sensitivity is genetically determined. The identification of such a genetic marker in man would be of enormous potential value in the prevention of human disease. Unfortunately no such marker has at present been identified in humans.

Identification and elimination of the responsible antigen is the most important goal in management. Unfortunately antigens commonly causing allergic dermatitis are often ubiquitous and antigen avoidance may be difficult to achieve. As in atopic eczema, topical and occasionally systemic corticosteroids are useful suppressive agents together with antibacterial measures where indicated.

Specific immunological unresponsiveness has been studied extensively in animals[195]. Two patterns of unresponsiveness are of particular potential relevance to human allergic contact eczema: (1) induction of tolerance to sensitizing chemicals so that sensitivity does not develop following subsequent exposure which would normally sensitize, and (2) specific inhibition of contact sensitivity such that sensitivity which has already been established is suppressed. Both these aspects of specific unresponsiveness have received limited attention in humans.

Early attempts[196-198] in man to induce immunological tolerance were unsuccessful. However some attenuation of sensitivity to DNCB occurred following prior application of DNCB to the buccal mucosa[199, 200] or prior feeding[201] of the allergen. Tolerance to nitrogen mustard was achieved in patients undergoing topical treatment for mycosis fungoides lymphoma by prior intravenous injection of small amounts of the drug[202]. These findings could not be reproduced in patients with mycosis fungoides[203] or psoriasis[204, 205]. These early observations indicate that the induction of tolerance in man may ultimately be possible. However the variable results achieved so far are a reflection of our ignorance of the mechanisms involved, the empirical nature of the dosage regimens and routes of administration and probably also of the differing immune status of patients in different diseases. Induction of tolerance is not at present a practical therapeutic proposition.

Specific inhibition of sensitivity would be especially applicable to the great majority of patients who present with established allergic eczema. Desensitization or hyposensitization to nitrogen mustard has been achieved in patients with mycosis fungoides by daily intravenous injections of the drug in increasing doses[202]. Limited confirmation of these results was obtained in nitrogen-mustard-sensitive patients with psoriasis[206]. Using this technique in three patients with mycosis fungoides, the author was able completely to desensitize one and to hyposensitize another. Desensitization or hyposensitization to nitrogen mustard[207] and to poison ivy[208] has also been reported following prolonged epicutaneous application of the allergen. However, successful desensitization to other common environmental contact allergens such as nickel has not been achieved and to date this approach remains of academic rather than practical interest.

Bacterial allergy in eczema

There are a variety of other clinical patterns of eczema which cannot be clearly related to atopic eczema or to allergic contact eczema. Descriptive terms such as discoid or flexural eczema are frequently applied in these circumstances. The term 'endogenous' is often used implying some unknown internal causation but 'idiopathic' would be more suitable since the mechanisms of such eczema are unknown.

It has long been considered that bacteria may play a more primary part in the pathogenesis of some types of eczema in addition to their obvious role in producing secondary infection. However previous attempts to incriminate bacteria on the basis of intradermal skin tests have been inconclusive. Interesting recent studies have provided further immunological evidence in favour of a more fundamental pathogenic role for skin surface bacteria. This evidence is as follows.

(1) Staphylococcal and micrococcal antigens can be identified in both the epidermis and dermis in some eczema patients. Some bacterial antigen appears to be firmly bound to epidermal cells[209].

(2) Patients with eczema have higher antibody levels against these bacteria compared with controls[210].

(3) Intradermal injections of bacterial antigens produce Arthus-like reactions irrespective of the serum levels of the appropriate antibody[211].

(4) Epidermal cell cultures which had adsorbed bacterial antigen were severely damaged following the addition of serum from eczema patients which contained the appropriate bacterial antibody[212].

These observations, especially the latter, provide evidence in support of the concept that allergic reactions to skin surface bacteria may at least aggravate if not initiate some types of endogenous eczema.

References

1. O'Laughlin, S., Schroeter, A. L. and Jordan, R. E. (1978). Chronic urticaria-like lesions in systemic lupus erythematosus. *Arch. Dermatol.*, **114**, 879
2. Soter, N. A. and Austen, K. F. (1976). The diversity of mast cell-derived mediators: implications for acute, subacute and chronic cutaneous inflammatory disorders. *J. Invest. Dermatol.*, **67**, 313
3. Zeiger, R. S., Yurdin, D. L. and Colten, H. R. (1976). Histamine metabolism. II. Cellular and subcellular localization of the catabolic enzymes, histaminase, and histamine methyl transferase, in human leukocytes. *J. Allergy Clin. Immunol.*, **58**, 172
4. Wasserman, S. I., Goetzl, E. J. and Austen, K. F. (1975). Inactivation of slow reacting substance of anaphylaxis by human eosinophil arylsulphatase. *J. Immunol.*, **114**, 645
5. Champion, R. H., Roberts, S. O. B., Carpenter, R. G. and Roger, J. H. (1969). Urticaria and angio-oedema. A review of 544 patients. *Br. J. Dermatol.*, **81**, 588
6. Lieberman, P., Siegle, R. L., Kaplan, R. J. and Hashimoto, K. (1976). Chronic urticaria and anaphylaxis. Reactions to iophendylate. *J. Am. Med. Assoc.*, **236**, 1495
7. Juhlin, L., Johansson, G. V., Bennich, H., Högmann, C. and Thyresson, N. (1969). Immunoglobulin E in dermatoses. Levels in atopic dermatitis and urticaria. *Arch. Dermatol.*, **100**, 12
8. Graul, E. H., Borelli, S., Muller, H. and Gehrken, H. (1973). Immunoglobulin E Bestimmung bei Dermatosen. *Hautarzt*, **24**, 235
9. Wüthrich, B., Kopper, E. and Virchow, C. (1973). IgE Bestimmung bei Neurodermatitis und anderen Dermatosen. *Hautarzt*, **24**, 381
10. Chodirker, W. B., Bauman, W. and Komar, R. R. (1979). Immunological parameters and α_1-antitrypsin in chronic urticaria. *Clin. Allergy*, **9**, 201
11. McDuffie, F. C., Sams, W. M., Maldonado, J. E., Andreini, P. H., Conn, D. L. and Samayoa, E. A. (1973). Hypocomplementaemia with cutaneous vasculitis and arthritis. *Mayo Clin. Proc.*, **48**, 340
12. Sissons, J. G. P., Williams, D. G., Peters, D. K., Boulton-Jones, J. M. and Goldsmith, H. J. (1974). Skin lesions, angio-oedema and hypocomplementaemia. *Lancet*, **2**, 1350
13. Ballow, M., Ward, G. W., Gershwin, E. M. and Day, N. K. (1975). C1-bypass complement-activation pathway in patients with chronic urticaria and angio-oedema. *Lancet*, **2**, 248
14. May, J. E. and Frank, M. M. (1973). A new complement-mediated cytolytic mechanism – the C1-bypass activation pathway. *Proc. Natl. Acad. Sci.*, **70**, 649
15. Laurell, A.-B., Martensson, U. and Sjöholm, A. G. (1977). Studies of C1 subcomponents in chronic urticaria and angioedema. *Int. Arch. Allergy Appl. Immunol.*, **54**, 434
16. Soter, N. A., Mihm, M. C., Gigli, I., Dvorak, H. F. and Austen, K. F. (1976). Two distinct cellular patterns in cutaneous necrotizing angiitis. *J. Invest. Dermatol.*, **66**, 344
17. Braverman, I. M. and Yen, A. (1975). Demonstration of immune complexes in spontaneous

and histamine induced lesions and in normal skin of patients with leukocytoclastic angiitis. *J. Invest. Dermatol.*, **64**, 105

18. Gower, R. G., Sams, W. M., Thorne, G. and Claman, H. N. (1976). Immune complex deposition in leukocytoclastic vasculitis. *J. Invest. Dermatol.*, **66**, 271

19. Kaplan, A. P., Horakova, Z. and Katz, S. I. (1978). Assessment of tissue fluid histamine levels in patients with urticaria. *J. Allergy Clin. Immunol.*, **61**, 350

20. Greaves, M. W., Plummer, V. M., McLaughlin, P. and Stanworth, D. R. (1974). Serum and cell bound IgE in chronic urticaria. *Clin. Allergy*, **4**, 265

21. Kern, F. and Lichtenstein, L. M. (1976). Defective histamine release in chronic urticaria. *J. Clin. Invest.*, **57**, 1369

22. Juhlin, L. and Michaelsson, G. (1969). Cutaneous reactions to kallikrein, bradykinin and histamine in healthy subjects and in patients with urticaria. *Acta Dermatovenereol.*, **49**, 26

23. Doeglas, H. M. G. and Bluemink, E. (1975). Protease inhibitors in plasma of patients with chronic urticaria. *Arch. Dermatol.*, **111**, 979

24. Hauser, D. D., Arbesman, C. E., Ito, K. and Wicher, K. (1970). Cold urticaria. Immunological studies. *Am. J. Med.*, **49**, 23

25. Kaplan, A. P., Gray, L., Shaff, R. E., Horakova, Z. and Beavan, M. A. (1975). *In vivo* studies of mediator release in cold urticaria and cholinergic urticaria. *J. Allergy Clin. Immunol.*, **55**, 394

26. Soter, N. A., Wasserman, S. I. and Austen, K. F. (1976). Cold urticaria: Release into the circulation of histamine and eosinophil chemotactic factor of anaphylaxis during cold challenge. *N. Engl. J. Med.*, **294**, 687

27. Bentley-Phillips, C. B., Black, A. K. and Greaves, M. W. (1976). Induced tolerance in cold urticaria caused by cold-evoked histamine release. *Lancet*, **2**, 63

28. Wasserman, S. I., Soter, N. A., Center, D. M. and Austen, K. F. (1977). Cold urticaria. Recognition and characterization of a neutrophil chemotactic factor which appears in serum during experimental cold challenge. *J. Clin. Invest.*, **60**, 189

29. Juhlin, L. and Shelley, W. B. (1961). Role of mast cell and basophil in cold urticaria with associated systemic reactions. *J. Am. Med. Assoc.*, **177**, 371

30. Wanderer, A. A., Maselli, R., Ellis, E. F. and Ishizaka, K. (1971). Immunologic characterization of serum factors responsible for cold urticaria. *J. Allergy Clin. Immunol.*, **48**, 13

31. Constanzi, J. J. and Coltman, C. A. (1967). Kappa chain cold precipitable immunoglobulin G (IgG) associated with cold urticaria. *Clin. Exp. Immunol.*, **2**, 167

32. Rawnsley, H. M. and Shelley, W. B. (1968). Cold urticaria with cryoglobulinaemia. *Arch. Dermatol.*, **98**, 12

33. Villacorte, G. V. (1970). Immunologic studies in a case of acquired cold urticaria associated with cryoglobulinaemia and allergic cutaneous vasculitis. *J. Allergy*, **45**, 122

34. Soter, N. A., Joshi, N. P., Twarog, F. J., Zeiger, R. S., Rothman, P. M. and Colten, H. R. (1977). Delayed cold-induced urticaria: A dominantly inherited disorder. *J. Allergy Clin. Immunol.*, **59**, 294

35. Kaplan, A. P. and Beaven, M. A. (1976). *In vivo* studies of the pathogenesis of cold urticaria, cholinergic urticaria and vibration induced swelling. *J. Invest. Dermatol.*, **67**, 327

36. Greaves, M. W., Sneddon, I. B., Smith, A. K. and Stanworth, D. R. (1974). Heat urticaria. *Br. J. Dermatol.*, **90**, 289

37. Daman, L., Lieberman, P., Ganier, M. and Hashimoto, K. (1978). Localized heat urticaria. *J. Allergy Clin. Immunol.*, **61**, 273

38. Harber, L. C., Holloway, R. M., Wheatly, V. R. and Baer, R. L. (1963). Immunologic and biophysical studies in solar urticaria. *J. Invest. Dermatol.*, **39**, 439

39. Kirby, J. D., Matthews, C. N. A., James, J., Duncan, E. H. L. and Warin, R. P. (1971). The incidence and other aspects of factitious wealing (dermographism). *Br. J. Dermatol.*, **85**, 331

40. Aoyama, H., Katsumata, Y. and Ozawa, T. (1970). Dermographism – inducing principles of urticaria factitia. *Jpn. J. Dermatol.*, **80**, 122
41. Newcomb, R. W. and Nelson, H. (1973). Dermatographia mediated by immunoglobulin E. *Am. J. Med.*, **54**, 174
42. Rose, B. (1941). Studies on blood histamine in cases of allergy; blood histamine during wheal formation. *J. Allergy*, **12**, 327
43. Warin, R. P. and Champion, R. H. (1974). *Urticaria*, p. 125. (London: Saunders)
44. Levine, M. I. and Winkler, L. (1966). *J. Montefiore Hosp.*, **1**, 25
45. James, J. and Warin, R. P. (1969). Factitious wealing at the site of previous cutaneous response. *Br. J. Dermatol.*, **81**, 882
46. Kalz, F. and Pritchard, H. (1952). Investigations of some side-effects in patients treated with penicillin. *Arch. Dermatol.*, **65**, 568
47. Paver, W. K. (1970). Cholinergic urticaria with systemic presentation. *Aust. J. Dermatol.*, **11**, 97
48. Warin, R. P. and Champion, R. H. (1974). *Urticaria*, pp. 139–140. (London: Saunders)
49. Herxheimer, A. (1956). The nervous pathway mediating cholinergic urticaria. *Clin. Sci.*, **15**, 194
50. Morgan, J. K. (1953). Observations on cholinergic urticaria. *J. Invest. Dermatol.*, **21**, 173
51. Illig, L. and Heinicke, A. (1967). Zur Pathogenese der Cholinergischen Urticaria. II. *Arch. Klin. Exp. Dermatol.*, **229**, 285
52. Commens, C. A. and Greaves, M. W. (1978). Tests to establish the diagnosis in cholinergic urticaria. *Br. J. Dermatol.*, **98**, 47
53. Commens, C. A. and Greaves, M. W. (1978). Cimetidine in chronic idiopathic urticaria: a randomized double-blind study. *Br. J. Dermatol.*, **99**, 675
54. Kennes, B., De Maubenge, J. and Delespesse, G. (1977). Treatment of chronic urticaria with a beta$_2$-adrenergic stimulant. *Clin. Allergy*, **7**, 35
55. Moore-Robinson, M. and Warin, R. P. (1967). Effect of salicylates in urticaria. *Br. Med. J.*, **4**, 262
56. Lockey, S. D. (1971). Reactions to hidden agents in foods, beverages and drugs. *Ann. Allergy*, **29**, 461
57. Michaelson, G. and Juhlin, L. (1973). Urticaria induced by preservatives and dye additives in food and drugs. *Br. J. Dermatol.*, **88**, 525
58. Warin, R. P. and Champion, R. H. (1974). *Urticaria*, p. 142. (London: Saunders)
59. Moore-Robinson, M. and Warin, R. P. (1968). Some clinical aspects of cholinergic urticaria. *Br. J. Dermatol.*, **80**, 794
60. Donaldson, V. H. and Evans, R. R. (1963). A biochemical abnormality in hereditary angioneurotic edema: absence of serum inhibitor of C1 esterase. *Am. J. Med.*, **35**, 37
61. Frank, M. M., Gelfand, J. A. and Atkinson, J. P. (1976). Hereditary angio-oedema: the clinical syndrome and its management. *Ann. Intern. Med.*, **84**, 580
62. Gigli, I. (1979). Complement system and related cutaneous disorders. In Safai, B. and Good, R. A. (eds.) *Immunodermatology*. (New York: Plenum Press)
63. Donaldson, V. H., Rosen, F. S. and Bing, D. H. (1977). Role of the second component of complement (C2) and plasmin in kinin release in hereditary angioneurotic edema (H.A.N.E.) plasma. *Trans. Am. Assoc. Phys.*, **90**, 174
64. Rosen, F. S., Charache, P., Pensky, J. and Donaldson, V. H. (1965). Hereditary angioneurotic oedema: two genetic variants. *Science*, **148**, 957
65. Hadjiyannaki, K. and Lachmann, P. J. (1971). Hereditary angio-oedema: a review with particular reference to pathogenesis and treatment. *Clin. Allergy*, **1**, 221
66. Pickering, R. J., Kelly, J. R., Good, R. A. and Gewurz, H. (1969). Replacement therapy in hereditary angioedema. Successful treatment of two patients with fresh frozen plasma. *Lancet*, **1**, 326

67. Schulz, K.-H. (1974). Hereditares Quincke-Oedem. Neure Wege der Therapie. *Hautarzt*, 25, 12
68. Nilsson, I. M., Andersson, L. and Bjorkman, S. E. (1966). Epsilon-aminocaproic acid (E-ACA) as a therapeutic agent based on 5 years clinical experience. *Acta Med. Scand.* (Suppl.), 448, 1
69. Champion, R. H. and Lachmann, P. J. (1969). Hereditary angio-oedema treated with ε-aminocaproic acid. *Br. J. Dermatol.*, 81, 763
70. Sheffer. A. L., Austen, K. F. and Rosen. F. S. (1972). Tranexamic acid therapy in hereditary angioneurotic edema. *N. Engl. J. Med.*, 287. 452
71. Blohme, G. (1972). Treatment of hereditary angioneurotic oedema with tranexamic acid: a random double-blind cross-over study. *Acta Med. Scand.*, 192. 293
72. Naish. P. and Barratt, J. (1979). Hereditary angio-oedema. *Lancet*, 1. 611
73. Charytan, C. and Purtilo, D. (1969). Glomerular capillary thrombosis and acute renal failure after epsilon-aminocaproic acid therapy. *N. Engl. J. Med.*, 280, 1102
74. Korsan-Bengtsen, K., Ysander, L., Blohme, G. and Tibbin, E. (1969). Extensive muscle necrosis after long-term treatment with aminocaproic acid (EACA) in a case of hereditary periodic edema. *Acta Med. Scand.*, 185, 341
75. Frank, M. M., Sergeant, J. S., Kane, M. A. and Alling, D. W. (1972). Epsilon aminocaproic acid therapy of hereditary angioneurotic edema. A double blind study. *N. Engl. J. Med.*, 286, 808
76. Spaulding. W. B. (1960). Methyltestosterone therapy for hereditary episodic oedema. *Ann. Intern. Med.*, 53. 739
77. Potts. G. O. (1977). Pharmacology of danazol. *J. Int. Med. Res.*, 5 (Suppl. 3). 1
78. Gelfand. J. A., Sherins. R. J., Alling. D. W. and Frank. M. M. (1976). Treatment of hereditary angio-oedema with danazol: reversal of clinical and biochemical abnormalities. *N. Engl. J. Med.*, 295. 1444
79. Blackmore, W. P. (1977). Danazol in the treatment of hereditary angio-oedema. *J. Int. Med. Res.*, 5 (Suppl. 3), 38
80. Tappeinner, G., Hintner, H., Glatzl, J. and Wolff, K. (1979). Hereditary angio-oedema: treatment with danazol. *Br. J. Dermatol.*, 100, 207
81. Fraser, I. S. and Allen, J. K. (1979). Danazol and cholesterol metabolism. *Lancet*, 1, 931
82. Zeek, P. M. (1953). Periarteritis nodosa and other forms of necrotizing angiitis. *N. Engl. J. Med.*, 248, 764
83. Copeman, P. W. M. and Ryan, T. J. (1970). The problems of classification of cutaneous angiitis with reference to histopathology and pathogenesis. *Br. J. Dermatol.*, 82 (Suppl. 5), 2
84. Cream. J. J. (1973). Immune complex disease and mixed cryoglobulinaemia. In Beutner. E. H., Chorzelski. T. P., Bean. S. F. and Jordan, R. E. (eds.) *Immunopathology of the Skin: Labelled Antibody Studies.* p. 148. (Stroudsburg: Dowden. Hutchinson and Ross)
85. Shuster, S. (1978). *Dermatology in Internal Medicine*, p. 177. (Oxford: Oxford University Press)
86. Sams, W. M., Thorne, E. G., Small, P., Moss, M. F., McIntosh, R. M. and Stanford, R. E. (1976). Leukocytoclastic vasculitis. *Arch. Dermatol.*, 112, 219
87. Gairdner, D. (1948). The Schönlein–Henoch syndrome (anaphylactoid purpura). *Q. J. Med.*, 17, 95
88. Cream, J. J. (1970). Schönlein–Henoch purpura in the adult: a study of 77 adults with anaphylactoid or Schönlein–Henoch purpura. *Q. J. Med.*, 39, 461
89. Soter, N. A., Austen, K. F. and Gigli, I. (1974). Urticaria and arthralgia as manifestations of necrotizing angiitis (vasculitis). *J. Invest. Dermatol.*, 63, 485
90. Elias, P. M. and Fritsch, P. O. (1979). Erythema multiforme. In Fitzpatrick, T. B., Eisen, A. Z., Wolff, K., Freedberg, I. M. and Austen, K. F. (eds.) *Dermatology in General Medicine*, p. 295. (New York: McGraw-Hill)
91. Graham, J. H. and MacVicar, D. N. (1972). Bullous dermatoses. In Graham, J. H.,

Johnson, W. C. and Helwig, E. B. (eds.) *Dermal Pathology*, p. 312. (Hagerstown: Harper and Row)

92. De Moragas, J. M. (1979). Panniculitis. In Fitzpatrick, T. B., Eisen, A. Z., Wolff, K., Freedberg, I. M. and Austen, K. F. (eds.) *Dermatology in General Medicine*, p. 784. (New York: McGraw-Hill)

93. Lever, W. F. and Schaumberg-Lever, G. (1975). Erythema nodosum. In *Histopathology of the Skin*, p. 226. (Philadelphia: Lippincott)

94. Perry, H. O. and Winkelmann, R. K. (1964). Subacute migratory nodular panniculitis. *Arch. Dermatol.*, **89**, 170

95. Wolff, K. (1979). Mycobacterial diseases: tuberculosis. In Fitzpatrick, T. B., Eisen, A. Z., Wolff, K., Freedberg, I. M. and Austen, K. F. (eds.) *Dermatology in General Medicine*, p. 1485. (New York: McGraw-Hill)

96. Lever, W. F. and Schaumberg-Lever, G. (1975). Erythema induratum. In *Histopathology of the Skin*, p. 230. (Philadelphia: Lippincott)

97. Zeek, O. M. (1952). Periarteritis nodosa: a critical review. *Am. J. Pathol.*, **22**, 777

98. Fisher, I. and Orkin, M. (1964). Cutaneous form of periarteritis nodosa. *Arch. Dermatol.*, **89**, 180

99. Diaz-Perez, J. L. and Winkelmann, R. K. (1974). Cutaneous periarteritis nodosa. *Arch. Dermatol.*, **110**, 407

100. Churg, J. and Strauss, L. (1951). Allergic granulomatosis, allergic angiitis, and periarteritis nodosa. *Am. J. Pathol.*, **27**, 277

101. Cream, J. J. (1972). Cryoglobulins in vasculitis. *Clin. Exp. Immunol.*, **10**, 117

102. Cream, J. J. (1973). Anticomplementary sera in cutaneous vasculitis. *Br. J. Dermatol.*, **89**, 55

103. McDuffie, F. C. (1970). Serum complement levels in cutaneous diseases. *Br. J. Dermatol.*, **82** (Suppl. 5), 20

104. Soter, N. A., Austen, K. F. and Gigli, I. (1974). The complement system in necrotizing angiitis of the skin: Analysis of complement component activities in patients with concomitant collagen-vascular diseases. *J. Invest. Dermatol.*, **63**, 219

105. Asghar, S. S., Faber, W. R. and Cormane, R. H. (1975). C1q precipitin in the sera of patients with allergic vasculitis (Gougerot-Ruiter syndrome). *J. Invest. Dermatol.*, **64**, 113

106. Schroeter, A. L., Copeman, P. W. M., Jordan, R. E., Sams, W. M. and Winkelmann, R. K. (1971). Immunofluorescence of cutaneous vasculitis associated with systemic disease. *Arch. Dermatol.*, **104**, 254

107. Sams, W. M., Claman, H. N., Kohler, P. F., McIntosh, R. M., Small, P. and Moss, M. F. (1975). Human necrotizing vasculitis: immunoglobulins and complement in vessel walls of cutaneous lesions and normal skin. *J. Invest. Dermatol.*, **64**, 441

108. Wolff, H. H., Maciejewski, W., Scherer, R. and Braun-Falco, O. (1978). Immunoelectron-microscopic examination of early lesions in histamine induced immune complex vasculitis in man. *Br. J. Dermatol.*, **99**, 13

109. Lockwood, C. M., Worlledge, S., Nicholas, A., Cotton, C. and Peters, D. K. (1979). Reversal of impaired splenic function in patients with nephritis or vasculitis (or both) by plasma exchange. *N. Engl. J. Med.*, **300**, 524

110. Dodman, B., Cunliffe, W. J. and Roberts, B. E. (1973). Observations in tissue fibrinolytic activity in patients with cutaneous vasculitis. *Br. J. Dermatol.*, **88**, 231

111. Jasin, H. E., Lo Spolluto, J. and Ziff, M. (1970). Rheumatoid hyperviscosity syndrome. *Am. J. Med.*, **49**, 23

112. Spector, W. G. and Heesom, N. (1969). The production of granulomata by antigen–antibody complexes. *J. Pathol.*, **98**, 31

113. Goeck, D. J., Hsu, K., Morgan, C., Bombardieri, S., Lockshin, M. and Christian, C. L. (1971). *J. Exp. Med.*, **134**, 330

114. Parish, W. E. and Rhodes, E. L. (1967). Bacterial antigens and aggregated gamma globulin in the lesions of nodular vasculitis. *Br. J. Dermatol.*, **79**, 131

115. Parish, W. E. (1971). Studies on vasculitis: II. Some properties of complexes formed of antibacterial antibodies with or without cutaneous vasculitis. *Clin. Allergy*, 1, 111

116. Parish, W. E. (1971). Studies on vasculitis: III. Decreased formation of antibody to M protein, group A polysaccharide and to some exotoxins in persons with vasculitis after streptococcal infection. *Clin. Allergy*, 1, 295

117. Parish, W. E. (1971). Studies on vasculitis: IV. The low incidence of antibacterial anaphylactic antibodies in the sera of persons with cutaneous vasculitis following bacterial infection. *Clin. Allergy*, 1, 433

118. Wells, G. C. (1969). Allergic vasculitis (Tri-sympton of Gougerot) treated with dapsone. *Proc. R. Soc. Med.*, 62, 665

119. Cream, J. J., Levene, G. M. and Calnan, C. D. (1971). Erythema elevatum diutinum: an unusual response to streptococcal antigen and response to dapsone. *Br. J. Dermatol.*, 84, 393

120. Thompson, D. M., Main, R. A., Beck, J. S. and Albert-Recht, F. (1973). Studies on a patient with leucocytoclastic vasculitis 'pyoderma gangrenosum' and paraproteinaemia. *Br. J. Dermatol.*.

121. Stendahl, O., Molin, L. and Dahlgren, C. (1978). The inhibition of polymorphonuclear leukocyte cytotoxicity by dapsone. *J. Clin. Invest.*, 62, 214

122. Cunliffe, W. J. (1968). An association between cutaneous vasculitis and decreased blood fibrinolytic activity. *Lancet*, 1, 1226

123. Isacson, S., Linell, F., Moller, H. and Nilssun, I. M. (1970). Coagulation and fibrinolysis in chronic panniculitis. *Acta Dermatovenereol.*, 50. 213

124. Cunliffe, W. J. and Menon, S. (1971). The association between cutaneous vasculitis and decreased blood fibrinolytic activity. *Br. J. Dermatol.*, 84, 99

125. Meenan, F. O. C. (1959). Prognosis in infantile eczema. *Ir. J. Med. Sci.*, 398, 79

126. Burrows, D. and Penman, R. W. B. (1960). Prognosis in the eczema–asthma syndrome. *Br. Med. J.*, 2, 825

127. Roth, H. L. and Kierland, R. R. (1964). The natural history of atopic dermatitis. *Arch. Dermatol.*, 89, 209

128. Rajka, G. (1975). *Atopic Dermatitis*. (London: Saunders)

129. Musgrove, K. and Morgan, J. K. (1976). Infantile eczema: a long-term follow-up study. *Br. J. Dermatol.*, 95, 365

130. Hanifin, J. M. and Lobitz, W. C. (1977). Newer concepts of atopic dermatitis. *Arch. Dermatol.*, 113, 663

131. Kaufman, H. S. and Hobbs, J. R. (1970). Immunoglobulin deficiencies in an atopic population. *Lancet*, 2, 1061

132. Taylor, B., Norman, A. P., Orgel, H. A., Stokes, C. R., Turner, M. W. and Soothill, J. F. (1973). Transient IgA deficiency and pathogenesis of infantile atopy. *Lancet*, 2, 111

133. Kaufman, H. S. and Frick, O. L. (1976). Immunological development in infants of allergic parents. *Clin. Allergy*, 6, 321

134. Matthews, D. J., Taylor, B., Norman, A. P., Turner, M. W. and Soothill, J. F. (1977). Prevention of eczema. *Lancet*, 1, 321

135. Juhlin, L., Johansson, S. G. O., Bennich, H., Högman, C. and Thyresson, N. (1969). Immunoglobulin E in dermatoses: Levels in atopic dermatitis and urticaria. *Arch. Dermatol.*, 100, 12

136. Rajka, G. (1961). Prurigo Besnier (atopic dermatitis) with special reference to the role of allergic factors: II. The evaluation of skin reactions. *Acta Dermatovenereol.*, 41, 1

137. Stone, S. P., Muller, S. A. and Gleich, G. J. (1973). IgE levels in atopic dermatitis. *Arch. Dermatol.*, 108, 806

138. Jones, H. E., Inouye, J. C., McGerity, J. L. and Lewis, C. W. (1975). Atopic disease and serum immunoglobulin E. *Br. J. Dermatol.*, 92, 17

139. Ogawa, M., Berger, P. A., McIntyre, O. R., Clendenning, W. E., Hanover, N. H. and Ishizaka, K. (1971). IgE in atopic dermatitis. *Arch. Dermatol.*, 103, 580

140. Gurevitch, A. W., Heiner, D. C. and Reisner, R. (1973). IgE in atopic dermatitis and other common dermatoses. *Arch. Dermatol.*, **107**, 712
141. Wüthrich, B. (1978). Serum IgE in atopic dermatitis. Relationship to severity of cutaneous involvement and course of disease as well as coexistence of atopic respiratory diseases. *Clin. Allergy*, **8**, 241
142. Cormane, R. H., Husz, S. and Hammerlinck, F. F. (1974). Immunoglobulin- and complement-bearing lymphocytes in allergic contact dermatitis and atopic dermatitis (eczema). *Br. J. Dermatol.*, **90**, 597
143. Carapeto, F. J., Winkelmann, R. J. and Jordan, R. E. (1976). T and B lymphocytes in contact and atopic dermatitis. *Arch. Dermatol.*, **112**, 1095
144. Ohman, S. and Johansson, S. G. O. (1974). Immunoglobulins in atopic dermatitis. *Acta Dermatovenereol.*, **54**, 193
145. Clendenning, W. E., Clack, W. E., Ogawa, M. and Ishizaka, K. (1973). Serum IgE studies in atopic dermatitis. *J. Invest. Dermatol.*, **61**, 233
146. Stone, S. P., Gleich, G. J. and Muller, S. A. (1976). Atopic dermatitis and IgE. *Arch. Dermatol.*, **112**, 1254
147. Shakib, F., McLaughlan, P., Stanworth, D. R., Smith, E. and Fairburn, E. (1977). Elevated serum IgE and IgG$_4$ in patients with atopic dermatitis. *Br. J. Dermatol.*, **97**, 59
148. Currie, J. M., Wright, R. C. and Miller, O. W. (1971). The frequency of warts in atopic patients. *Cutis*, **8**, 244
149. Solomon, L. M. and Telner, P. (1966). Eruptive molluscum contagiosum in atopic dermatitis. *Can. Med. Assoc. J.*, **95**, 978
150. Pauly, C. R., Artis, W. M. and Jones, H. E. (1978). Atopic dermatitis, impaired cellular immunity and molluscum contagiosum. *Arch. Dermatol.*, **114**, 391
151. Hanifin, J. M., Ray, L. F. and Lobitz, W. C. (1974). Immunological reactivity in dermatophytosis. *Br. J. Dermatol.*, **90**, 1
152. Palacios, J., Fuller, E. W. and Blaylock, W. K. (1966). Immunological capabilities of patients with atopic dermatitis. *J. Invest. Dermatol.*, **47**, 484
153. Jones, H. E., Lewis, C. and McMartin, S. L. (1973). Allergic contact sensitivity in atopic dermatitis. *Arch. Dermatol.*, **107**, 217
154. Uehara, M. (1977). Atopic dermatitis and tuberculin reactivity. *Arch. Dermatol.*, **113**, 1226
155. Elliott, S. T. and Hanifin, J. M. (1979). Delayed cutaneous hypersensitivity and lymphocyte transformation. *Arch. Dermatol.*, **115**, 36
156. Byrom, N. A. and Timlin, D. M. (1979). Immune status in atopic eczema: a survey. *Br. J. Dermatol.*, **100**, 491
157. Braathen, L. R., Førre, Ø., Natvig, J. B. and Eeg-Larsen, T. (1979). Predominance of T lymphocytes in the dermal infiltrate of atopic dermatitis. *Br. J. Dermatol.*, **100**, 511
158. Byrom, N. A., Staughton, R. C. D., Campbell, M.-A., Timlin, D. M., Chooi, M., Lane, A. M., Copeman, P. W. M. and Hobbs, J. R. (1979). Thymosin-inducible null cells in atopic eczema. *Br. J. Dermatol.*, **100**, 499
159. Gorski, A. J., Dupont, B., Hansen, J. A. and Good, R. A. (1975). Leukocyte migration inhibitory factor (LMIF) induced by conconavalin A. Standardized microassay for production *in vitro*. *Proc. Natl. Acad. Sci.*, **72**, 3197
160. Gorski, A. J., Dupont, B., Hansen, J. A., O'Reilly, R., Smithwick, E., Gorska, R. and Good, R. A. (1976). Leukocyte migration inhibitory factor (LMIF) profile in primary and secondary immunodeficiency diseases. *Clin. Exp. Immunol.*, **26**, 505
161. Horsmanheimo, M. and Horsmanheimo, A. (1979). Leukocyte migration inhibition factor in atopic dermatitis: induction by concanavalin A *in vitro*. *J. Invest. Dermatol.*, **72**, 128
162. Aldrich, R. A., Steinberg, A. G. and Campbell, D. C. (1954). Pedigree demonstrating a sex-linked recessive condition characterized by draining ears, eczematoid dermatitis and bloody diarrhoea. *Paediatrics*, **13**, 133

163. Rostenberg, A. and Solomon, L. M. (1968). Infantile eczema in systemic disease. *Arch. Dermatol.*, **98**, 41
164. Tada, T., Okumura, K. and Taniguchi, M. (1973). Cellular and humoral controls of reaginic antibody synthesis in the rat. In Goodfriend, L., Sehon, A. H. and Orange, R. P. (eds.) *Mechanisms in Allergy*, pp. 43–61. (New York: Marcel Dekker)
165. Juto. P. and Strannegård. Ö. (1979). T-lymphocytes and blood eosinophils in early infancy in relation to heredity for allergy and type of feeding. *J. Allergy Clin. Immunol.*, **64**, 38
166. Leyden, J. J., Marples, R. R. and Kligman, A. M. (1974). *Staphylococcus aureus* in the lesions of atopic dermatitis. *Br. J. Dermatol.*, **90**, 525
167. Eaglestein, W. H., Feinstein, R. J., Halprin, K. M., Bergstresser. P. R. and Mertz, P. M. (1977). Systemic antibiotic therapy of secondarily infected dermatitis. *Arch. Dermatol.*, **113**, 1378
168. White, C. R. and Hanifin, J. M. (1978). Levamisole therapy in atopic dermatitis. Randomized double-blind evaluation. *Arch. Dermatol.*, **114**, 1314
169. Alomar, A., Gimenez Camarasa, J. M. and De Moragas, J. M. (1978). The use of levamisole in atopic dermatitis. A prospective study. *Arch. Dermatol.*, **114**, 1316
170. Saarinen, U., Kojossari, M., Backman, A. and Siimes, M. (1979). Prolonged breast-feeding as prophylaxis for atopic disease. *Lancet*, **2**, 163
171. Halpern, S. R., Sellars, W. A.. Johnson, R. B., Anderson, D. W., Saperstein, S. and Reisch, J. S. (1973). Development of childhood allergy in infants fed breast, soy or cow milk. *J. Allergy Clin. Immunol.*, **51**, 139
172. Eastham, E. J., Lichauco, T., Grady, M. I. and Walker, W. A. (1978). Antigenicity of infant formulas: role of immature intestine on protein permeability. *J. Paediatr.*, **93**, 561
173. Atherton, D. J., Sewell, M., Soothill, J. F., Wells, R. S. and Chilvers, C. E. D. (1978). A double-blind controlled crossover trial of an antigen-avoidance diet in atopic eczema. *Lancet*, **1**, 401
174. Fisher, A. A. (1973). *Contact Dermatitis*. (Philadelphia: Lea and Febiger)
175. Cronin. E. (1980). *Contact Dermatitis*. (Edinburgh: Churchill Livingstone)
176. Dupuis. G. (1979). Studies on poison ivy. *In vitro* lymphocyte transformation by urushiol-protein conjugates. *Br. J. Dermatol.*, **101**, 617
177. Milner, J. E. (1974). *In vitro* lymphocyte responses in contact hypersensitivity. *J. Invest. Dermatol.*, **62**, 591
178. Miller, A. E. and Levis, W. R. (1973). Studies on the contact sensitization of man with simple chemicals. I. Specific lymphocyte transformation in response to dinitrochlorobenzene sensitization. *J. Invest. Dermatol.*, **61**, 261
179. Turk, J. L. (1975). The passive transfer of delayed hypersensitivity. In *Delayed Hypersensitivity*. pp. 75–88. (Amsterdam: North Holland)
180. Turk, J. L. (1975). The significance of changes in lymphoid tissue during the induction of delayed hypersensitivity. In *Delayed Hypersensitivity*. pp. 181–210. (Amsterdam: North Holland)
181. Shelley. W. B. and Juhlin. L. (1978). The Langerhans cell: its origin. nature. and function. *Acta Dermatovenereol.* (Suppl.). **79**. 7
182. van Haelst, U. J. (1969). Light and electron microscopic studies of the normal and pathological thymus of the rat. III. A mesenchymal histiocytic type of cell. *Z. Zellforsch..* **99**. 198
183. Jimbow, K., Sato, S. and Kukita, A. (1969). Cells containing Langerhans granules in human lymph nodes of dermatopathic lymphadenopathy. *J. Invest. Dermatol.*, **53**, 295
184. Nezelof, C., Basset, F. and Rousseau, M. F. (1973). Histiocytosis X. Histiogenetic arguments for a Langerhans cell origin. *Biomedicine*, **18**, 365
185. Rowden, G., Lewis, M. G. and Sullivan, A. K. (1977). Ia antigen expression on human epidermal Langerhans cells. *Nature (London)*, **268**, 247
186. Klareskog, L., Malmnäs-Tjernlund, U., Forsum, U. and Peterson, P. A. (1977). Epidermal Langerhans cells express Ia antigens. *Nature (London)*, **268**, 248

187. Stingl, G., Wolff-Schreiner, E. C., Pichler, W. J., Gschnait, F., Knapp, W. and Wolff, K. (1977). Epidermal Langerhans cells bear Fc and C3 receptors. *Nature (London)*, **268**, 245

188. Katz, S. I., Kunihiko, T. and Sachs, D. H. (1979). Epidermal Langerhans cells are derived from cells originating in bone marrow. *Nature (London)*, **282**, 324

189. Silberberg, I. (1973). Apposition of mononuclear cells to Langerhans cells in contact allergic reactions. *Acta Dermatovener.*, **53**, 1

190. Silberberg, I., Baer, R. L. and Rosenthal, S. A. (1974). The role of Langerhans cells in contact allergy. *Acta Dermatovenereol.*, **54**, 321

191. Silberberg, I., Baer, R. L. and Rosenthal, S. A. (1976). The role of Langerhans cells in allergic contact hypersensitivity. A review of findings in man and guinea-pig. *J. Invest. Dermatol.*, **66**, 210

192. Sagabiel, R. W. (1972). *In vivo* and *in vitro* uptake of ferritin by Langerhans cells of the epidermis. *J. Invest. Dermatol.*, **58**. 47

193. Shelley, W. B. and Juhlin, L. (1977). Selective uptake of contact allergens by the Langerhans cell. *Arch. Dermatol.*, **113**, 187

194. Stingl, G., Katz, S. I., Clement, L., Green, I. and Shevach, E. (1978). Immunologic functions of Ia-bearing epidermal Langerhans cells. *J. Immunol.*, **121**, 2005

195. Turk, J. L. (1975). Immunological unresponsiveness. In *Delayed Hypersensitivity*, pp. 129–136. (Amsterdam: North Holland)

196. White, W. A. and Baer, R. L. (1950). Failure to prevent experimental eczematous sensitization. *J. Allergy*, **21**, 344

197. Grolnick, M. (1951). Studies in contact dermatitis. VIII. The effect of feeding antigen on the subsequent development of skin sensitization. *J. Allergy*, **22**, 170

198. Kligman, A. M. (1958). Poison ivy (Rhus) dermatitis. *Arch. Dermatol.*, **77**, 149

199. Lowney, E. D. (1968). Immunological unresponsiveness to a contact sensitizer in man. *J. Invest. Dermatol.*, **51**, 411

200. Lowney, E. D. (1971). Tolerance of dinitrochlorobenzene, a contact sensitizer, in man. *J. Allergy Clin. Immunol.*, **42**, 28

201. Lowney, E. D. (1973). Suppression of contact sensitization in man by prior feeding of antigen. *J. Invest. Dermatol.*, **61**, 90

202. Van Scott, E. J. and Kalmanson, J. D. (1973). Complete remissions of mycosis fungoides lymphoma induced by topical nitrogen mustard (HN_2). Control of delayed hypersensitivity to HN_2 by desensitization and by induction of specific immunologic tolerance. *Cancer*, **32**, 18

203. Leshaw, S., Simon, R. S. and Baer, R. L. (1977). Failure to induce tolerance to mechlorethamine hydrochloride. *Arch. Dermatol.*, **113**, 1406

204. Baer, R. L., Michaelides, P. and Prestia, A. E. (1972). Failure to induce immune tolerance to nitrogen mustard. *J. Invest. Dermatol.*, **58**, 1

205. Breza, T. S., Kechijian, P. and Taylor, J. R. (1975). Mechlorethamine in psoriasis. Further attempts to induce immunological tolerance. *Arch. Dermatol.*, **111**, 1438

206. Pariser, D. M., Childers, R. C., Kechijian, P., Halprin, K. M. and Taylor, J. R. (1976). Intravenous desensitization to mechlorethamine in patients with psoriasis. *Arch. Dermatol.*, **112**, 1113

207. Constantine, V. S., Fuks, Z. Y. and Farber, E. M. (1975). Mechlorethamine desensitization in therapy for mycosis fungoides. Topical desensitization to mechlorethamine (nitrogen mustard) contact hypersensitivity. *Arch. Dermatol.*, **111**, 484

208. Kligman, A. M. (1958). Hyposensitization against Rhus dermatitis. *Arch. Dermatol.*, **78**, 47

209. Welbourn, E., Champion, R. H. and Parish, W. E. (1976). Hypersensitivity to bacteria in eczema. I. Bacterial culture, skin tests and immunofluorescent detection of immunoglobulins and bacterial antigens. *Br. J. Dermatol.*, **94**, 619

210. Parish, W. E., Welbourn, E. and Champion, R. H. (1976). Hypersensitivity to bacteria in

eczema. II. Titre and immunoglobulin class of antibodies to staphylococci and micrococci. *Br. J. Dermatol.*, **95**, 285

211. Welbourn, E., Champion, R. H. and Parish, W. E. (1976). Hypersensitivity to bacteria in eczema. III. Arthus-like responses to bacterial antigens without specific antibody. *Br. J. Dermatol.*, **95**, 379

212. Parish, W. E., Welbourn, E. and Champion, R. H. (1976). Hypersensitivity to bacteria in eczema. IV. Cytotoxic effect of antibacterial antibody on skin cells acquiring bacterial antigens. *Br. J. Dermatol.*, **95**, 493

7
Respiratory Allergy

R. J. DAVIES

INTRODUCTION

In 1698, Sir John Floyer outlined in the preface to his *Treatise of the Asthma* those aspects which he hoped to illuminate and, with regard to respiratory allergy, they remain as pertinent today as they were almost three centuries ago (Figure 7.1). Allergy, meaning in its broadest sense an altered state of re-activity in the host following exposure to an allergen, is involved in a very wide range of lung diseases. Allergic factors are probably of considerable import-ance in the development of the localized pneumonia that follows infection with *Streptococcus pneumoniae* and delayed hypersensitivity mechanisms play a prominent role in both the disease produced by *Mycobacterium tuberculosis* and its immunity. However, allergic mechanisms are perhaps more obvious in the precipitation of acute attacks of rhinitis and asthma in the atopic child or in the development of sudden episodes of breathlessness and fever in a farmer some hours after handling mouldy hay. As allergy is involved in the pro-duction of so many diseases in the respiratory tract it is necessary to concen-trate in this chapter on those in which allergic factors are of prime importance.

ATOPY

In 1916, Cooke and Vander Veer[1] recognized a tendency to develop a sensi-tivity to common environmental agents in subjects with a personal and family history of hay fever, asthma and eczema. Some years later Coca[2] introduced the term 'atopy', derived from the Greek meaning 'no place', to cover 'a type of hypersensitiveness peculiar to man, subject to hereditary influence, present-ing the characteristic immediate-wealing type skin reactions, having circu-lating reagin and manifesting peculiar clinical syndromes such as asthma and hay fever'. This was a compound definition which linked the clinical diseases to immediate skin sensitivity and circulating reagin–immunoglobulin E antibody (IgE). Many patients with asthma and rhinitis show no evidence of Type I allergy. although this may be present in other subjects without clinical evidence of disease. For this reason, Pepys[3] in 1975 suggested that the term atopy should be used more precisely to describe the capacity of an individual to develop Type I allergy to common environmental materials demonstrable by skin or serological tests without being linked to the presence of clinical

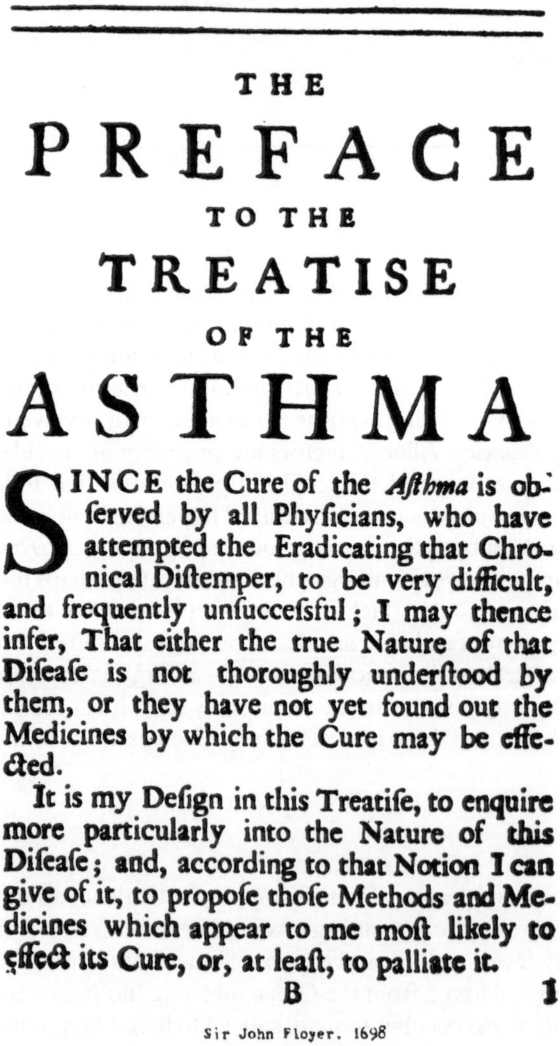

THE
PREFACE
TO THE
TREATISE
OF THE
ASTHMA

SINCE the Cure of the *Asthma* is observed by all Physicians, who have attempted the Eradicating that Chronical Distemper, to be very difficult, and frequently unsuccefsful; I may thence infer, That either the true Nature of that Difeafe is not thoroughly underftood by them, or they have not yet found out the Medicines by which the Cure may be effected.

It is my Defign in this Treatife, to enquire more particularly into the Nature of this Difeafe; and, according to that Notion I can give of it, to propofe thofe Methods and Medicines which appear to me moft likely to effect its Cure, or, at leaft, to palliate it.

B   1

Sir John Floyer. 1698

Figure 7.1 The preface to the *Treatise of the Asthma*, by Sir John Floyer. 1698

manifestations. Atopy can best be detected by skin prick testing with a number of allergens known to be common to a particular environment and individuals are considered atopic if they show one or more positive tests. Asthma, rhinitis and eczema can then be considered as diseases which may be associated with the atopic state in some patients.

Skin test studies on large, unselected populations from different parts of the world have shown that up to 25–35% of individuals are atopic. The peak prevalence of positive skin tests was found to occur during the third decade and to fall rapidly in populations aged over 50 years. Furthermore, the frequency of positive skin tests has been found to be significantly higher amongst those with a history of asthma and rhinitis[4, 5]. In one of the studies 17% of the population was found to have positive skin tests but no respiratory symptoms, underlining the fact that atopy can occur without overt allergic respiratory disease. Nevertheless prospective studies have shown that as many as half the subjects with positive skin tests to pollen, but without symptoms at the time of testing, developed rhinitis within 5 years[6]. Indeed the incidence of hay fever was ten times higher in those subjects who showed strong skin test reactions to grass pollen in a 3-year follow-up of previously asymptomatic subjects[7]. Hospital investigations in patients with asthma and their first degree relatives have indicated that the higher the atopic status, that is the greater the number of positive results in response to a battery of allergen extracts, the earlier the age of onset of asthma and the greater the incidence of hay fever, perennial rhinitis and eczema[8]. Prospective studies on the development of positive immediate skin tests and symptoms to protein allergens, such as the enzymes from *Bacillus subtilis*, used in the detergent industry, indicated that the incidence of sensitization was higher in atopic workers, although both positive skin tests and symptoms did develop in workers who were non-atopic[9]. This emphasizes the fact that the atopic and non-atopic states are unlikely to be mutually exclusive, particularly when individuals are extensively exposed to potent allergens. It remains to be determined whether the ready facility of atopic individuals to produce IgE antibodies is the result of a quantitative or qualitative deficiency in the production of other classes of antibody, particularly secretory immunoglobulin A antibody[10] (IgA), or to a functional or numerical deficiency in T lymphocytes or one of their sub-populations, suppressor T cells[11].

SKIN TESTING

Skin testing with allergen extracts continues to play a very important role in the immunological investigation of patients with respiratory allergy. It is necessary, however, to realize both the implications and the limitations of the tests.

Immediate skin reactions

The characteristics of the immediate skin reaction are a weal with surrounding erythema and accompanying pruritis which develop within 2–3 minutes, reach their maximum at about 15 minutes and then gradually wane over the subsequent 1–2 hours. The reaction results from the combination of at least a divalent allergen with adjacent antibody molecules on the surface of mast cells. Usually the mast cell sensitizing antibody is of IgE class, although there is evidence in man that similar sensitization may be produced by an antibody of immunoglobulin G class (IgG). This appears to sensitize mast cells in the skin for a shorter time, hence its description as short-term sensitizing IgG or IgG-STS[12]. It has been shown that whilst positive test reactions in man to purified cytoplasmic protein allergens from *Candida albicans* are mediated by long-term sensitizing antibody (IgE), similar skin test reactions to the poly-saccharide mannan from this fungus are mediated by heat-stable short-term sensitizing antibody (IgG-STS)[13]. IgG-STS antibodies have been found in the sera of patients with allergy to foods[12] and against common allergens in a significant number of patients with cryptogenic non-atopic asthma[14].

In one study specific IgE antibodies were found in the serum of the majority of 49 asthmatic patients who showed immediate asthmatic reactions on

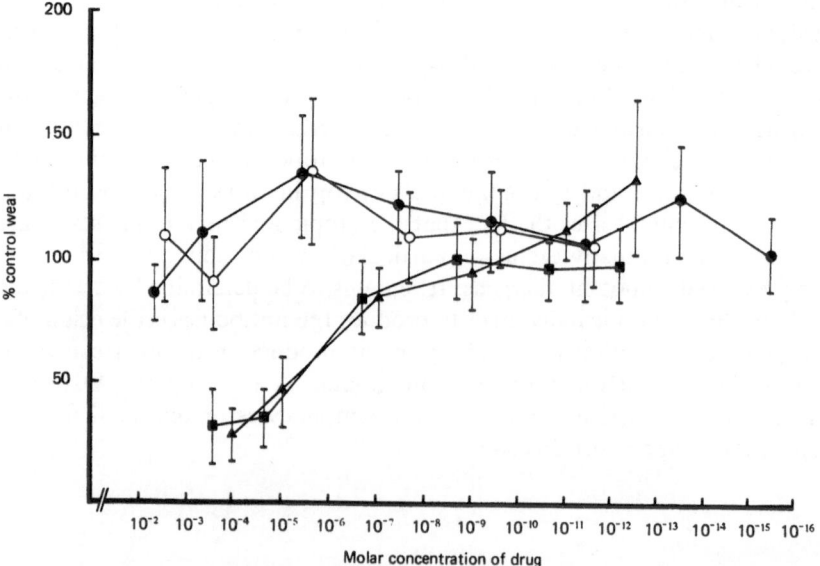

Figure 7.2 Dose–response curves showing the inhibitory effects of clemastine and ketotifen but not sodium cromoglycate or chlorpheniramine on the immediate weal response to skin prick testing with allergens in ten subjects. The results are shown as the mean ± standard error. The pharmacological agents were administered by intracutaneous injection 30 minutes prior to the allergen skin prick tests. Sodium cromoglycate, o———o; chlorpheniramine, ●———●; clemastine, ■———■; ketotifen, ▲———▲.

bronchial provocation testing. However, in some of the patients with lower levels of total IgE, the immediate asthma was not inhibited by sodium cromoglycate and these individuals had specific IgG-STS present in their serum against the provoking allergens[15]. These results require confirmation and the exact role played by IgG-STS in clinical disease remains to be determined.

Studies using antibodies directed against IgE have suggested that the capacity of the skin to react and produce immediate skin tests develops about 3 weeks after birth. Immediate skin reactions can be inhibited by antihistamines, but not usually by β-adrenoceptor agonists, corticosteroids or even injections of sodium cromoglycate into the test site[16-18] (Figure 7.2). Whether antihistamines with anti-H_2 activity have any additional role in the inhibition of immediate skin reactions has still to be evaluated.

The frequency with which positive skin prick tests occur with different allergens in both unselected populations[19] and asthmatic patients attending an allergy clinic[20] is shown in Table 7.1. Analysis of these results showed that 99% of the subjects giving one or more positive skin reactions could have been identified by skin testing with only three allergens together with the appropriate animal extract if the subject kept pets. These allergens were *Dermatophagoides farinae* or *Dermatophagoides pteronyssinus*, grass pollen and *Aspergillus fumigatus*. When the purpose of the skin tests is solely to screen for the presence of atopy only these allergens together with appropriate control solutions need to be used.

Table 7.1 The frequency of positive immediate skin prick tests to common allergens in an atopic asthmatic population attending an asthma and allergy clinic and in an adult population (aged 40–64) invited to attend a general practice health screening programme

Allergen	Percentage with positive immediate skin prick tests	
	Atopic asthmatics (n = 554)	'Unselected' adult population (n = 1300)
House dust	70	16
Dermatophagoides farinae	69	—
Dermatophagoides pteronyssinus	—	14
Grass, tree and shrub pollens	66	—
Grass pollen	—	10
Cat, dog, horse danders	38	—
Foods (egg, milk, wheat, fish, nuts)	16	—
Aspergillus fumigatus	16	4
Other moulds	21	—
Any allergen	100	25

Late skin reactions

About 75% of immediate weals induced by allergen skin testing that are greater than 8–10 mm in diameter are followed by late skin reactions[21, 22]. In the fully developed form these consist of oedematous. tender. reddened areas up to 10 cm or more in diameter. The lesion reaches a maximum size 4–16 hours after the immediate skin reaction and usually subsides within 36 hours. This type of late reaction does not follow histamine weals of similar size. Radioactive isotope studies have shown that a similar degree of exudation occurs at the site of histamine and allergen induced wealing reactions over the first hour, but exudation only continues thereafter at the site of the allergen test[23].

Biopsy studies of late skin reactions resulting from injection of extracts of *Aspergillus fumigatus* showed infiltration with mononuclear cells together with some eosinophilic polymorphonuclear leukocytes. Aggregates of immunoglobulin and the third component of complement were shown in and around the vascular endothelium and tissue spaces on immunofluorescence[24]. On this evidence, the authors suggested that immune complex Type III allergic reactions might be involved in the pathogenesis. However, similar studies of late skin reactions following injections of ragweed pollen failed to demonstrate any consistent deposition of immunoglobulin or complement components[25]. Further late skin reactions have been shown to develop after injection of whole antihuman IgE antibody, or indeed its pepsin digest $F(ab)^2$ which, without its Fc fragment, would be unlikely to take part in the formation of immune complexes[26]. This suggests that the development of late skin reactions following injection of some allergens may be more directly linked to IgE mediated Type I allergy. Whilst corticosteroids have little effect on the immediate skin reaction they do prevent development of the late response and the nature of the mediators involved in its pathogenesis has still to be determined. Although late cutaneous responses are of considerable immunopharmacological interest, particularly because they may result from the same mechanisms as those involved in late asthma, they have little importance in clinical practice.

TOTAL AND SPECIFIC IgE ANTIBODIES

Since Type I allergic reactions play such an important role in the development of many of the allergic diseases of the respiratory tract, levels of both total and specific IgE antibody in serum and secretion have been extensively investigated. In general these studies have been of much greater importance in elucidating mechanisms rather than in clinical practice.

Total and specific IgE in serum

The distribution of serum levels of IgE antibody has a skewed distribution and a number of studies have indicated that the geometric mean for non-atopic 'normal' individuals is between 20 and 40 units/ml. In one study of 102 'normal' subjects, the mean level was found to be 36 units/ml and 96 of the subjects[27] had a level below 178 units/ml. A study of an unselected population of over 12 000 individuals aged between 45 and 70 years showed a level of IgE antibody of $34 \pm ^{84}_{26}$ (geometric mean $\pm$ one standard deviation). Analysis of variance showed that the presence of positive skin tests or a personal or family history of atopic diseases each contributed significantly and separately to the differences in levels of this antibody. The presence of a family history together with a personal history of atopic diseases had a further independent effect[5]. Patients with atopic asthma have a raised level of total IgE antibody and those with allergic bronchopulmonary aspergillosis have extremely high levels. In this disease both total serum levels of IgE and levels of specific IgE against antigens from *Aspergillus fumigatus* rise during episodes of symptoms associated with new pulmonary shadows and increased eosinophilia. For this reason it has been suggested that serial determinations of total and specific IgE may be of value in the clinical management of the disease[28, 29, 38]. Conversely, in patients with cryptogenic pulmonary eosinophilia there is a disproportionate increase in blood eosinophils[30] as compared with only minor elevations in the total serum levels of IgE.

Radioallergosorbent testing (RAST) for the presence of specific IgE antibodies is virtually never positive when the total IgE level is less than 20 units/ml. It is arguable whether measurement of serum levels of specific IgE antibody has any advantage over allergen skin prick testing. Some patients may prefer venepuncture to a series of skin prick tests, whilst others may have such widespread eczema that skin testing is precluded. In general there is good correlation, particularly with more purified allergens, between the weal diameter of the skin prick test and the amount of circulating IgE antibodies specifically directed against the same allergens[31]. This relationship becomes closer with larger weal diameters, but even small weals have been found to correlate with specific IgE antibody and the results of history and provocation tests[32].

Levels of both total and specific IgE may rise during the pollen season[33].

Total and specific IgE in secretions

IgE antibody present in serum is thought to represent overflow from antibody production by plasma cells in tissues throughout the body. Although serum levels of specific IgE antibody may reflect local production in response to a particular allergen, it is possible that measurement of locally produced IgE may more closely reflect the degree of sensitization in that organ. For example, it has been demonstrated that some individuals with rhinitis, proven by provocation tests, may have negative skin tests and serum RAST for specific IgE antibody against the provoking agent but measurable amounts of the antibody in nasal secretions[34]. Further, IgE antibody can be measured in the sputum from patients with asthma and indeed with bronchitis[35]. Whether this antibody is actively produced within the respiratory tract or whether it results from transudation from plasma during an inflammatory process requires confirmation. At the present time no studies have shown the specificity of the secretory antibodies in patients with asthma. Recent evidence has shown that nearly all atopic patients with allergic rhinitis have significant amounts of specific IgA and specific IgE antibody against ragweed antigen E in their nasal secretions, whilst secretions from most non-allergic individuals contain no measurable levels[36]. The authors suggest that these results are in keeping with the hypothesis that hay fever occurs in a 'high antibody responder' population genetically able to respond to low doses of inhalant allergens. This underlines the need for further studies on levels of total and specific antibodies in nasal secretions and sputum in patients with respiratory allergy and the possibility remains that such measurements might correlate better with symptomatology.

PRECIPITINS AND CIRCULATING ANTIBODIES

The pulmonary diseases caused by *Aspergillus fumigatus* are characterized by different patterns of serological reactions. Typically, sera from patients who develop aspergillomata show strong multiple lines on agar double diffusion tests with antigens from *Aspergillus fumigatus* whilst patients with allergic bronchopulmonary aspergillosis in general show only one to three lines[37]. Precipitins can be found in up to 84% of patients with allergic broncho-pulmonary aspergillosis by double gel diffusion, provided the serum is concentrated up to four-fold. However, they can also be found in about 20% of patients with positive skin prick tests to *Aspergillus fumigatus* but no clinical evidence of the disease, though it is rare to find positive tests in individuals with negative skin prick tests to the fungus. More sensitive methods such as the enzyme-linked immunosorbent assay (ELISA) can be used to look for the presence of specific IgG antibody against *Aspergillus fumigatus*, but this test gives a similar percentage of positive results as double gel diffusion using concentrated serum. Since the ELISA is quantitative it can be used to follow antibody levels and a significant association has been found between levels of specific IgG antibodies against *A. fumigatus* and radiographically diagnosed exacerbations of pulmonary eosinophilia. Repeated measurements using this test may be of greater value in the diagnosis of clinical undetectable episodes of pulmonary eosinophilia than serial chest radiographs[38, 39].

Precipitating antibodies, usually of IgG class, against the appropriate antigens can regularly be demonstrated by double gel diffusion in the serum of all patients with extrinsic allergic bronchio-alveolitis. Precipitin tests against *Micropolyspora faeni* are positive in about 80–90% of acute cases of farmer's lung, though they may also be positive in approximately one-fifth of exposed but apparently unaffected farmers and in the same number of those suffering from other lung diseases[40]. The ELISA test for specific IgG antibodies against *M. faeni* has shown that patients with farmer's lung have significantly higher levels of antibody than exposed but asymptomatic farmers and there is some evidence to suggest that levels of the antibody may vary with the severity of the disease[41]. Nevertheless, the disease cannot be diagnosed solely on the presence of precipitins in serum, nor on the absolute level of circulating antibody. Similarly, precipitins to pigeon antigens may be found in the serum of 20–50% of otherwise healthy pigeon breeders[42]. Budgerigar fanciers remain an exception because nearly all the patients who show precipitins to antigens from budgerigar serum have evidence of the disease. In spite of the fact that precipitating antibodies can be found in the serum of apparently healthy, exposed individuals, the test remains of considerable importance. It confirms that antigen is entering the body in amounts sufficient to induce antibody production and suggests the possibility of an allergic disease. Careful serological studies with extracts from possible causative materials can lead to identification of the major antigens involved. Surveys of exposed populations will identify those who have precipitating antibodies and indicate individuals who may be at risk for eventual development of extrinsic allergic bronchioalveolitis.

PROVOCATION TESTS – PATTERNS OF RESPIRATORY RESPONSE

The techniques, measurement and interpretation of provocation tests in the respiratory tract are fully outlined in Chapter 3.III.

Nasal provocation tests

The patterns of nasal airway response following provocation with histamine and allergen have not been as extensively studied as the reactions occurring in the lung after administration of these agents. This is partly due to the need for more complicated equipment to measure nasal airway resistance and also because significant variations in the patency of each nostril occur spontaneously throughout the day. The typical time course of the immediate nasal response following provocation with allergen and histamine is shown in Figure 7.3. The maximum increase in nasal airways resistance is reached slightly sooner with histamine than allergen, but in both cases the reaction is complete in 1–2 hours. This response is almost identical to that seen in the lower respiratory tract and similarly immediate nasal reactions induced by allergen may be followed by late responses. In a study of 54 grass pollen-sensitive patients with rhinitis, provocation tests[43] lead to a dual response in 37. The time course of a late nasal response is shown in Figure 7.4. The nasal airway resistance reaches a maximum between 4 and 6 hours after the provocation test and may remain high for up to 36 hours. The effect of therapeutic agents on the two basic responses in the nose has not been as extensively studied as in the lower respiratory tract, but the available evidence suggests that the reactions in the nose and the bronchi respond in a similar fashion.

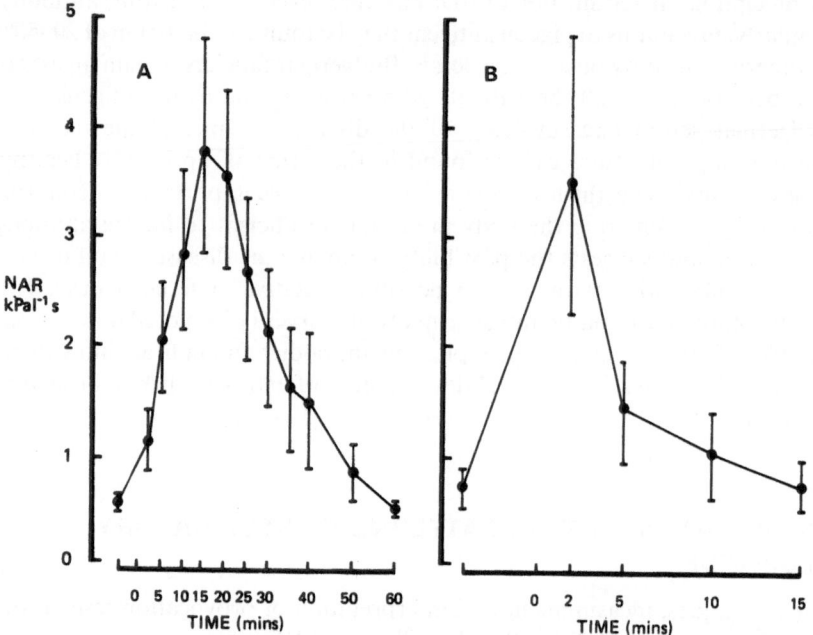

Figure 7.3 The time course of the immediate nasal response following provocation testing with allergen (A) and histamine (B). (NAR = nasal airway resistance). The results are shown as the mean and standard errors of the mean for 20 patients

Bronchial provocation tests

Bronchial provocation tests can provoke transient reactions in the respiratory tract which develop either within minutes of exposure – immediate reactions – or one or more hours later – late reactions. The respiratory response may affect the airways of the lungs only as in asthma, or involve both the airways and lung parenchyma as in bronchio-alveolitis.

Asthma

Immediate asthmatic reactions may be provoked by allergens, pharmacological agents and non-specific stimuli such as exercise. Figure 7.5 shows the results of bronchial provocation testing with extracts of *Dermatophagoides pteronyssinus* and grass pollen in seven subjects and the effect of exercise testing in the same individuals. In this study similar initial falls in forced expiratory volume in 1 second (FEV_1) occurred after both types of provocation, but those following allergen inhalation became more profound and

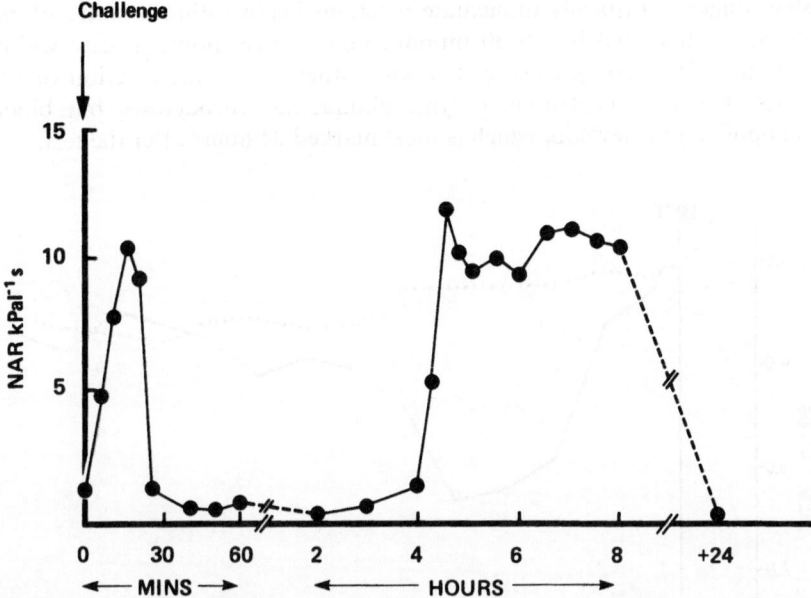

Figure 7.4 A dual (immediate and late) nasal reaction in a patient with allergic rhinitis following a nasal allergen challenge. (NAR = nasal airway resistance)

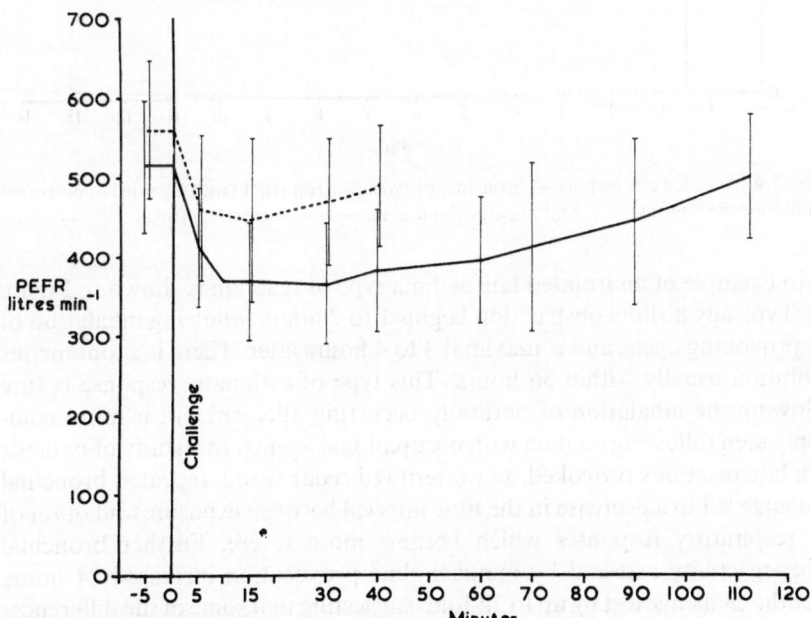

Figure 7.5 A comparison of immediate asthmatic reactions produced by allergen and exercise in the same seven subjects. Results expressed as the mean ± standard deviation. Exercise test. ------; allergen bronchial provocation test. ———

lasted longer[44]. Typically immediate reactions begin within minutes of exposure, are maximal by 15–30 minutes and resolve spontaneously within 1–2 hours. They are not associated with either a systemic reaction or the development of a neutrophil polymorphonuclear leucocytosis, but blood eosinophilia may develop, which is most marked 24 hours after the test.

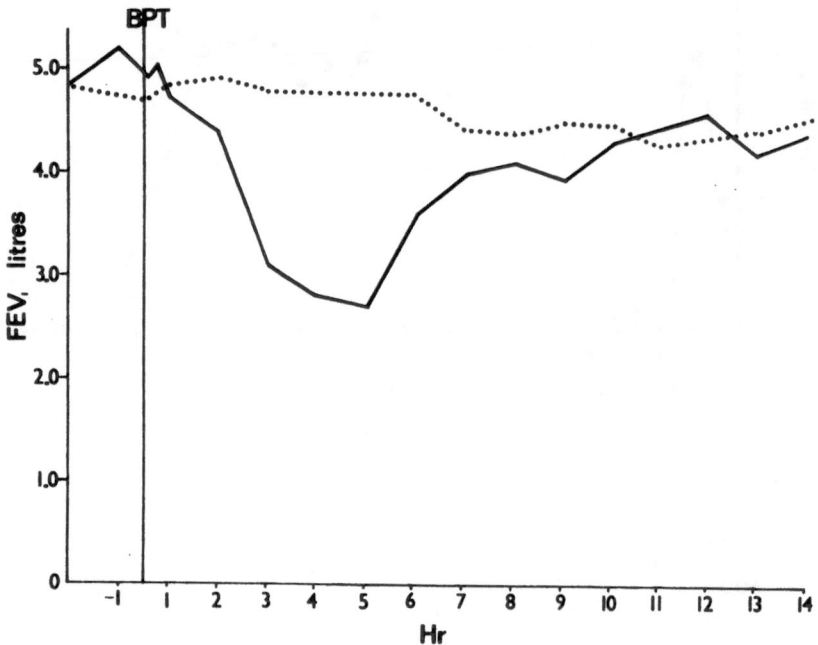

Figure 7.6 Isolated late asthma. A bronchial provocation test (BPT) with a penicillin precursor (6-aminopenicillanic acid). 6-Amino-penicillanic acid, ———; lactose control, ··········

An example of an isolated late asthma type of reaction is shown in Figure 7.6. Typically airflow obstruction begins 1 to 2 hours following inhalation of the provoking agent and is maximal 3 to 4 hours later. There is spontaneous resolution usually within 36 hours. This type of asthmatic response is rare following the inhalation of naturally occurring allergens but is more commonly seen following contact with occupational agents. In a study of patients with late reactions provoked by western red cedar wood, repeated bronchial challenge led to a decrease in the time interval between exposure and onset of the respiratory responses which became more severe. Further bronchial hyper-reactivity assessed by methacholine provocation increased 24 hours after the challenge test by up to 30-fold, suggesting that some of the differences in the timing and severity of late asthmatic reactions may be a reflection of the degree of hyper-reactivity at the time of the test[45, 46].

More sensitive methods of assessing airflow obstruction, such as maximal expiratory flow rates at 50% of vital capacity or 60% of total lung capacity, have detected abnormalities during the asymptomatic period immediately after the provocation test before the onset of the otherwise isolated late asthmatic reaction in individuals developing asthma following inhalation of western red cedar[47]. This does not occur in all patients and is not due to the

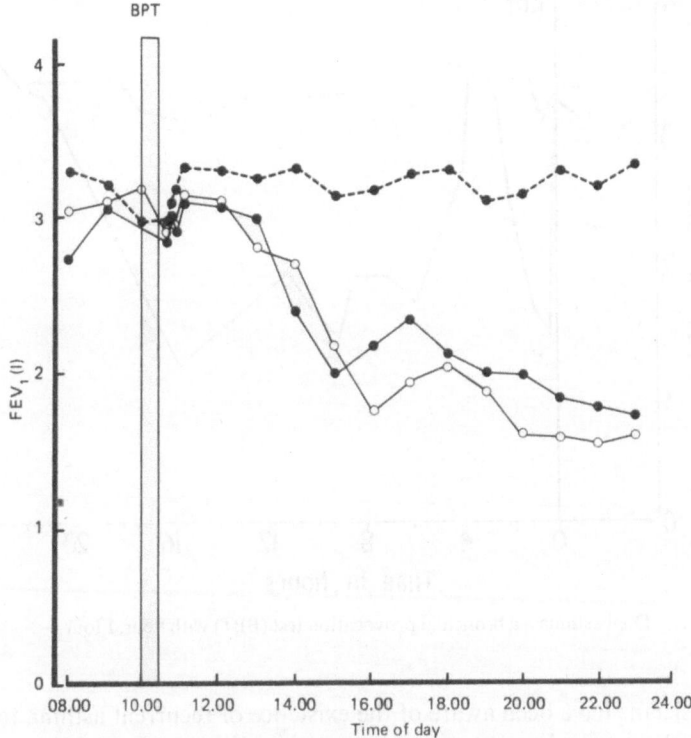

Figure 7.7 Comparison of the isolated late asthmatic reactions following the inhalation of western red cedar in dust form, o———o, and as an aqueous extract,   in a patient with occupational asthma. Control dust is shown by

fact that the patient is inhaling the allergen in dust form. Figure 7.7 illustrates a bronchial provocation test in a wood worker who developed occupational asthma following exposure to red cedar. The same pattern of isolated late asthma occurred on challenge with the dust and an aqueous extract of western red cedar. Further, no abnormalities in airflow were detected during the initial phase immediately after the provocation test on analysis of maximum expiratory flow rates[48].

Dual asthmatic reactions have been shown in carefully performed bronchial provocation tests with extracts from the house dust mite and ragweed pollen which have indicated that about half of the immediate asthmatic reactions are followed by late asthmatic responses. The characteristics of this type of dual asthmatic reaction are shown in Figure 7.8. Respiratory function returns towards the pre-challenge level after the immediate asthmatic response but falls 1–2 hours later with the same characteristics as the isolated late response[49, 50].

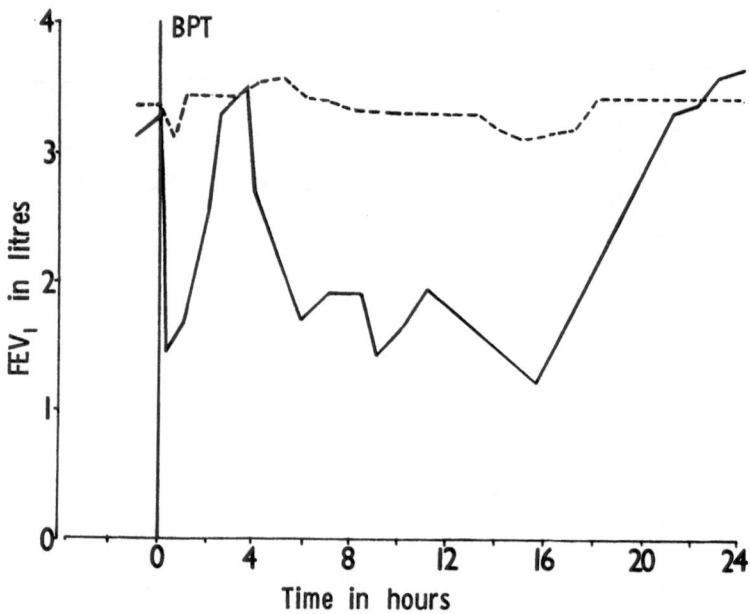

Figure 7.8   Dual asthma – a bronchial provocation test (BPT) with flour. Flour, ————; lactose control, - - - - - -

Physicians have been aware of the existence of recurrent asthma for some time and nocturnal symptoms were recognized[51] as an important feature of bronchial asthma as early as 1882. Lung function measurements in asthmatic patients have confirmed the tendency for airflow obstruction to increase during the night and early morning[52]. Carefully controlled bronchial provocation tests with grain dust in a farmer showed that a single exposure led to asthma which recurred on several nights with maintenance of relatively normal lung function during the intervening days[53]. This is illustrated in Figure 7.9. Similar recurrent asthmatic reactions have been reported in workers handling western red cedar[54] and after bronchial provocation tests with penicillin, formalin, ampicillin and budgerigar serum[55, 56]. Recurrent nocturnal asthmatic reactions almost certainly occur after inhalation of common environmental allergens, but as yet these have not been assessed following bronchial provocation tests.

Important studies in the electronics industry have demonstrated that the patterns of asthma following bronchial provocation tests in hospital do reflect the type of respiratory response noted by the patients at work[57]. Investigations in woodworkers have shown that the first symptoms of asthma noted by the patients usually occurred after working hours and bronchial provocation tests performed at that time revealed the development of late asthmatic reactions. With continued exposure, the same individuals also complained of symptoms immediately on starting work and inhalation tests done at that time frequently showed the presence of dual asthmatic reactions[58].

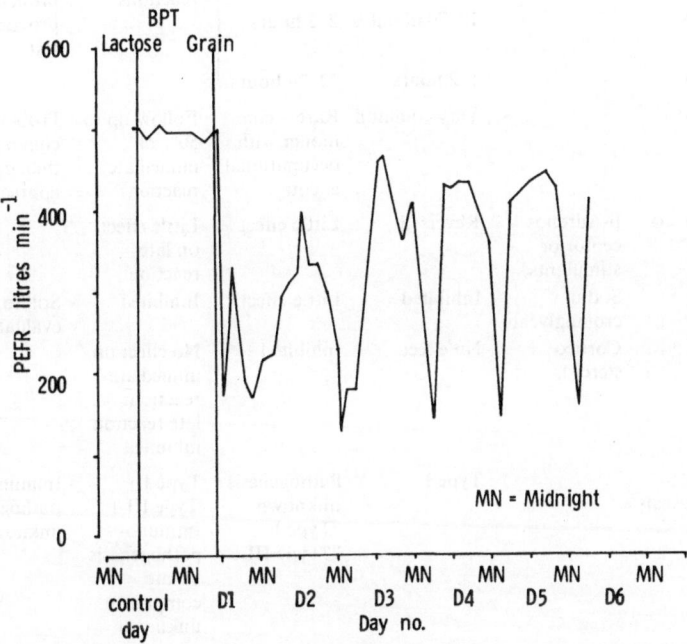

Figure 7.9   Recurrent asthma in a farmer following bronchial provocation testing (BPT) with lactose and grain dust

The characteristics of these different types of asthmatic reactions following bronchial provocation tests are outlined in Table 7.2, as is their response to therapy, the possible allergic pathogenesis and their clinical importance. In general, immediate asthmatic reactions respond well to treatment with β-adrenoceptor stimulants, but the administration of these drugs prior to immediate asthmatic reactions has no subsequent effect on the development of late asthma. Inhalation of sodium cromoglycate before the bronchial provocation test can inhibit both immediate asthma and the late component of dual asthma, whereas the administration of corticosteroids either by inhalation or systemically does not influence the development of immediate asthma but will inhibit the late response[59–61]. The effect of these drugs on the development of recurrent asthmatic reactions has still to be evaluated.

Table 7.2 The characteristics of the different types of asthmatic reactions following bronchial provocation tests

		Type of asthmatic reaction			
		Immediate	*Late*	*Dual*	*Recurrent*
TIME OF ONSET	Start	Within minutes	After 1–2 hours	Combination of immediate and late reactions	May persist for days or weeks after a single bronchial provocation test
MAXIMUM CHANGE		10–20 minutes	2–3 hours		
DURATION		1–2 hours	12–24 hours		
FREQUENCY		Very common	Rare – commoner with occupational agents	Follow-up to 50% of immediate reactions	Probably commoner than currently appreciated
RESPONSE TO THERAPY	β-Adrenoceptor or stimulants	Reversed	Little effect	Little effect on late reaction	
	Sodium cromoglycate	Inhibited	Little effect	Inhibited	Still to be evaluated
	Corticosteroids	No effect	Inhibited	No effect on immediate reaction; late reaction inhibited	
ALLERGIC PATHOGENESIS		Type I	Pathogenesis unknown ?Type I ??Type III	Type I ± Type III + Immunopathogenesis of late component unknown	Immuno-pathogenesis unknown
CLINICAL IMPORTANCE		Very important in minor attacks	Probably very important in hospital practice	Probably very important in hospital practice	Probably very important in hospital practice

Immediate asthmatic reactions are probably the cause of much morbidity in everyday life, but late and recurrent asthmatic reactions which respond only partially to therapy with β-adrenoceptor stimulants may well result in the more prolonged and severe episodes of asthma that lead to hospital admission.

Bronchio-alveolitis

The exact nature of the mechanical changes in the lungs of patients with extrinsic allergic bronchio-alveolitis following bronchial provocation testing remains to be fully elucidated and may well differ from that seen in the established form of the disease. In a study of patients with established bird fancier's lung, lung volumes, diffusing capacity (DL_{CO}) and transfer co-efficient (K_{CO}) were all reduced, indicating the presence of a restrictive defect in lung function with additional parenchymal disease. Peak expiratory flow rate (PEFR) and the ratio of forced expiratory volume (FEV_1) to forced vital capacity (FVC) were normal and total lung resistance was low, suggesting that the large airways were normal. The changes seen in lung elastic recoil, closing volume and closing capacity could all be accounted for by the reduction in lung volumes and provided no mechanical evidence for involvement of small airways. These results were considered compatible with a disease having a patchy involvement. Areas of the lung which were extensively involved would contribute little to the overall lung function, whilst other areas remained physiologically normal[62]. Indeed this is exactly the picture which is seen pathologically. However, respiratory function tests in established cases of farmer's lung have shown that the larger airways may be narrowed[63]. It is perhaps not surprising that the inhalation of organic dust, much of which has

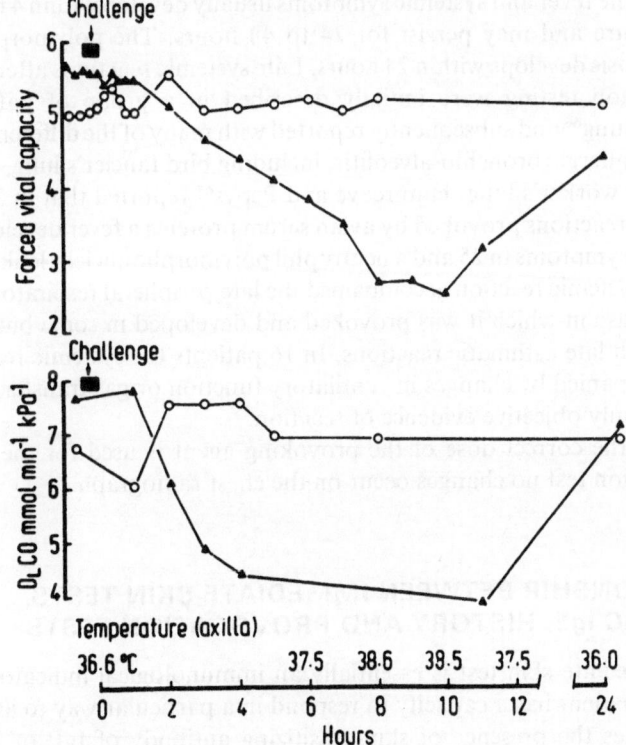

Figure 7.10 A bronchial provocation test with an extract of contaminated water in a patient with 'humidifier fever'. The changes in forced vital capacity, transfer factor (DL_{CO}) and body temperature (axilla) are shown. Control solution, O————O ; extract of contaminated water, ▲————▲

a particle size of below 5 μm, might involve all parts of the respiratory tract and for this reason the disease is best referred to as bronchio-alveolitis.

Unfortunately, studies of respiratory function following bronchial provocation in patients with extrinsic allergic bronchio-alveolitis have not been sufficiently extensive to clarify the relative degree of involvement of large airways, small airways and lung parenchyma. The results of a typical provocation test in a patient with 'humidifier fever' are shown in Figure 7.10. Both the vital capacity and carbon monoxide transfer factor show significant falls maximal 4 to 6 hours after the test[64]. This type of physiological change could well be explained by closure of small airways rather than involvement of the alveoli. Indeed, in a study of patients with bird fancier's lung, the majority showed an asthmatic response after bronchial provocation testing[65].

An important feature of the reaction that follows bronchial provocation tests in patients with extrinsic allergic bronchio-alveolitis is a systemic response characterized by fever often associated with malaise, shivers, myalgia and headache and the development of a neutrophil polymorphonuclear leukocytosis. The fever and systemic symptoms usually develop within 4 to 10 hours of exposure and may persist for 24 to 48 hours. The polymorphonuclear leukocytosis develops within 24 hours. Late systemic reactions after bronchial provocation testing were initially described in a group of patients with farmer's lung[66] and subsequently reported with many of the different causes of extrinsic allergic bronchio-alveolitis, including bird fancier's lung, bagassosis and malt worker's lung. Hargreave and Pepys[65] reported that in 31 patients with late reactions provoked by avian serum proteins a fever developed in 29, systemic symptoms in 25 and a neutrophil polymorphonuclear leukocytosis in 22. The systemic reaction accompanied the late peripheral respiratory reaction in each case in which it was provoked and developed in some but not all of those with late asthmatic reactions. In 16 patients the systemic reaction was unaccompanied by changes in ventilatory function or gas transfer, and fever was the only objective evidence of reaction.

When the correct dose of the provoking agent is used for the bronchial provocation test no changes occur on the chest radiograph.

RELATIONSHIP BETWEEN IMMEDIATE SKIN TESTS, SPECIFIC IgE, HISTORY AND PROVOCATION TESTS

The immediate skin test is essentially an immunological indicator showing that the patient has a capacity to respond in a particular way to an allergen. It identifies the presence of skin-sensitizing antibody of IgE or IgG class. Whether this type of allergic reaction will occur in the respiratory tract following a natural everyday exposure to a particular allergen or, indeed, whether it will result in disease depends on many other factors as yet not fully identified. However, there is a significant correlation between the presence of positive skin prick tests to allergens and a positive history of provocation by them, at least in patients with asthma and rhinitis[20]. Furthermore, when the patient has both a positive history of provocation and a positive skin test to the same allergen, agreement with results of challenge tests has been shown to be as high as 90%[67]. In general the measurement of specific IgE, at least in serum, has little advantage over skin prick testing. High levels of specific IgE correlate better with the clinical history, as do weals with large diameters. All the methods currently available for identifying the causative role of a particular allergen in respiratory disease have their faults. The clinical history can be very unreliable, particularly with such allergens as the house dust mite, since the hyper-reactive nose or bronchial tree may respond in a non-specific manner to contact with any dust. Both skin tests and serum measurements of specific IgE antibody reflect sensitization rather than disease, and even the results of provocation tests may be misleading. Bronchial provocation tests with pollen extracts have shown similar results, at least in terms of changes in airway conductance, in asthmatic subjects and in those with hay fever who deny any lower respiratory tract symptoms[68]. Bronchial provocation testing is usually performed with allergen extracts rather than with pollen particles and the dose given is considerably greater than that encountered in everyday life. It is highly likely that clinical symptoms develop after repeated low dose exposure which probably leads to the development of bronchial hyper-reactivity. Indeed, it is possible to show substantial differences in terms of bronchial hyper-reactivity between symptomatic individuals and allergic individuals with no lower respiratory tract symptoms[69].

These results emphasize the fact that several test procedures may be required to reach the correct diagnosis of allergic respiratory disease resulting from contact with a particular allergen.

HYPER-REACTIVITY

Nasal

Nasal symptoms in patients with rhinitis are often provoked by exposure to non-allergenic substances in the ambient air and changes in temperature. The severity of the resulting symptoms depends on the reactivity of the nasal mucosa.

Animal experiments and microscopic studies of the human nasal mucosa have shown that the submucous glands of the nose are innervated by the parasympathetic nervous system, whereas the capacitance blood vessels (veins and sinusoids) are controlled mainly by the sympathetic system. Intranasal application of the cholinergic agent, methacholine, produces hypersecretion with only slight blockage of the nose. In a recent study, methacholine challenge was shown to produce measurable secretions in all 'normal' subjects, but no sneezing and only insignificant blockage, a response that could be inhibited by prior treatment with ipratropium. Examination of patients with severe perennial rhinitis showed a much increased secretory response to methacholine challenge. again inhibited by ipratropium. suggesting a much higher degree of non-specific reactivity. Similarly, nasal provocation with histamine, which leads predominantly to sneezing and nasal blockage but only slight hypersecretion, has a much greater effect in patients with perennial rhinitis compared to controls. Clearly the outcome of allergen provocation tests in the nose reflects not only the degree of specific nasal sensitization but also the level of non-specific hyper-reactivity[70, 71].

Bronchial

The increased reactivity of the airways of the lung in patients with asthma has been recognized since the seventeenth century. It can be demonstrated by a variety of stimuli, including exercise[72], exposure to cold air[73], inhalation of histamine[74], or cholinergic drugs[75]. Townley and co-workers[69] have extensively studied the response of the bronchial airways to methacholine in patients with asthma, allergic rhinitis and 'normal' individuals from families with a history of atopic disease. Their studies show that the airways of virtually all patients with asthma have a marked response to the inhalation of methacholine and are 100 to 1000 times more sensitive than those of 'normal' subjects. Most asthmatics who cease to have attacks retain their response to methacholine for several years, although the degree of their sensitivity is only a tenth that of current asthmatics. Less than 5% of individuals with allergic rhinitis or non-atopic normal subjects show a high level of methacholine responsiveness, but 'normal' subjects from families with atopic disease have more positive responses to methacholine than 'normals' from families without any history of asthma, rhinitis or eczema. Indeed, the methacholine responsiveness of the airways of people with allergic rhinitis is not significantly different from that of 'normal' subjects from families with atopic disease[69]. A number of studies have shown that the airway response to inhaled histamine is similar to that found after inhalation of methacholine. In addition, methacholine sensitivity and exercise-induced asthma have been found to be significantly related, especially in those asthmatics with the more reactive airways[76]. Indeed, in a study of the response of the lung airways to exercise testing in patients with asthma and rhinitis compared to control subjects, no difference was shown between subjects with allergic rhinitis and non-allergic controls, whilst patients with asthma were significantly different. Further, there was no relationship between the degree of exercise-induced asthma and atopic status as judged by the number or sum of the weal diameters to common allergens or circulating levels of IgE antibody[77]. Studies of cumulative dose–response curves to inhaled carbachol in asthmatic and non-asthmatic subjects have shown wide variation in the dose required to cause a 25% decrease in specific airway conductance (bronchial sensitivity) and in the slopes of the curves (bronchial reactivity). The mean dose–response curves of the asthmatic and normal subjects were widely divergent. indicating that the asthmatic subjects differed from normal subjects more in terms of bronchial reactivity than in bronchial sensitivity[78].

Exercise and infections

Exercise-induced asthma has been shown to occur in over 85% of asthmatic children and in the majority of adults with this disease. Exercise provokes acute obstruction to airflow which is maximal shortly after the exercise ceases. The severity depends upon the type of exercise, with running provoking the greatest degree of asthma, swimming and walking the least, and cycling having an intermediate effect. The duration and severity of the exercise also affect the degree of exercise-induced asthma, the maximum bronchoconstriction occurring after 6 to 8 minutes of running hard enough to raise the heart rate to 180 beats/minute in children or 140 beats/minute in adults. Exercise-induced asthma can be prevented by premedication with β-adrenoceptor

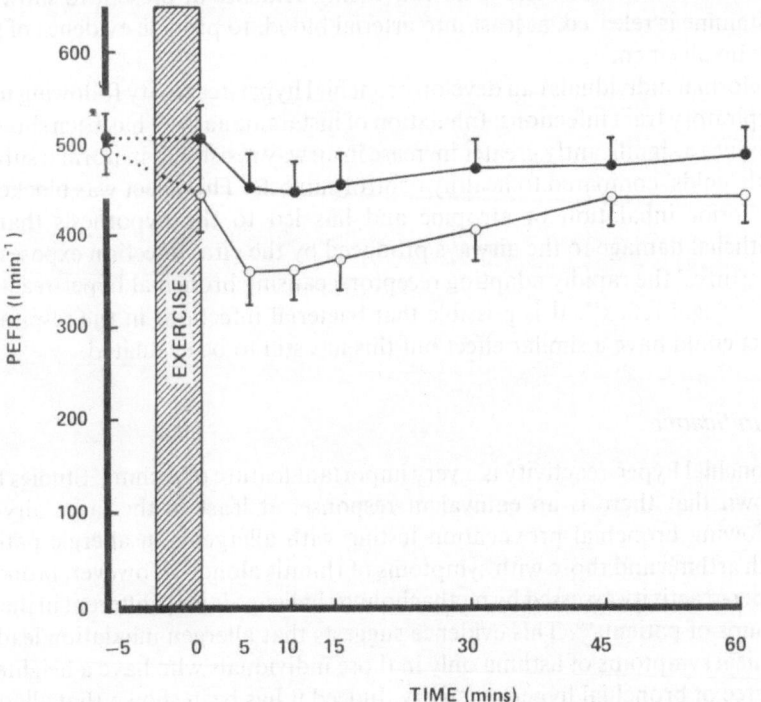

Figure 7.11 The effect of a slow release preparation of aminophylline, ●———●, and placebo, ○———○, on exercise-induced asthma in nine subjects with asthma. Results expressed as the mean ± standard error

stimulants and sodium cromoglycate inhibits the response in most subjects if given before the test. Atropine can also inhibit exercise-induced asthma, but steroids are only effective in a minority of cases[72]. The response of the airways to exercise can be used as a method for testing drugs thought to be of value in the management of asthma. Figure 7.11 shows such a study in which a slow-release preparation of aminophylline is significantly more effective than placebo in inhibiting the airflow obstruction produced by exercise[79]. Until recently it was not clear why different types of exercise should vary in the degree of asthma that they produce and, indeed, the mechanisms leading to this phenomenon have been much disputed. Recently, McFadden and co-workers[80] have shown that exercise induces asthma by causing the patient to hyperventilate, and the critical factor is the temperature and humidity of the inspired air. Cold dry air leads to a marked degree of airflow obstruction in asthmatic subjects, whereas the inhalation of moist warm air is far less effective. The authors argue that exercise-induced asthma is initiated by the heat flux across the respiratory tract mucosa, but how this leads to airflow obstruction has still to be fully determined.

There have been a number of studies of mediator release during exercise-induced asthma but there is no convincing evidence at present to show that histamine is released, at least into arterial blood, to provide evidence of mast cell involvement[81].

Normal individuals can develop bronchial hyper-reactivity following upper respiratory tract infections. Inhalation of histamine aerosol has been shown to produce a significantly greater increase in airway resistance in normal subjects with 'colds' compared to healthy control subjects. This effect was blocked by the prior inhalation of atropine and has led to the hypothesis that the epithelial damage to the airways produced by the viral infection exposes and 'sensitizes' the rapidly adapting receptors, causing bronchial hyper-reactivity via a vagal reflex[82]. It is possible that bacterial infections in the respiratory tract could have a similar effect but this has still to be evaluated.

Significance

Bronchial hyper-reactivity is a very important feature of asthma. Studies have shown that there is an equivalent response, at least in the large airways, following bronchial provocation testing with allergens, in allergic patients with asthma and those with symptoms of rhinitis alone[68]. However, bronchial hyper-reactivity assessed by methacholine challenge is very different in the two groups of patients[69]. This evidence suggests that allergen inhalation leads to clinical symptoms of asthma only in those individuals who have a heightened degree of bronchial hyper-reactivity. Indeed it has been shown that allergens induce asthma more easily as the level of non-specific bronchial hyper-reactivity increases[83]. Further, it has been shown that the degree of non-specific bronchial hyper-reactivity increases for up to 7 days following bronchial provocation challenge tests with allergen, particularly in those individuals who develop late asthmatic reactions[84]. Follow-up studies of patients with occupational asthma have shown that the level of bronchial hyper-reactivity, assessed by methacholine dose–response curves, decreases in symptomatic patients with asthma when they are removed from exposure to the causative material[46]. This information suggests that allergic reactions in the respiratory tract can lead to the development of bronchial hyper-reactivity which decreases if exposure is avoided. An attractive hypothesis to explain the phenomenon of bronchial hyper-reactivity is that the release of neutrophil chemotactic factor (NCF), eosinophil chemotactic factor (ECF–A) and other mediators which have still to be identified, can lead to gradual development of an inflammatory response in the bronchial airways after initial degranulation of the mast cells causing sensitization of rapidly adapting receptors. This explanation has a number of defects, in particular that bronchial hyper-reactivity is also a feature of patients with cryptogenic non-atopic asthma in whom, at present, no known immunological mechanisms are involved. Further, there are conflicting reports of the effectiveness of atropine-like agents in the inhibition of both experimentally produced and naturally occurring asthma. Not surprisingly, anticholinergic compounds such as ipratropium bromide inhibit the bronchial response to methacholine but have little or no effect in inhibiting histamine-induced bronchoconstriction[69]. Neither is atropine particularly effective in inhibiting allergen-induced bronchoconstriction[85], though this is contested[86]. Nevertheless since bronchial hyper-reactivity appears to play such a central role in the clinical development of asthma therapeutic agents which can inhibit release of mediators from mast cells should be very effective, since not only would the immediate response be inhibited but also the subsequent late asthmatic reactions and the development of hyper-reactivity in the airways of the lung.

THE CLASSIFICATION OF ASTHMA AND RHINITIS

Asthma and rhinitis can be divided into atopic and non-atopic according to the results of skin prick testing. Although this classification implies the presence or absence of Type I IgE-mediated allergic reactions in the development of the disease, this is not absolute. It is possible to have atopic asthma or atopic rhinitis with no clearly identifiable allergic provoking factors. The disease usually starts earlier in life in patients with atopic asthma, is more likely to be associated with rhinitis and eczema, often has a more favourable prognosis and may respond better to certain types of therapy, namely sodium cromoglycate. Whilst most children with asthma have positive skin tests, large-scale community studies of adult asthmatics who have had asthma at some time in their life suggest that only half are atopic. Rhinitis has not in general been investigated in groups classified as atopic and non-atopic.

Nevertheless, the majority of cases of hay fever develop during the second decade of life, a later age of onset than for atopic asthma. Almost by definition patients with seasonal allergic rhinitis are atopic but studies in patients with so-called perennial rhinitis have shown that positive skin tests are present in just under one half[87]. Asthma and rhinitis can be divided on the basis of history or results of provocation tests into extrinsic, in which there is an identifiable allergen or occupational agent provoking the attack and crypto-genic. when no such factor can be identified. As illustrated in Table 7.3 patients with extrinsic asthma are usually atopic but they can be non-atopic

Table 7.3   Classification of asthma and rhinitis

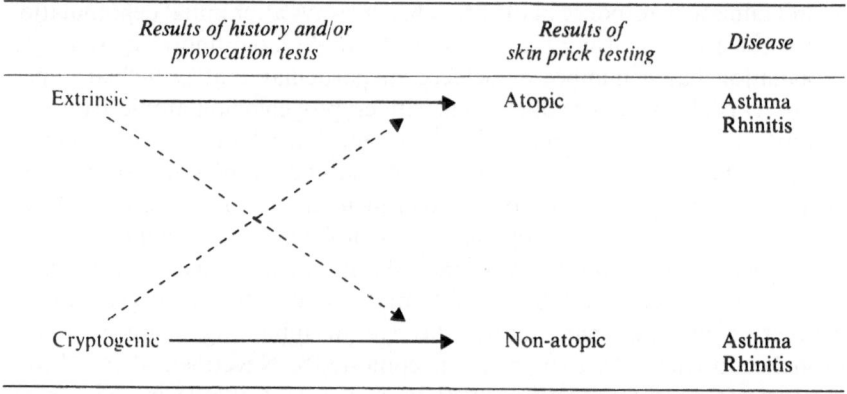

Results of history and/or provocation tests	Results of skin prick testing	Disease
Extrinsic	Atopic	Asthma Rhinitis
Cryptogenic	Non-atopic	Asthma Rhinitis

particularly when the provoking factor is an occupational agent. Type I IgE-mediated allergic reactions may be involved in the pathogenesis of extrinsic non-atopic asthma. particularly after extensive exposure to proteins from *Bacillus subtilis* in the detergent trade, or exposure in the plastics industry to small, highly reactive molecules such as phthalic anhydride or trimellitic anhydride, which act as haptens[88]. Alternatively this type of asthma may result from other varieties of allergic reaction which have still to be defined or from non-immunological mechanisms. for example the possible development of β-adrenoceptor blockade following exposure to toluene di-isocyanate[89]. Similarly, extrinsic non-atopic rhinitis may occur in patients exposed to occu-pational materials. in particular to the dust of western red cedar[45].

Cryptogenic asthma usually occurs in non-atopic individuals but as indicated in Table 7.3, no extrinsic factor may be identified in some asthmatics who have positive skin tests, that is, cryptogenic atopic asthma. The presence of atopy should alert the clinician to a careful review of the history, looking for extrinsic provoking factors such as household pets or chemical agents encountered either at work or in the home. In these circumstances bronchial provocation tests with allergens or chemical materials may be required to reach the correct diagnosis.

Traditionally, rhinitis has been classified as allergic or perennial but many cases of perennial rhinitis result from allergy, particularly to the house dust mite. The term cryptogenic rhinitis should be used for those cases in which no external provoking agent can be defined and like cryptogenic asthma, the majority will be non-atopic on skin testing. Cryptogenic rhinitis can be subdivided into those cases in which nasal eosinophilia can be demonstrated (resembling cryptogenic asthma) and cryptogenic rhinitis in which no nasal eosinophilia can be found. These two types of cryptogenic rhinitis differ in their response to therapy. Cryptogenic rhinitis with nasal eosinophilia responds to treatment with corticosteroids but not sodium cromoglycate, whilst cryptogenic rhinitis with no nasal eosinophilia is very difficult to treat since neither systemic nor topical steroids have much effect.

RHINITIS AND NASAL POLYPS

Extrinsic atopic rhinitis

Patients with this disease may have seasonal or perennial symptoms. Total serum IgE levels and blood eosinophil counts are usually normal provided there is no associated asthma or eczema. Whilst it may be relatively easy to recognize the provoking allergen in cases of seasonal extrinsic atopic rhinitis this can be more difficult when the symptoms are perennial. Indeed in a recent study of patients referred with perennial rhinitis thought to be due to house dust mite allergy, nasal provocation tests using the technique of anterior rhinomanometry were only positive in about 75% of the cases.

Seasonal

This disease, often called seasonal allergic rhinitis or hay fever, is the most common of all allergic diseases and studies from around the world have shown a prevalence rate varying from 2–20% of the population, giving a reasonable average prevalence of 10%. It appears to be particularly common in the United States, possibly due to the widespread occurrence of ragweed[91]. There is a particularly high prevalence in young adults, and in a study of Danish medical students hay fever was present in 15% and latent pollen allergy[92] in an additional 6%.

Nasal irritation. sneezing and watery rhinorrhoea are the most troublesome symptoms in the majority of patients with hay fever but some may also suffer from itching of the eyes and an association with asthma is frequent. Intense itching of the soft palate may occur, indicating that allergens have been carried to the rhino-pharynx by the muco-ciliary system. Occasionally patients experience referred pain such as itching in the ears, which is due to common innervation of the pharyngeal mucosa and the ear.

Clinical experience has shown that even without treatment the severity of symptoms gradually decreases with age though many still suffer late in life. Complete remissions have been recorded. In a five-year follow-up of seasonal allergic rhinitis, without asthma, in untreated children, 9% had become symptom-free[93] and improvement had occurred in a further 29%. In general patients with seasonal allergic rhinitis have more chance of remission than those with perennial symptoms and hay fever patients have a two- to threefold increased risk of developing perennial asthma[94].

Perennial

Less is known about patients who have extrinsic atopic rhinitis with perennial symptoms. Almost all individuals suffer on occasions from attacks of sneezing and nasal blockage and perennial rhinitis has been defined as a disease giving rise to two or three of the following symptoms which occur for more than an hour on most days.

1. Sneezing attacks – more than five sneezes,
2. Serous or seromucous hypersecretion,
3. Nasal blockage due to a swollen nasal mucosa.

Apart from the typical hay fever symptoms, patients with perennial rhinitis may complain of a permanent cold in the head and malaise. Total nasal obstruction may be followed by headaches, disturbed sleep and mouth breathing with loss of smell and taste.

Cryptogenic non-atopic rhinitis

Patients with this disease can be divided into two groups on the basis of the presence of eosinophil cells in nasal smears, collected by scraping the mucous membranes with a cotton applicator. This simple test can be very informative in the assessment of nasal disease. Nasal eosinophilia has been shown in virtually all patients with hay fever during the grass pollen season[95]. Eosinophilia can be demonstrated in nasal smears from the challenged but not the unchallenged nostril within three hours of allergen provocation testing. Patients with perennial symptoms and nasal eosinophilia but negative skin tests correspond closely to cryptogenic non-atopic asthmatics who frequently have peripheral blood eosinophilia. The clinician must be careful to exclude any occupational cause for this type of rhinitis. Further it is possible that some of these individuals may have become sensitized to particular allergens without systemic manifestations in the skin or serum.

The second group of patients with cryptogenic rhinitis are those who have both negative skin tests and no eosinophilia in nasal smears. It has been suggested that these individuals have non-specific nasal hyper-reactivity due to autonomic inbalance but further investigations are required to fully elucidate the mechanisms involved in this disease.

Nasal polyps

Nasal polyps are smooth, round, soft, yellow or pale glistening structures usually attached to the nasal or sinus mucosa by a relatively narrow stalk. They can be broadly divided into two groups. (1) those characterized by neutrophil infiltration on biopsy and associated with a purulent nasal secretion and lack of response to treatment with corticosteroids; and (2) those associated with nasal eosinophilia, seromucous secretion and responsiveness to corticosteroids. These have been termed 'neutrophil polyps' and 'eosinophil polyps' by Mygind[96].

The initial symptoms of nasal polyps are a sensation of secretion which cannot be expelled. Sneezing is rare. The paranasal sinuses are always affected in nasal polyposis and this leads to many of the clinical effects. Sustained low grade infection in the sinuses with accumulation of viscid secretions and pressure from the polyps are factors which give a constant sensation of pressure over the nasal bridge and give rise to frontal headaches. The early formation of polyps can distort the nasomaxillary suture resulting in broadening of the nasal bridge, lateral displacement of the eyes and widening of the nasal cavity.

Neutrophil polyps

These account for 10–15% of the more severe cases of polyposis in adults, association with chronic purulent rhinosinusitis; 25% of children with cystic fibrosis have polyps infiltrated with neturophils[97] and the finding of polyposis in children should always lead to a sweat test for the diagnosis of cystic fibrosis.

Apart from periodic antibiotic treatment, surgery on the nose and paranasal sinuses is the only effective treatment for neutrophil polyps.

Eosinophil polyps

These polyps are often found in association with asthma and perennial rhinitis and the eosinophil leukocyte is the dominant cell in both the polyp and nasal smears. Their aetiology remains obscure. Type I allergic reactions may be a causal factor in the development of eosinophil polyps but they seldom occur in children and young adults with asthma and eczema. Rather they predominate in middle-aged patients with cryptogenic non-atopic asthma. Nasal polyps may occur in up to one half of the patients with aspirin intolerance[98]. On the other hand marked local IgE synthesis has been demonstrated in these polyps[99], and levels of IgE in nasal secretions may be more elevated in patients with nasal polyps than in hay fever patients, although their serum IgE is normal[100].

Eosinophil polyps respond well to oral steroid therapy and more recently the effect of topically applied corticosteroids in the form of aerosols has been assessed. One double-blind short-term trial demonstrated the beneficial effect of beclomethasone dipropionate in about 80% of patients suffering from nasal polyps. Obviously the aerosol must be able to enter the nostril for this type of therapy to be effective and the patient with a totally obstructed nose may need either oral corticosteroids or surgical removal before treatment with beclomethasone dipropionate is started[101]. The effect of aerosol treatment is slow and the patient needs to take this therapy for at least a month before the therapeutic result can be fully assessed. The effect of long-term application of local corticosteroids on the nasal mucosa has been carefully studied over 5 years. There is no evidence that such side-effects as nasal bleeding, increased rate of infection or atrophy, assessed by light or scanning electron microscopy, have been induced by this type of treatment[102].

Treatment of rhinitis

For many years oral agents having antihistaminic activity were the standard treatment for rhinitis. Many of these drugs also possess anticholinergic and sedative effects and some also antagonize 5-hydroxytryptamine. Although these drugs are very useful in the symptomatic treatment of nasal allergy and are able to inhibit sneezing and rhinorrhoea, they have less effect on nasal obstruction and are seldom helpful in the treatment of polyposis. The majority of antihistamines have marked sedative effects though this is thought to be less with azatadine. Phenindamine is said to have a stimulatory rather than sedative action.

Direct intranasal drug application is advantageous since it allows a higher local concentration to be achieved with reduced risk of systemic effects. Decongestants, such as ephedrine and pseudo-ephedrine are frequently used in conjunction with antihistamines adding a vasoconstrictor effect to the competitive inhibition of histamine. Adrenaline is a potent vasoconstrictor but it has a very rapid and short-lasting effect and tachyphylaxis is common. It has been largely replaced by xylometazoline or oxymetazoline, both of which have more prolonged activity. These drugs are effective in the treatment of nasal obstruction but the vasoconstriction is followed by secondary hyperaemia which can lead to severe obstruction some hours after administration of the spray. Patients often consider that this is a feature of the disease and increase therapy which only leads to further secondary hyperaemia, nasal irritability and tachyphylaxis. In spite of these side-effects, these drugs are of value provided they are prescribed for limited periods.

The intranasal application of sodium cromoglycate has been shown by some investigators to inhibit allergen-induced nasal blockage[103], but this has not been found in other studies[104]. Controlled clinical trials using either intranasal sodium cromoglycate powder applied four times a day or a 2% solution 3-hourly, have shown a variable effect for this drug in the management of rhinitis[105, 103]. It seems that although sodium cromoglycate can reduce symptoms in rhinitis its clinical usefulness is limited. In a double-blind comparison of a corticosteroid, betamethasone valerate and sodium cromoglycate, both administered nasally, only two of 18 patients receiving the corticosteroid found the treatment unsuccessful, compared to 12 of the 19 patients taking sodium cromoglycate[106]. Indeed the topical application of corticosteroids has become the treatment of choice for rhinitis. Corticosteroids prescribed orally or by injection as depot preparations can be very effective and may be indicated for the treatment of severe rhinitis which is unresponsive to other forms of therapy; 5 mg of prednisolone given daily substantially relieves symptoms and can safely be used over short periods of time, for example in students taking exams during the summer months.

In 1954, Frankland and Augustin carried out the first placebo-controlled trial of hyposensitization employing both crude and partially purified grass pollen extracts in patients with hay fever and hay asthma and showed that pollen extracts were significantly more effective than placebo in relieving symptoms[107]. Similar results were obtained in a placebo-controlled study of ragweed-sensitive children with autumn rhinitis and asthma[108]. This method of treatment is clinically as well as immunologically specific and the efficacy of pre-seasonal courses of injections depends on the dose administered[109].

There is little doubt that hyposensitization therapy is of value in the treatment of extrinsic atopic rhinitis due to contact with grass and ragweed pollen but at the present time there is little evidence on which to assess the value of this form of treatment with extracts of the house dust mite in perennial rhinitis.

ASTHMA

Asthma is a disease characterized by wide variations in resistance to flow in intrapulmonary airways over short periods of time. Respiratory function tests are necessary for the diagnosis and must be performed either during an acute episode or after bronchodilator therapy. For this reason it is difficult to be sure of the true prevalence of asthma in the community. Further, in both adults and children there is a very significant difference between the proportion of the population who state that they have wheezing compared to those who are regarded as having asthma. Studies of schoolchildren in Birmingham over a ten-year period have suggested that there has been an increase in the prevalence of diagnosed asthma from 1.8% to 2.3% and a further 3.2% of children had wheezing not regarded as asthma[110]. Worldwide studies have shown that asthma is more common in boys and in the United Kingdom, negro children born in England have a similar prevalence of asthma compared to European children whereas Asian children have a lower incidence, even when born in this country. It is difficult to separate wheezing attacks resulting from respiratory infections or bronchitis from what is recognized as asthma. Indeed in a survey of adults aged between 45 and 70 years in southeast London, 28.1% of men and 22.1% of women gave a history of having wheezed at some time[19] and very similar results were found in a survey carried out in three different areas in the Netherlands where 31.5% of men and 19.6% of women aged 40–64 years gave a history of wheezing at some time in their lives. Only a small proportion of both adults and children who report the liability to wheeze are regarded as having asthma and prevalence rates for this disease vary considerably throughout the world. The population of Tristan da Cunha is highly inbred and in 1961 consisted of 286 islanders of whom at least 32% had asthma. Asthma is virtually unknown in children from the Papua New Guinea highlands and in adults the prevalence was recently estimated to be only about 0.3%. Recent evidence suggests that a reasonable cumulative prevalence rate for asthma in the United Kingdom[19, 111] is around 5%.

Presentation

Everybody is familiar with the presentation of asthma as attacks of wheeze in a child following exposure to a provoking allergen and when the disease presents with these symptoms there is no difficulty in the diagnosis. It is now well recognized that perhaps the most common presenting feature of asthma in its early stages is cough, particularly at night, which may be followed later by wheezing on exercise and finally by attacks of wheezing and shortness of breath. Nocturnal attacks of cough and breathlessness closely mimic the symptoms of left ventricular failure and the diagnosis from history alone may be difficult. Asthma may develop for the first time in middle-aged smokers and in these individuals who may suffer from productive cough and breathlessness, the diagnosis is frequently confused with chronic obstructive bronchitis. Since effective therapy is available for patients with asthma, i.e. reversible airways disease, it is essential to consider this diagnosis in all individuals presenting with cough, sputum production, wheeze or breathlessness.

Diagnosis

It is essential, because of the different ways in which asthma can present, to confirm the diagnosis by demonstrating reversible obstruction to airflow in the intrathoracic airways. This may be achieved by sequential measurements of PEFR, FEV_1 and FVC with time or following treatment with bronchodilators such as β-adrenoceptor stimulants or corticosteroids. An improvement of 15% or more in these measurements has become accepted as the degree of reversibility separating patients with asthma from the normal population. It may be necessary to perform an exercise test to demonstrate reversible obstruction to airflow and dose–response curves following the inhalation of methacholine or histamine are increasingly being used to diagnose asthma. Often measurements of respiratory function in patients thought to have asthma may be within the normal range when seen in the clinic, and it may be necessary to provide the patient with a peak flow meter to record lung function at different times during the day. The value of such measurements of PEFR recorded on waking, at lunchtime and in the evening in a 55-year-old non-atopic man thought to have chronic bronchitis is illustrated in Figure 7.12. Recordings made over a two-week period showed

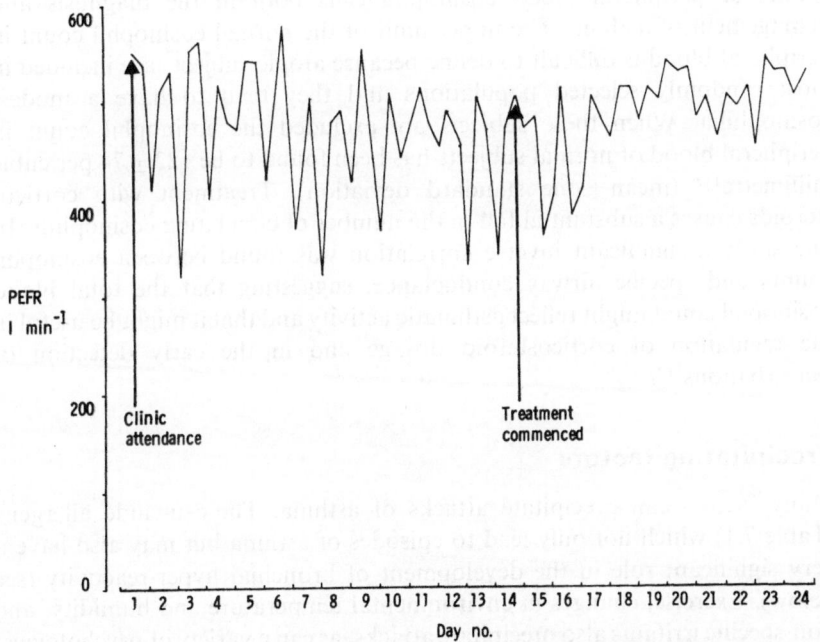

Figure 7.12 Peak flow measured throughout the day in a 55-year-old atopic man thought to have chronic bronchitis

the regular occurrence of airflow obstruction in the late evening whilst peak flows measured in the morning and at lunchtime were often within the normal range. Regular treatment with salbutamol and sustained release aminophylline rapidly led to relief of symptoms and peak flow recordings no longer showed significant episodes of airflow obstruction. In order to confirm variable obstruction to airflow it may be necessary to institute a trial of corticosteroids given orally; 30 to 45 mg of prednisolone should be given daily for two weeks with measurements of respiratory function before and after this therapy. Since there is no effective treatment for the basic abnormalities occurring in chronic obstructive bronchitis and emphysema it is essential to discover whether any part of the airflow obstruction is reversible, i.e. due to asthma. In the view of the author, all patients with obstructive airways disease should therefore have a trial of corticosteroids to discover any asthmatic element in their disease.

Microscopic examination of sputum can be a very useful test. The presence of eosinophils in sputum is strongly suggestive of a diagnosis of asthma, in individuals with airflow obstruction. Curschmann's spirals and Charcot–Leyden crystals may also be seen and in cases of severe and prolonged airway narrowing the sputum itself may be expectorated in threads presumably coming from the narrowed bronchi. Increasing emphasis has been placed on counts of peripheral blood eosinophil cells both in the diagnosis and management of asthma. The upper limit of the normal eosinophil count in peripheral blood is difficult to define because atopic subjects are included in most randomly selected populations and they tend to have a modest eosinophilia. When these subjects are excluded the eosinophil count in peripheral blood of normal subjects has been found to be 122 ± 74 per cubic millimetre[112] (mean $\pm$ one standard deviation). Treatment with corticosteroids causes a substantial fall in the number of circulating eosinophils. In one study a significant inverse correlation was found between eosinophil counts and specific airway conductance, suggesting that the total blood eosinophil count might reflect asthmatic activity and that it might be useful in the regulation of corticosteroid dosage and in the early detection of exacerbations[112].

Precipitating factors

Many factors can precipitate attacks of asthma. These include allergens (Table 7.1) which not only lead to episodes of asthma but may also have a very significant role in the development of bronchial hyper-reactivity (see below). Exercise, changes in environmental temperature and humidity, and non-specific irritants also precipitate attacks, as can a variety of psychological stimuli presumably via a vagal reflex[113]. The administration of β-adrenoceptor blocking drugs such as propranolol[114] can induce severe episodes of airflow obstruction in patients with asthma by altering the control exerted by the autonomic nervous system and circulating hormones from the adrenal medulla upon smooth muscle contraction and mediator release for mast cells. It is well recognized that the majority of anti-inflammatory analgesic drugs, in particular aspirin, can precipitate asthma in up to 5% of patients with this disease probably by interference with the balance of prostaglandin biosynthesis[115]. Artificial colouring agents, especially azo-dyes such as tartrazine which are found in many foods and even pharmaceutical products, can precipitate asthma attacks, often in patients wih aspirin idiosyncrasy.

Whether immunological or non-immunological mechanisms are involved in the aetiology of these reactions has still to be elucidated[116, 117].

Viral and bacterial infections

There is now little doubt that viral infections of the respiratory tract can precipitate attacks of asthma. Studies by Gregg in general practice in London showed that rhino-viruses were the most commonly isolated infective agents during episodes of wheezing in both children and adults. In children with a history of asthma or recurrent wheezy bronchitis, rhino-virus infections were more often associated with wheezy bronchitis than with the symptoms of an upper respiratory tract illness alone and in asthmatic adults such infections were usually associated with wheezing[118]. In a prospective study of asthmatic children admitted to hospital, 42% of the episodes of wheezing were associated with identifiable viral infections, the most common being respiratory syncytial virus[119] followed by para-influenza type II. Although it has been shown that viral infections can lead to the development of bronchial hyper-reactivity and so precipitate attacks of wheezing, it is possible that infection, particularly by respiratory syncytial virus may initiate asthma. In one study 56% of infants who had suffered an attack of acute bronchiolitis subsequently developed episodes of asthma[120]. However it is equally possible that these children were already asthmatic and that acute bronchiolitis was the first manifestation of the underlying bronchial hyper-reactivity.

In 1933 Cook used the term 'infective' in his classification of patients with asthma to describe those who had intrinsic (cryptogenic) asthma due, he thought, to bacterial infection. In spite of the absence of any convincing evidence that demonstrates any role for bacteria in the development or precipitation of this disease the term 'infective asthma' continues to be used. In one study, nose and throat swabs from 97 asthmatic children were examined and compared with those from 32 normal non-hospitalized children. There was no qualitative or quantitative difference in the incidence of pathogenic organisms isolated from asthmatic children who were clinically well or unwell at the time of examination when compared with non-asthmatic children[121]. The significance of bacteria isolated from sputum is often in doubt since specimens can readily be contaminated by the flora of the oropharynx and mouth. This problem can be avoided by the use of transtracheal aspiration and this technique has been used to study the micro-organisms present in the lower respiratory tract of patients with asthma. In a study by Berman and co-workers small numbers of pathogenic bacteria were isolated from patients with asthma but also from control subjects and in only one out of 27 asthmatics did the authors suggest the possibility that bacterial infection had contributed to exacerbation of the disease[122]. In spite of the lack of any evidence to implicate bacterial infection in the development or precipitation of asthma, antibiotics are frequently prescribed. Indeed in England as many as

50% of exacerbations of asthma are treated with antibiotics[123]. Bacterial vaccines continue to be administered as a form of hyposensitization therapy in patients presumed to have 'infective asthma'. There is no evidence whatsoever from the reported literature to suggest that this treatment is of any value[124].

Pathogenesis

Type I allergy predominates in the immunological mechanisms that cause asthma. The cross-linking of adjacent IgE molecules on the surface of mast cells by allergen results in a series of as yet poorly defined intracellular biochemical reactions which by mechanisms involving calcium, energy metabolism and intact microtubules, lead to fusion of granules with the cell membrane and release of histamine and the formation and release of other mediators. Initially this reaction may occur in mast cells free in the bronchial lumen and the resulting mediator release may make the mucosa more permeable to allergens with resulting involvement of mast cells in the lining of the respiratory tract[125]. Evidence from allergen-induced skin responses has suggested that both the immediate and late reaction may be related to the release of vasoactive and smooth muscle reactive mediators, chemotactic factors, structural proteoglycans and enzymes from mast cells. The release of these compounds may be considered in (1) an early phase, essentially involving vasoactive mediators and (2) a late cellular phase, involving chemotactic mediators[126]. It must be remembered that nearly all the information about mast cell reactions and mediator release has come from numerous *in vitro* studies using animal preparations, human chopped lung, or basophil-rich fractions from peripheral blood. There is as yet surprisingly little information from *in vivo* studies in man to substantiate these findings.

The early phase involves the release of histamine which can cause both direct and reflex contraction of the smooth muscle of large and small airways and dilatation of small vessels with separation of the endothelium of venules allowing transudation of serum and extravasation of leukocytes. The biological activities of histamine are expressed by interaction with both H_1 receptors causing bronchoconstriction, vasodilation and increased intracellular levels of cyclic guanosine monophosphate (cyclic GMP) and H_2 receptors leading to inhibition of lymphocyte-mediated cytotoxicity and IgE-mediator release of histamine as well as an increase in intracellular levels of cyclic adenosine monophosphate (cyclic AMP). SRS-A is a vasodilator and is thought to have a preferential effect in constricting peripheral airways[127]. Arachidonic acid mobilized from phospholipids of the cell membrane can be converted to prostaglandins and thromboxanes by cyclo-oxygenase, and prostaglandin $F_{2\alpha}$ ($PGF_{2\alpha}$) is a potent bronchoconstrictor whilst prostaglandin E_2 causes dilation of the airways. Platelet activation factors (PAFs) are also released during the early phase. These are as yet chemically undefined and although they are not directly bronchoconstricting or vasoactive, they can induce aggregation of platelets and release of serotonin. Release of these mediators provides an adequate explanation for the development of immediate asthmatic reactions following allergen interaction with IgE-coated mast cells, and there is some evidence at least for release of histamine *in vivo* following allergen provocation. Bhat and co-workers have shown that venous plasma histamine increases four-fold during asthma induced by allergen inhalation[128]. Animal experiments of a similar nature have shown that not only does plasma venous histamine increase significantly during asthma induced by allergen inhalation but that the change in arterial plasma histamine is four- to five-fold greater[129]. Further, raised plasma histamine levels have been found in patients admitted to hospital with severe asthma and these fall to normal following successful therapy[130]. However, antihistamines administered orally have not been found to be effective in the treatment of asthma, although the aerosol administration of clemastine, which is an antihistamine with H_1 blocking activity, has been found in one study to be as effective a bronchodilator as salbutamol in patients with asthma[131]. These results have not been confirmed by others[132] casting some doubt on the role of histamine released *in vivo* from mast cells in the pathogenesis of asthma. Although mast cell mediators have been characterized as isolated factors, they do interact. Histamine and SRS-A are synergistic in producing bronchoconstriction and both induce the generation of prostaglandin. Additionally, histamine in high concentration inhibits and in low concentration enhances ECF-A-induced chemotaxis, whereas prostaglandin E_1 enhances and $PGF_{2\alpha}$ inhibits neutrophil chemotaxis. Other interactions which may be critical in the development of asthma await elucidation.

At the present time there is considerable interest in the development of the late phase of the asthmatic reaction which is not only of considerable importance in the clinical manifestations of asthma but is also likely to be important in the development of bronchial hyper-reactivity. Histological studies of late skin reactions have shown the influx of both neutrophil and eosinophil polymorphonucleocytes and lymphocytes as well as fibrin deposition and some vascular damage which can result, it appears, solely from an IgE-mediated reaction[25]. Recent evidence suggests that these pathological changes can at least in part be explained by the release of chemotactic mediators from mast cells. As yet the picture is incomplete and the discovery of further mediators is awaited. ECF-A was the first chemotactic factor from the mast cell to be characterized. It has a molecular weight of 400 and is preformed in both human lung and mast cell. It is preferentially chemotactic for eosinophils which may participate in the inflammatory reaction in two ways. On the one hand these cells can phagocytose immune complexes and inactivate histamine, SRS-A and PAFs by the release of histaminase, arylsulphatase and phospholipase respectively. On the other hand, release of constituents from granules in eosinophils which contain cationic protein can lead to generation of substances that potentiate the inflammatory reaction which, in the airways of the lung, could increase obstruction to airflow[133] More recently a high molecular weight compound has been identified in mast cells and leukaemic basophils which is specifically chemotactic for neutrophils – high molecular weight neutrophil chemotactic factor (HMW-NCF). *In vivo* studies in man have demonstrated the presence of neutrophil chemotactic activity (NCA) in the serum of patients with allergic asthma, following specific bronchial provocation with allergen[134]. Neutrophil chemotactic activity appears in the circulation within minutes of antigen challenge and may persist for up to 24 hours[135]. Its release is antigen-dose-dependent and NCA may be found in the circulation following stimulation with concentrations which have proved insufficient to cause significant alterations in airflow obstruction. The release of NCA is inhibited by sodium cromoglycate[136] but the effects of other drugs used in the treatment of asthma, in particular the β-adrenoceptor agonists on the release of this mediator have still to be fully evaluated. This is of considerable theoretical and clinical consequence. β-Adrenoceptor agonists have been shown *in vitro* to prevent release of mediators from chopped human lung preparations following allergen challenge by a mechanism thought to involve increased levels of intracellular cyclic AMP but whether this applies to the administration of the drug *in vivo* is as yet unknown. The presence of NCA at the site of the allergic reaction in the airways of the lung can attract polymorphonuclear leukocytes and contribute significantly to the development and prolongation of the inflammatory reaction. The therapeutic benefits of corticosteroids in the treatment of asthma may be explained on the basis that they have a powerful anti-inflammatory action.

In 1968 Szentivanyi[137] suggested that β-adrenoceptor blockade might be the factor responsible for the hyper-reactivity of the airways in all asthmatics. According to this theory, mediators released as a result of allergic reactions cause bronchoconstriction because their action is not opposed by stimulation of intact β-adrenoceptors which normally serve to maintain broncho-dilatation. There is much evidence to show that patients with asthma do have a decreased adrenergic response and studies on peripheral blood lymphocytes from asthmatic patients have demonstrated a decreased basal level of cyclic AMP and a smaller increase in the amount of this nucleotide following stimulation with catecholamines[138]. Although these findings are not contested there is a considerable argument as to whether they represent an inherent defect in atopic or asthmatic individuals or whether they result from the effects of recent treatment with adrenergic agents or excessive release of endogenous cathecholamines. *In vivo* and *in vitro* studies on alterations of plasma and urinary cyclic AMP and the cyclic AMP responses of isolated peripheral blood lymphocytes to adrenergic stimulation have shown similar results in asthmatic patients who are not taking adrenergic agonist drugs when compared to control subjects[139]. Indeed leukocyte cyclic AMP response becomes depressed within hours of treatment with adrenergic agonists, remains suppressed during the period of treatment and gradually recovers within a number of days after withdrawal from drug therapy[140]. Observations in patients have suggested that abuse of inhaled bronchodilators may lead to a state of unresponsiveness to further adrenergic medication and may result in death[141]. Recent evidence has shown that the response to an adrenergic agonist involves a complex series of events. These include binding of the agonist to a specific receptor on the external surface of the cell membrane followed by coupling of the complex to membrane bound adenylate cyclase. This enzyme becomes activated through a process which involves a regulatory guanine nucleotide and then converts adenosine triphosphate (ATP) to cyclic AMP. Cyclic AMP interacts with protein kinases to mediate the intracellular effects of the adrenergic agonist. Current evidence suggests that agonist-induced adrenergic desensitization primarily involves a change in the specific receptor or cognitive moiety of the sequence. Studies using radio-labelled β-adrenoceptor agonist ligands have shown that the process of desensitization involves the selective loss of high affinity β-adrenergic receptor binding sites and that the remaining receptors bind agonist with lower affinity, a type of binding not associated with stimulation of adenylate cyclase[142]. However in one recent study evidence was obtained to suggest that atopic patients have a decreased number of β-adrenergic receptors even in the absence of treatment with adrenergic drugs, suggesting that the mechanisms responsible for loss of β-adrenoceptors have still to be fully elucidated[143]. Clinical studies have shown that administration of corticosteroids can restore responsiveness to adrenergic bronchodilators in tolerant patients[144]. Recent preliminary reports using radio-labelled antagonists have indicated that treatment with corticosteroids produces this effect by increasing the number of available β-adrenergic receptors[145].

Management

Environmental control and immunotherapy

The importance of altering the environment in which the asthmatic patient lives was first recognized in the seventeenth century by Sir Thomas Brown who wrote: 'The ancient inhabitants of this Island were less troubled by coughs when they went naked and slept in caves and woods than men now in chambers and feather beds'. The efficacy of environmental control in relieving asthma or indeed extrinsic allergic bronchio-alveolitis is clear when one considers the effect of removing such patients from exposure to provoking agents at work or from contact with animals (such as horses, dogs, cats, rodents, and birds).

Similarly it is logical to try to reduce the affected person's contact with environmental allergens such as grass pollen and the house dust mite. Mite counts in mattresses can be reduced by regular vacuuming[146] and they can be virtually eliminated by enclosing the mattresses in plastic covers[147]. Indeed the low or zero levels of mite infestation in mattresses in residential schools, hospitals, and asthma clinics, particularly those situated at high altitude, may acount for the reduction in symptoms in mite-sensitive asthmatics. In two trials of mite-avoidance measures one indicated a beneficial effect[148] while the other did not[149]. Although it is more difficult to avoid contact with grass pollen, simple measures such as keeping the bedroom windows closed and avoiding outdoor activity in the evening when grass pollen counts at ground level are high can help to reduce symptoms.

The term immunotherapy is preferable to hyposensitization when considering therapy aimed at altering allergic responses. The mode of action of the currently available allergen injections is far from clear and attempts are now being made to specifically inhibit IgE responses by induction of suppressor mechanisms or the development of specific immunological tolerance. In the latter method allergens have been coupled covalently to a synthetic copolymer of D-glutamic-D-lysine (D-GL) and experimental evidence in animals has suggested that selective and specific suppression of IgE antibody responses can be achieved possibly by inhibition of helper T cells[150]. The results of clinical trials using ragweed D-GL conjugates in patients with extrinsic atopic rhinitis due to ragweed are awaited.

Since the first use of allergen injections by Noon and Freeman in 1911 this technique has been widely used throughout the world. Unfortunately most studies designed to assess its value have been largely unsatisfactory because of poor selection of patients or lack of appropriate randomization and placebo control.

Immunotherapy for pollen-induced asthma is clinically useful[151] but the value of this form of treatment with the house dust mite has been much disputed. In a recent controlled study of children with asthma a beneficial effect was noted; of particular interest was the fact that the injection treatment with *D. pteronyssinus* extract appeared to inhibit the development of late bronchial reactions in almost half the subjects[152]. Asthma resulting from contact with animals has been largely unresponsive to immunotherapy but a recent report indicated that such treatment with purified cat-pelt antigen may be effective[153]. There is little doubt that the success of immunotherapy depends upon the correct identification and purification of the allergens involved in the disease and it is likely that the lack of success of many allergen preparations was due to the fact that the necessary antigens were absent. The clearer understanding of the antigens involved in the provocation of asthma, together with increased knowledge of the control mechanisms for IgE antibody production, may well herald a new era for effective immunotherapy in asthma.

Drug therapy

With the notable exception of occupational asthma it is rare for patients with extrinsic atopic asthma to be adequately controlled solely by measures designed to alter environmental contact with the precipitating allergen. Similarly immunotherapy, though often helpful, rarely brings complete relief of symptoms. For this reason it is necessary to institute drug therapy. The general principal in the management of asthma is to administer sufficient therapy not only to relieve symptoms and allow the patient as far as possible to carry out a normal life, but also to try and maintain respiratory function near to or within the normal range. If these conditions are met, the patient is less likely to have disabling attacks of asthma and the risk of death during a severe exacerbation should be greatly reduced. Many patients under the age of 35 still die from asthma every year and in many cases this can be related to inadequate therapy. Where possible inhalant treatment using aerosol or powder forms of the drug are to be preferred since higher concentrations can be achieved in the respiratory tract with less likelihood of unwanted side-effects when compared to systemic therapy.

Relatively selective β_2-adrenoceptor agonist drugs such as salbutamol and terbutaline are widely used in the management of asthma throughout the world. These drugs and many others like them have been derived from the basic isoprenaline molecule in which substitution or rearrangement of existing groups have rendered the compounds more resistant to the effect of catechol-O-methyl-transferase. thus prolonging their action and making them more specific for the β_2 or bronchial as opposed to the β_1 or cardiac receptors. Comparative studies have shown little difference between the majority of these agents, which are effective bronchodilators[154]. Tremor is the main unwanted side-effect but this is much less noticeable when these drugs are administered as aerosols rather than in the oral form. Stimulation of β-adrenoceptors can lead to a rise in intracellular levels of cyclic AMP and this can explain the mechanism of their action in bronchial smooth muscle. *In vitro*, such drugs have been shown to be effective in diminishing histamine release from suitably sensitized and challenged human leukocytes and chopped human lung[155]. However, the concentration of the drug required for this effect is high and it is doubtful whether this can be achieved by oral doses of these drugs that can be tolerated in man[156]. It remains possible however, that the necessary concentration may be achieved following aerosol administration. At the present time there is insufficient *in vivo* evidence in man to determine whether β-adrenoceptors agonists have a therapeutic action solely on bronchial smooth muscle or whether in addition they have an 'anti-allergic' effect by inhibiting release of mediators from mast cells. These drugs should be administered regularly throughout the day, save in asthmatics who have only very infrequent isolated episodes of asthma. This latter situation may be relatively infrequent. Careful symptomatic and respiratory function studies are required throughout the day to assess the severity of disease in patients with asthma before deciding upon the frequency of administration of drugs including β-adrenoceptor agonists. Ipratropium bromide is an anticholinergic agent which can be administered by aerosol. In general it has not been found to be quite as effective as salbutamol in the treatment of patients with asthma, though the two drugs show fairly equivalent results in patients with chronic bronchitis. There is some evidence to suggest that additional bronchodilatation may be achieved in patients with asthma when both drugs are administered concomitantly[157].

Cyclic AMP is catalysed to 5′ AMP by a phosphodiesterase enzyme. Methyl xanthines, particularly theophylline, inhibit the action of this enzyme, thus sustaining any beneficial increase in cellular cyclic AMP produced by β-adrenergic stimulation. Although this effect can be shown *in vitro*, it is arguable as to whether or not this mechanism explains the beneficial effect of administration of theophyllines in patients with asthma. The most commonly used form of theophylline is aminophylline (theophylline ethylene diamine). A number of studies have shown that therapeutic levels of theophylline are between 10–20 μg/ml. Ideal therapy requires measurement of blood levels. More recently slow release preparations have been introduced which allow adequate blood levels and therapeutic efficacy to be achieved on twice daily dosage[79]. There is some evidence that β-adrenoceptor agonist drugs and theophyllines may act synergistically when administered together[158]. The important unwanted effect of theophylline is gastrointestinal disturbance with nausea and vomiting.

In 1965 sodium cromoglycate was isolated and found to be among the most active of the synthetic bischromones in its ability to inhibit certain anaphylactic reactions in animals and bronchial reactions to inhaled allergens in man. It has no direct bronchodilator action and has no antihistamine, anti-inflammatory or steroid-like properties[159]. There have been numerous trials which have indicated a definite superiority for sodium cromoglyate over placebo in the suppression of asthmatic symptoms reported by adults and children with asthma, though usually the clinical improvement is not matched by appropriate changes in tests of respiratory function[160, 161]. Although clinical experience suggests that sodium cromoglycate is most effective in allergen-induced asthma, it has been shown to inhibit exercise-induced asthma in which there is little evidence for mast cell involvement. Further, sodium cromoglycate effectively blocks airflow obstruction produced by the inhalation of sulphur dioxide. Experiments in man have shown two quite different dose–response curves for the effect of sodium cromoglycate on inhibition of asthma induced by allergen and on that induced by sulphur dioxide suggesting that the drug may indeed have two distinct modes of action[162]. The concept that sodium cromoglycate inhibits release of mediators from mast cells is supported by the studies of Atkins and co-workers[136] who showed that the drug inhibits release of NCA following allergen challenge in man. More recently evidence has accumulated to suggest that sodium cromoglycate may also inhibit bronchoconstriction following stimulation of irritant receptors by some action on the nervous reflex arc, but the exact mechanism remains to be determined[162]. *In vitro* and *in vivo* evidence from studies on mediator release and from direct bronchial provocation tests suggests that sodium cromoglycate ought to be a very effective drug in the management of asthma. By preventing release of mediators from mast cells, it ought not only to inhibit the effects of allergen challenge in everyday life but also inhibit the development of late inflammatory responses in the bronchial airways, possibly preventing the development of bronchial hyper-reactivity. However, in clinical practice throughout the world many physicians have not found this drug to be a particularly effective therapy for asthma.

Until the late 1960s administration of corticosteroids by aerosol had no advantage over oral administration because a similar dose was required for adequate control of asthma. However, the introduction of synthetic corticosteroids with a high index of topical activity provided a major therapeutic advance in the management of this disease. Many studies have shown the efficacy of such drugs and administration of 400 µg of beclomethasone dipropionate daily has been shown to permit a 50% reduction in the oral dosage of prednisolone in patients taking up to 15 mg. No evidence of adrenal suppression has been found at a daily dose of 400 µg of beclomethasone dipropionate and although *Candida albicans* can frequently be isolated from the oropharynx it rarely becomes of clinical significance[163]. These results have been confirmed throughout the world and the effectiveness of beclomethasone dipropionate has been found to be sustained for as long as 2 years and under these circumstances administration was not associated with any abnormal chest X-ray findings or endocrine suppression. In this study *C. albicans* was isolated from the oropharynx in approximately one third of the subjects but this was usually transient[164].

Asthma can be most effectively treated by prescribing drugs regularly. It is sensible to start with an inhaled β-adrenoceptor agonist drug. If this is insufficient to control the disease then either theophylline or sodium cromoglycate can be added. Inadequate control of symptoms requires replacement of sodium cromoglycate by an inhaled corticosteroid such as beclomethasone dipropionate. Some asthmatics may not be controlled on this therapy and will require oral administration of prednisolone. Generally administration of this drug at doses less than 10 mg per day is rarely accompanied by unwanted effects. Much has been written about the mechanisms of action of corticosteroids in asthma but this is still very poorly understood. The longheld belief that these drugs act by stabilizing lysosomal membranes probably does not apply *in vivo*. Glucocorticoids cause a neutrophil leukocytosis but reduction in circulating levels of eosinophils, monocytes and lymphocytes. Whilst the function of granulocytes is relatively refractory to corticosteroids, monocyte and macrophage function is particularly sensitive to treatment with these drugs[165] and perhaps the principle mechanism of their effectiveness in asthma is by suppression of the inflammatory response.

OCCUPATIONAL ASTHMA

Occupational asthma can be defined as the occurrence of episodes of reversible obstruction to airflow following exposure to materials encountered at the workplace. Exposure to many highly reactive chemicals such as toluene di-isocyanate (TDI) which were once only encountered in factories, may now occur in the home or in the course of hobbies. Contamination of the atmosphere by industrial pollution can lead to outbreaks of asthma in neighbouring communities and industrial materials can be brought to the home in clothes and hair or on the skin. Common environmental materials such as pollens and animal danders may be important occupational allergens to people such as gardeners, florists, veterinarians and animal handlers. In any study of respiratory disease it is essential to enquire about the patient's occupation as a cause for disease. In his book, *De Morbis Artificum Diatriba* published in 1713, Ramazzini stressed the importance of this history when he stated, 'To the questions recommended by Hippocrates one more should be added, "What is your occupation?".'

The first scientific accounts of industrial disease were published by Agricola and Paracelsus in the sixteenth century but it is Bernardino Ramazzini who has become generally regarded as the father of occupational medicine. He was the first to focus attention on the shortness of breath and urticaria that occurred in workers following exposure to grain dust. Amongst his many contributions to occupational disease was his philosophy that medicine, like law, should contribute to the well-being of workers. He exhorted the medical profession to take an interest in the many industrial processes that were leading to disability and death amongst their patients. Since that time an increasing number of dusts, gases, vapours and fumes have been incriminated in the aetiology of occupational asthma. In 1911 in Chicago, Karasek and Karasek[166] recognized the harmful effect of platinum salts on the respiratory system of photographic workers, but it was many years later before Hunter emphasized the frequent occurrence of sneezing, wheezing and running of the eyes amongst metal refinery workers in London exposed to the complex salts of platinum[167]. He and his co-workers pointed out the important phenomenon of symptoms of asthma occurring during the night away from the factory, a feature which can confuse the occupational origin of the disease. Recent studies have stressed the importance of these nocturnal symptoms as a presenting feature of occupational asthma[55].

The development of the plastics industry has created new hazards at work. Although toxicity to TDI was suspected during the Second World War, it was first reported to the medical profession in 1951 when 9 out of 12 men employed mixing TDI were found to have persistent respiratory symptoms. In spite of extensive research, the pathogenesis of the occupational asthma that may follow contact with TDI remains to be elucidated. In 1969, asthma was found to develop in employees involved in the production of 'biological' washing powders[168] and reversible airflow obstruction has been described in those manufacturing antibiotics[56]. The process of soldering wires, so important in the electrical industry, is not without hazard. Recent studies have incriminated colophony resin, which has been used for many centuries in this process, as the cause of the respiratory disease[57]. Asthma has been found to develop in workers employed in an increasingly wide variety of occupations and the more closely the industrial processes are scrutinized the more frequently this disease is found.

Prevalence

At the present time there is unfortunately little reliable information about the proportion of cases of asthma caused by contact with materials at work though it has been claimed that up to 15% of all male cases of asthma in Japan result from exposure to industrial dusts, gases, vapours or fumes[169]. In the absence of adequate large scale epidemiological surveys, it is possible to get some idea of the prevalence of occupational asthma from studies in individual industries.

Worldwide prospective studies in the detergent industry have indicated that about 2% of all exposed employees developed symptoms due to inhalation of enzymes from *Bacillus subtilis* used in the production of washing powders[170]. In the colour printing trade, when gum acacia was used as a powder to separate printed sheets, between 20 and 50% of employees were found to develop respiratory symptoms varying from mild rhinitis to severe asthma[171]. Roberts, in a prospective study of workers in the metal refining industry, suggested that almost all developed respiratory tract symptoms of varying severity[172]. The prevalence of asthma amongst those employed in the manufacture or use of toluene di-isocyanate has been estimated from co-operative industrial surveys to be about 5%[173]. In the United States over 100 000 people are employed in this industry indicating that there may be in excess of 5000 cases of asthma resulting from exposure to this chemical. A recent study in the electronics industry has shown that 22% of those involved in the process of soldering develop asthmatic symptoms[174].

The prevalence of byssinosis varies between countries and with the type of cotton used. It may affect between 20 and 80% of those spinning coarse cotton but is much less prevalent in mills using fine cotton yarns[175]. It is important to appreciate that most studies on the prevalence of occupational lung disease inevitably concentrate on individuals at work. These represent a 'survivor' population in that affected workers may well have left the industry. For this reason cross-sectional studies may indicate a low point prevalence of the disease whereas the cumulative prevalence may be very much higher. Bouhuys and co-workers discovered a much greater prevalence of chronic cough, breathlessness and reduced respiratory function in retired hemp workers in a

Spanish village compared to suitably matched control subjects who had worked in other industries[176].

Occupational asthma has been described in a number of important industries, for example, the pharmaceutical industry and the wood and lumber trade, in which satisfactory epidemiological studies have still to be performed to indicate the extent of this problem.

It is of particular importance, not least from the medico-legal aspect, to discover whether asthma induced by a particular occupational agent continues to occur when all exposure to the offending agent has ceased. This emphasizes the need for careful studies of individuals who have left industries for health reasons.

Atopy

Atopic subjects differ from non-atopics in the ready development of Type I allergy following exposure to inhalant allergens, and as might be expected it has been shown that atopic individuals more readily develop positive skin tests to the enzymes from *Bacillus subtilis* than do non-atopics[9]. However this difference may be lost if the degree of exposure is particularly heavy. In a retrospective study of printers, the time to development of asthma from first contact with gum acacia was half as long in atopic subjects compared to those with a non-atopic background. A prospective study of workers processing platinum salts indicated that a higher proportion of those who were atopic developed positive immediate skin tests to these salts as well as symptoms which developed more rapidly. However, occupational asthma is not confined to those who are atopic. Indeed non-atopic individuals appear to predominate in many of the selected studies presented in the literature. For example 19 of 22 woodworkers who developed asthma after inhalation of the dust from western red cedar were non-atopic[45] as were 15 of 16 symptomatic workers in the platinum industry. A possible explanation for this contradiction is that atopic workers may have rapidly developed severe symptoms making them leave their jobs early, leaving behind an essentially non-atopic 'survivor' population which may develop hypersensitivity and symptoms at a later date. Preliminary studies in the platinum industry lend support to this hypothesis. On the other hand, when exposure levels are particularly high or because Type I allergic mechanisms are not involved, atopy may not be an important predisposing factor.

Pathogenesis

Irritant mechanisms

Amongst the several processes that may be involved in the production of airflow obstruction is stimulation of irritant and cough receptors by inhaled materials. This reflex is mediated by the vagus nerve and is one of the ways in which many air pollutants are thought to precipitate attacks of asthma. The increase in airway resistance that follows inhalation of sulphur dioxide can be inhibited in animals by cervical block of the vagus nerve, and in man by the prior inhalation of atropine[177]. Accidental exposure to ammonia, hydrochloric acid or sulphur dioxide in the petroleum or chemical industries can lead to episodes of asthma, particularly in those individuals who have preexisting bronchial hyper-reactivity. The inhalation of an irritant gas such as chlorine can lead to a severe inflammatory reaction and an asthma-like syndrome which can occur on subsequent days on contact with concentrations of gas previously regarded as trivial. This indicates the possible induction of non-specific bronchial hyper-reactivity by inflammatory agents[178]. Exposure to nitrogen dioxide in silo filler's disease is of particular interest since the inflammatory reaction in the lung develops some hours after inhaling the gas when it has been slowly hydrolysed to nitric acid. The timing of this reaction in the lung after inhalation of the gas mimics the late respiratory reaction caused by allergic mechanisms. Formaldehyde vapour is a strong respiratory irritant, but a small number of people develop severe prolonged attacks of asthma following its inhalation. Similarly, while toluene di-isocyanate leads to airway irritation in the majority of subjects exposed to high concentrations (greater than 0.5 ppm) a small proportion develop asthma at concentrations as low as 0.001 ppm. This underlines the difficulty of separating irritant from allergic mechanisms and suggests that certain industrial materials may act as irritants in some workers but sensitize others.

Pharmacological mechanisms

The inhalation of cotton dust or its aqueous extract can lead to airway responses in healthy previously non-exposed subjects as well as in affected workers. Although this response is not synonymous with byssinosis it is clear that some subjects can react to dust exposure with symptoms and decreases in maximum expiratory flow rates while others have no symptoms but their airway conductance decreases[179]. This universal effect on the lung on first inhalation of cotton dust argues strongly against the involvement of allergic mechanisms in the pathogenesis of this disease. Indeed under appropriate experimental conditions, extracts from cotton, flax and hemp can, in high concentrations, release histamine from non-sensitized chopped human lung[180]. The exact role of this histamine-liberating agent in the development of byssinosis remains to be elucidated. Several cases of acute asthma have been described in farmworkers who have sprayed crops with organic phosphorous insecticides[181]. The substances act as anticholinesterases and probably precipitate asthma by allowing an increase in the local concentration of acetyl choline in the bronchial airways. Aqueous extracts of western red cedar wood have been shown to release histamine directly from guinea-pig and human lung tissue *in vitro*[182] and the complex salts of platinum have been reported to cause similar release of histamine after intra-cardiac injection in experimental animals[183]. *In vitro* experiments with TDI have shown that this chemical has an inhibitory action at β-adrenoceptors at least in human lymphocytes[89]. Whether or not these pharmacological reactions have any role in the development of clinical disease remains to be established.

Allergic mechanisms

The investigation of both atopic and non-atopic individuals with occupational asthma has been dominated by the search for Type I allergic mechanisms. Evidence for this type of reaction has been increasingly found even in occupational asthma caused by highly reactive low molecular weight chemicals and in this respect RAST has been of particular value[184].

Aetiological agents

There are a considerable number of dusts, gases, vapours and fumes of industrial origin which cause asthma. Some of these materials can also be encountered in the urban environment, in homes or in the course of hobbies. Dust from castor bean mills or grain elevators[185] and TDI in 'do-it-yourself', polyurethane foams and varnishings[186] and soldering fluxes used in home electronics[187] are examples of some of the agents which can lead to asthma outside the confines of the factory. Much of the evidence linking the development of asthma to a variety of industrial materials has come from bronchial provocation testing. Information about the pathogenesis of the disease has been derived from skin testing, passive antibody transfer tests to man or monkey and more recently identification of specific IgE antibody in serum. This kind of information has implicated immunological mechanisms in many cases of occupational asthma, but in others this evidence is lacking or incomplete and other mechanisms may be important in the pathogenesis.

The commoner and more important forms of occupational asthma and the industrial in which the materials may be met are outlined in Table 7.4. The possible immunological, irritant or pharmacological pathogenesis is indicated in the table, as are the results of skin and passive transfer tests to man or monkey, bronchial provocation tests and the results of radioimmunoassay for specific IgE in the serum of affected workers.

Prevention and treatment

The primary objective in the management of asthma of occupational origin must be prevention. This may be achieved by precise identification of causal agents, reduction in levels of exposure to potentially harmful industrial materials and selection and monitoring of those employed. Bronchial provocation tests of the occupational type may be necessary to define the precise nature of the material leading to asthma and information from this type of investigation can help to define the levels of exposure which lead to disease. It is important to realize that in sensitized workers the concentration of the occupational material needed to precipitate episodes of asthma may be much lower than the dose necessary to cause initial sensitization. The latter information can only come from long-term studies in particular industries.

Environmental control

Control of the industrial environment requires creation of and adherence to standards of maximum levels of exposure. Work exposure to potentially sensitizing or irritant substances should be kept at the lowest practicable levels by careful design and maintenance of the work environment. In this respect it is very important to ensure that 'area' monitoring of levels of industrial dusts, gases, vapours or fumes, adequately reflects the personal exposure received by individuals at their work-place. Lowering exposure levels to the enzymes from *Bacillus subtilis* in the detergent industry led to a decreased sensitization rate as judged by the development of positive skin tests and fewer cases of occupational asthma. This indicates that it is possible to prevent sensitization by lessening exposure.

It has become apparent that short-term and/or peak exposures may represent a particularly important aspect of disease production. Improvements in the techniques for accurate monitoring of levels of exposure will lead to a clearer understanding of the dose–response relationship both for development of sensitization and production of disease. This will allow the maximum allowable levels of exposure to be assessed on the basis of valid information.

The size of dust particles may itself be critically important in determining whether occupational asthma occurs. In byssinosis, the risk of developing disease is extremely low if the particles are greater than 7 µm in diameter. However with particles below this size the development of acute symptoms is likely even if the concentration in the air is as low as 0.2 mg per cubic metre of air[179].

In general face masks of the filtering type are neither efficient nor well tolerated. However positive pressure air hoods which prevent inhalation of contaminated air from the factory floor can be effective. Special attention must be paid to the disposal of extracted industrial materials into the atmosphere, making sure that exhaust systems do not lie in close proximity to air intakes and the extracted material is not allowed to affect the local community.

Selection of employees

There is evidence from certain industries, particularly the enzyme industry and the metal refining trade, that atopic individuals are more likely to develop

Table 7.4 Outline of occupational asthma

Industrial material	Industry	Pathogenesis (+ = probable; ? = possible)			Results of				Reference
		Irritant	Pharma-cological	Allergic	Bronchial provocation tests	Skin tests (prick or intra-cutaneous)	Passive transfer tests to man or monkey	Specific IgE in serum	
Ammonia. sulphur dioxide. hydrochloric acid, chlorine, nitrogen dioxide	Chemical and petroleum industry, silo fillers	+			+				178
Formalin	Medical	?		?	+				190
Animal, bird, fish and insect-serum, dander secretions	Veterinarians, animal and poultry breeders, laboratory workers, fishermen, sericulture			+	+	+	+	+	203
Castor bean	Oil, food and pharmaceutical industry			+	+	+		+	204
Soybean				+	+	+	+	+	192
Green coffee bean				+	+	+			205
Papain	pharmaceutical industry			+	+	+		+	206
Bromelin				+	+	+		+	193
Pancreatic extracts				+	+	+	+		207
Enzymes from *Bacillus subtilis*	Detergent industry			+	+	+	+	+	168
Hog trypsin				+	+	+	+		207
Ethylene diamine	Plastics, rubber and resin industry			+	+	+	+		208
Phthalic anhydride				+	+	+		+	198
Trimellitic anhydride				+	+	+	+	+	88
Reactive dyes	Textile industry			+	+	+	+		194
Phenylglycine acid chloride	Pharmaceutical industry			+	+	+	+	+	212
Sulphonechloramides									197

Complex salts of	Metal refining		?	+	+	+	+	+	167
platinum									200
Salts of nickel	Metal plating			?	+	+			209
Flour	Bakers, farmers, grain			+	+	+		+	188
	elevator operators								189
Grain	Bakers, farmers, grain			+	+	+		+	53
	elevator operators								199
Wood dusts	Wood mills,			?	+	+			45
	carpenters								
Vegetable gums (acacia,	Printers			+		+	+		171
karaya)									
Carmine dyes	Textile industry			?	+				201
Ampicillin				?	+				56
Spiramycin	Pharmaceutical			?	+				202
Tetracycline	industry			?	+	+			191
Piperazine				?	+				196
Amprolium hydro-				?	+				210
chloride				?	+				
Dimethyl ethanolamine	Paint, plastics, rubber								195
Toluene di-isocyanate	and resin industry	?	?	?	+				89
Pyrolysis products of	Polyurethane industry	?		?	+				211
PVC price labels	Meat wrappers								
Soldering fluxes	Electrical trade	?		?	+				174
Organic phosphorus	Farm workers		?						181
insecticides									
Cotton dusts	Textile industry,		?	?	+	+			179
	vegetable oil								

asthma. For this reason it would be sensible to exclude such workers from occupations in which there is a high risk of exposure to sensitizing dusts, vapours or fumes. This should be done at the pre-employment stage, preferably on the basis of the results of skin testing with a battery of relevant common inhalant allergens. Clearly those individuals with asthma should also be excluded and this may require some test of bronchial hyper-reactivity. Routine lung function testing of those at risk should be an indispensable part of any adequate prevention and control programme.

The development of any respiratory symptoms should be investigated looking particularly for evidence of reversible airways disease. In those industries in which the development of sensitivity and asthma are related to the production of specific IgE antibody, there is evidence to suggest that both positive skin tests and measurable levels of specific IgE antibody may develop before respiratory symptoms. The routine performance of these tests could provide a method of monitoring those at risk and preventing the onset of respiratory disease.

Management

The most important aspect of treatment of occupational asthma is to remove the affected person from the site of exposure to the offending industrial material. This may be possible by transferring the affected worker to other parts of the factory though unfortunately it may often be necessary to terminate the individual's employment. Under certain circumstances, when pressing social or financial considerations are paramount, other forms of therapy may be considered. Asthma of occupational origin responds in a similar fashion to that resulting from other causes. Indeed bronchial challenge tests with occupational agents have shown the effectiveness of pre-treatment with such pharmaceutical agents as sodium cromoglycate or beclomethasone dipropionate in the different types of asthmatic reaction[59]. Although specific hyposensitization has been performed successfully with the complex salts of platinum[213] it is unlikely that this therapeutic procedure will be applicable on a widespread basis. Appropriate treatment may make it possible for the affected worker to remain in his job. It is essential that such individuals should be kept under careful longterm observation with repeated tests of respiratory function to identify any deterioration at the earliest stage. Further, the situation should be carefully explained to the patient who should be aware of the possible risks involved.

Medicolegal aspects

Occupational asthma has been recognized by law as a disease of occupational origin with rights of compensation in very few countries. In 1960 the first occupational asthma to be recognized by law in France was that associated with the manufacture and handling of penicillin. This was followed in 1967 by asthma related to contact with the dust of tropical woods. Since that time a number of chemical agents including paraphenylene diamine, ethanolamine, isocyanates, biological enzymes and organic phosphates and pyrophosphates have been added to the list. In Germany in 1961, a law was passed concerned with reference to 'Bronchial asthma enforcing the cessation of a professional occupation or any other paid employment'. A great number of cases have been referred for investigation under this law and some accepted for industrial injury, particularly those caused by contact with flour dust and TDI. At the present time consideration is being given in many other countries to the acceptance of occupational asthma as an occupational disease with rights of compensation.

PULMONARY DISEASES CAUSED BY *Aspergillus fumigatus*

Moulds of the genus *Aspergillus* are hardy and ubiquitous organisms which can be found in such diverse sources as fertile soil, decaying vegetation, swimming-pool water and flour. In addition, *Aspergillus* species are the moulds most commonly cultured from houses, in particular from basements, bedding and housedust. Many species of *Aspergillus* may infect humans, but one of the most commonly encountered in *Aspergillus fumigatus*. Indeed, pulmonary disease due to this fungus was first recognized in the nineteenth century when an aspergilloma was found in the lung cavity of a woman, but the first report of an association between *A. fumigatus* and respiratory tract allergy was by Van Leeuwen[214] in 1925.

    A. fumigatus can lead to the development of five different lung diseases and the type of disease is influenced by the immunological reactivity of the host. In a series of 107 consecutive patients attending hospital with chronic chest disease three were found to have aspergilloma, five allergic broncho-pulmonary aspergillosis and one invasive aspergillosis[215].

Asthma

In atopic individuals the inhalation of *Aspergillus* spores can lead to the development of asthma with positive immediate skin tests to its extracts, causing disease in a similar way to other common inhalant allergens.

Extrinsic allergic bronchio-alveolitis

This disease can occur in both atopic and non-atopic individuals. The spores of *Aspergillus* species are about 3 μm in diameter and can readily reach the peripheral parts of the lung very occasionally giving rise to extrinsic allergic bronchio-alveolitis. This most commonly occurs in malt workers following inhalation of the spores of *A. clavatus*[216].

Aspergilloma

This disease typically occurs in non-atopic individuals though occasionally it can occur in patients who are atopic. Damaged parts of the lung become infested with *A. fumigatus* leading to the development of a fungal ball or mycetoma. This has a characteristic appearance on the chest radiograph being surrounded by a translucent halo (Figure 7.13). Aspergillomata have been

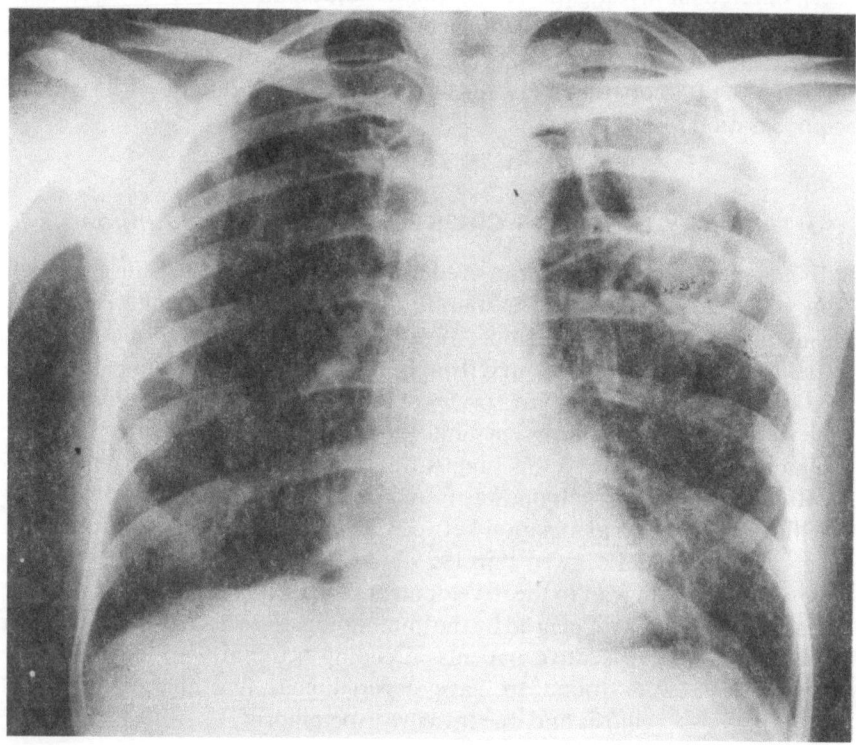

Figure 7.13 Two mycetoma in the upper and middle zones of the left lung, due to *Aspergillus fumigatus*. Note the halo of air around the fungal balls

found to develop in about 15% of healed post-tuberculous cavities. Although they do not influence overall mortality, aspergillomata may cause considerable morbidity by giving rise to persistent cough and frequent episodes of haemoptysis which may be severe[217]. Patients with this disease may show weak positive skin tests to extracts of *A. fumigatus* but their serum characteristically contains large quantities of antibodies against extracts of the fungus which on double diffusion in agar-gel give rise to as many as 15 to 20 precipitin lines. Aspergillomata may occasionally be due to other members of the genus, namely *A. nidulans*, *A. terreus* and *A. flavus* as well as *Allescheria boydii*.

Invasive aspergillosis

This disease occurs in patients who are immunosuppressed either by diseases such as lymphoma or as a result of therapy with cytotoxic or immunosuppressive drugs. This disease can be associated with the development of precipitating antibody which can be demonstrated on agar-gel diffusion but unfortunately invasive aspergillosis often remains unrecognized until post mortem.

Allergic bronchopulmonary aspergillosis

In 1952 Hinson, Moon and Plummer described a condition in the respiratory tract caused by *A. fumigatus* and characterized by pulmonary eosinophilia,

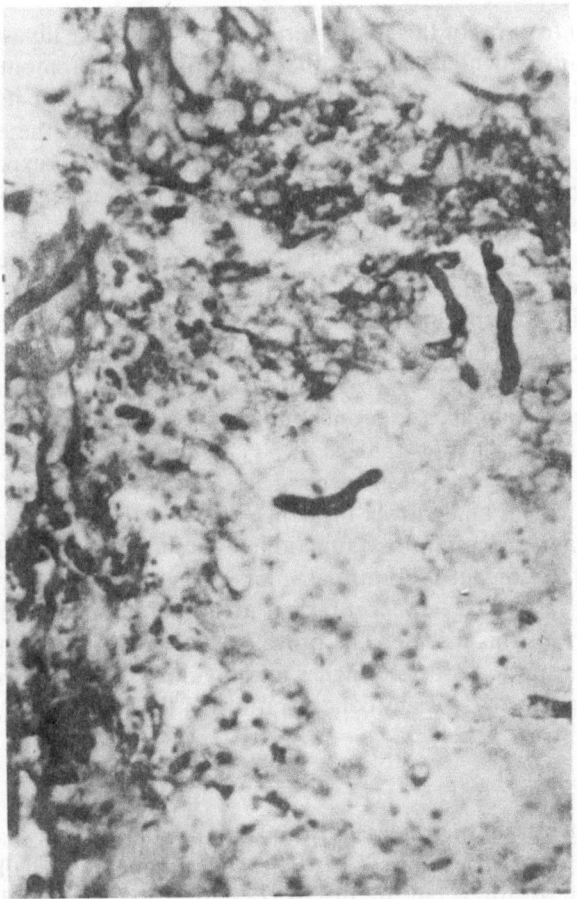

Figure 7.14 Section of a sputum plug in a patient with allergic bronchopulmonary aspergillosis showing the presence of fungal mycelium

that is pulmonary infiltrates with a peripheral blood and/or sputum eosinophilia[218]. Allergic bronchopulmonary aspergillosis is the commonest form of
pulmonary eosinophilia in the United Kingdom and patients with this disease
are almost always atopic and have a history of bronchial asthma. The criteria
for diagnosis were established by McCarthy and Pepys[219, 220] as the presence of
asthma, a previous episode of transient shadowing on the chest radiograph
with blood and/or sputum eosinophilia and an immediate positive skin prick
test to an extract of *A. fumigatus*. Supportive evidence for the diagnosis of the
disease comes from the demonstration of late skin or bronchial reactions to
extracts of the fungus, the culture of *A. fumigatus* from sputum plugs and the
demonstration in most cases of specific precipitating antibodies in serum.

Clinical features and respiratory function tests

The clinical features of this disease are typical. A 'flu-like illness' develops in
an asthmatic patient usually in the autumn or winter months when the
concentration of *Aspergillus* spores in the atmosphere is at its highest and
analysis of peak expiratory flow rates measured during these periods has
shown deterioration in respiratory function. Many patients expectorate large
quantities of sputum (up to an egg-cupful or more) and approximately 50%
cough up surprisingly large sputum plugs which on section and suitable
staining show both eosinophils and the presence of fungal mycelium (Figure
7.14). These plugs which may be up to 1–2 cm in size and come from medium
sized ectatic bronchi, are related to areas of pulmonary infiltration and
collapse, a condition referred to in the past as 'mucoid impaction'. There may
be a time interval of up to 25 years in patients whose asthma starts early in life
before they develop allergic bronchopulmonary aspergillosis, whereas those
whose asthma starts after the age of 30 can develop the disease within 3–5
years. This latter group is in general less atopic with fewer skin tests to
common allergens and a lower incidence of a personal and family history of
atopic disease[219]. Respiratory function tests show the typical features of
airflow obstruction but a substantial number of patients[221] also have a reduced
gas transfer factor (D_{LCO}). Host factors are of paramount importance in the
development of this disease. The prevalence of allergic bronchopulmonary
aspergillosis appears to be no higher in individuals such as farmers who are
exposed to particularly heavy concentrations of the spores of *A. fumigatus*[222].

Chest radiographs

The characteristic of this disease is the occurrence of transient shadows in any
part of the lung fields (Figure 7.15). Their development is usually associated
with clinical features but in up to 25% of cases the shadows remain
asymptomatic. About half of the acute episodes of consolidation are followed
by permanent changes on the chest radiograph most often in the form

of ring shadows. Band shadows may occur which may later be replaced by tubular shadows and these may result from transient filling of dilated bronchi with secretions and fungal material. Proximal rather than distal bronchiectasis typically occurs in this disease (Figure 7.16) and these findings on the radiograph[223] have been shown to be associated with a decrease in D_{LCO}.

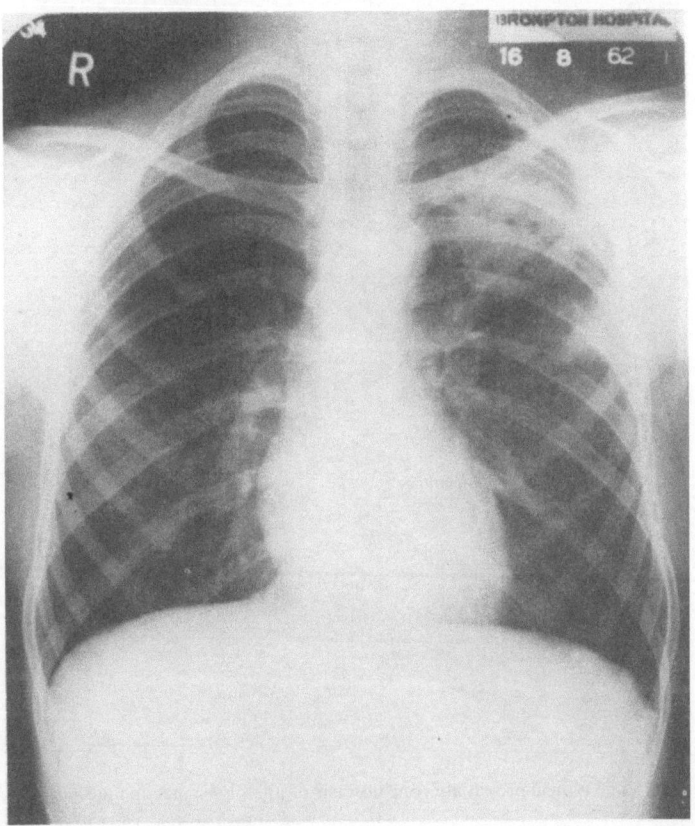

Figure 7.15 Pulmonary infiltrates in a patient with allergic bronchopulmonary aspergillosis

Precipitins and IgE antibody

Patients with allergic bronchopulmonary aspergillosis frequently have extremely high levels of total serum IgE antibody which become elevated during or shortly after episodes of pulmonary infiltration. However, most of this IgE antibody is not specifically directed against *A. fumigatus*. The marked elevation is thought to be the result of non-specific stimulation of IgE-producing plasma cells[224]. The presence of precipitating antibody is not diagnostic of allergic bronchopulmonary aspergillosis. Indeed circulating

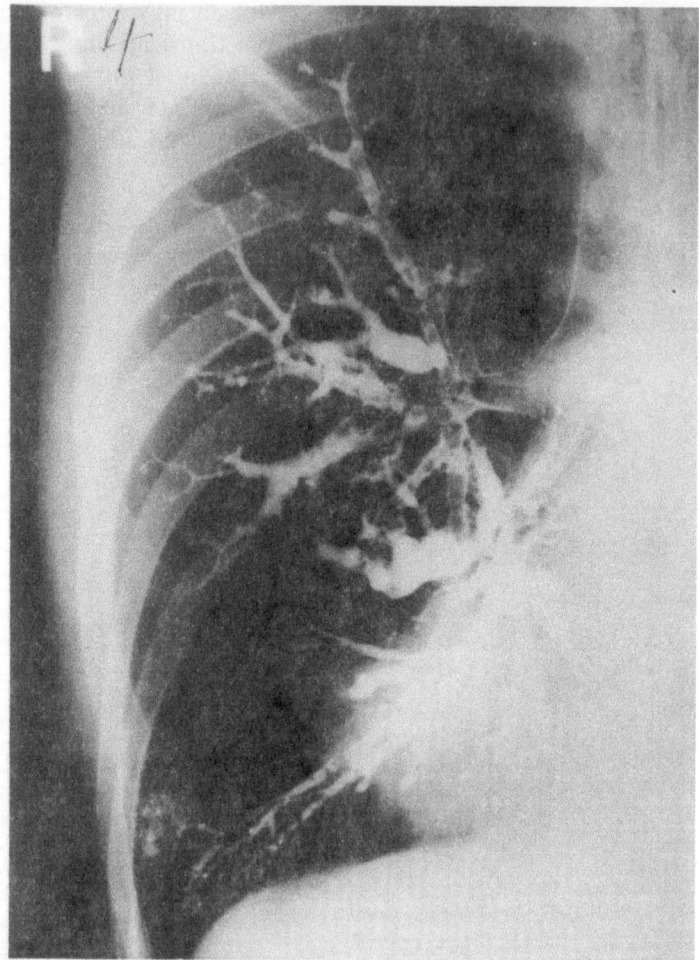

Figure 7.16 The typical proximal bronchiectasis of allergic bronchopulmonary aspergillosis

antibody against *Aspergillus* can be found in almost all sera if a highly sensitive primary antigen binding test is used[225].

Immunopathology

The inhaled spores of *A. fumigatus* grow well in viscid secretions in the large subsegmental bronchi of patients with asthma. A cardinal feature of patients with allergic bronchopulmonary aspergillosis that distinguishes the disease from other examples of allergy to inhaled materials is that the allergenic source can grow in the bronchial lumen and continually shed antigens into the tissues. Their combination with IgE and IgG antibody sets in motion a chain of immunological reactions culminating in bronchial wall damage and surrounding eosinophilic consolidation. Indeed pathological studies have indicated the presence of many eosinophils in the areas of infiltration confirming the importance of the IgE-mediated response in the production of the disease. However, mononuclear cells and granuloma are also found suggesting involvement of cellular immunity but there is little evidence of vasculitis and immunofluorescent studies have not regularly indicated deposits of immune complexes[28]. Nevertheless, the importance of precipitating antibody in the pathogenesis of the disease is supported by the successful serum transfer of pulmonary lesions from man to monkey. The inhalation of *Aspergillus* extract by monkeys was shown to lead to the development of infiltration only in those animals previously sensitized with serum containing both IgE and precipitating antibody against the fungus[226].

Treatment

In general, treatment with antifungal agents has been disappointing in the management of respiratory disease caused by *A. fumigatus*. Pulmonary aspergilloma causing severe symptoms are best treated by resection. Antifungal agents such as amphotericin have been used with some success in patients who have invasive aspergillosis but successful management of this disease relies primarily on treatment of the underlying immunodeficiency[227]. The cornerstone of treatment of allergic bronchopulmonary aspergillosis is the use of corticosteroids. Not only does this lead to improvement in the airflow obstruction but also to expectoration of mucus plugs and resolution of the pulmonary infiltrates. In the long term there is some evidence to suggest that a dose of prednisolone of 7.5 mg per day or greater is necessary to reduce the number of episodes of fever and pulmonary infiltrations[228]. A double-blind multicentre study of the efficacy of beclomethasone dipropionate aerosol in the control of asthmatic symptoms and the development of pulmonary infiltrates showed that although asthma was improved, the occurrence of infiltrates was not reduced. In general, therefore, it is preferable to manage the asthmatic element of the disease on its merits, which may necessitate the use of systemic corticosteroids, and diagnosed episodes of pulmonary eosinophilia should be treated with high doses of prednisolone over a period of 2–3 weeks.

EXTRINSIC ALLERGIC BRONCHIO-ALVEOLITIS

In his book *De Morbis Artificum Diatriba*, published in 1713, Ramazzini stated that, 'whenever it is necessary to sift wheat and barley or other kinds of grain, the men who sift and measure are so plagued by the dust that when the work is finished they heap·a thousand curses on their calling'. This almost certainly was the first description of what we now call extrinsic allergic bronchio-alveolitis. In 1967 the generic name fibrosing alveolitis was suggested for conditions which were characterized by an inflammatory process in the lung beyond the terminal bronchioles having as their essential features cellular thickening of the alveolar walls showing a tendency to fibrosis and the presence of large mononuclear cells, presumably of alveolar origin, within the alveolar spaces[229]. It is now recognized that this disease can be divided into two broad groups.

(1) Cryptogenic fibrosing alveolitis in which the cause remains unknown and which is associated in many cases with the presence of circulating autoantibodies, and

(2) Extrinsic allergic bronchio-alveolitis where the cause has been recognized and in which the disease may remit following successful cessation of exposure to the provoking agent.

In recent years it has become apparent that a wide variety of inhaled organic dusts can lead to this disease, and histological and physiological studies have indicated that the disease may also affect the terminal bronchioles and even the larger airways. For this reason these diseases are perhaps best described as examples of extrinsic allergic bronchio-alveolitis or hypersensitivity pneumonitis (a term favoured by the North Americans).

Clinical features and radiographic changes

The disease may present in an acute or chronic form. In the acute form cough, breathlessness and fever occur after an interval of 4–6 hours following exposure to the particular causative agent. Frequent episodes may be associated with weight loss and a feeling of malaise, whilst in the chronic form patients complain mainly of the gradual development of breathlessness. On examination fine crackles may be heard over the lung fields but this is less frequent in extrinsic allergic bronchio-alveolitis when compared to the cryptogenic form of the disease. Similarly, finger clubbing may occur but this is more frequent in cryptogenic fibrosing alveolitis. Acute episodes of extrinsic allergic bronchio-alveolitis are associated with a peripheral blood leukocytosis. Initially the chest radiograph may be normal but with continuing exposure fine, nodular shadowing can be seen throughout the lung fields (Figure 7.17). As the disease progresses, line shadowing and contraction of the lung fields may occur. The physiological changes in the lungs in established cases of extrinsic allergic bronchio-alveolitis are essentially those of a restrictive ventilatory defect. There is reduction in static lung volumes together with reduced carbon monoxide transfer and coefficient[62]. However, in many established cases irreversible obstruction to airflow can also be shown indicating the bronchial involvement[63].

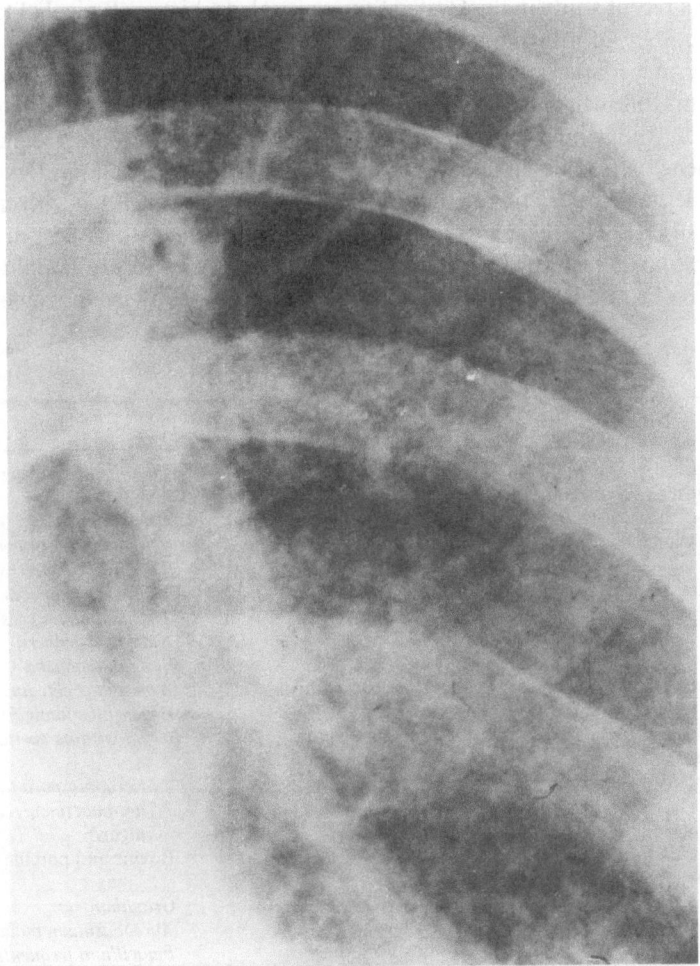

Figure 7.17 A chest radiograph showing the soft nodular shadowing in the lung of a patient with farmer's lung

Aetiology

The list of organic dusts leading to extrinsic allergic bronchio-alveolitis is continually increasing and some of the more important causes, together with the exposure that leads to the disease and the responsible agents are shown in Table 7.5. Overall, extrinsic allergic bronchio-alveolitis is a relatively rare disease, though its prevalence amongst certain communities can be high. The commonest form of the disease is almost certainly farmer's lung which has been described in countries throughout the world. In the wetter areas of the United Kingdom it has been shown to affect up to 8% of farm workers[230] whilst a recent study in the United States revealed a history typical of farmer's lung in 3.9% of a farming population[231]. The clinical manifestations of this disease are characteristic of the acute form of extrinsic allergic bronchio-alveolitis following heavy but intermittent exposure. Farmers handling hay or grain in the winter months that has been stored in damp conditions, experience a 'flu-like' illness which starts abruptly 4–6 hours later. Dry cough, breathlessness and chills with a fever of 38.3–40 °C, together with malaise, predominate. The fever subsides in 24 hours but the breathlessness and early fatigue may persist for several weeks. With repeated exposure, weight loss of 10–20 lbs is usual. During the acute febrile episodes there is a neutrophil

Table 7.5 The commoner causes of extrinsic allergic bronchio-alveolitis

Disease	Exposure	Agent
Bagassosis	Mouldy sugarcane	*Thermoactinomyces sachari*
Bird fancier's disease	Avian dust	Avian proteins
Cheesewasher's disease	Cheese mould	*Penicillium casie*
Farmer's lung	Mouldy hay	*Micropolyspora faeni*
		Thermoactinomyces vulgaris
Humidifer or forced-air system lung	Fungal spores	*Thermoactinomyces candidus*
		Thermoactinomyces vulgaris
		Naegleria gruberi,
		Acanthomoeba
Malt worker's disease	Malt and barley dusts	*Aspergillus clavatus*
		Aspergillus fumigatus
Maple bark stripper's disease	Mouldy maple bark	*Cryptostroma corticale*
Mushroom worker's disease	Mushroom compost	? *Micropolyspora faeni*
		? *Thermoactinomyces vulgaris*
Pituitary snufftaker's disease	Pituitary powder	Bovine and porcine proteins
Sequoiosis	Mouldy redwood sawdust	*Graphium*
		Aureobasidium pullulans
Suberosis	Mouldy cork dust	*Penicillium frequentans*

polymorphonuclear leukocytosis of 15 000–20 000 per mm³, though eosino-philia is rare. Occasionally the rheumatoid factor may be positive. Eventually the chest radiograph becomes abnormal and the typical physiological changes in lung function occur. The most important cause of farmer's lung is the inhalation of the spores of *Micropolyspora faeni* which are less than 5 μm in diameter allowing them to penetrate to the periphery of the lung. Studies have been carried out on haystacks to determine the characteristics of the mould flora that develop during storage. Thermophilic actinomycetes are rare in good and mouldy hay baled with less than 28% water but become abundant in wet baled hay with the number present being related to the water content and the degree of spontaneous heating. Although bacteria predominate in the first 2 days during which hay has been stored, increasing numbers of *Thermo-*

actinomyces vulgaris and *Micropolyspora faeni* are found from 4–7 days onwards particularly when the hay contains 40% of water. Mouldy hay is only one of numerous sources of thermophilic actinomycetes and other sources include piles of straw, corn stacks, sawdust or other waste material that can be used for bedding in the dairy farm, and damp mouldy oats, corn fodder or any organic material that has become mouldy and then warmed up to between 50–60 °C will provide a suitable source of the antigen. Acute episodes of farmer's lung occur most often in the late winter when the farmer, having used up his supply of good fodder or bedding, throws down the mouldy material. The barn is closed tight against the cold and clouds of spores are inevitably inhaled. Indeed, it has been calculated that up to 750 000 spores per minute may be retained in the lungs[232].

Extrinsic allergic bronchio-alveolitis has been described amongst pigeon fanciers, chicken farmers, turkey breeders and budgerigar owners, following inhalation of the dry dust of bird droppings. Studies of members of pigeon breeding clubs have indicated that 6–21% may develop the disease[233]. In America there are approximately 75 000 pigeon breeders and therefore up to 15 000 people could be at risk from developing irreversible lung damage.

Although budgerigars are extremely popular pets in the United Kingdom the frequency of the disease amongst their owners is very much lower. Whilst pigeon breeders develop an acute illness like farmer's lung, budgerigar fanciers typically develop their disease insidiously, as they have a more frequent but lower dose exposure. They usually present with shortness of breath on exercise and radiographic and physiological studies often show that the disease is already far advanced. The antigens leading to bird fancier's lung are present in both bird serum and droppings. Macro- and γ-globulin components in pigeon serum were found to react specifically only with pigeon fancier's sera and budgerigar γ-globulin and β-globulin reacted specifically only with budgerigar fancier's sera[234]. Further, it has been shown that antigens present in the pigeon alimentary tract cross-react with pigeon serum proteins, notably pigeon γ-globulins[235]. More recently precipitins have been found in the sera of patients with coeliac disease, which cross-react with an antigen found in the sera of several avian species, leading to the suggestion that bird fancier's lung and coeliac disease might be associated. However, the precipitins present in the blood of patients with coeliac disease did not cross-react with those avian serum antigens commonly associated with the development of bird fancier's lung[236].

Approximately 500 of the 600 cases of bagassosis referred to in the literature have been reported from Louisiana. Nevertheless the disease is of world-wide distribution and occurs wherever sugar cane is processed. Several cases have been seen in non-occupationally exposed individuals, including those using the material as a garden fertilizer, housewives residing in homes several miles downwind from sugarcane fields and processing areas and employees working in air-conditioned offices at or near a sugarcane processing plant. The acute form of the disease presents with the characteristic features of extrinsic allergic bronchio-alveolitis. Dyspnoea, fever, cough, chills, weakness, anorexia and malaise develop after repeated exposure to organic dust derived from stored bagasse, which is the residual sugarcane fibre. It has been demonstrated that *Thermoactinomyces sacchari* is the major source of antigen in mouldy bagasse. In the last few years the method of storage and processing of bagasse has been altered in order to retard decay due to microbial growth during storage. These changes have aso resulted in reduction of organic dusts generated during the mechanical processing. A recent study in a Louisiana paper mill, which in the past had considerable numbers of workers with the disease, indicated that bagassosis was no longer occurring[237]. This finding is of very considerable importance because it shows that suitable alteration in the way in which the basic material is handled can lead to conditions unsuitable for growth of thermophilic actinomycetes, leading to elimination of the disease.

Recently attention has been focused on individuals who developed a respiratory disease exhibiting the features of extrinsic allergic bronchio-alveolitis and caused by contamination of domestic cold mist vapourizers with fungi and contamination of ducted air-heating and air-conditioning systems with thermophilic actinomycetes. Studies in North America have indicated that the disease may develop in up to 15% of workers in some offices[238]. However in the United Kingdom there have been a number of outbreaks of a disease which has been termed 'humidifier fever' in which the individuals developed an influenza-like illness without the typical radiographic changes of extrinsic allergic bronchio-alveolitis. The episodes usually occurred after absence from work for a few days and have been termed 'Monday sickness'. Affected workers are often able to return to work the following day and appear refractory to further exposure. In addition if they work over the weekend then 'Monday sickness' does not occur. In 1977 this disease was reported in a large modern stationery factory in Aberdeen, where three vacuum pumps and two air-compressors were being used to provide air and vacuum facilities for the machines. The vacuum pumps were of the 'liquid ring' type in which a rotating turbine created a vacuum using circulating water. The effluent from these pumps consisted of an air/water mixture of approximately 9000 litres of air and 600 litres of water per minute, which was discharged into two vertical separating tanks. The water fell to the bottom for subsequent recirculation, and the air was discharged into the atmosphere of the pump room. Twenty-four workers were affected with symptoms of chest tightness, shivering and dyspnoea at rest. None had abnormal chest X-rays. The water from the pump was found to contain a wide range of micro-organisms and amoeba, and the affected workers showed precipitins against a filtrate of this material which also reproduced symptoms in two affected workers who volunteered for inhalation challenge tests. Subsequent studies have suggested that the important antigen may be *Acanthamoeba*[64]. The recognition of the possible cause of the illness made it possible to affect a cure by ducting the air effluent through the factory roof, rather than into the atmosphere of the factory itself. Another amoeba, *Naegleria gruberi* has been implicated as a possible source of the antigen in a similar illness occurring in workers in a factory in South Wales.

Recently an epidemic of fever, cough and breathlessness occurring in over 100 people in an industrial community in Finland has been described. The symptoms occurred 3–6 hours after sauna or bathing. The water source of the community was found to be a small lake which was contaminated with several bacteria, fungi and algae. Bronchial provocation tests with the water led to recrudescence of symptoms and a fall in the lung transfer factor for carbon monoxide. However, no precipitating antibodies were found in the serum of these individuals and although the clinical picture resembled the 'humidifier fever' described in the United Kingdom it is possible that bacterial endotoxins may be the cause of the symptoms and alterations in lung physiology[239].

Immunopathogenesis

Histological studies in the acute form of the disease have shown interstitial pneumonia, sarcoid-like granulomata, bronchiolitis and vasculitis. A prominent mononuclear cell infiltration is present consisting largely of lymphocytes and plasma cells together with lymphoid collections containing antibody-secreting germinal follicles. Further, large numbers of alveolar cells with the characteristics of activated macrophages are found within the pulmonary lesions. Unlike sarcoidosis, the multinucleate giant cells in the non-caseating granuloma often have characteristic clefts that have been shown to contain refractile foreign material which appears to be of vegetable origin and many represent material from the inhaled organic dusts (Figure 7.18). In general, the perivascular neutrophil polymorphonuclear infiltration and fibrinoid necrosis of vessel walls typical of the experimental Arthus reaction are not seen. However, lung biopsy specimens obtained very early in the onset of the disease or following bronchial provocation challenge tests have revealed the presence of antigens, immunoglobulins and complement deposition by immunofluorescence as well as necrotizing vasculitis. In the chronic form of the disease, interstitial pulmonary fibrosis predominates with fine fibrosis throughout the alveolar wall and destruction of the lung architecture by larger areas of fibrosis leading to irregular honeycombing. Bronchioles are often involved and demonstrate a necrotizing process which destroys portions of their mural structure and occludes the bronchiolar lumens with macrophages, inflammatory cells and tissue debris. The bronchiolar epithelium may be destroyed and replaced by a flat regenerating epithelium. The involved adjacent alveoli are lined by hypertrophied cuboidal epithelial cells[242, 243].

The factors whoch predispose towards the development of extrinsic allergic

though there may be elevated serum levels of IgG, IgA and IgM. There is some
evidence of a genetically determined susceptibility. HLA BW 40 and HLA B 8
have been found with increased frequency in patients with pigeon fancier's
and farmer's lung[244, 245].

Many of the aetiological agents in this disease can induce non-specific
pulmonary inflammation via activation of the alternative complement
pathway, or by a non-specific adjuvant effect[246, 247]. Further, the induction of
prior inflammation in the lung by agents such as BCG, followed by challenge
with organic dust can induce granulomatous pulmonary lesions which

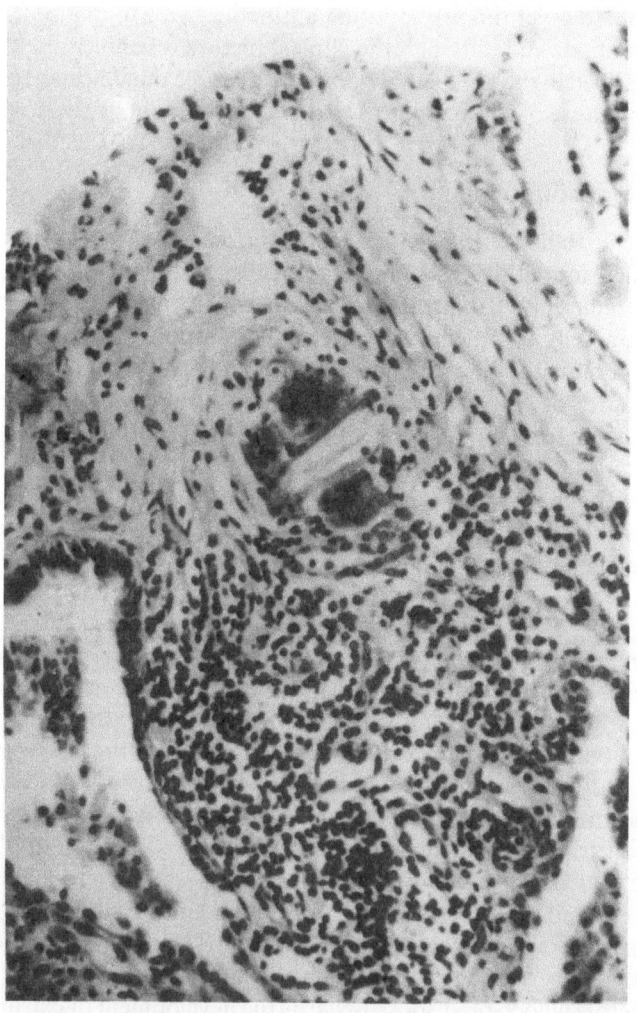

Figure 7.18   Histopathology of extrinsic allergic bronchio-alveolitis showing a granuloma with a
multinucleate giant cell containing a characteristic 'cleft'

resemble those of extrinsic allergic bronchio-alveolitis in association with demonstrable local pulmonary cell mediated hypersensitivity. If these same antigens are administered in a non-particulate form or without prior induction of pulmonary inflammation, lesions are not produced[248]. Activation of complement by the alternative pathway can lead to the formation of split products such as C3B which is known to induce macrophage lysosomal enzyme release. This may explain some of the early non-specific lesions of this disease and indeed complement deposits, not associated with any immune complexes, are sometimes found in lung biopsies[249]. Lysosomal enzymes can in turn further cleave C3, leading to a mechanism for continued macrophage activation in an 'amplification loop' process. It is conceivable that pulmonary granulomata containing macrophages with ingested organic dust antigen may evolve at least in part through this non-specific mechanism[250].

Although many patients with certain forms of extrinsic allergic bronchio-alveolitis, such as pigeon breeders or bird fanciers, demonstrate immediate weal and flare skin reactions to crude avian antigens, IgE-mediated allergic reactions are probably not of great significance in the development of the typical granulomatous lesions of this disease. However, as has already been stated, many of these patients do show immediate asthmatic reactions following bronchial provocation tests and in this sense Type I allergy is important in the development of the lung disease association with the inhalation of these organic allergens. Pepys[251] suggested that extrinsic allergic bronchio-alveolitis might be the result of a Type III immune complex reaction occurring in the lung following the inhalation of the organic allergen. The evidence for this was based on:

(1) The presence in the sera of circulating antibodies specific to these antigens,
(2) The demonstration in the skin of late reactions,
(3) The typical time course of the acute respiratory reaction beginning 4–8 hours after inhalation of the organic material.

Although the immunopathology of the early stages of the disease reveals the presence of antigen, immunoglobulins and complement deposition as well as necrotizing vasculitis, the mononuclear cell and granulomatous infiltrates seen in most cases of allergic bronchio-alveolitis are substantially different from the vasculitic lesions seen in other immune complex diseases in man. However it is possible that immune complexes can activate alveolar macrophages to secrete hydrolytic enzymes and it is known that insoluble antigen–antibody complexes, not readily digested by lysosomal enzymes, may lead to the formation of granulomata[252].

The pulmonary histopathology in extrinsic allergic bronchio-alveolitis greatly resembles that of cell-mediated hypersensitivity reactions, suggesting an important role for Type IV allergic reactions. Studies in man have demonstrated that lymphokine production occurs after peripheral blood or bronchio-alveolar lymphocytes are exposed to both avian and/or actino-mycete antigens. Indeed in some forms of the disease lymphokine production appears to correlate with disease activity. Studies in bird breeders have shown both lymphocyte transformation and the production of macrophage inhi-bition factor following *in vitro* tests with avian antigens in a significant percentage of patients with the disease but not in their asymptomatic counterparts[253].

Animal studies have been widely used in attempts to elucidate the underlying immunological mechanisms involved in the production of this disease. It is possible to produce a disease in rabbits that is histologically very similar to extrinsic allergic bronchio-alveolitis following suitable immuniz-ation and challenge. usually by intratracheal injection of the antigen. Using such techniques, Bice *et al.*[254] were able to produce the typical pulmonary lesions in unimmunized rabbits on challenge with the antigen following the administration of lymph node cells from sensitized animals. Unimmunized animals that had only received donor hyperimmune serum did not generally produce pulmonary lesions after similar respiratory antigenic challenge.

Recently it has become apparent that local organ-restricted immune mechanisms may be operative at the pulmonary level with or without systemic manifestations of sensitization. In a study of extrinsic allergic bronchio-alveolitis in man, lymphokine production was demonstrated by bronchio-alveolar cells while peripheral cells failed to demonstrate reactivity to the same antigen[255]. Increasing importance is being attached to these bronchio-alveolar cells, and Salvaggio[256] has suggested that the focal point in the pathogenesis of extrinsic allergic bronchio-alveolitis is the activated alveolar macrophage. He postulates that both non-specific and allergic mechanisms may act together in the development of the pathological lesions. Activation of the alternative complement pathway by organic dust, formation of local immune complexes and specifically sensitized bronchio-alveolar T lymphocytes can all lead to the activation of macrophages, causing inflammation and eventual fibrosis via a macrophage-mediated influence on fibroblasts by soluble mediators.

Diagnosis and management

The diagnosis of extrinsic allergic bronchio-alveolitis is based on the typical clinical history with appropriate exposure to the allergen, together with demonstration of precipitating antibody against the causal agent in the serum. This may be confirmed by an appropriate chest radiograph and pulmonary function tests. In cases of diagnostic difficulty, when, for example, precipi-tating antibody cannot be detected, it may be necessary to perform bronchial provocation tests. It is very important to recognize the extrinsic nature of this disease so that continued inhalation of the organic material by the patient can be prevented. This may necessitate a change in occupation or hobby or the removal of a budgerigar or air-conditioning system from the home. Following this the progression of the disease is usually but not always arrested. Left unrecognized, with continued exposure to the allergen, the disease may progress to pulmonary fibrosis and death. Indeed in a study of 50 patients with farmer's lung over an average period of 6 years, there was a mortality rate of 10%. and a further one-third had persistent respiratory symptoms and physiological abnormalities with pulmonary fibrosis being the major problem[257]. In a study in England which included 200 patients diagnosed between 1939 and 1975, there were four deaths from farmer's lung and severe disability was present in approximately one-third[258].

The oral administration of corticosteroids may help in resolution of the disease, but antigen avoidance remains the mainstay of clinical management. As yet, no efficacious or universally acceptable mask has been developed which will prevent inhalation of the organic material. Once recognized these diseases can be prevented. The most effective way of achieving this is to alter the working conditions in such a way that the causative agent is no longer present, or cannot be inhaled by man. This has already proved possible with bagassosis and alteration in farming practice could also make farmer's lung a disease of the past.

Acknowledgements

Figures 7.6, 7.8 and 7.9 are reproduced with the permission of the editors of *Asthma: Theory and Practice*, Chapman and Hall, London.
Figures 7.14, 7.15 and 7.16, with permission of the editor of the *British Journal of Hospital Medicine*.
Figure 7.10, with the permission of the authors and editor of the *Lancet*. (Friend, J. A. R., Gaddie, J., Palmer, K. N. V., Pickering, C. A. C., and Pepys, J. (1977). Extrinsic allergic alveolitis and contaminated cooling water in a factory machine. *Lancet*, **1**, 297)

References

1. Cooke. R. A. and Vander Veer, A. (1916). Human sensitization. *J. Immunol.*, **1**, 201
2. Coca. A. F. and Cooke, R. A. (1923). On the classification of the phenomena of hypersensitiveness. *J. Immunol., Balt.*, **2**, 383
3. Pepys. J. (1975). Atopy. In Gell, P. G. H., Coombes, R. R. A. and Lackmann, P. J. (eds.) *Clinical Aspects of Immunology*, pp. 877–902 (Oxford: Blackwell Scientific)
4. Barbee, R. A., Lebowitz, M. D., Thomson, H. C, and Burrows, B. (1976). Immediate skin-test reactivity in the general population sample. *Ann. Intern. Med.*, **84**, 129
5. D'Souza. M. F. and Davies. R. J. (1977). The distribution of allergic disorders and atopy in the community and their relationship to total levels of serum IgE antibody. *Am. Rev. Resp. Dis.* (annual meeting Supplement), 211
6. Chambers, V. V. and Glazer, J. (1958). The incidence of subsequent ragweed pollinosis in symptom-free persons having positive reactions to ragweed pollen extract. *J. Allergy.* **29**, 249

7. Hagy, G. W. and Settipane, G. A. (1971). Prognosis of positive allergy skin tests in an asymptomatic population. A 3-year follow-up of college students. *J. Allergy Clin. Immunol.*, **48**, 200

8. Pepys, J. (1973). Types of allergic reaction. *Clin. Allergy*, **3**, 491

9. Newhouse, M. L., Tagg, B., Pocock, S. J. and McEwan, A. C. (1970). An epidemiological study of workers producing enzyme washing powders. *Lancet*, **1**, 689

10. Leskowitz, S., Salvaggio, J. E. and Schwartz, H. J. (1972). An hypothesis for the development of atopic allergy in man. *Clin. Allergy*, **2**, 237

11. Tada, T. (1975). Regulation of reaginic antibody formation in animals. *Prog. Allergy*, **19**, 122

12. Parish, W. W. (1973). A human heat-stable anaphylactic or anaphylactoid antibody which may participate in pulmonary disorders. In Austin, K. F. and Lichtenstein, L. M. (eds.) *Asthma; Physiology, Immuno-pharmacology and Treatment*, p. 72 (New York: Academic Press)

13. Longbottom, J. L., Brighton, W. D., Edge, G. E. and Pepys, J. (1976). Antibodies mediating Type I skin test reactions to polysaccharide and protein antigens of *Candida albicans*. *Clin. Allergy*, **6**, 41

14. Pepys, J., Parish, W. E., Stenius, B. and Wide, L. (1975). Long-term and short-term sensitizing antibodies to common allergens in extrinsic and cryptogenic asthma. *Clin. Allergy*, **4**, 237

15. Bryant, D. H., Burns, M. W. and Lazarus, L. (1973). New type of allergic asthma due to IgG 'reaginic' antibody. *Br. Med. J.*, **4**, 589

16. Cox, J. S. (1971). Disodium cromoglycate. Mode of action and its possible relevance to the clinical use of the drug. *Br. J. Dis. Chest*, **65**, 189

17. Shipps, B. E., Sobotka, A. K., Sanders, J. P., Teets, K. C., Norman, P. S. and Lichtenstein, L. M. (1980). Effect of theophylline and terbutaline on immediate skin tests. *J. Allergy Clin. Immunol.*, **65**, 61

18. Phillips, M. J., Thomas, R. M. and Davies, R. J. (1980). A comparison of drug dose relationships on the allergen- and histamine-induced skin weal. (In press)

19. D'Souza, M. F., Davies, R. J. and Swann, A. V. (1980). Factors associated with reported asthma in middle age. (In press)

20. Hendrik, D. J., Davies, R. J., D'Souza, M. F. and Pepys, J. (1975). An analysis of skin prick test reactions in 656 asthmatic patients. *Thorax*, **30**, 2

21. Davies, R. J. (1978). Serological and skin test responses to allergens from *Staphylococcus aureus*, *Streptococcus pneumoniae* and *Haemophilus influenzae* in asthma and chronic bronchitis. RhD Thesis, University of Cambridge

22. Umemoto, L., Poothullil, J., Dolovich, J. and Hargreave, F. E. (1976). Factors which influence late cutaneous allergic responses. *J. Allergy Clin. Immunol.*, **58**, 60

23. Jan, K., Nahmias, C., Coates, G., Hargreave, F. E., Davis, C. and Dolovich, J. (1980). The use of radioactive isotopes for analysis of cutaneous allergic responses. *Clin. Allergy*, **10**, 25

24. Pepys, J., Turner-Warwick, M., Dawson, P. L. and Hinson, K. F. W. (1968). Arthus (Type III) skin test reactions in man: clinical and immunopathological features. In Rose, B., Richter, M., Sehon, A. and Frankland, A. W. (eds.) *Allergology*, p. 221 (Amsterdam; Excerpta Medica)

25. Solley, G. O., Gleich, G. J., Jordan, R. E. and Schroeter, A. L. (1976). The late phase of the immediate weal and flare skin reaction. Its dependence upon IgE antibodies. *Clin. Invest.*, **58**, 408

26. Dolovich, J., Hargreave, F. E., Chalmers, S., Shier, K. J., Gauldie, J. and Bienenstock, J. (1973). Late cutaneous allergic responses in isolated IgE-dependent reactions. *J. Allergy Clin. Immunol.*, **52**, 38

27. Nye, L., Merret, T. E., Landon, J. and White, R. J. (1975). A detailed investigation of circulating IgE levels in a normal population. *Clin. Allergy*, **1**, 13

28. Slavin, R. G., (1978). Allergic broncho-pulmonary aspergillosis. In Middleton, E., Reed, C. R. and Ellis, E. F. (eds.) *Allergy: Principles and Practice*, pp. 843–2854. (St Louis: C. V. Mosby)

29. Malo, J. L., Longbottom, J., Mitchell, J., Hawkins, R. and Pepys, J. (1977). Studies in chronic allergic bronchopulmonary aspergillosis. 3. Immunological findings. *Thorax*, **32**, 269

30. Turner-Warwick, M., Assem, E. S. K. and Lockwood, M. (1976). Cryptogenic pulmonary eosinophilia. *Clin. Allergy*, **6**, 135

31. Davies, R. J. and Pepys, J. (1976). Egg allergy, influenza vaccine and immunoglobulin E antibody. *J. Allergy Clin. Immunol.*, **57**, 373

32. Stenius, B., Wide, L., Seymour, W. M., Holford-Strevens, V. and Pepys, J. (1971). Clinical significance of specific IgE to common allergens. 1. Relationship of specific IgE against *Dermatophagoides* spp. and grass pollen to skin and nasal tests and history. *Clin. Allergy*, **1**, 37

33. Yunginger J. W. and Gleich, G. J. (1973). Seasonal changes in IgE antibodies and their relationship to IgG antibodies during immunotherapy for ragweed hay fever. *J. Clin. Invest.*, **52**, 1268

34. Huggins, K. G. and Brostoff, J. (1975). Local production of specific IgE antibodies in allergic rhinitis patients with negative skin tests. *Lancet*, **2**, 148

35. Turnbull, L. S., Turnbull, L. W., Leitch, A. G., Crofton, J. W. and Kay, A. B. (1977). Mediators of immediate-type hypersensitivity in sputum from patients with chronic bronchitis and asthma. *Lancet*, **2**, 526

36. Platts-Mills, T. A., von Maur, R. K., Ishizaka, K., Norman, P. S. and Lichtenstein, L. M. (1976). IgA and IgG anti-ragweed antibodies in nasal secretions. Quantitative measurements of antibodies and correlation with inhibition of histamine release. *J. Clin. Invest.*, **57**, 1041

37. Longbottom, J. L. and Pepys, T. (1974). Diagnosis of fungal diseases. In Gell, P. G. H. and Coombs, R. R. A. (eds.) *Clinical Aspects of Immunology*, p. 71. (Oxford: Blackwell Scientific)

38. Report to the Research Committee of the British Thoracic Association (1979). Inhaled beclomethasone dipropionate in allergic bronchopulmonary aspergillosis. *Br. J. Dis. Chest*, **73**, 349

39. Sepulveda, R., Longbottom, J. L. and Pepys, J. (1979), Enzyme-linked immunosorbent assay (ELISA) for IgG and IgE antibodies to protein and polysaccharide antigens of *Aspergillus fumigatus*. *Clin. Allergy*, **9**, 359

40. Pepys, J. and Jenkins, P. A. (1965). Precipitin (FLH) tests in farmer's lung. *Thorax*, **20**, 21

41. Barndad, S. (1980). Enzyme-linked immunosorbent assay (ELISA) for IgG antibodies in farmer's lung disease. *Clin. Allergy*, **10**, 161

42. Elgefors, B., Belin, L. and Hansen, L. A. (1971). Pigeon breeder's lung. *Scand. J. Resp. Dis.*, **52**, 167

43. Taylor, G. and Shivalkar, P. R. (1971). Arthus-type reactivity in the nasal airways and skin in pollen-sensitive subjects. *Clin. Allergy*, **1**, 407

44. Green, M., Schofield, N. McC. and Davies, R. J. (1976). Comparison in the same asthmatic subjects of airway responses to exercise and allergen inhalation. *Eur. J. Clin. Invest.*, **6**, 322

45. Chan-Yeung, M., Barton, G. M., McLean, L. and Grzybowsky, S. (1973). Occupational asthma and rhinitis due to western red cedar (*Thuja plicata*). *Am. Rev. Resp. Dis.*, **108**, 1094

46. Lam, S., Wong, R. and Yeung, M. (1979). Non-specific bronchial reactivity in occupational asthma. *J. Allergy Clin. Immunol.*, **63**, 28

47. Chan-Yeung, M. (1973). Maximum expiratory flow and airways resistance during induced broncho-constriction in patients with asthma due to western red cedar (*Thuja plicata*). *Am. Rev. Resp. Dis.*, **108**, 1103

48. Graham, V. A. L. and Davies, R. J. (1980). Provocation tests with an aqueous extract and the dust of western red cedar in a wood worker. (In press)
49. Booij-Noord, H., de Vries, K., Sluiter, H. J. and Orie, N. G. M. (1972). Late bronchial obstructive reaction to experimental inhalation of housedust extract. *Clin. Allergy*, **2**, 43
50. Robertson, D. G., Kerrigan, A. T., Hargreave, F. E., Chalmers, R. and Dolovich, J. (1974). Late asthmatic responses induced by rag-weed pollen and allergen. *J. Allergy Clin. Immunol*, **54**, 244
51. Salter, H. H. (1882) *Asthma, Pathology and Treatment*, p. 33. (London: William Wood)
52. Clark, T. J. and Hetzel, M. R. (1977). Diurnal variation of asthma. *Br. J. Dis. Chest*, **71**, 87
53. Davies, R. J., Green, M. and Schofield, N. McC. (1976). Recurrent nocturnal asthma after exposure to grain dust. *Am. Rev. Resp. Dis.*, **114**, 1011
54. Gandevia, J. and Milne, J. (1970). Occupational asthma and rhinitis with western red cedar (*Thuja plicata*) with special reference to bronchial reactivity. *Br. J. Indust. Med.*, **27**, 235
55. Newman Taylor, A. E. W., Davies, R. J., Hendrick, D. J. and Pepys, J. (1979). Recurrent nocturnal asthmatic reactions to bronchial provocation tests. *Clin. Allergy*, **9**, 213
56. Davies, R. J., Hendrick, D. J. and Pepys, J. (1974). Asthma due to inhaled chemical agents: ampicillin, benzyl penicillin, 6-amino penicillanic acid and related substances. *Clin. Allergy*, **4**, 227
57. Burge, P. S., O'Brien, I. M. and Harries, M. G. (1979). Peak flow rate records in the diagnosis of occupational asthma due to colophony. *Thorax*, **34**, 308
58. Chan-Yeung, M. (1977). Fate of occupational asthma. A follow-up study of patients with occupational asthma due to western red cedar (*Thuja plicata*). *Am. Rev. Resp. Dis.*, **116**, 1023
59. Pepys, J., Davies, R. J., Breslin, A. B., Hendrick, D. J. and Hutchcroft, B. J. (1974). The effects of inhaled beclomethasone dipropionate (Becotide) and sodium cromoglycate on asthmatic reactions to provocation tests. *Clin. Allergy*, **4**, 13
60. Booij-Noord, H., de Vries, K., Sluiter, H. J. and Orie, N. G. M. (1972). Late bronchial obstructive reaction to experimental inhalation of house dust extract. *Clin. Allergy*, **2**, 43
61. Orie, N. G. M., van Lookeren, Campagne, N. G., Knal, J., Booij-Noord, H. and de Vries, K. (1973). In Pepys, J. and Yamamura, Y. (eds.). *Intal in Bronchial Asthma*.
62. Schofield, N. McC., Davies, R. J., Cameron, I. R. and Green, M. (1976). Small airways in fibrosing alveolitis. *Am. Rev. Resp. Dis.*, **113**, 729
63. Hapke, E. J., Seal, R. M. E., Thomas, G. O., Hayes, M. and Meek, J. C. (1968). Farmer's lung: a clinical, radiographic, functional and serological correlation of acute and chronic stage. *Thorax*, **23**, 451
64. Friend, J. A., Gaddie, J., Palmer, K. N., Pickering, C. A. C. and Pepys, J. (1977). Extrinsic allergic alveolitis and contaminated cooling-water in a factory machine. *Lancet*, **1**, 297
65. Hargreave, F. E. and Pepys, J. (1972). Allergic respiratory reactions in bird fanciers provoked by allergen inhalation provocation rests. Relation to clinical features and allergic mechanisms. *J. Allergy Clin. Immunol.*, **50**, 157
66. Williams, J. V., (1963). Inhalation and skin tests with extract of hay and fungi in patients with farmer's lung. *Thorax*, **18**, 182
67. Eriksson, N. E. (1977). Diagnosis of reaginic allergy with house dust, animal dander and pollen allergen in adult patients, IV. *Int. Arch. Allergy Appl. Immunol.*, **53**, 450
68. Fish, J. E., Ankis, M. G., Kelly, J. F. and Peterman, V. I. (1980). Comparison of responses to pollen extract in subjects with allergic asthma and non-asthmatic subjects with allergic rhinitis. *J. Allergy Clin. Immunol.*, **65**, 154
69. Townley, R. G., Bewtra, A. K., Nair, N. M., Brodkey, F. D., Watt, G. D. and Burke, K. M. (1979). Methacholine inhalation challenge studies. *J. Allergy Clin. Immunol.*, **64**, 569
70. Borum, P. (1979). Nasal methacholine challenge. A test for the measurement of nasal reactivity. *J. Allergy Clin. Immunol.*, **63**, 253

71. Borum, P. (1979). Reactivity of the nasal mucosa. In Pepys, J. and Edwards, A. M. E. (eds.), *The Mast Cell: its Role in Health and Disease*, pp. 761–766 (Bath: The Pitman Press)

72. Godfrey, S. (1976). Exercise-induced asthma, clinical, physiological and therapeutic implications. *J. Allergy Clin. Immunol.*, **56**, 1

73. Wells, R. E., Walker, J. E. and Nickler, R. B. (1960). Effects of cold air on respiratory airflow resistance in patients with respiratory-tract disease. *N. Engl. J. Med.*, **263**, 268

74. Curry, J. J. (1946). The action of histamine on the respiratory tract in normal and asthmatic subjects. *J. Clin. Invest.*, **25**, 785

75. Dubois, A. B. and Dautreband, L. (1958). Acute effects of breathing inert dust particles and carbachol aerosol on the mechanical characteristics of the lungs in man; changes and response after inhaling sympathomimetic aerosols. *J. Clin. Invest.*, **37**, 17

76. Eggleston, P. A., (1979). A comparison of the asthmatic response to methacholine and exercise. *J. Allergy Clin. Immunol.*, **63**, 104

77. Schofield, N. McC., Green, M. and Davies, R. J. (1980) Response of the lung airways to exercise testing in asthma and rhinitis. *Br. J. Dis. Chest.*, **74**, 163

78. Oretrek, J., Gay, R. A. R. D., Smith, A. P., Grimaud, C. and Charpin, J. (1977). Airways response to carbachol in normal and asthmatic subjects; distinction between bronchial sensitivity and reactivity. *Am. Rev. Resp. Dis.*, **115**, 937

79. Phillips, J. J., Ollier, S., Trembath, P. W., Boobis, S. W., and Davies, R. J. (1980). Sustained release aminophylline (Phyllocontin): plasma levels and effect on exercise-induced asthma. (In press)

80. Deal, E. C., McFadden, E. R., Ingram, R. H. Jr., Strauss, R. H. and Jaegar, J. J. (1979). Role of respiratory heat exchange in production of exercise-induced asthma. *J. Appl. Physiol.*, **46**, 467

81. McFadden, E. R. and Soter, N. A. (1977. A search for chemical mediators or immediate hypersensitivity and humoral factors in the pathogenesis of exercise-induced asthma. In Lichtenstein, L. M. and Austen, K. F. (eds.) *Asthma*, pp. 351–364 (London: Academic Press)

82. Empey, D. W., Laitinen, L. A., Jacobs, L., Gold, W. M. and Nadel, J. A. (1976). Mechanisms of hyper-reactivity in normal subjects after upper respiratory tract infection. *Am. Rev. Resp. Dis.*, **113**, 131

83. Killian, D., Cockroft, D. W., Hargreave, F. E. and Dolovich, J. (1976). Factors in allergen-induced asthma; relevance of the intensity of the airways' allergic reaction and the non-specific bronchial reactivity. *Clin. Allergy*, **6**, 219

84. Cockroft, D. W., Ruffin, R. E., Dolovich, J. and Hargreave, F. E. (1977). Allergen-induced increase in non-allergic bronchial reactivity. *Clin. Allergy*, **7**, 503

85. Fish, J. E., Rosenthal, R. R., Sumner, W. R., Menices, H., Norman, P. S. and Permutt, S. (1977). The effect of atropine on acute antigen-mediated airway constriction in subjects with allergic asthma. *Am. Rev. Resp. Dis.*, **115**, 371

86. Yu, D. Y., Galant, S. P. and Gold, W. M. (1972). Inhibition of antigen-induced broncho-constriction by atropine in asthmatic patients. *J. Appl. Physiol.*, **32**, 823

87. Mygind, N. (1978). *Nasal Allergy*, p. 230 (Oxford: Blackwell Scientific)

88. Zeiss, C. R., Patterson, R., Pruzansky, J. J., Miller, M. M., Rosenberg, M. and Levitz, D. (1977). Trimellitic anhydride-induced airway syndromes: clinical and immunologic studies. *J. Allergy Clin. Immunol.*, **60**, 96

89. Davies, R. J., Butcher, B. T., O'Neill, C. E. and Salvaggio, J. E. (1977). The *in vitro* effect of toluene di-isocyanate on lymphocyte and cyclic adenosine monophosphate production by isoproteronal, prostaglandin, and histamine. A possible mode of action. *J. Allergy Clin. Immunol.*, **60**, 223

90. Davies, R. J., Penketh, A. R. L. and Phillips, M. J. (1980). The value of nasal provocation tests using the technique of anterior rhinomanometry in the diagnosis of perennial rhinitis caused by allergy to the house dust mite. (In press)

91. Broder, I., Higgins, M. W., Mathews, K. P. and Keller, J. B. (1974). Epidemiology of asthma and allergic rhinitis in a total community: Tecumseh, Michigan. 3, Second survey of the community. *J. Allergy*, **53**, 127

92. Mygind, N. (1978). *Nasal Allergy*, p. 219 (Oxford: Blackwell Scientific)

93. Smith, J. M. (1971). A five-year prospective survey of rural children with asthma and hay-fever. *J. Allergy*, **47**, 23

94. Edfors-Lubs, M. L. (1971). Allergy in 7000 twin pairs. *Acta Allergol.* (Kbh), **26**, 249

95. Murray, A. B. (1971). Nasal secretion eosinophilia in children with grass pollen hay fever. *Can. Med. Assoc. J.*, **104**, 599

96. Mygind, N. (1978). *Nasal Allergy*, p. 233 (Oxford: Blackwell Scientific)

97. Lanoff, G., Daddono, A. and Johnson, E. (1973). Nasal polyps in children: a ten-year study. *Ann. Allergy*, **31**, 551

98. Samter, M. and Beers, R. F. Jr. (1967). Concerning the nature of intolerance to aspirin. *J. Allergy*, **40**, 281

99. Donovan, R., Johansson, S. G. O., Bennich H. and Soothill, J. F. (1970). Immunoglobulins in nasal polyp fluid. *Int. Arch. Allergy*, **37**, 154

100. Mygind, N., Weeke, B. and Ullman, S. (1975). Quantitative determination of immuno-globulins in nasal secretions. *Int. Arch. Appl. Immunol.*, **49**, 99

101. Mygind, N., Brahe Pedersen, C. B., Prytzs, S. and Sørensen, H. (1975). Treatment of nasal polyps with intranasal beclamethasone dipropionate aerosol. *Clin. Allergy*, **5**, 159

102. Mygind, N. (1978). *Nasal Allergy*, p. 323 (Oxford: Blackwell Scientific)

103. Taylor, G. and Schwalkar, P. R. (1971). Di-sodium cromoglycate: laboratory studies and clinical trial in allergic rhinitis. *Clin. Allergy*, **1**, 189

104. Phillips, M. J., Ollier, S. and Davies, R. J. (1980). Anterior rhinometry in the evaluation of the effects of ketotifen, clemastine, cromoglycate and placebo in nasal allergen provocation. *Respiration*. (In press)

105. Blair, H. and Herbert, R. L. (1973). Treatment of seasonal allergic rhinitis with 2% sodium cromoglycate (BP) solution. *Clin. Allergy*, **3**, 283

106. Frankland, A. W. and Walker, S. R. (1975). A comparison of intranasal betamethasone valerate and sodium cromoglycate in seasonal allergic rhinitis. *Clin. Allergy*, **5**, 295

107. Frankland, A. W. and Augustin, R. (1954). Prophylaxis of summer hay-fever and asthma; controlled trial comparing crude grass-pollen extracts with isolated main protein com-ponent. *Lancet*, **1**, 1055

108. Johnstone, D. E., (1957). Study of the role of antigen dosage in the treatment of pollenosis and pollen asthma. *J. Dis. Child.*, **94**, 1

109. Norman, P. S., (1980). An overview of immunotherapy: implications for the future. *J. Allergy Clin. Immunol.*, **65**, 87

110. Morrison-Smith, J., Harding, L. K. and Cumming, G. (1971). The changing prevalence of asthma in schoolchildren. *Clin. Allergy*, **1**, 57

111. Gregg, I. (1977). Epidemiology. In Clark, T. J. H. and Godfrey, S. (eds.) *Asthma: Theory and Practice*, pp. 214–240 (London: Chapman and Hall)

112. Horn, B. R., Kabin, E. D., Theodore, J. and van Kessel, A. (1975). Total eosinophil counts in the management of bronchial asthma. *N. Eng. J. Med.*, **292**, 1152

113. McFadden, G. R., Luparello, T., Lyons, H. A. and Bleeker, E. (1969). The mechanism of action of suggestion in the induction of acute asthma attacks. *Psychosomatic Med.*, **31**, 134

114. McNeill, R. S. (1964). Effect of a beta-adrenergic blocking agent, propranolol, on asthmatics. *Lancet*, **2**, 1101

115. Harnett, J. C., Spector, S. L. and Farr, R. S. (1978). Aspirin idiosyncrasy, asthma and urticaria. In Middleton, E., Reed, C. E. and Ellis, E. F. (eds.) *Allergy: Principles and Practice*, p. 1002 (St Louis: C. V. Mosby)

116. Stenius, B. S. M. and Lemola, M. (1976). Hypersensitivity to acetylsalicylic acid (ASA) and tartrazine in patients with asthma. *Clin. Allergy*, **6**, 119

117. Weber, R. W., Hoffman, M., Raine, D. A. and Nelson, H. S. (1979). Incidence of bronchoconstriction due to aspirin, azo dyes, non-azo dyes and preservatives in a population of perennial asthmatics. *J. Allergy Clin. Immunol.*, **64**, 32

118. Gregg, I. (1977). Infection. In Clarke, T. J. H. and Godfrey, S. (eds.) *Asthma*, pp. 162–176 (London: Chapman and Hall)

119. McIntosh, K., Ellis, E. F., Hoffman, L. S., Lybass, T. G., Eller, J. J. and Fulginiti, V. A. (1973). The association of viral and bacterial respiratory infections with exacerbations of wheezing in young asthmatic children. *J. Paediatr.*, **82**, 578

120. Rooney, J. C. and Williams, H. (1971). The relationship between proved viral bronchiolitis and subsequent wheezing. *J. Paediatr.*, **79**, 744

121. Sanders, S. and Norman, A. P. (1968). The bacterial flora of the upper respiratory tract in children with severe asthma. *J. Allergy*, **41**, 319

122. Berman, S. Z., Mathison, D. A., Stevenson, D. D., Tarn, E. M. and Vaughan, J. H. (1975). Transtracheal aspiration studies in asthmatic subjects in relapse with 'infective asthma' and in subjects without respiratory disease. *J. Allergy Clin. Immunol.*, **56**, 206

123. Davies, R. J. (1978). Serological and skin test responses to allergens from *Staphylococcus aureus, Streptococcus pneumoniae* and *Haemophilus influenzae* in asthma and chronic bronchitis. p. 205. *MD Thesis.*, University of Cambridge

124. Frankland, A. W., Hughes, W. H. and Gorrill, R. H. (1955). Autogenous bacterial vaccines in treatment of asthma. *Br. Med. J.*, **2**, 941

125. Tomita, Y., Patterson, R. and Suszko, I. M. (1974). Respiratory mast cells and basiliphoid cells. *Int. Arch. Allergy Appl. Immunol.*, **47**, 261

126. Wasserman, S. I. (1979). The mast cell and the inflammatory response. In Pepys, J. and Edwards, A. M. (eds.). *The Mast Cell: its Role in Health and Disease*, p. 9 (Bath: The Pitman Press)

127. Drazen, J. M., Lewis, R. A., Wasserman, S. I., Orange, R. P. and Austen, K. F. (1979). Differential effects of a partially purified preparation of slow-reaching substance of anaphylaxis of guinea-pig tracheal spirals and parenchymal strips. *J. Clin. Invest.*, **63**, 1

128. Bhat, K. N., Arroyave, C. M., Marney, S. R., Stevenson, D. D. and Tan, E. M. (1976). Plasma histamine changes during provoked bronchospasm in asthmatic patients. *J. Allergy Clin. Immunol.*, **58**, 647

129. Chiesa, A., Dain, G. D., Meyers, G. L., Kessler, G.-F. and Gold, W. M. (1975). Histamine release during antigen inhalation in experimental asthma in dogs. *Am. Rev. Resp. Dis.*, **111**, 148

130. Bruce, C., Weatherstone, R., Seaton, A. and Taylor, W. H. (1976). Histamine level in plasma, blood and urine in severe asthma, and the effect of corticosteroid treatment. *Thorax*, **31**, 724

131. Nogrady, S. G., Hartley, J. P. R., Handslip, P. D. J. and Hurst, N. P. (1978). Bronchodilatation after inhalation of the antihistamine clemastine. *Thorax*, **33**, 479

132. Partridge, M. R. and Saunders, K. B. (1979). Effect of an inhaled antihistamine (clemastine) as a bronchodilator and as a maintenance treatment in asthma. *Thorax*, **34**, 771

133. Dahl, R. (1979). The eosinophil cell and eosinophil cationic protein in bronchial asthma. In Pepys, J. and Edwards, A. M. (eds.) *The Mast Cell: its Role in Health and Disease*, p. 101 (Bath: The Pitman Press)

134. Atkins, P. C., Norman, M. and Weiner, H. (1977). Release of neutrophil chemotactic activity during immediate hypersensitivity reaction in humans. *Ann. Intern. Med.*, **86**, 415

135. Wasserman, S. I. and Center, D. M. (1979). The relevance of neutrophil chemotactic factors to allergic disease. *J. Allergy Clin. Immunol.*, **64**, 231

136. Atkins, P. C., Norman, M. E. and Zweiman, B. (1978). Antigen-induced neutrophil chemotactic activity in man. Correlation with bronchospasm and inhibition by disodium cromoglycate. *J. Allergy Clin. Immunol.*, **62**, 149

290 IMMUNOLOGICAL ASPECTS OF ALLERGY

137. Szentivanyi, A. (1968). The beta-adrenergic theory of the atopic abnormality in bronchial asthma. *J. Allergy*, **42**, 203
138. Parker, C. W. and Smith, J. W. (1973). Alterations in cyclic adenosine monophosphate metabolism in human bronchial asthma. 1. Leukocyte responsiveness to β-adrenergic agents. *J. Clin. Invest.*, **52**, 48
139. Connolly, M. E. and Greenacre, J. K. (1976). The lymphocyte β-adrenoceptor in normal subjects and patients with bronchial asthma. The effect of different forms of treatment on receptor function. *J. Clin. Invest.*, **58**, 1307
140. Morris, H. G. (1980). Drug-induced desensitization of beta-adrenergic receptors. *J. Allergy Clin. Immunol.*, **65**, 83
141. Connolly, M. E., George, C. F., Davies, D. S. and Dollery, C. T. (1973). Acquired resistance to beta stimulants—a possible explanation for the rise in the asthma death rate in Britain. *Chest*, **63** (Suppl.), 16
142. Wessels, M. R., Mullikin, D. and Lefkowitz, R. J. (1979). Selective alteration in high affinity agonist binding. A mechanism for beta-adrenergic receptor desensitization. *Mol. Pharmacol.*, **16**, 10
143. Brooks, S. M., McGowan, K., Bernstein, I. L. Altenau, P. and Peagler, J. (1979). Relationship between numbers of beta-adrenergic receptors in lymphocytes and disease severity in asthma. *J. Allergy Clin. Immunol.*, **63**, 401
144. Tattersfield, A. F. and Holgate, S. T. (1976). Intravenous prednisolone in asthma. *Lancet*, **1**, 422
145. Mano, K., Akbarzadeh, A., Koesnadi, K., Sano, Y., Bewtra, A. and Townley, R. (1979). The effect of hydrocortisone on beta-adrenergic receptors in tissue. *J. Allergy Clin. Immunol.*, **63**, 147
146. Hughes, A. M. and Maunsell, K. (1973). A study of a population of house dust mite in its natural environment. *Clin. Allergy*, **3**, 127
147. Blythe, M. E., Al Ubaydi, F., Williams, J. D. and Morrison Smith, J. (1975). Study of dust mites in three Birmingham hospitals. *Br. Med. J.*, **1**, 62
148. Sarsfield, J. K., Gowland, G., Toy, R. and Norman, A. L. E. (1974). Mite-sensitive asthma of childhood. Trial of avoidance measures. *Arch. Dis. Child.*, **49**, 716
149. Burr, M. L., St. Leger, A. S. and Neale, E. (1976). Anti-mite measurements in mite-sensitive adult asthma. A controlled trial. *Lancet*, **1**, 333
150. Katz, D. H. (1979). New concepts concerning the clinical control of IgE synthesis. *Clin. Allergy*, **9**, 609
151. Lichtenstein L. M. (1978). An evaluation of the role of immunotherapy in asthma. *Am. Rev. Resp. Dis.*, **117**, 191
152. Warner, J. O., Price, J. F., Soothill, J. F. and Hey, E. N. (1978). Controlled trial of hyposensitization to *Dermatophagoides pteronyssinus* in children with asthma. *Lancet*, **2**, 912
153. Taylor, W. M., Ohman, J. L. and Lowell, F. C. (1978). Immunotherapy in cat-induced asthma. Double-blind trial with evaluation of bronchial responses to cat allergen and histamine. *J. Allergy Clin. Immunol.*, **61**, 283
154. Legge, J. S., Caddie, J. and Palmer, K. N. V. (1971). Comparison of two oral selective β₂-adrenergic stimulant drugs in bronchial asthma. *Br. Med. J.*, **1**, 637
155. Assem, E. S. K. and Schild, H. O. (1969). Inhibition by sympathomimetic amines of histamine release induced by antigen in passively sensitised human lung. *Nature (London)*, **224**, 1028
156. Jack, D., Harris, D. M. and Middleton, E. (1978). Adrenergic agents. In Middleton, E., Reed, C. E. and Ellis, E. F. (eds.) *Allergy: Principles and Practice*, pp. 404–433 (St Louis: C. V. Mosby)
157. Lightbody, I. M., Ingram, C. C., Legge, J. S. and Johnston, R. N. (1978). Ipratropium bromide, salbutamol and prednisolone in bronchial asthma and chronic bronchitis. *Br. J. Dis. Chest*, **72**, 181

158. Campbell, I. A., Middleton, W. G., Mackenzie, R., Shotter, M. V., McHardy, G. J. R. and Kay, A. B. (1976). Interaction between isoprenaline and aminophylline in asthma. *Thorax*, **31**, 488

159. Cox, J. S. (1967). Disodium cromoglycate (FPL 670) (Intal): A specific inhibitor of reaginic antibody–antigen mechanisms. *Nature (London)*, **216**, 1328

160. Brompton Hospital/Medical Research Council collaborative trial. (1972). Longterm study of disodium cromoglycate in treatment of severe extrinsic or intrinsic bronchial asthma in adults. *Br. Med. J.*, **4**, 383

161. Silverman, M., Connolly, N. M., Balfour-Lynn, L. and Godfrey, S. (1972). Long-term trial of disodium cromoglycate and isoprenaline in children with asthma. *Br. Med. J.*, **3**, 378

162. Altounyan, R. F. C. (1979). Review of the clinical activity and modes of action of sodium cromoglycate. In Pepys, J. and Edwards, A. M. (eds) *The Mast Cell*, pp. 199–216. (Bath: The Pitman Press)

163. Preliminary report of the Brompton Hospital, Medical Research Council collaborative trial. (1974). Double-blind trial comparing two dosage schedules of beclomethasone dipropionate aerosol in the treatment of chronic bronchial asthma. *Lancet*, **2**, 303

164. Davies, G., Thomas, P., Broder, I., Mintz, S., Silverman, F., Leznoff, A. and Trotman, C. (1977). Steroid-dependent asthma treated with inhaled beclomethasone dipropionate. A longterm study. *Ann. Intern. Med.*, **86**, 549

165. Fauci, A. S., Dale, D. C. and Balow, J. E. (1976). Glucocorticosteroid therapy: mechanisms of action and clinical considerations. *Ann. Intern. Med.*, **84**, 304

166. Karasek, S. R. and Karasek, M. (1911). Preliminary report of the injurious effect of metal platinum chromates, cyanides, hydrofluoric acid and/or materials used in silvering mirrors. Report of the Illinois State Commission on occupational disease.

167. Hunter, D., Milton, R. and Perry, K. M. A. (1945). Asthma caused by the complex salts of platinum. *Br. J. Indust. Med.*, **2**, 92

168. Flindt, M. L. H. (1969. Pulmonary diseases due to inhalation of derivatives of *Bacillus subtilis* enzyme preparations. *Lancet*, **1**, 1177

169. Kobayashi, S. (1974). Occupational asthma due to inhalation of pharmacological dusts and other occupational asthmas in Japan. In Yamamura, Y., Frick, O. L., Harinchi Y., Kishimoto S., Miyamoto T., Naranjo, P. and De Weck, A. L. (eds.) *Allergology* (Amsterdam: Excerpta Medica)

170. Biological effects of proteolytic enzyme detergents (1976). *Thorax*, **31**, 621

171. Fowler, P. B. S. (1952). Printer's asthma. *Lancet*, **2**, 755

172. Roberts, A. E. (1951). Platinosis: A 5-year study of the effects of soluble platinum salts on employees in platinum laboratory and refinery. *Arch. Industr. Hyg.*, **4**, 549

173. U.S. Department of Health, Education and Welfare (1973). Occupational exposure to toluene di-isocyanate. (Washington DC: US Government Printing Office)

174. Burge, P. S., Perks, W. H., O'Brien, I. M., Hawkins, R. and Green, M. (1979). Occupational asthma in an electronics factory. *Thorax*, **34**, 13

175. Schilling, R. S. F. (1956). Byssinosis in cotton and other textile workers. *Lancet*, **2**, 261 and 319

176. Bouhuys, A., Barbero, A., Lindell, S. E., Roach, S. A., and Schilling, R. S. F. (1967). Byssinosis in hemp workers. *Arch. Environ. Health*, **14**, 533

177. Nadel, J. S., Salem, H., Tamplin, B. and Tokiwa, Y. (1965). Mechanism of bronchoconstriction during the inhalation of sulphur dioxide. *J. Appl. Physiol.*, **20**, 164

178. Gandevia, B. (1970). Occupational asthma. *Med. J. Aust.*, **2**, 332 and 372

179. Bouhuys, A. (1974). *Breathing, Physiology, Environment and Lung Disease*. p. 416 (New York: Grune and Stratton)

180. Bouhuys, A. and Lindell, S. E. (1961). Release of histamine by cotton dust extracts from human lung tissue *in vitro*. *Experientia*, **17**, 211

181. Weiner, A. (1961). Bronchial asthma due to the organic phosphate insecticides. *Ann. Allergy*, **19**, 397

182. Evans, E. and Nicholls, P. J. (1974). Histamine release by western red cedar (*Thuja plicata*) from lung tissue *in vitro*. *Br. J. Industr. Med.*, **31**, 28

183. Parrot, J. L., Hebert, R., Saindelle, A. and Ruff, F. (1969). Platinum and platinosis: allergy and histamine release due to some platinum salts. *Arch. Environ. Health*, **19**, 685

184. Davies, R. J., Butcher, B. T. and Salvaggio, J. E. (1977). Occupational asthma caused by low molecular weight chemical agents. *J. Allergy Clin. Immunol.*, **60**, 93

185. Cowan, D. W., Thompson, H. J., Paulus, H. J. and Mielke, P. W. (1963). Bronchial asthma associated with air pollutants from the grain industry. *J. Air Pollution Central Assoc.*, **13**, 546

186. Peters, J. M. and Murphy, R. L. M. (1971). Hazards to health: do-it-yourself polyurethane foam. *Am. Rev. Resp. Dis.*, **104**, 432

187. Fawcett, I. W., Taylor, A. J. and Pepys, J. (1976). Asthma due to inhaled chemical agents – fumes from Multicore soldering flux and colophony resin. *Clin. Allergy*, **6**, 57

188. Björkstén, F., Backman, A., Järvinen, K. A. J., Lehti, H., Salvilahti, E., Syvänen, P. and Kärkkäinen, T. H. (1977). Immunoglobulin E specific to wheat and rye flour proteins. *Clin. Allergy*, **7**, 473

189. Hendrick, D. J., Davies, R. J. and Pepys, J. (1976). Bakers' asthma. *Clin. Allergy*, **6**, 241

190. Hendrick, D. J. and Lane, D. J. (1975). Formalin asthma in hospital staff. *Br. Med. J.*, **1**, 607

191. Menon, M. P. S. and Das, A. K. (1977). Tetracycline asthma – a case report. *Clin. Allergy*, **7**, 285

192. Bush, R. K. and Cohen, M. (1977). Immediate and late-onset asthma from occupational exposure to soybean dust. *Clin. Allergy*, **7**, 369

193. Galleguillos, F. and Rodriguez, J. C. (1978). Asthma caused by bromelin inhalation. *Clin. Allergy*, **8**, 21

194. Alanko, K., Keskinen, H., Björkstén, F. and Ojanen, S. (1978). Immediate-type hypersensitivity to reactive dyes. *Clin. Allergy*, **8**, 25

195. Vallieres, M., Cockcroft, D. W., Taylor, D. M., Dolovich, J. and Hargreave, F. E. (1977). Dimethyl ethanolamine-induced asthma. *Am. Rev. Resp. Dis.*, **115**, 867

196. Pepys, J., Pickering, C. A. C. and Loudon, H. W. (1972). Asthma due to inhaled chemical agents – piperazine dihydrochloride. *Clin. Allergy*, **2**, 189

197. Feinburg, S. M. and Watrous, R. M. (1945). Atopy to simple chemical compounds – sulfonechloramides. *J. Allergy*, **16**, 209

198. Maccia, C. A., Bernstein, I. L., Emmet, E. A. and Brooks, S. M. (1976). *In vitro* demonstration of specific IgE in phthalic anhydride hypersensitivity. *Am. Rev. Resp. Dis.*, **113**, 701

199. Cuthbert, O. D., Brostoff, J., Wraith, D. G. and Brighton, W. D. (1979). 'Barn allergy': asthma and rhinitis due to storage mites. *Clin. Allergy*, **9**, 229

200. Cromwell, O., Pepys, J., Parish, W. E. and Hughes, E. G. (1979). Specific IgE antibodies to platinum salts in sensitized workers. *Clin. Allergy*, **9**, 109

201. Burge, P. S., O'Brien, I. M., Harries, M. G. and Pepys, J. (1979). Occupational asthma due to inhaled carmine. *Clin. Allergy*, **9**, 185

202. Davies, R. J. and Pepys, J. (1975). Asthma due to inhaled chemical agents – the macrolide antibiotic spiramycin. *Clin. Allergy*, **5**, 99

203. Lincoln, T. A., Bolton, N. E. and Garrett, A. S. Jr. (1974). Occupational allergy to animal dander and sera. *J. Occup. Med.*, **16**, 465

204. Figley, K. D. and Elrod, R. M. (1928). Endemic asthma due to castor bean dust. *J. Am. Med. Assoc.*, **90**, 79

205. Karr, R. M., Lehrer, S. B., Butcher, B. T. and Salvaggio, J. E. (1978). Coffee workers' asthma: a clinical appraisal using the radioallergosorbent test. *J. Allergy Clin. Immunol.*, **62**, 143

206. Dolovich, J., Shaikh, W., Tarlo, S., Bell, B. and Hargreave, F. E. (1977). Human exposure and sensitization to airborne papain. *Ann. Allergy*, **38**, 94

207. Colten, H. R., Polakoff, P. L., Weinstein, S. F. and Strider, D. (1975). Immediate hypersensitivity to hog trypsin resulting from industrial exposure. *N. Eng. J. Med.*, **292**, 1050

208. Gelfand, H. H. (1963). Respiratory allergy due to chemical compounds encountered in the rubber, lacquer, shellac and beauty culture industries. *J. Allergy*, **34**, 374

209. McConnell, L. H., Fink, J. N., Schlueter, D. P. and Schmidt, M. G. (1973). Asthma caused by nickel sensitivity. *Ann. Intern. Med.*, **78**, 888

210. Greene, S. A. and Freedman, S. (1976). Asthma due to inhaled chemical agents – amprolium hydrochloride. *Clin. Allergy*, **6**, 105

211. Andrasch, R. H., Coster, F., Lawson, W. H. and Bardona, E. J. (1975). Meat wrappers asthma and reappraisal of a new occupational syndrome. *J. Allergy Clin. Immunol.*, **55**, 130

212. Kammermeyer, J. K. and Mathews, K. P. (1973). Hypersensitivity to phenylglycine acid chloride. *J. Allergy Clin. Immunol.*, **52**, 73

213. Levene, G. M. and Calnan, C. D. (1971). Platinum sensitivity: treatment by specific hyposensitization. *Clin. Allergy*, **1**, 75

214. van Leeuwen, W. S., Bren, Z., Kremer, W. and Varekamp, H. (1925). On the significance of small spored types of aspergilli in the aetiology of bronchial asthma. *Z. Immunitätsforsch.*, **44**, 1

215. Henderson, A. H., English, M. P. and Vecht, R. J. (1968). Pulmonary aspergillosis. A survey of its occurrence in patients with chronic lung disease and a discussion of the significance of diagnostic tests. *Thorax*, **23**, 513

216. Channell, S., Blyth, W., Lloyd, M., Weir, D. M., Amos, W. M. G., Littlewood, A. P., Riddle, H. F. V. and Grant, I. W. B. (1969). Allergic alveolitis in malt workers. A clinical, mycological and immunological study. *Q. J. Med.*, **38**, 351

217. British Tuberculosis Association Research Committee (1968). Aspergillosis in persistent lung cavities after tuberculosis. *Tubercle*, **49**, 1

218. Hinson, K. F. W., Moor, A. J. and Plummer, N. S. (1952). Broncho-pulmonary aspergillosis; review and report of eight new cases. *Thorax*, **7**, 317

219. McCarthy, D. S. and Pepys, J. (1971). Allergic broncho-pulmonary aspergillosis: clinical immunology. (1) Clinical features. *Clin. Allergy*, **1**, 261

220. McCarthy, D. S. and Pepys, J. (1971). Allergic broncho-pulmonary aspergillosis: clinical immunology. (2) Skin, nasal and bronchial tests. *Clin. Allergy*, **1**, 415

221. Malo, J. L., Hawkins, R. and Pepys, J. (1977). Studies in chronic allergic broncho-pulmonary aspergillosis. 1. Clinical and physiological findings. *Thorax*, **32**, 254

222. Vernon, D. R. H. and Allen, F. (1980). Environmental factors in allergic broncho-pulmonary aspergillosis. *Clin. Allergy*, **10**, 217

223. Malo, J. L., Pepys, J. and Simon, G. (1977). Studies in chronic allergic broncho-pulmonary aspergillosis. 2. Radiological findings. *Thorax*, **32**, 262

224. Patterson, R. and Roberts, M. (1974). IgE and IgG antibodies against *Aspergillus fumigatus* in sera of patients with broncho-pulmonary allergic aspergillosis. *Int. Arch. Allergy Appl. Immunol.*, **46**, 150

225. Bardana, E. J. Jr., McClatchy, J. K. and Farr, R. S. (1972). The primary interaction of antibody to components of aspergilli. II. Antibodies in sera from normal persons and from patients with aspergillosis. *J. Allergy Clin. Immunol.*, **50**, 222

226. Golbert, T. M. and Patterson, R. (1970). Pulmonary allergic aspergillosis. *Ann. Intern. Med.*, **72**, 395

227. Aisner, J., Schimoff, S. C. and Wiernik, P. H. (1977). Treatment of invasive aspergillosis: relation of early diagnosis and treatment to response. *Ann. Intern. Med.*, **86**, 539

228. Safirstein, B. H., D'Souza, M. F., Simon, G., Tai, E. H.-C. and Pepys, J. (1973). Five-year follow-up of allergic broncho-pulmonary aspergillosis. *Am. Rev. Resp. Dis.*, **108**, 450

229. Scadding, J. C., Hinson, K. F. (1967). Diffuse fibrosing alveolitis (diffuse interstitial fibrosis of the lungs). Correlation of histology at biopsy with prognosis. *Thorax*, **22**, 291
230. Grant, I. W. B., Blyth, W., Wardrop, B. E., Gordon, R. M., Pearson, J. C. G. and Mair, A. (1972). Prevalance of farmers' lung in Scotland: a pilot survey. *Br. Med. J.*, **1**, 530
231. Madsen, D., Klock, L. E., Wenzel, F. J., Robbins. J. L. and Schmidt, D. C. (1976). The prevalence of farmers' lung in an agricultural population. *Am. Rev. Resp. Dis.*, **113**, 171
232. Lacey, J. and Lacey, M. E. (1964). Spore concentrations in the air of farm buildings. *Trans. Br. Mycol. Soc.*, **47**, 547
233. Christensen, L. T., Schmitt, C. D. and Robbins, L. (1975). Pigeon breeder's disease – a prevalence study and review. *Clin. Allergy*, **5**, 417
234. Faux, J. A., Wells, I. D. and Pepys, J. (1971). Specificity of avian serum proteins in tests against sera of bird fanciers. *Clin. Allergy*, **1**, 159
235. Edwards, J. H., Barboriak, J. J. and Fink, J. N. (1970). Antigens in pigeon breeders' disease. *Immunology*, **19**, 729
236. Faux, J. A., Hendrick, D. J. and Anand, N. S. (1978). Precipitins to different avian serum antigens in bird fancier's lung and coeliac disease. *Clin. Allergy*, **8**, 101
237 Lehrer, S. B., Turer, E., Weill, H. and Salvaggio, J. E. (1978). Elimination of bagassosis in Louisiana paper manufacturing plant workers. *Clin. Allergy*, **8**, 15
238. Banaszak, E. F., Thiede, W. H. and Fink, J. N. (1970). Hypersensitivity pneumonitis due to a contamination of an air conditioner. *N. Eng. J. Med.*, **283**, 271
239. Muittari, A., Kuusisto, P., Virtanen, P., Sovijärvi, A., Grönvoos, P., Haemoinen, K. A., Antila, P. and Kellomaki, L. (1980). An epidemic of extrinsic allergic alveolitis caused by tap water. *Clin. Allergy*, **10**, 77
240. Ghose, T., Landrigan, P., Killeen, R. and Dill, J. (1974). Immunopathological studies in patients with farmer's lung. *Clin. Allergy*, **1**, 119
241. Barrowcliff, D. F. and Arblaster, P. G. (1968). Farmers' lung: a study of an early acute fatal case. *Thorax*, **23**, 490
242. Seal, R. M., Hapke, E. J. and Thomas, G. O. (1968). The pathology of the aute and chronic stages of farmers' lung. *Thorax*, **23**, 469
243. Emanuel, D. A., Wenzel, F. J., Bowerman, C. I. and Lawton, B. R. (1964). Farmers' lung. Clinical, pathological and immunologic study of 24 patients. *Am. J. Med.*, **37**, 392
244. Allen, D. H., Basten, A., Williams, G. V. and Woolcock, A. J. (1975). Familial hypersensitivity pneumonitis. *Am. J. Med.*, **59**, 505
245. Flaherty, D. K., Iha, T., Chemlik, F., Dickie, H. and Reed, C. E. (1975). HL-A and farmers' lung. *Lancet*, **2**, 507
246. Bice, D. E., McCarron, K., Hoffman, E. O. and Salvaggio, J. E. (1977). Adjuvant properties of *Micropolyspora faeni*. *Int. Arch. Allergy Appl. Immunol.*, **55**, 267
247. Edwards, J. H., Baker, J. T. and Davies, B. H. (1974). Precipitin test negative farmers' lung – activation of the alternative pathway of complement by mouldy hay dust. *Clin. Allergy*, **4**, 379
248. Moore, V. L., Hensley, G. T. and Fink, J. N. (1975). An animal model of hypersensitivity pneumonitis in the rabbit. *J. Clin. Invest.*, **56**, 937
249. Edwards, J. H. (1976). A quantitative study on the activation of the alternative pathway of complement by mouldy haydust and thermophilic actinomycetes. *Clin. Allergy*, **6**, 19
250. Schorlemmer, H. U., Edwards, J. H., Davies, P. and Allison, A. C. (1977). Macrophage responses to mouldy hay dust. *Micropolyspora faeni* and zymozan, activators of complement by the alternative pathway. *Clin. Exp. Immunol.*, **27**, 198
251. Hypersensitivity diseases of lungs due to fungi and organic dusts. *Monographs in Allergy*. Vol. 4 (Basle: J. Karger)
252. Spector, W. G. and Heesom, W. (1969). The production of granulomata by antigen–antibody complexes. *J. Pathol.*, **98**, 31

253. Moore, V. L., Fink, J. N., Barboriak, J. J., Ruff, L. L., Schluter, D. P. (1974). Immunologic events in pigeon breeder's disease. *J. Allergy Clin. Immunol.*, **53**, 319
254. Bice, D. E., Salvaggio, J. and Hoffman, E. (1976). Passive transfer of experimental hypersensitivity pneumonitis with lymphoid cells in the rabbit. *J. Allergy Clin. Immunol.*, **58**, 250
255. Schuyler, M. R., Thigpen, T. P. and Salvaggio, J. E. (1978). Local pulmonary immunity in pigeon breeder's disease. A case study. *Ann. Intern. Med.*, **88**, 355
256. Salvaggio, J. E. (1979). Immunological mechanisms in pulmonary disease. *Clin. Allergy*, **9**, 659
257. Barbee, R. A., Callies, Q., Dickie, H. A. and Rankin, J. (1966). The long-term prognosis in farmers' lung. *Am. Rev. Resp. Dis.*, **97**, 223
258. Smyth, J. T., Adkins, G. E., Margaret, L., Lloyd, M., Moore, B. and McWhite, E. (1975). Farmers' lung in Devon. *Thorax*, **30**, 197

8
Hyposensitization Therapy

J. F. PRICE

'I do not want to boast, but I think I am quite done with the accursed thing for this year. There can be no sort of doubt, seeing the kind of season it has been, that I should have suffered, and that severely, if I had not had these inoculations.'

Patient with hay fever, 1911

Patients with hay fever and asthma have been treated with injections of allergen extract for almost 70 years. However there is still no satisfactory method for standardizing the extracts used. The early reports of benefit were based on the anecdotal impressions of patient and physician; it was 43 years after the original descriptions[1,2] that the first placebo controlled trial was published[3]. The initial work was founded on unsound theory and we still do not fully understand the changes in the immune system brought about by hyposensitization. It is not surprising that immunotherapy remains a controversial subject and its use varies greatly in different parts of the world.

ALLERGEN EXTRACTS

Extracts made commercially available for hyposensitization should contain concentrations of allergen, constant from batch to batch, which are sufficient to stimulate a beneficial immune response without provoking dangerous side-effects. Many extracts are prepared using weight by volume methods. A given weight of raw material is extracted, dialysed, concentrated, then reconstituted to the original extraction volume. The standardization of the material depends on standardization of the extraction process and quality control tests such as measurement of the protein nitrogen content. The latter may be unreliable when the principal allergenic protein in the crude extract forms only a small proportion of the total protein (for example antigen E in ragweed). Commercial extracts of ragweed and grass pollen manufactured in this way show considerable variation in their capacity to elicit skin reactions in allergic subjects. This variation is found not only with extracts produced by different companies but with different batches produced by the same firm[4, 5]. Attempts have been made to improve standardization by isoelectric focusing. This allows a more sophisticated analysis of the proteins present in the extract, but precise measurement of individual protein concentrations is not possible. The most direct but also the most time consuming way to improve the quality of an extract is to identify and isolate the allergenic proteins. These can then be assayed against specific precipitating antisera raised in animals. To some extent the major allergens in ragweed (antigen E)[6], Group 1 of rye grass[5], and *Dermatophagoides pteronyssinus*[7] have been isolated, but most allergen extracts are crude mixtures. Two techniques have been devised to bypass the isolation process. In the first, crude extracts are compared by their capacity to inhibit the radioallergosorbent test (RAST) using serum from atopic patients containing a known concentration of specific IgE antibody[8]. In the second, individual allergens in an extract are identified by crossed immunoelectrophoresis using ^{125}I-labelled anti-IgE[9]. Though both methods are promising, further assessment is needed before they can be generally accepted.

The problem of standardization makes it difficult to compare dosage schedules in clinical trials, but there is some evidence that low dose regimes are ineffective[10]. The doses of crude aqueous extracts which appear to be therapeutic frequently provoke adverse allergic reactions, and much experimental work has been done to produce safer extracts which still give clinical benefit. Allergens were first modified by precipitation with alum. Alum, although not a good adjuvant, slows the rate of absorption of the allergen, so larger doses can then be given with each injection, and the number of injections reduced. The same therapeutic effect is possible with half the number of injections of an alum precipitated ragweed as with an aqueous extract[11]. The incidence of adverse reactions can be reduced if the allergen is extracted with puridine, an organic solvent, before precipitation. Alum-precipitated pyridine extracts give clinical benefit[12] but have not been compared with aqueous extracts in controlled studies. The rate of absorption can also be reduced by treatment of the allergen with glutaraldehyde to form polymers. Polymers of ragweed antigen E do not lose their antigenicity and will stimulate the production of blocking antibody[13]. Grass pollen polymers have been further modified by absorption on to 1-tyrosine, which acts as an adjuvant[14]. Side-effects are uncommon with both alum-precipitated pyridine extracts and glutaraldehyde-treated tyrosine absorbed preparations, and subjective assessment by patient questionnaire suggests that clinical benefit can be achieved with only three injections of the latter[15].

Mild treatment of certain allergens with formaldehyde reduces their capacity to provoke IgE and histamine mediated responses. These 'allergoids', as they have been called. still stimulate good IgG antibody responses[16]. The regulation of antibody production by B lymphocytes (to protein antigens) depends on the interaction of several subpopulations of T cells – helper cells, suppressor cells and amplifier cells. Several groups, using animal models, have investigated the possibility of modifying allergens in such a way that they specifically inactivate IgE-producing B lymphocytes. Ishizaka and Ishizaka[17] found that weekly injections of urea-denatured ragweed antigen E suppressed IgE production to ragweed in normal mice and in mice that have been primed with antigen E. Injections of urea-denatured ovalbumen in primed mice inhibited IgE responses to ovalbumen and to sensitizing doses of dinitrophenylated ovalbumen. Adoptive transfer experiments indicated that this property resided in splenic T-cell fractions from mice that have been treated with urea-denatured ovalbumen. It was concluded that injections of the urea-denatured antigen preparations generated suppressor T cells[17].

Sehon and Lee[18] showed that injections of ovalbumen conjugated with mouse γ-globulin specifically suppressed primary and secondary IgE antibody responses to ovalbumen in mice. Their experiments suggested that protein antigens. when conjugated with isologous γ-globulins, also generated suppressor T cells. Further studies were done with conjugates derived from monomethoxypolyethylene glycol and such antigens as ovalbumen, ragweed antigen E and Timothy grass pollen. These conjugates did not show the antigenic capacity of the unmodified antigen, and their injection reduced or abolished IgE antibody response. In the doses given there was, however, no significant effect on the response in terms of IgM or IgG antibody[18].

This work suggests that antigen in a non-immunogenic form promotes the proliferation of suppressor T cells. Perhaps IgE-producing B cells are more sensitive to the suppressor cells than the B lymphocytes which produce IgG and IgM. The mechanism for this effect is unknown but, in future such modified antigens may prove to be valuable in the treatment of IgE mediated hypersensitivity in man.

CLINICAL TRIALS

Since the introduction of hyposensitization therapy a wide range of extracts of pollens, dust, moulds, animal danders and bacteria have been used, sometimes in combination, to treat allergic rhinitis and asthma. Anaphylactic reactions to insect stings have also been treated by immunotherapy, and this is discussed in Chapter 10. Unfortunately most of the published trials have not been controlled and the assessment has been based on subjective impression. The patients taking part in a trial of hyposensitization must be shown by history and provocation testing to be sensitive to the allergen, the trial should be double-blind placebo controlled, and objective physiological and immuno-logical measurements are necessary, as well as clinical assessment. It is perhaps not surprising that few allergen extracts have been investigated in this way. The methods available for the assessment of hyposensitization therapy are listed below:

Clinical: patient questionnaire
daily diary card scores

Physiological: respiratory function tests of airflow obstruction and lung volume
nasal airflow measurement

Immunological: leukocyte histamine release
measurement of allergen-specific IgE, IgG and IgA antibodies in serum and secretions
allergen provocation tests to skin, nose and lung

Allergic rhinitis

The seasonal recurrence of hay fever was recognized in 1819[19] and later, Blackley[20] and Dunbar[21] showed that the mucous membranes and skin of hay fever sufferers were sensitive to pollen in a way not shown by normal individuals. Hyposensitization therapy was first used for hay fever by Noon in 1911 and has been the main form of treatment since. It became well established before the importance of a 'placebo effect' was recognized, but during the last 25 years a number of controlled studies have been published showing benefit in patients sensitive to grass pollen and ragweed.

Hay fever due to grass pollen allergy causes symptoms in June and July in Europe. Frankland and Augustin in 1954 carried out the first controlled trial in patients allergic to grass pollen, and found a significant improvement in symptoms after preseasonal injections of both crude and partially purified pollen extract[3]. Alum-precipitated pyridine extracts of pollen have also been shown to reduce symptoms of hay fever in placebo-controlled trials[12]. With alum-precipitated extracts and with glutaraldehyde pollen tyrosine adsorbate, clinical improvement occurs in 70–80% of patients, and adverse reactions to the injections are uncommon[15, 22].

Ragweed allergy is said to affect about 5% of the population in the United States; symptoms develop in August and September. Comprehensive clinical and immunological studies have been made of this disease, partly because it is common and partly because the major allergen in ragweed has been clearly identified. This is antigen E, a protein with a molecular weight of 38 000, which comprises about 6% of the total protein in ragweed pollen. During the past 15 years detailed studies have been carried out at the Johns Hopkins University School of Medicine. In order to assess the response to immunotherapy, a diary card scoring system was developed which correlated well with changes in the pollen count during the ragweed season and with objective laboratory measurements of cell sensitivity. Using this assessment, the relatively low antigen dose regimes, which on clinical impression had been considered to be beneficial, were shown to be no more effective than placebo. However, further studies using larger doses of antigen provided firm evidence that immunotherapy leads to a statistically significant, if moderate, relief of symptoms in adult patients[23-25]. A more striking improvement was noted in children with ragweed hay fever after preseasonal injections, in a separate controlled trial[26].

The only other pollen which has been studied in a controlled way is mountain cedar; this causes hay fever in the south-western United States. Hyposensitization was shown to control seasonal symptoms due to this pollen[27].

Local hyposensitization using intranasal grass pollen extract is an attractive prospect, and one placebo-controlled trial has suggested that improvement in symptoms after nasal hyposensitization may be comparable to that with preseasonal injection therapy. The results of this trial were assessed subjectively and no immunological studies were reported[28], but this form of immunotherapy merits further investigation.

The role of immunotherapy in the treatment of perennial rhinitis is less clear. Dust contains the main allergens responsible for perennial rhinitis, and the house mite, *Dermatophagoides pteronyssinus*, is thought to be the most important allergen in dust. There are few satisfactory controlled trials of hyposensitization to dust or dust mite in patients with perennial rhinitis, and the results of the studies are in some ways conflicting. One trial of immunotherapy with house mite in adults showed reduced nasal sensitivity on provocation testing but no improvement in nasal symptoms judged by diary card and questionnaire[29]. The converse was found in a study of Chinese patients with rhinitis in Hong Kong, which demonstrated a significant improvement in symptoms assessed by diary cards but no consistent change in the skin or nasal challenge tests[30]. Both trials were placebo controlled and done on carefully selected patients, and in both an aqueous extract of *Dermatophagoides* was used. It is difficult to explain the discrepancy in the results.

In the Hong Kong study an initial course of 18–22 weekly injections was followed by a monthly maintenance course for a year. No improvement was detected at the end of the weekly course, and benefit occurred later during maintenance. The suggestion that prolonged immunotherapy with mite is necessary for clinical benefit is supported by some studies in asthma. Hyposensitization to mite in children with perennial asthma and rhinitis resulted in subjective improvement in nasal as well as bronchial symptoms[31]. In this study the assessment was made after 1 year of treatment.

In summary, immunotherapy brings about an improvement in symptoms but not a cure of seasonal allergic rhinitis. The injections have to be repeated before each pollen season but there is some evidence, from studies done over several years, of a cumulative effect[25, 32]. There is no conclusive evidence of benefit from hyposensitization to dust or mite in perennial rhinitis, though there is a strong suggestion of improvement in symptoms in both adults and children when treatment is maintained for more than a year. Disodium cromoglycate[36] and betamethazone valerate[34], applied topically during the pollen season, have been shown to be effective in controlling nasal symptoms and they are reasonable alternatives to hyposensitization.

Asthma

Asthma, a more complex disease than hay fever, has many causes. The disease runs in families, indicating genetic susceptibility, but environmental factors may be important, particularly in the newborn period. Patients with asthma have abnormal bronchial lability which can be demonstrated by their response to exercise or the inhalation of histamine. Several hypotheses have been proposed for a common pathogenic mechanism; β-adrenergic blockade[35] and over-responsiveness of the cholinergic nervous system are likely to be important, but they do not satisfy the requirements for a single basic defect. Some but not all asthmatics have evidence of allergy, demonstrated by immediate positive prick tests to common allergens, and in a proportion there is a causal relationship between symptoms and contact with a specific allergen. Traditionally, asthma is divided into extrinsic and intrinsic depending on whether the patient shows signs of allergy. In adults, intrinsic asthma is important, but in childhood it is rare. Of children presenting with asthma 90% give positive immediate skin reactions to inhalant allergens[37].

Immunotherapy is used extensively in the treatment of asthma, both extrinsic and intrinsic. We believe, however, that there is no place for the use of immunotherapy in asthmatic patients when no allergen of clinical importance can be identified by history, provocation tests and laboratory investigation. The case for hyposensitization in extrinsic asthma is less well proven than that for hay fever. Only a small proportion of asthmatic patients show sensitivity to one allergen – most give positive skin and bronchial provocation tests to several. This has led to the use of mixtures of allergens for immunotherapy, a practice which has never been validated scientifically. Hyposensitization therapy began to be used for asthma when allergists expressed the view that pollen-sensitive patients showed an improvement in bronchial as well as nasal symptoms. Frankland and Augustin reported beneficial effects in adults sensitive to grass pollen[3] and Johnstone and Dutton suggested that high dose therapy was effective in ragweed-sensitive asthmatic children[38]. Both these trials were controlled to some extent but response was judged solely on clinical impression. In 1967, McAllen observed increased tolerance to bronchial provocation with grass pollen after immunotherapy; some patients showed clinical improvement but the provocation tests did not correlate well with symptoms[39]. A recent placebo-controlled trial of carefully selected ragweed-sensitive asthmatics showed no change in clinical symptoms or in sensitivity on bronchial provocation as a result of treatment[40]. So in the small group of asthmatic patients who are exclusively pollen sensitive, the results of trials of immunotherapy are contradictory and even in those where treatment appeared effective, there was only moderate improvement in symptoms.

For three centuries[41] exposure to dust has been recognized as a cause of wheezing in patients with perennial asthma, but the link between house dust and house mite allergy was not described until 1964[42]. Skin and bronchial provocation tests, measurement of IgE antibodies and leukocyte histamine release tests all indicate that the house dust mite, *Dermatophagoides pteronyssinus*, is one of the commonest allergens to which asthmatics become sensitized in Europe. It is still difficult to determine the clinical importance of any one allergen in perennial asthmatics who, in most cases, have multiple sensitivities, and it follows that asthmatic patients who take part in trials of hyposensitization to house dust or house mite need careful selection if the results are to be interpreted correctly. The British Tuberculosis Association supervised a placebo-controlled trial of hyposensitization to house dust in 1968; 33 adult asthmatics showed no improvement in symptoms after 15 injections[43]. Trials with house dust mite extracts have been slightly more encouraging. Immunotherapy using *Dermatophagoides farinae*[44] and *Dermatophagoides pteronyssinus*[45] resulted in moderate improvement in small numbers of patients, although another trial failed to demonstrate any difference in response to treatment with extracts of house mite when compared with house dust[46]. A carefully controlled study of the clinical and immunological effects of immunotherapy with an aqueous extract of *Dermatophagoides*, at the Brompton Hospital in 1973, showed less asthma, less use of drugs and an increased clinical tolerance to household dust in the treatment group. Clinical improvement was greatest in the most allergic patients and not different from controls in those with small skin and nasal reactions to *Dermatophagoides*[29]. In contrast, treatment of 45 patients with tyrosine-absorbed *Dermatophagoides pteronyssinus* failed to produce improvement in symptoms, lung function, or skin and nasal challenge tests[47].

More consistent results have been obtained in children. Aas conducted a double blind study of hyposensitization with house dust extract in 80 asthmatic children and noted clinical improvement with reduced sensitivity on bronchial provocation after 2½ to 3 years of treatment. Clinical and bronchial provocation results correlated well[48]. Hyposensitization with tyrosine absorbed *Dermatophagoides pteronyssinus*, administered for 12 months, was also effective in children. Compared to controls, treated children used fewer drugs while maintaining clinical and lung function improvements. Unlike the trial with house dust extract, no change was observed in the immediate response on bronchial provocation, but the late reaction to *Dermatophagoides* was lost in half the treated patients and these showed the greatest improvement in symptoms[30]. It may be significant that the trial periods, 3 years and 1 year, were considerably longer in the studies in children than in any of the studies in adults.

There are a very large number of allergens in the environment which may from time to time cause symptoms of asthma, but there are no satisfactory studies of hyposensitization to any other than pollens, dust and dust mite. There are no placebo-controlled trials with moulds or animal danders. Twenty years ago immunotherapy with bacterial vaccines was assessed in two controlled trials, using extracts prepared from cultures of bacteria commonly found in the upper respiratory tract[49, 50]. Both trials showed no therapeutic effect and subsequent trials have confirmed these negative results. We now know that most respiratory infections which precipitate wheezing in asthmatic patients are in fact caused by viruses.

MECHANISMS

The original rationale for treating hay fever with inoculations of pollen extract was that the symptoms were caused by a toxin released from pollen, and the injections would stimulate the synthesis of antitoxin. This premise was disproved when the serum of allergic patients was found to passively sensitize the skin of normal subjects[51]. Coca and Grove discovered heat-labile antibodies in the serum of allergic individuals, which were capable of giving prolonged sensitization. They called them 'reagins'[52]. Most reagins have been identified as antibodies of the IgE class, a group of homocytotropic antibodies which are present in minute amounts in serum and which have an affinity for basophils and mast cells. Divalent IgE molecules attach to these cells by their FC footpiece, and the bridging of the molecules by allergen triggers the rapid release of histamine and other vasoactive substances[53, 54].

Although the rational basis for immunotherapy has been confuted, the practice continued because clinicians felt it was beneficial. Then in 1935, Cooke and others investigated the effects of blood transfusion, using hay fever patients treated with immunotherapy as donors. When untreated patients with the same sensitization were transfused at the beginning of the pollen season, it was found that the donor serum contained a transferable protective substance. These authors suggested that inhibiting or blocking antibody coexisted with sensitizing antibody, in patients given immunotherapy, and prevented allergen from reacting with sensitized cells[55]. Their conclusions were based on passive transfer experiments in skin. Sensitizing and blocking antibodies can be assayed in vitro by the leukocyte histamine release test. A patient's sensitivity to an allergen can be estimated by measuring the release of histamine from suspensions of the patient's leukocytes, when they are challenged with the allergen. By using different concentrations of allergen a dose–response curve is obtained, and the concentration of allergen which provokes 50% histamine release can be determined. Sensitivity to ragweed measured in this way correlates well with severity of hay fever during the pollen season. Blocking antibodies in patients receiving immunotherapy can be assessed by the capacity of the serum to inhibit allergen-provoked histamine release. Their presence results in a shift of the dose–response curve to the right and an increase in the concentration of allergen needed to stimulate 50% histamine release.

Blocking antibodies belong mainly to the IgG class of immunoglobulins[56]. All patients with ragweed hay fever who are treated with sufficient doses of allergen show a rise in blocking antibody. Those with very high antibody levels do significantly better than those with low levels, but neither symptom relief nor the relationship between severity of symptoms and leukocyte histamine release can be predicted accurately from the blocking antibody titres[23, 57].

The results of leukocyte histamine release studies do not prove that improvement in symptoms is the direct result of blocking antibody production. When patients are given hyposensitization therapy their leukocytes show changes in their response to allergen challenge, which are independent of blocking antibody synthesis. At first an increased dose of allergen is required to elicit the release of histamine – that is the cells become less sensitive. Later, the histamine released at optimum allergen concentration is reduced, in other words the cells become less reactive. In a few patients the release of histamine is abolished completely[58]. While there is a tendency for patients with reduced cell reactivity to show improvement in symptoms, this change does not invariably predict a good clinical outcome. It has been suggested that hyposensitization causes a general reduction in cell reactivity. Patients who have reduced leukocyte reactivity to ragweed after specific treatment also show reduced reactivity to other allergens. This non-specific effect on the leukocytes is not however reflected in the clinical response. Ragweed hyposensitization in patients who are also sensitive to grass pollen results in improvement during the ragweed season but not during the grass season[59].

Several techniques have been developed to measure allergen-specific IgE reaginic, and IgG blocking antibodies in the serum. IgE antibodies are usually estimated by the RAST technique but other methods include an antigen-binding assay and a modification of the red cell linked antigen – antiglobulin reaction (RCLAAR). IgG antibodies can be measured by the antigen-binding assay and the RCLAAR, and also by an indirect radio-immunoelectrophoresis (RIEP), or a method based on the absorption of IgG on to a Sepharose protein A complex to which is added ^{125}I-labelled allergen.

Serum of allergic individuals contains IgE and low levels of specific IgG antibody. Hay fever patients show a rise in IgE antibody during the pollen season; the titre then gradually falls during the winter months and reaches its lowest level just before the start of the next pollen season. It is now generally accepted that allergen-specific IgE and IgG antibodies rise during the first few months of immunotherapy[32, 60]. The true rise in IgE antibody is probably higher than that observed, because IgG interferes with the binding of IgE to the solid-phase allergen in the RAST. Conversely, IgG antibody may be overestimated, as some IgE activity is likely to be included. There is less agreement about the changes in antibody levels with long-term immuno-therapy. Some investigators found that the seasonal rise in IgE antibody, which is characteristic of hay fever, was reduced or abolished[61, 62], but this was not confirmed in other studies[60, 63]. Though most reports describe a fall in skin sensitizing antibody activity when hyposensitization is continued for more than a year, the proportion of patients who show this decrease varies considerably. One group noted a fall in IgE antibody titre in 18 out of 19 patients who had received ragweed immunotherapy for 15 months[61], but another group found IgE antibody levels were decreased below the initial levels in only 50% of patients after 2–6 years of treatment[32]. IgG antibody may remain high during maintenance therapy or decrease with time[26, 32]. The discrepancies in the results from different centres might be explained by different methods of antibody measurement but are more likely to be due to the lack of standardization of allergen extracts and dose schedules used for hyposensitization. In spite of the rise in IgE antibody during the early stages of immunotherapy, patients do not become more sensitive. This has been attributed to the action of IgG-blocking antibody combining with free allergen in serum to lower the allergen concentration below that required to elicit a hypersensitivity reaction. Decreased sensitivity over a longer period of time might be explained by the competitive inhibition of allergen binding to cells which stimulate B lymphocytes to become IgE antibody producing cells. The major weakness in the 'blocking antibody' hypothesis is the persistent failure to demonstrate a significant correlation between clinical improvement and the titre of IgG antibody, the titre of IgE antibody, or the IgG/IgE antibody ratio. Another suggestion put forward is that blocking-antibody activity might reside in one of the IgG subclasses. In support of this, IgG$_4$ myeloma protein was found to block passive sensitization by IgE antibodies in baboon skin[64]. During immunotherapy with grass pollen, a disproportionate increase in specific IgG$_4$ antibody is observed, but again this does not correlate with clinical improvement[65].

Antibodies in secretions are also stimulated by immunotherapy. Allergen specific IgG and IgA antibodies can be detected by double antibody radioimmunoassay in the nasal secretions of most allergic subjects but are rarely found in normals. The levels of both classes of antibody in secretions rise during immunotherapy. The IgG titres in nasal secretions are not related to the IgG titres in the serum, and no allergen-specific IgA antibody is detected in the blood. This indicates that the secretory antibodies are produced locally. Their action might be to block allergens at the site of entry and prevent them combining with IgE on mast cells lying free in secretions. Both the IgG and

IgA antibodies have been shown to inhibit the release of histamine from leukocytes *in vitro*, but it remains to be seen whether secretory antibody production correlates with treatment response[66].

Recently it has been suggested that IgG antibodies may control IgE responses by feedback inhibition through 'suppressor T cells'. Hay fever patients frequently show altered *in vitro* lymphocyte function (blast transformation and MIF production) in the presence of allergen[67]. After immunotherapy these cellular responses are usually reduced[68]. Allergen-specific IgG antibodies induced by hyposensitization will suppress *in vitro* responses to grass pollen of lymphocytes from untreated hay fever patients[69]. In rats and rabbits soluble T-cell factors have been shown to control the synthesis of IgE antibodies, but these substances do not appear to be immunoglobulins[70, 71]. It is not unreasonable to propose that immunotherapy stimulates suppressor T-cell activity, thus specifically reducing IgE production, but it is improbable from the evidence of animal experiments that IgG antibody has a direct suppressor effect on IgE-producing B cells.

Finally, allergen provocation tests have been used to evaluate the response to immunotherapy. Aas found that clinical benefit in asthmatic children receiving hyposensitization to house dust was associated with a reduction in bronchial sensitivity[48], but most investigations have failed to show a convincing correlation between improvement in symptoms and response to bronchial, nasal or skin provocation. This lack of correlation is surprising, and while errors in technique might be partly responsible, patients with clear-cut relief of symptoms frequently give immediate reactions to the same concentration of allergen before and after hyposensitization. Experimental studies of the effects of immunotherapy have been directed mainly towards IgE and mast cell mediated reactions, but other allergic mechanisms, possibly triggered by immediate reactions, may contribute to the symptoms of hay fever and asthma. Late (4–8 hour) reactions have been described after cutaneous, bronchial and nasal provocation. In a controlled trial of hyposensitization to house mite in perennial asthma, clinical improvement was significantly associated with the loss of late bronchial reactions, but no change was seen in the immediate responses. Late bronchial reactions were lost in half the treated patients, and these showed the greatest improvement in symptoms[31]. This observation, if it is confirmed, introduces new possibilities for research into the mechanisms of hyposensitization therapy.

References

1. Noon, L. (1911). Prophylactic inoculation for hay fever. *Lancet*, 1, 1572
2. Freeman, J. (1911). Further observations on the treatment of hay fever by hypodermic inoculations of pollen vaccine. *Lancet*, 2, 814
3. Frankland, A. W. and Augustin, R. (1954). Prophylaxis of summer hay fever and asthma. Controlled trial comparing crude grass-pollen extracts with isolated main pollen component. *Lancet*, 1, 1055

4. Baer, H., Godfrey, H., Maloney, C. J., Norman, P. S. and Lichtenstein, L. M. (1970). The potency and antigen E content of commercially prepared ragweed extracts. *J. Allergy*, **45**, 347

5. Baer, H., Maloney, C. J., Norman, P. S. and Marsh, D. G. (1974). The potency and Group 1 content of six commercially prepared grass pollen extracts. *J. Allergy Clin. Immunol.*, **54**, 157

6. King, T. P., Norman, P. S. and Lichtenstein, L. M. (1967). Isolation and characterisation of allergens from ragweed pollen. IV. *Biochemistry*, **6**, 1992

7. Chapman, M. D. and Platts-Mills, T. A. E. (1978). Measurement of IgG, IgA and IgE antibodies to *Dermatophagoides pteronyssinus* by antigen-binding assay using a partially purified fraction of mite extract (F_4P_1). *Clin. Exp. Immunol.*, **34**, 126

8. Foucard, T., Johansson, S. G. O., Bennich, H. and Berg, T. (1972). *In vitro* estimation of allergens by a radioimmune antiglobulin technique using human IgE antibodies. *Int. Arch. Allergy Appl. Immunol.*, **43**, 360

9. Weeke, B. and Lowenstein, H. (1975). Quantitative immunoelectrophoresis (QIE) used in analysis of allergen extracts and diagnosis of allergy. *Int. Arch. Allergy Appl. Immunol.*, **49**, 74

10. Johnstone, D. E. (1957). Study of the role of antigen dosage in the treatment of pollenosis and pollen asthma. *J. Dis. Child.*, **94**, 1

11. Norman. P. S., Winkerwerder, W. L. and Lichtenstein, L. M. (1972). Trials of alum-precipitated pollen extracts in the treatment of hay fever. *J. Allergy Clin. Immunol.*, **50**, 31

12. Kerr, J. W. and Murchison. L. E. (1963). A controlled trial of pollen adsorbate in the treatment of hay fever. *Scot. Med. J.*, **8**, 485

13. Patterson. R., Suszko. I. M. and McIntire, F. C. (1973). Polymerised ragweed antigen E. Preparation and immunological studies. *J. Immunol.*, **110**, 1402

14. Miller, A. C. M. and Tees, E. C. (1974). A metabolizable adjuvant clinical trial of grass pollen – tyrosine adsorbate. *Clin. Allergy*, **4**, 49

15. Miller, A. C. M. L. (1976). A comparative trial of hyposensitisation in 1973 in the treatment of hay fever using Pollinex and Alavac-P. *Clin. Allergy*, **6**, 551

16. Marsh. D. G., Lichtenstein. L. M. and Campbell, D. H. (1970). Studies on 'allergoids' prepared from naturally occurring allergens. 1. Assay of allergenicity and antigenicity of formalised rye Group 1 allergen. *Immunology*, **18**, 705

17. Ishizaka, K. and Ishizaka, T. (1978). Mechanisms of reaginic hypersensitivity and immunotherapy. *Lung*, **155**, 3

18. Sehon, A. H. and Lee, W. Y. (1979). Suppression of immunoglobulin E antibodies with modified allergens. *J. Allergy Clin. Immunol.*, **64**, 242

19. Bostock, J. (1819). *Med. Chir. Trans.*, **10**, 161

20. Blackley, C. H. (1873). *Experimental Researches on the Causes and Nature of Catarrhus aestivus*. London

21. Dunbar, W. P. (1903). *Zur Ursache and specifischen Hellung des Heufiebers*. München

22. Miller, A. C. M. L. (1976). A trial of hyposensitisation in 1974/5 in the treatment of hay fever using glutaraldehyde-pollen tyrosine adsorbate. *Clin. Allergy*, **6**, 557

23. Lichtenstein, L. M., Norman, P. S. and Winkerwerder, W. L. (1968). Clinical and *in vitro* studies on the role of immunotherapy in ragweed hay fever. *Am. J. Med.*, **44**, 514

24. Lichtenstein, L. M., Norman, P. S. and Winkerwerder, W. L. (1971). A single year of immunotherapy for ragweed hay fever. Immunologic and clinical studies. *Ann. Intern. Med.*, **75**, 663

25. Norman, P. S. and Winkerwerder, W. L. (1971). Maintenance immunotherapy in ragweed hay fever. *J. Allergy*, **47**, 273

26. Sadan, N., Rhyne, M. B., Mellits, E. D., Goldstein, E. O., Levy, D. A. and Lichtenstein, L. M. (1969). Immunotherapy of pollinosis in children. *N. Engl. J. Med.*, **280**, 623

27. Pence, H. L., Mitchell, D. Q., Greely, R. L. Updegraff, B. R. and Selfridge, H. A. (1976). Immunotherapy for mountain cedar pollinosis. *J. Allergy Clin. Immunol.*, **58**, 39

28. Mehta, S. B. and Smith, J. M. (1975). Nasal hyposensitisation and hay fever. *Clin. Allergy*, **5**, 279

29. D'Souza, M. F., Pepys, J., Wells, I. D., Tai, E., Palmer, F., Overall, B. G., McGrath, I. T. and Megson, M. (1973). Hyposensitisation with *Dermatophagoides pteronyssinus* in house dust allergy: a controlled study of clinical and immunological effects. *Clin. Allergy*, **3**, 177

30. Gabriel, M., Ng, H. K., Allan, W. G. L., Hill, L. E. and Nunn, A. J. (1977). Study of prolonged hyposensitisation with *Dermatophagoides pteronyssinus* extract in allergic rhinitis. *Clin. Allergy*, **7**, 325

31. Warner, J. O., Price, J. F., Soothill, J. F. and Hey, E. N. (1978). Controlled trial of hyposensitisation to *Dermatophagoides pteronyssinus* in children with asthma. *Lancet*. **2**. 912

32. Foucard, T. and Johansson, S. G. O. (1978). Allergen specific IgE and IgG antibodies in pollen allergic children given immunotherapy for 2–6 years. *Clin. Allergy*, **8**, 249

33. Knight, A., Underdown, B. J.. Demanuele, F. and Hargreave. F. E. (1976). Disodium cromoglycate in ragweed-allergic rhinitis. *J. Allergy Clin. Immunol.*, **58**. 278

34. Coffman, D. A. and Jenkins, M. (1975). Intranasal betamethasone valerate in seasonal rhinitis. *Practitioner*, **215**, 665

35. Szentivanyi, A. (1968). The β-adrenergic theory of the atopic abnormality in bronchial asthma. *J. Allergy Clin. Immunol.*, **42**, 203

36. Gold, M. (1973). Cholinergic pharmacology in asthma. In Austin, K. F. and Lichtenstein, L. M. (eds.) *Asthma, Physiology. Immunology and Treatment*, pp. 169–184. (New York: Academic Press)

37. Smith, M. J. (1973). Skin tests and atopic allergy in children. *Clin. Allergy*, **3**, 269

38. Johnstone. D. E. and Dutton. A. (1968). The value of hyposensitisation therapy for bronchial asthma in children: a 14 years study. *Paediatrics*, **42**. 793

39. McAllen, M. K., Heaf, P. J. D. and McInroy, P. (1967). Depot grass pollen injections in asthma. Effect of repeated treatment on clinical response and measured bronchial sensitivity. *Br. Med. J.*, **1**, 22

40. Lichtenstein, L. M., Norman, P. S., Bruce, C. A. and Rosenthal, R. R. (1975). Immunotherapy in extrinsic asthma. In Stein. M. (ed.) *New Directions in Asthma*, pp. 457–482. (American College of Chest Physicians)

41. Van Helmont. J. B. (1662). *Physick Refined*. (London: Lodwick Lloyd)

42. Voorhorst. R.. Spieksma-Boezeman. M. I. A. and Spieksma. F. T. M. (1964). Is a mite (*Dermatophagoides sp.*) the producer of the house dust allergen? *Allergie Asthma Forsch.*. **10**. 329

43. Forgacs, P. and Swan, A. D. (1968). Treatment of house dust allergy. A report from the Research Committee of the British Tuberculosis Association. *Br. Med. J.*, **3**, 774

44. Maunsell, K., Wraith, D. G. and Hughes, A. M. (1971). Hyposensitisation in mite asthma. *Lancet*, **1**, 967

45. Smith, A. P. (1971). Hyposensitisation with *Dermatophagoides pteronyssinus* antigen. Trial in asthma induced by house dust. *Br. Med. J.*, **4**, 204

46. Smith, M. J. and Pizarro, Y. A. (1972). Hyposensitisation with extracts of *Dermatophagoides pteronyssinus* and house dust. *Clin. Allergy*, **2**, 281

47. Gaddie, J., Skinner, C. and Palmer, K. N. (1976). Hyposensitisation with house dust mite vaccine in bronchial asthma. *Br. Med. J.*, **2**, 561

48. Aas, K. (1971). Hyposensitisation in house dust allergy asthma. *Acta Paediatr. Scand.*, **60**, 264

49. Frankland, A. W., Hughes, W. H. and Gorrill, R. H. (1955). Autogenous bacterial vaccines in treatment of asthma. *Br. Med. J.*, **2**. 941

50. Helander. E. (1959). Bacterial vaccines in the treatment of bronchial asthma. *Acta Allergol.*. **13**. 47

51. Prausnitz. C. and Kustner. H. (1921). Studien über die Ueberempfindlichkeit. *Zentralbl. Bakteriol.*. **86**. 160

52. Coca. A. F. and Grove. E. (1925). Studies in hypersensitiveness. XIII. A study of atopic reagins. *J. Immunol.*. **10**. 445

53. Ishizaka. K.. Ishizaka. T. and Hornbrook. M. M. (1966). Physico-chemical properties of reaginic antibody. IV. Presence of a unique immunoglobulin as a carrier of reaginic activity. *J. Immunol.*. **97**. 75

54. Ishizaka, T., Soto, C. S. and Ishizaka, K. (1973). Mechanisms of passive sensitisation. 3. Number of IgE molecules and their receptor sites on human basophil granulocytes. *J. Immunol.*, **111**, 500

55. Cooke, R. A., Barnard, J. H., Hebald, S. and Stull, A. (1935). Serological evidence of immunity with co-existing sensitisation in a type of human allergy (hay fever). *J. Exp. Med.*, **62**, 733

56. Lichtenstein, L. M., Holtzman, N. A. and Burnett, L. S. (1968). A quantitative *in vitro* study of the chromatographic distribution and immunoglobulin characteristics of human blocking antibody. *J. Immunol.*, **101**, 317

57. Lichtenstein. L. M.. Norman. P. S.. Winkerwerder. W. L. and Osler. A. G. (1966). *In vitro* studies of human ragweed allergy. Changes in cellular and humoral activity associated with specific desensitisation. *J. Clin. Invest.*, **45**, 1126

58. Pruzansky, J. J. and Patterson, R. (1967). Histamine release from leukocytes of hypersensitive individuals: II. Reduced sensitivity of leukocytes after injection therapy. *J. Allergy*. **39**, 44

59. Lichtenstein, L. M. and Levy, D. A. (1972). Is 'desensitisation' for ragweed hay fever immunologically specific? *Int. Arch. Allergy Appl. Immunol.*, **42**, 615

60. Yunginger, J. W. and Gleich, G. J. (1973). Seasonal changes in IgE antibodies and their relationship to IgG antibodies during immunotherapy for ragweed hay fever. *J. Clin. Invest.*, **52**, 1268

61. Levy, D. A., Lichtenstein, L. M., Goldstein, E. C. and Ishizaka, K. (1971). Immunologic and cellular changes accompanying the therapy of pollen allergy. *J. Clin. Invest.*, **50**, 360

62. Reisman, R. E., Wypych, J. I. and Arbesman, C. E. (1975). Relationship of immunotherapy, seasonal pollen exposure and clinical response to serum concentrations of total IgE and ragweed specific IgE. *Int. Arch. Allergy Appl. Immunol.*, **48**, 721

63. Foucard, T. and Johansson, S. G. O. (1976). Immunological studies *in vitro* and *in vivo* of children with pollenosis given immunotherapy with an aqueous and glutaraldehyde treated tyrosine adsorbed grass pollen extract. *Clin. Allergy*, **6**, 429

64. Stanworth, D. R. and Smith, A. K. (1973). Inhibition of reagin mediated PCA reactions in baboons by the human IgG$_4$ subclass. *Clin. Allergy*, **3**, 37

65. Devey, M. E., Wilson, D. V. and Wheeler, A. W. (1976). The IgG subclasses of antibodies to grass pollen allergens produced in hay fever patients during hyposensitisation. *Clin. Allergy*, **6**, 227

66. Platts-Mills, T. A. E., von Maur, R. K., Ishizaka, K., Norman, P. S. and Lichtenstein, L. M. (1976). IgA and IgG anti-ragweed antibodies in nasal secretions. Quantitative measurements of antibodies and correlation with inhibition of histamine release. *J. Clin. Invest.*, **57**, 1041

67. Rocklin, R. E., Pence, H., Kaplan, H. and Evans, R. (1974). Cell mediated immune response of ragweed sensitive patients to ragweed antigen E. *In vitro* lymphocyte transformation and elaboration of lymphocyte mediators. *J. Clin. Invest.*, **53**, 735

68. Evans, R., Pence, H., Kaplan, H. and Rocklin, R. E. (1976). The effect of immunotherapy on humoral and cellular responses in ragweed hay fever. *J. Clin. Invest.*, **57**, 1378

69. Romagnani, S., Biliotti, G. and Ricci, M. (1975). Depression of grass pollen induced lymphocyte transformation by serum from hyposensitised patients. *Clin. Exp. Immunol.*, **19**, 83

70. Okumura, K. and Tada, T. (1974). Regulation of homocytotropic antibody formation in the rat. IX. Further characterisation of the antigen-specific inhibitory T cell factor in hapten specific homocytotropic antibody response. *J. Immunol.*, **112**, 783

71. Kishimoto, T. and Ishizaka, K. (1974). Regulation of antibody response *in vitro*. VIII. Multiplicity of soluble factors released from carrier specific cells. *J. Immunol.*, **112**, 1685

9 PART I:
Allergic Disorders of the Eye

D. L. EASTY

INTRODUCTION

The eye and its adnexa offer a unique opportunity for the clinical and experimental observation of allergic reactions; the superficial tissues can be examined with the slit-lamp microscope and the optic media and the tissues of the posterior segment of the globe can be evaluated with the ophthalmoscope. The external eye may be examined by a less sophisticated technique with a simple pen torch and a × 8 magnifier. To examine the upper tarsal plate the upper lid is everted by taking the lashes with the finger tips of one hand using downwards pressure with a glass rod held in the other hand at the upper margin of the tarsal plate. Fluorescein and rose bengal drops (available in

Table 9.I.1 Target organs in allergic eye disease

Target organ	Disease
Lids	contact cutaneous allergy
Conjunctiva	allergic conjunctivitis
	contact conjunctivitis
Cornea	keratitis – peripheral
	– central
Episclera	episcleritis
Sclera	scleritis
Uvea iris	iritis ⎫
ciliary body	cyclitis ⎬ iridocyclitis
choroid	choroiditis
Lens	lens-induced uveitis
Retina	vasculitis – central
	– peripheral

unidose packs) are necessary to exclude epithelial deficits in the cornea such as in ulcerative herpetic keratitis. Signs of uveitis such as posterior synechiae can be seen with a loupe, but a flare or cells in the anterior chamber cannot be detected. Inflammatory disease in the deeper tissues may produce a haze in the optic media which can be seen with the ophthalmoscope, as can the manifestations of inflammatory disease of the retina and choroid if a careful search is made. Allergic disease of the target organs of the eye can therefore be observed and response to treatment can be accurately monitored (Table 9.I.1).

The conjunctiva possesses some of the features of a lymph node in the way in which it responds to infectious disease by the formation of lymphatic follicles which are capable of producing sensitized lymphocytes and antibody

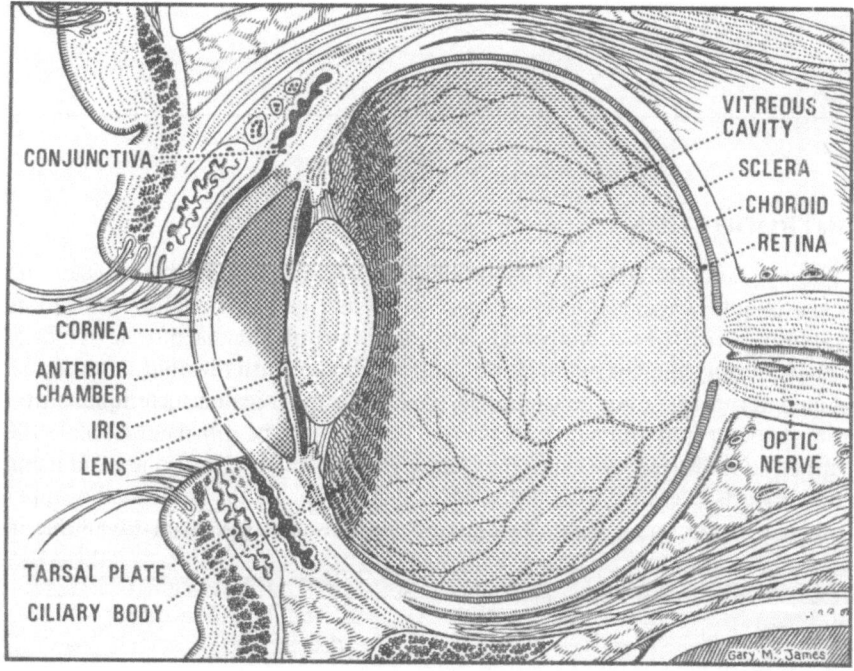

Figure 9.I.1   Corneal section of the eye in the orbit to demonstrate some of the target organs involved in immunological or allergic eye disease

in the immediate vicinity. The cornea has been thought to be a privileged tissue in the past, but it must be remembered that it is in intimate contact with the vascular system at the corneal–scleral junction (Figure 9.I.1) and is protected by the copious system of blood vessels in the tarsal plates. However, in spite of this it is the avascular cornea which is at risk of developing severe infective disease. In contrast the uveal tract is a vascular layer which has an intimate contact with the systemic immune system; it is therefore not uncommon for inflammatory disease of the uvea to be associated with systemic immuno-logical disease. The blood vessels of the anterior uvea in the iris and ciliary body and in the retina are similar to those in the central nervous system in that the vascular endothelium has tight intercellular junctions and it is the breakdown in this blood–aqueous and blood–vitreous barrier which is responsible for many of the well-known phenomena of inflammatory disease of the posterior or the anterior segments of the globe. It also accounts for the privileged nature of the internal optic media and explains the difficulties which are experienced in the management of intraocular infections.

Inflammatory eye disease has a special connotation because of the risks to the visual integrity of the eye. It is for this reason that a number of diseases in which an exogenous causal micro-organism is recognized are nevertheless known as hypersensitivity phenomena. Allansmith has suggested that the concept of allergic eye disease is dependent on evidence of specific antibody or sensitized cells in the blood or eye tissues, identifiable antigen, an appropriate animal model, and passive transfer of the disease accomplished with cells or serum. The possibility that an ocular disease may be allergic is suggested by the presence of specific antibody in higher quantities in the ocular fluids than elsewhere, the accumulation of plasma cell and lymphocytes at the site of the disease, the accumulation of immunoglobulins, together with the fixation of complement. Further indications of allergic disease rely on evidence such as inhibition of the disease by corticosteroid, the presence of eosinophils or degranulating mast cells, and the association of the eye disease with disease elsewhere for which an immune role has been proved or suggested[1].

The eyes and their adnexa therefore offer an important field of interest for the allergist or clinical immunologist because of the consequences that allergic diseases may have on visual function.

THE EXTERNAL EYE

The external eye, which is composed of the lids with their lining of conjunctiva and the transparent cornea, is protected from foreign materials by the blink reflex, irrigation by tears, and a barrier formed by the epithelial layers of the conjunctiva and corneal epithelium both of which possess tight intercellular junctions.

The transparency of the cornea is dependent upon a lattice of collagen fibrils which are arranged in layers in a matrix of glycoprotein and mucopolysaccharides. The fibrils are equidistant from each other and are of similar diameter. The concept of equidistant spacing between collagen fibrils is fundamental to the Maurice theory of transparency[2]. In contrast, the sclera, which is the continuation of the cornea, both of which form the outer coat of the eye, is non-transparent; the collagen fibrils vary in their distance between each other and in individual diameters, which is thought to be the reason why this layer is not transparent. The cornea is maintained in dehydration by a single layer of endothelium which acts as a bicarbonate ion pump[3] to remove excess fluid from the stroma and, when affected by disease, allows corneal swelling and loss of transparency. The curvature of the cornea refracts light and focuses it on the retina, the crystalline lens being responsible for accommodation or the precise focusing of light between infinity and near. It is because the integrity of the cornea is vital to vision that a knowledge of the allergic diseases which affect this layer is of value to the allergist or clinical immunologist who may occasionally be asked to help in investigation or management.

Protection of the ocular surface

In addition to mechanical factors, such as the blink reflex and the irrigating effect of tears, the eye surface is protected in its normal state by the presence of lysozyme and IgA in the tears[4] and by the presence of chronic inflammatory cells in the conjunctivae which have certain of the characteristics of a lymph node[5]. The presence of large numbers of lymphocytes, plasma cells, macrophages and neutrophils in the normal conjunctiva has been reported[6]; and the plasma cells have dilated rough endoplasmic reticulum indicating that they are involved in the production of local antibody in the tissues and possibly in the tears[7]. It may be shown in the laboratory that the corneal surface is protected by systemic immunization from invasion by micro-organisms such as the herpes simplex virus which has been experimentally inoculated in the corneal epithelium[8]. Although it has been demonstrated that tears contain specific antibody the tears are probably not the only mechanism for protection, there being a large amount of antibody in the local tissues as IgG[9], which may play a role and possibly represents a specific protective development against invasion of the privileged corneal surface[10].

ALLERGIC DISEASE OF THE EXTERNAL EYE

This takes a number of different forms which are dependent upon the target organ. The conjunctiva is capable of being sensitized by external allergens, or may respond to a number of micro-organisms to produce specific clinical pictures. In the avascular cornea, micro-organisms may cause hypersensitivity phenomena in the sense that inflammatory responses in this tissue will produce deterioration in vision, although it must be remembered that at the same time they inhibit proliferation. The corneal periphery seems to be particularly at risk of developing disease in association with a number of systemic disease processes which are thought to be caused by immunological mechanisms.

The skin of the lids can be affected by contact sensitivity, and several commonly used topical ophthalmic preparations are frequently the cause. The patient experiences itching and hypersensitivity to light, and the lids, particularly the lower ones, together with the upper part of the cheek in the case of drops, become erythematous and indurated. With chronic exposure to an offending allergen scaling and lichenification may occur.

Immediate hypersensitivity

Table 9.I.2 demonstrates the diseases of the external eye in which immediate hypersensitivity plays an important role in the immunopathogenesis, although it must be recognized that in the more complex forms such as vernal catarrh, other immunological processes are no doubt playing a part.

Table 9.I.2 Conjunctival and corneal responses to external allergens[7]

Infantile allergic conjunctivitis
Hay fever conjunctivitis
Vernal disease:
    (a) low grade; fine papillary reaction
    (b) moderate, with early cobblestone formation of the upper margin of the tarsal plate and a fine papillary reaction elsewhere
    (c) severe, with conglomerations of fine papillae forming 'cobblestones'
    (d) adult allergic conjunctivitis (fine papillae)
    (e) adult papillary (cobblestone)
Limbal vernal disease
    (a) transient hyperaemia and swelling, with cellular infiltration
    (b) limbitis with 'lace scarring'
    (c) Trantas' spots
    (d) pannus
Corneal vernal disease (secondary to conjunctival disease)
    (a) superficial punctate keratitis ⎰ upper half of cornea
    (b) superficial punctate erosions ⎱
    (c) pannus; occasionally deep stromal vascularization
    (d) massive epithelial deficit
    (e) chronic corneal ulceration with deposits of mucous plaque
    (f) possibility of permanent corneal scarring
    (g) possibility of secondary infections
Contact conjunctivitis
    (a) fine papillary ⎰ induced by plastic contact lens wear
    (b) cobblestone ⎱

Acute allergic conjunctivitis may occur as brief episodes in babies or infants when it presents as swelling of the conjunctiva without hyperaemia producing an elevated milky appearance.

Hay fever conjunctivitis is commonly associated with the nasal symptoms and follows the same seasonal incidence. During an attack there is itching and photophobia, the conjunctival blood vessels in the tarsal plates and bulbar conjunctivae become congested. Patients are aged between 10 and 25 years; occasionally the condition may persist for long periods.

The severity of allergic conjunctivitis in children or adults ranges between the mild and transient to the severe and persistent. Table 9.I.2 shows the diseases which may be encountered, some of which are not always easy to diagnose by clinical observation alone, particularly in the early stages, or in infants. Low grade conjunctivitis may present with mild itching and transient

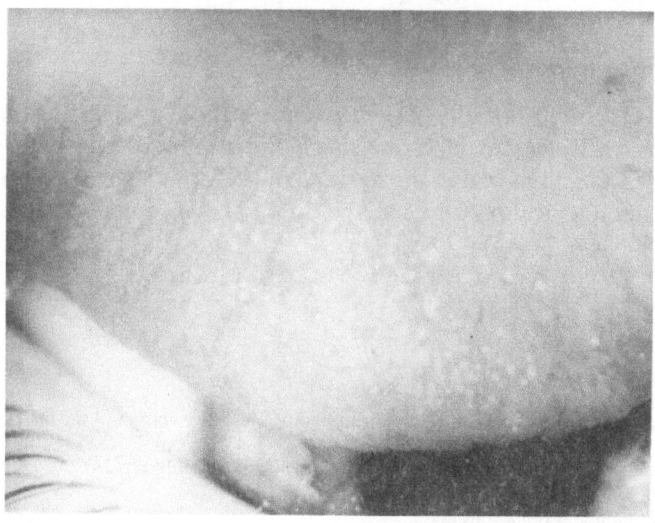

Figure 9.I.2 Everted upper tarsal plate in a patient with a mild papillary reaction due to low grade allergic conjunctivitis

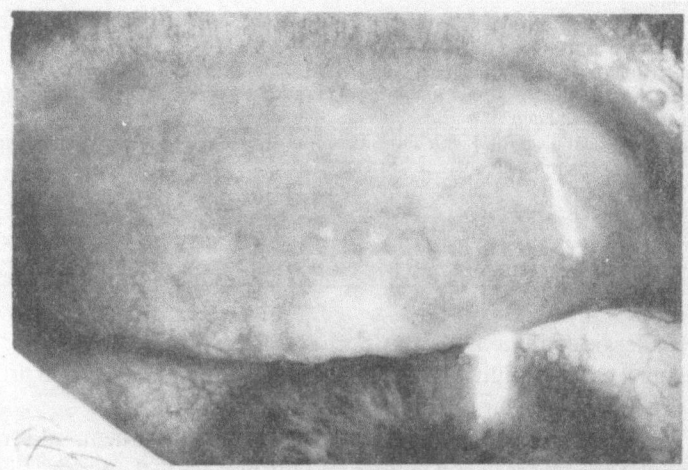

Figure 9.I.3 Everted upper tarsal plate in adult vernal disease, showing a fine papillary reaction, cellular infiltration, tissue hyperplasis and new vessel formation. Note that the vertical tarsal blood vessels are hidden by the reaction (compare with Figure 9.I.2)

soreness, ocular hyperaemia and chemosis, with changes in the tarsal plates which are barely distinguishable from the normal (Figure 9.I.2). With established disease fine papillae appear as minute excrescences composed of thickened epithelium with a central blood vessel and core of collagenous tissue (Figure 9.I.3). In the most severe disease, division of the micropapillae by downgrowths of hyperactive epithelium produces a cobblestone appearance

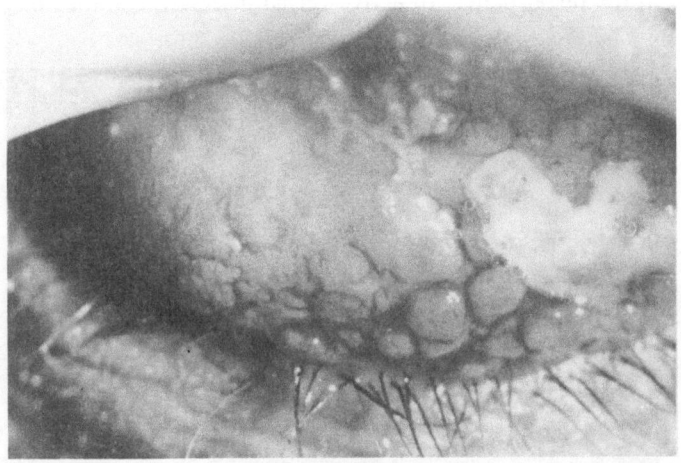

Figure 9.I.4 Everted upper lid in patient with vernal disease with massive cobblestone papillae which are swollen and hyperaemic, together with sticky mucous discharge, and lace-like scarring on the left side

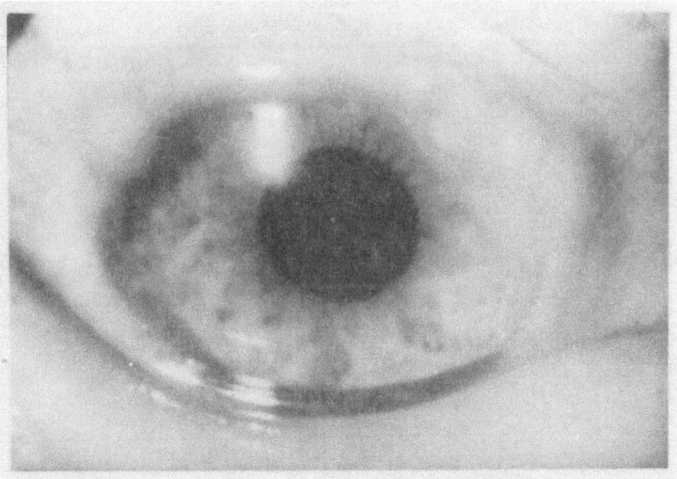

Figure 9.I.5 Limbal vernal disease in a 12-year-old boy with anhydrotic ectodermal dysplasia; there is a tendency for the limbal conjunctiva to extend on to the corneal surface

(Figure 9.I.4). During active disease the tarsal conjunctiva becomes hyper-aemic and there is diffuse oedema so that the papillae become swollen. In severe forms there is an increase in the number of mucous glands, which produce excessive amounts of thick and sticky discharge.

Though such syndromes are known as vernal or spring catarrh, the disease may occur throughout the year[11]. The disease may also affect the conjunctiva at the corneal–scleral junction (limbus) in isolation or in association with disease in the tarsal plates. In active vernal disease the limbus may become

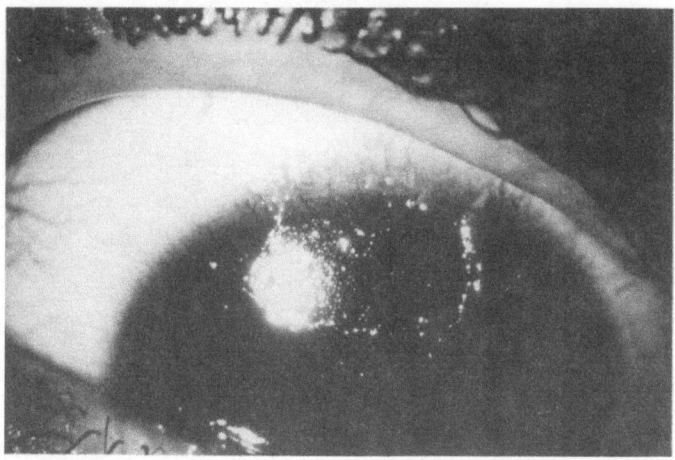

Figure 9.I.6   Large epithelial erosion in the upper portion of the cornea in a 10-year-old male with active vernal disease

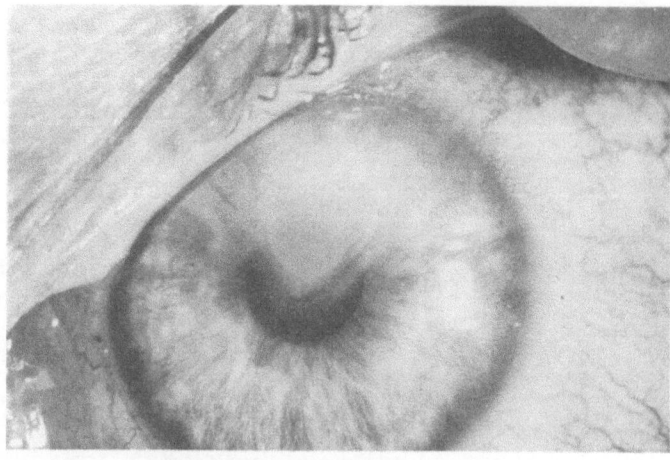

Figure 9.I.7   Mucous plaque formation in a 30-year-old male with adult vernal disease. Resolution occurred after surgical removal of the plaque

hyperaemic and oedematous, but also may respond by the production of epithelial hyperplasia, and excessive subepithelial collagen proliferation. A nodular appearance may be produced with a tendency towards overgrowth of the conjunctiva centrally across the corneal surface (Figure 9.I.5). Collections of cell debris may occur which form white spots on the surface of the limbal excrescences.

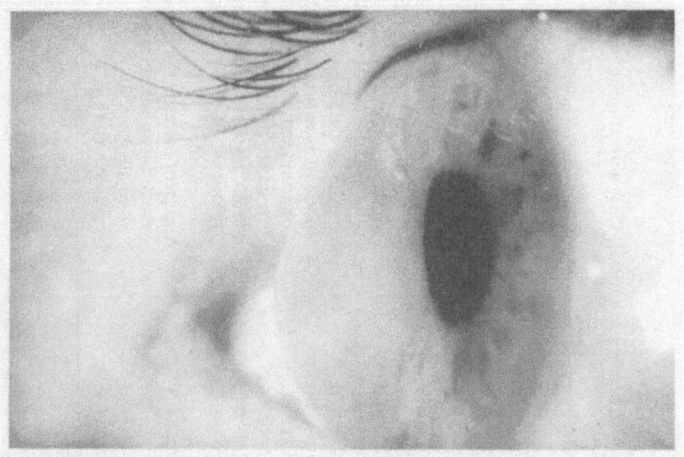

Figure 9.I.8 Keratoconus in a highly atopic male subject of 23 years with diffuse eczema and severe asthma (lateral view)

The cornea may become involved in its upper half with the appearance of a superficial punctate keratitis, the epithelium becoming necrotic and being shed in places to produced micro-erosions. The erosions eventually coalesce in untreated disease to produce a large abrasion (Figure 9.I.6) on to the base of which mucus may adhere in layers which result in a persistent plaque preventing regeneration of the epithelium (Figure 9.I.7). The resultant chronic ulcer is incapacitating and may lead to permanent scarring and loss of vision.

Eye disease in association with severe atopy

Vernal disease occurs in association with severe atopy in the form of eczema or asthma in approximately 70% of affected individuals[11] (Table 9.I.3). However, such disease is not the only ocular association: 30–40% of patients with keratoconus (Figure 9.I.8) suffer from severe atopic disease of some sort, including vernal catarrh, and atopic patients can suffer infective disease of the lids or the cornea, and in particular herpes simplex keratitis may occur in a primary form or recurrent form with increased severity[12] (Figure 9.I.9, Table 9.I.3). A further unexpected complication occurs in patients with corneal conditions requiring keratoplasty, including those with keratoconus

Table 9.1.3 Mean serum IgE levels in patients with vernal disease, keratoconus, herpetic keratitis (HSK) with atopic disease, and corneal graft failure in association with severe atopic disease[7]

Group	Mean age (years)	Number of male and female patients (M/F)	Percentage of patients with IgE > 200 u/ml	Serum RAST* for common allergens	Comments
Vernal disease	13.9	27/5	75%	Strongly +ve with common allergens	Associated with severe atopy in 70% of patients
Keratoconus	28.5	24/12	45%	Weakly +ve with common allergens	Associated with atopy in 30–40% of patients occasionally with vernal disease or conjunctival contact allergy
HSK + severe atopy	32	9/3	55%	Strongly +ve in severe disease	Even severe primary disease may be self-limited. In recurrent disease, the frequency of allergic reactions is increased
Graft failures	25	7/0	100%	Generally +ve	Apparent increased postoperative reactions to foreign tissue in those with +ve allergy tests
Controls	44	19/11	5%	Generally −ve	Negative history of atopic disease

* RAST = Radioallergosorbent test

not responding to conservative measures such as contact lenses, or patients who have undergone corneal scarring as a result of infectious disease (Figure 9.I.10). Table 9.I.3 shows some of the complications which have been met in a group of grafted patients all of whom had severe atopic disease, and in whom the serum IgE was grossly elevated[7].

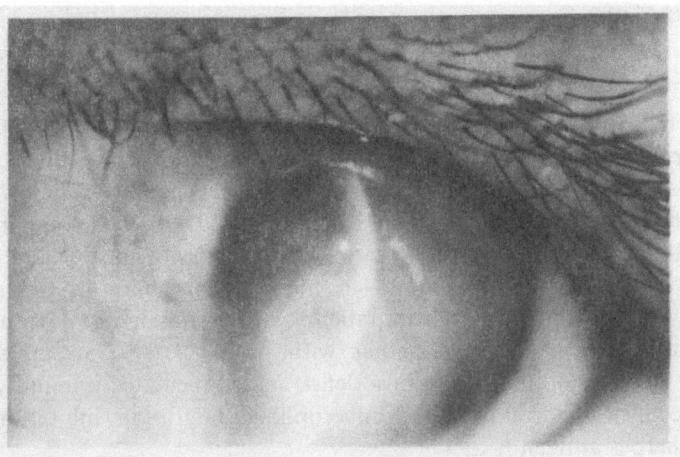

Figure 9.I.9 Corneal ulceration in a 25-year-old male patient with keratoconus, eczema, asthma and vernal disease. A keratoplasty was performed following eventual perforation

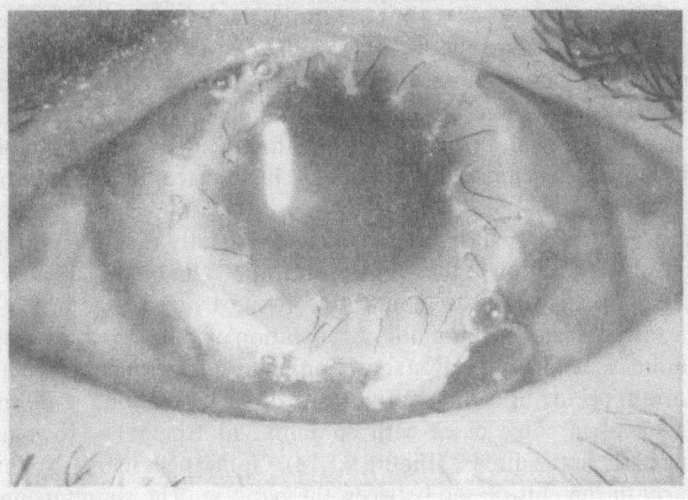

Figure 9.I.10 Corneal graft failure in a severely atopic subject with keratoconus. There is dense infiltration at the interface between donor and recipient with erosion through the stroma of fine suture material

A recurring feature in the atopic individual is the inability of corneal epithelium to regenerate; deficits which occur in vernal catarrh, herpetic keratitis, and in following keratoplasty, are persistent in this unfortunate group of patients.

Investigation

Patients with vernal catarrh and keratoconus demonstrate elevation of serum IgE in 75% and 45% of subjects respectively (Table 9.I.3). Serum RAST in small groups of vernal patients and keratoconus confirm the atopic status of these groups in that they both show positive responses to the common allergens as well as demonstrating in vernal subjects positive skin tests[11].

Tear fluid taken by capillary tubes can be assessed with RAST and it can be shown that scores found in the tears correspond with those found in the serum[7]. Histamine can be found in human tears both in the normal production but at higher levels in patients with vernal disease[13]. In patients with severe atopic disease together with primary or recurrent herpetic keratitis, there is no indication of a deficit in cell-mediated immunity using lymphocyte transformation and macrophage migration inhibition with specific herpes antigen[12].

Pathology

Biopsies taken from the upper tarsal plate indicate that there are a large number of inflammatory cells in *normal* conjuctiva which include lymphocyte infiltrations and plasma cells together with mast cells (Figure 9.I.11), but eosinophils are generally absent[6]. The degree of inflammatory response in biopsies in allergic conjunctivitis depends not only on the activity but also on treatment, together with the length of time that the disease has been present, the changes being less marked if the disease has existed for a short period of time.

The histology of vernal disease has been frequently described using light microscopy[14]. In addition to the cellular infiltration (Figures 9.I.12 and 9.I.13) there is a marked degree of connective tissue hyperplasia, which has a tendency towards later eosinophilic degeneration of collagen fibres. Capillary proliferation is seen in the early stages. Epithelial changes tend to occur early, proliferation occurring concomitantly with degeneration, with marked thickening and in some cases with columnar or triangular downgrowths appearing early in the disease (Figure 9.I.14). Goblet cells increase in number particularly in the culs-de-sac between the papillae. The simultaneous proliferation and degeneration of the epithelium results in the transformation of stratified columnar cells to stratified squamous cells, and keratinization may be present.

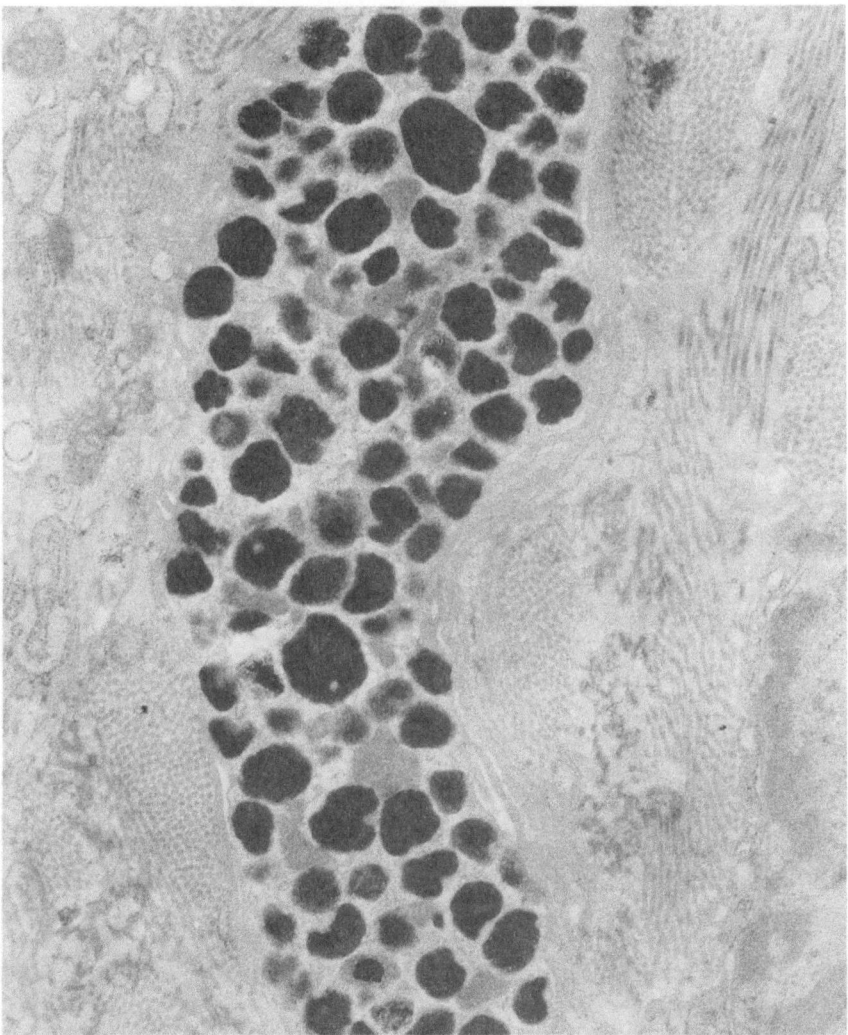

Figure 9.I.11   Mast cell with normal granular structure found in a conjunctival biopsy taken from a patient with a negative history of external eye disease (× 10 800). (Courtesy Dr Margaret Birkenshaw)

Electron microscopy (EM) of normal conjunctiva in patients with negative histories of external eye disease demonstrates a normal distribution of collagen fibres in the substantia propria, with normal epithelial cells. The majority of plasma cells are 'normal' with rough endoplasmic reticulum (RER) of flattened spaces parallel to each other and to the surface membrane. In many cells the RER can be active with dilated cisternae indicating the probable active production of local immunoglobulin[7]. Active Golgi regions

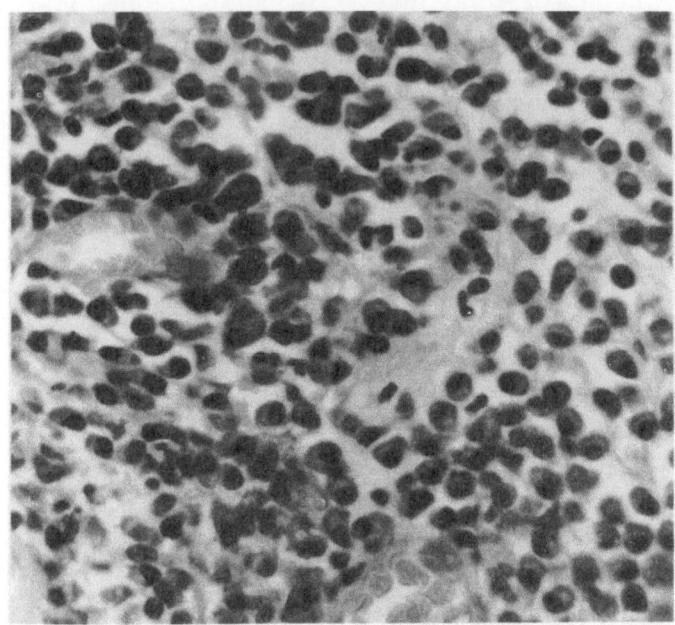

Figure 9.I.12 Infiltration with plasma cells, lymphocytes and eosinophils in a conjunctival biopsy taken from a subject with vernal disease (× 510). (Courtesy Dr Gwyn Morgan)

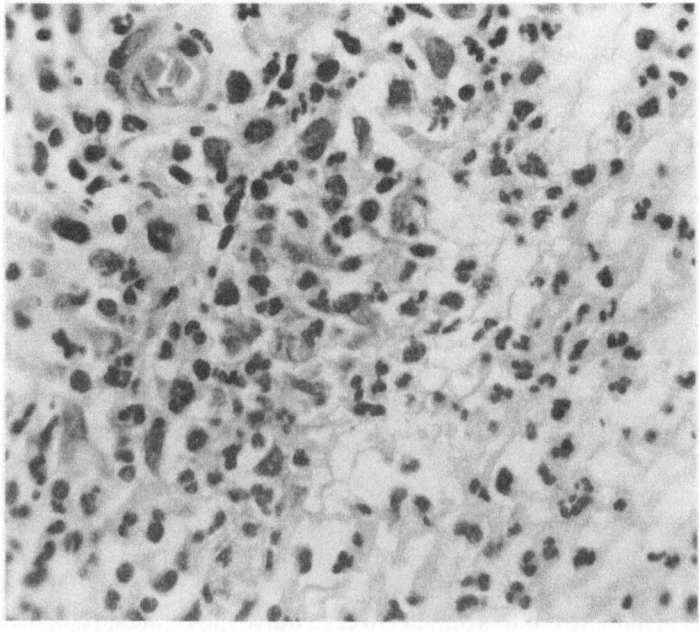

Figure 9.I.13 Eosinophil infiltration in a biopsy taken in vernal disease (× 570). (Courtesy Dr Gwyn Morgan)

can sometimes be pushed to the side of the cell. Numerous mast cells can be seen, most of which are entire, although a few can be seen to be degranulating. Plasma cells and mast cells are closely associated with each other and there are no eosinophils[7]. The conjunctiva even in the quiescent state therefore features many inflammatory cells and it seems likely these cells afford a degree of protection against external invasive organisms.

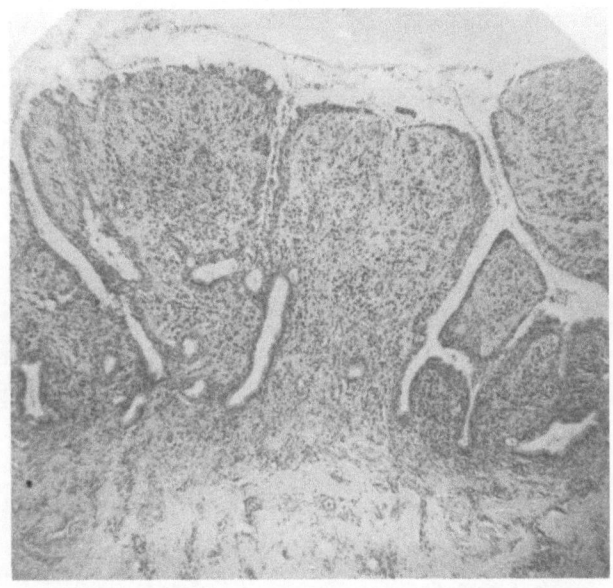

Figure 9.1.14 Cobblestone formation with infiltration with inflammatory cells and cyst formation (× 53). (Courtesy Dr Gwyn Morgan)

In early untreated vernal disease EM shows that the epithelial cells are separated by wide spaces containing cell debris and are infiltrated by neutrophils and eosinophils. Some of the epithelial cells may be stellated and have dendritic processes in contact with the subepithelial layer. The substantia propria may contain lymphocytes, eosinophils, mast cells, macrophages, neutrophils and plasma cells, the latter present in massive numbers. Both inactive and active plasma cells are found in association with mast cells, the basement membrane of the epithelium and encircling microvessels. Some of these cells, as would be expected, form IgE similar to those found in other mucous membranes[15, 16]. In patients undergoing active disease mast cells can be seen to be degranulating towards the surface (Figure 9.1.15) while those situated more deeply may be entire[7]. Degranulated mast cells may occasionally be found in the epithelium.

The important corneal complications which occur with active vernal disease are probably induced by the production of mediators by degranulating mast

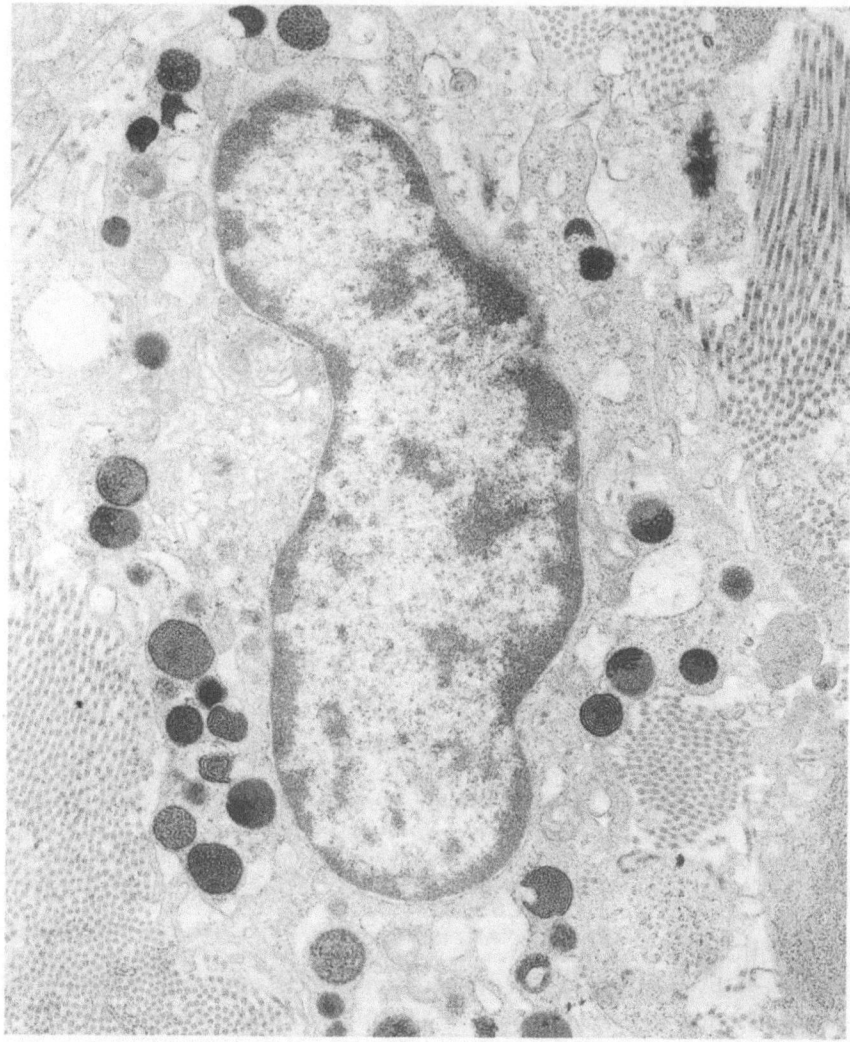

Figure 9.I.15 Degranulating mast cell from patient with active vernal disease (× 15 000).
(Courtesy Dr Margaret Birkenshaw)

cells in the upper tarsal plates. Such mediators which include histamine and 5-hydroxytryptamine cause foci of cell necrosis in the corneal epithelium, which coalesce to form a massive erosion on to the surface of which layers of mucus may adhere. The inability of corneal ulcers to heal in herpetic disease and the tendency towards prolonged corneal erosions following keratoplasty are again related to the degranulation of mast cells in the atopic subject. The continuing production of mediators in the tears is not provoked by external allergens alone and may occur as a result of a number of other triggers.

Vernal disease is not the only cause of giant papillary conjunctivitis, the prolonged use of contact lenses or artificial eyes produces a similar appearance[7]. Sarcoidosis may occasionally be associated with the occurrence of such papillae (Figure 9.1.16).

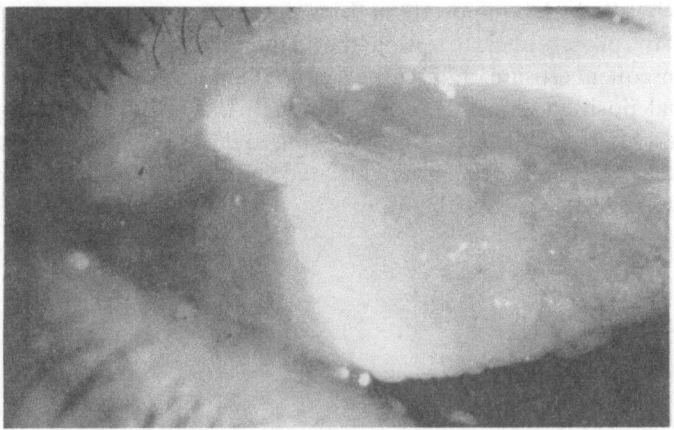

Figure 9.1.16 Papillary reaction in patient with sarcoidosis

Treatment

The symptoms of allergic eye disease may be disturbing, both in the patient with hay fever conjunctivitis or in vernal disease with its concomitant atopy and elevated serum IgE. In vernal subjects it has not been found helpful to desensitize to specific allergens, and treatment is prescribed according to symptoms, with antihistamine or disodium cromoglycate drops[18]. However severe exacerbations do not respond to such therapy, and resort to the use of topical steroid is necessary. The long-term use of such agents carries the risk of causing a cataract or a transient rise in intraocular pressure, both of which may lead to irreversible loss of vision (Table 9.1.8). Such risks are particularly evident in the subject with vernal disease where the use of steroids can effectively control the symptoms and it is in these patients that therapy should be used only for acute exacerbations where the integrity of the corneal surface is threatened. Where plaques of mucus have been laid down and there is poor regeneration of the epithelium, a simple surgical removal of the plaque can result in a rapid resolution of an incapacitating disease process[19].

Autoimmune diseases of the external eye

The diseases of the external eye which are thought to be autoimmune include cicatricial mucous membrane pemphigoid, peripheral corneal melting syndrome, Sjögren's syndrome, and Cogan interstitial keratitis.

Cicatricial mucous membrane pemphigoid is a rare disease of the conjunctiva, which undergoes shrinkage due to scarring, and the tarsal conjunctiva may become adherent to its bulbar counterpart, or to the surface of the cornea (Figure 9.I.17). The conjunctival fornices become shallow, and the epithelium becomes keratinized and loses many goblet cells which normally produce the mucous layer which is important in the maintenance of a stable tear film. As a result of the process of cicatrization, the lid margins become distorted inwards with consequent erosion of the corneal epithelium. In addition, lashes grow in abnormal position along the lids – although this is difficult to appreciate without adequate magnification. As a consequence of all these factors, the cornea may eventually become vascularized and develop epithelial defects and scarring in the stroma, leading to loss of vision and sometimes to complete blindness.

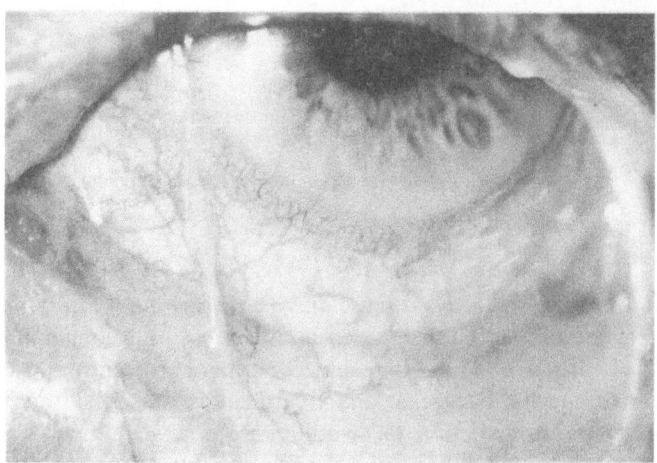

Figure 9.I.17 Lower conjunctival fornix in a patient with cicatricial mucous membrane pemphigoid. The conjunctiva becomes stretched forming an elevated fold in depression of the lower lid

Although it is a rare disease it is of importance because of its chronicity and relentless course requiring frequent hospital visits to maintain therapeutic control. The disease provides one of the most serious problems with which the ophthalmologist has to contend. It may present as a desquamative gingivitis with oral and nasal ulceration frequently present, together with skin and genital ulcers[20]. Immunofluorescent studies of conjunctival biopsies taken from such patients show basement membrane deposits of IgG or IgA in 40% of patients[21]. Circulating IgG antibodies have been demonstrated in a small percentage of patients against conjunctival basement membrane[22].

Treatment depends upon the replacement of the tears with artificial substitutes, and protection from infection with antibiotics. The use of topical corticosteroid can be damaging and is liable to lead on to corneal infections unless used in a dilute form. However, at an early stage of the disease, where staining with fluorescein drops may demonstrate ulceration of the conjunctiva, there may be a considerable therapeutic effect[23]. The use of systemic immunosuppressive agents has not proved to be successful.

The practolol ocular toxicity syndrome is somewhat reminiscent of cicatricial mucous membrane pemphigoid in which, by means of indirect immunofluorescence, autoantibody has been identified directed against the intercellular determinants of epithelial substrates[24]. Antibody could also be found in tears[25] and in biopsy material[26].

CORNEAL ALLERGIC DISEASE

Immune complex disease of the cornea may be produced experimentally in passively sensitized animals following injection of protein antigen into the corneal stroma. Antigen–antibody precipitation may be induced, located concentrically around the site of injection[27, 28]. Similar rings may be seen in certain corneal infections such as herpetic keratitis (Figure 9.1.18).

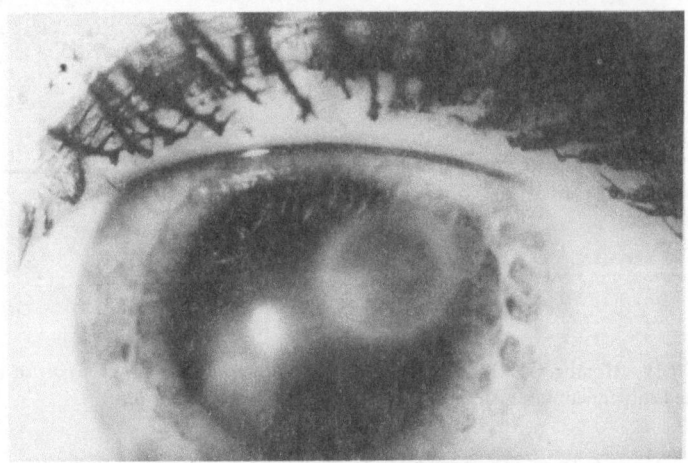

Figure 9.1.18 Corneal immune ring formation following primary herpes simplex keratitis. (Courtesy Editor. *The Practitioner*)

The success of corneal transplants was for long thought to be due to the lack of antigenicity of the corneal elements, the rapid death of donor cellular layers and their replacement by those of the host before an immune response could be initiated. It was postulated that an adaptation of the graft within the host rendered it less susceptible to specific rejection even in the presence of active sensitization in the host, another factor being the existence of the cornea as a privileged site[29, 30]. Following the demonstration that the corneal graft might be subject to immunological rejection[31, 32], it was found that an important feature deciding the success or failure of a transplant was the avascularity of the cornea. The prognosis for transplants performed in vascularized corneas is less good than in the avascular cornea[33], but it is not clear whether it is the afferent or the efferent limb of sensitization which is primarily responsible.

That the afferent limb is important was shown in experiments which demonstrated that some 90% of hitherto clear penetrating corneal allografts would undergo rejection following sensitizations of the host with a skin graft[34], which suggests that avascularity does not in itself present a barrier to graft rejection. It has been shown that the corneal epithelium, stroma, and endothelium can each be selectively rejected[35] and it is apparent that the corneal graft site enjoys a certain degree of privilege but is not exempt from rejection probably because the barrier of avascularity is not absolute.

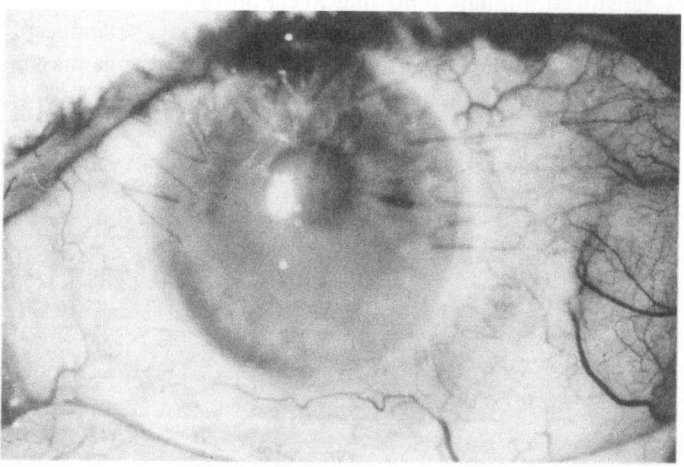

Figure 9.I.19 Homograft reaction producing stromal oedema in the lower part of the donor tissue, and subsequent visual deterioration

Rejection of the corneal endothelium is serious, because it is thought that this single cell layer fails to regenerate in the human, so that once stromal swelling recurs due to loss of endothelial function, urgent therapeutic measures must be taken if graft failure is to be avoided (Figure 9.I.19). Although the precise mechanism of such rejection is not understood, it has been shown that lymphocytes can reach the endothelium via the scar of the interface between recipient and host, or from the uveal tissue of the anterior segment (Figures 9.I.19–9.I.21).

There is now a certain amount of evidence which suggests that the sharing of two or more HLA antigens between the donor and recipient will reduce the

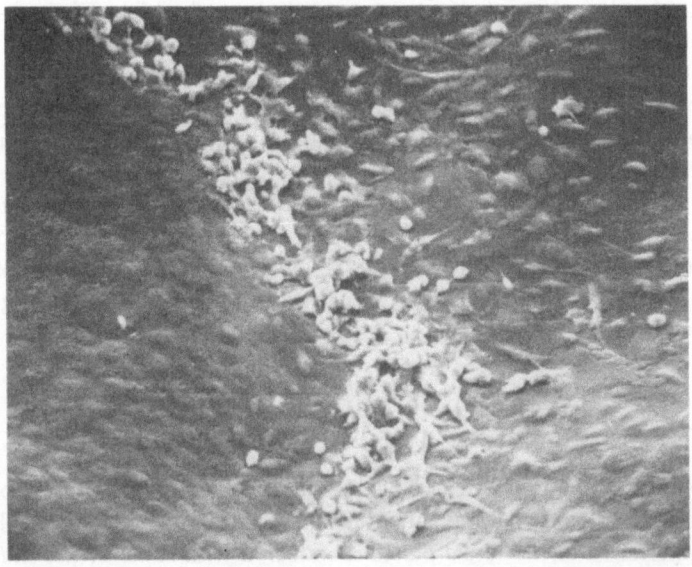

Figure 9.1.20 Line of lymphocytes and inflammatory cells causing cell death in their wake (SEM × 180). (Courtesy Dr Frank Pollack)

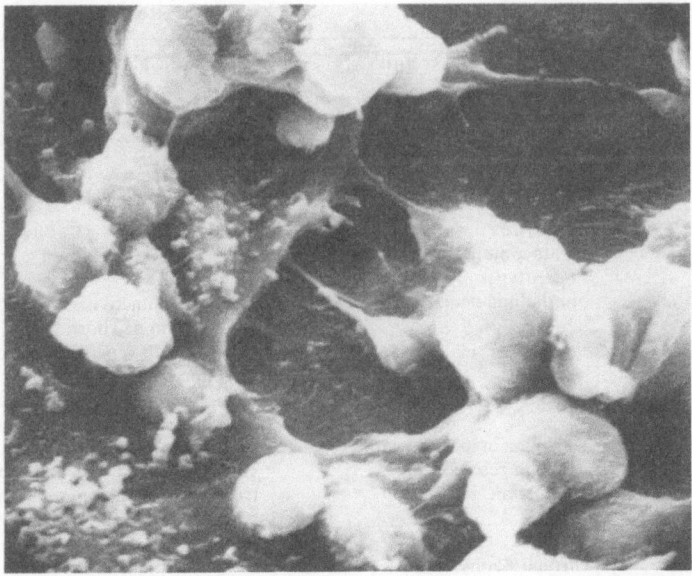

Figure 9.1.21 Scanning electron microscopy of lymphocytes involved in active endothelial rejection (SEM × 1800). (Courtesy Dr Frank Pollack)

incidence and severity of rejection particularly in the high-risk patient with active inflammatory disease of the anterior segment, or with corneal vessels present in the recipient at the time of the transplant[37]. Routine use of postoperative topical steroid medication can lessen the chances of such reactions, by reducing corneal vascularization, closing the junctions in between the endothelial cells of the iris vasculature, and inhibiting the spread of lymphocytes via the corneal stroma and through the anterior chamber. However, in such patients the risk of cataract or glaucoma from the continuing use of such medication is always present, which makes the necessity of careful matching of host and recipient using the HLA antigens the more important.

INFECTIVE DISEASE OF THE EXTERNAL EYE

The common infectious diseases of the external eye in which immunological mechanism may cause permanent tissue injury are demonstrated in Table 9.I.4. The conjunctiva of the tarsal plates is endowed with some of the character-istics of a lymphatic gland, and it may react to invasive organisms by the local production of antibody in the tears and serous exudation into the conjunctival sac, but also may produce lymphocyte follicles with germinal

Table 9.I.4 Infective diseases of the external eye where immunological mechanisms cause tissue damage in the cornea

Viral	herpes simplex keratitis	epithelial (ulcerative) stromal keratouveitis
	herpes zoster ophthalmicus	corneal stromal scarring nodular scleritis anterior uveitis vasculitis (iris)
	adenovirus keratoconjunctivitis (serotypes 8, 10, 19)	punctate keratitis
Chlamydial	ophthalmia neonatorum	follicular conjunctivitis and chronic discharge in newborn associated with venereal reservoir of infection
	inclusion conjunctivitis	follicular conjunctivitis and punctate epithelial keratitis
	trachoma associated with ocular reservoir of infection	follicular conjunctivitis producing conjunctival scarring and subsequent trichiasis and entropion; corneal vascularization (pannus) and opacification may occur
Bacterial	chronic staphylococcal infection	recurrent blepharitis marginal corneal ulceration rosacea keratitis phlyctenular keratitis

centres, which may easily be differentiated by the clinician (Figure 9.I.22). The inflammatory reaction in the tarsal plates will depend on the nature of the organism, cell-mediated responses occurring in diseases in which the organism is situated inside the cell, such as viral or chlamydial disease, which will therefore be associated with the appearance of follicles in the tarsal plates. By way of contrast, humoral processes will inhibit extracellular organisms, as in the case of bacterial infection, where the follicle formation seen in virus disease no longer occurs.

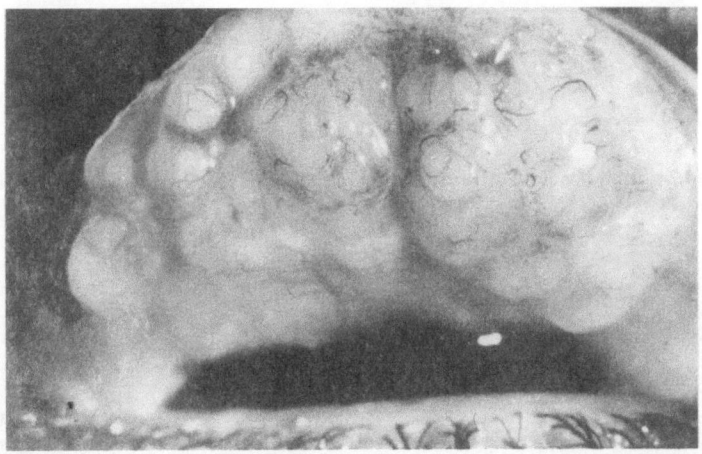

Figure 9.I.22 Massive follicles in the upper conjunctival fornix in a patient with hyperendemic trachoma. (Courtesy Dr Sorab Darougar)

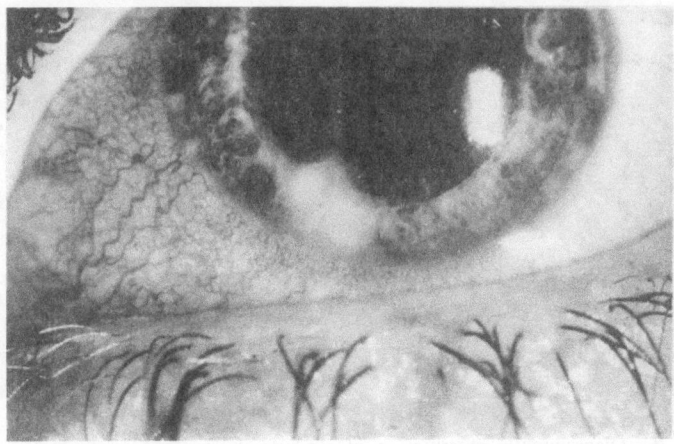

Figure 9.I.23 Peripheral corneal infiltrate in association with recurrent staphylococcal blepharitis. (Courtesy Editor, *The Practitioner*)

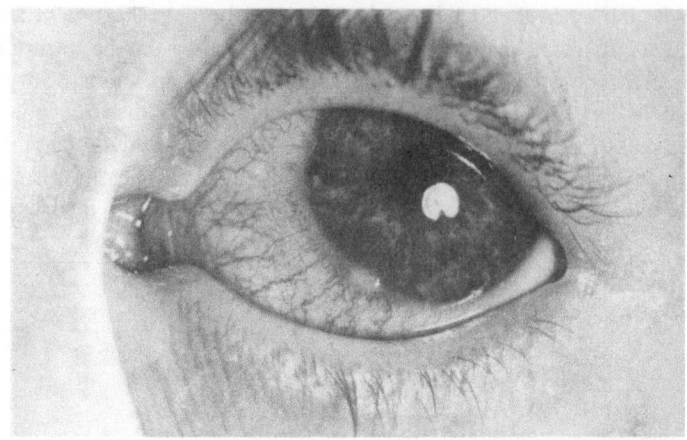

Figure 9.I.24 Phlyctenulosis of the conjunctiva in an 8-year-old boy. (Courtesy Editor, *The Practitioner*)

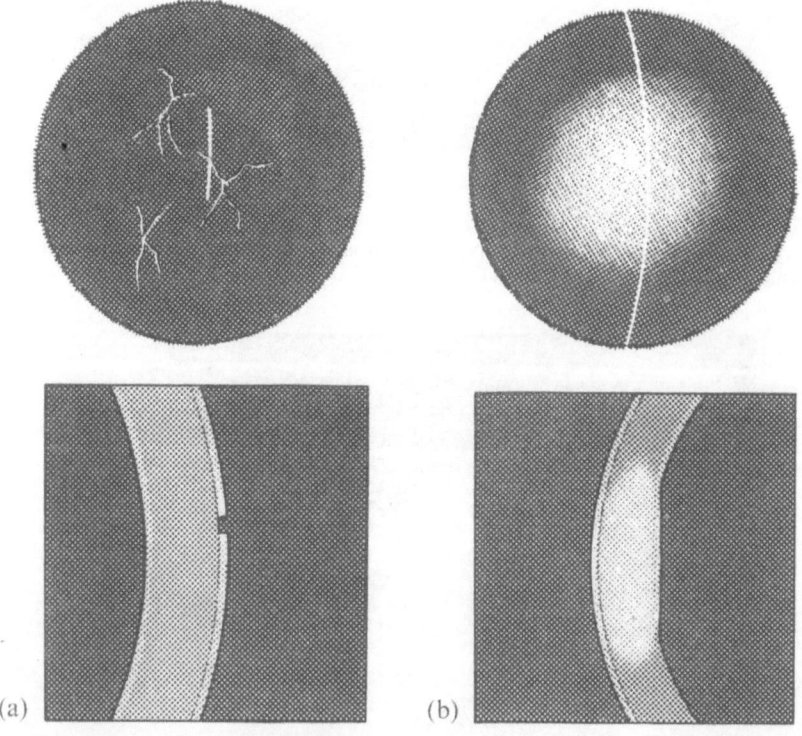

(a)   (b)

Figure 9.I.25 Diagrammatic presentation of slit-lamp microscope views of two corneal manifestations of herpes simplex infection; (a) ulcerative disease of the epithelium to form dendritic ulcers; (b) stromal disease following penetration of virus or viral antigen into the stroma where a chronic inflammatory process is set up

The staphylococcus is encountered as a pathogen in a number of diseases of the external eye and is a frequent cause of blepharitis, marginal corneal infiltrates or ulcers (Figure 9.I.23), and keratoconjunctivitis[38]. Catarrhal infiltrates occur at the limbus and are considered to be due to immune complex deposition at this position[20]. A similar but more aggressive allergic response occurs in phlyctenulosis (Figure 9.I.24), where an elevated limbal lesion may invade the corneal surface accompanied by a leash of blood vessels and leading to scarring. It is associated with severe photophobia which appears to be due to diffuse punctate epithelial erosions similar to those found in vernal disease, but involving the entire corneal surface. The presence of degranulating mast cells in conjunctival biopsies taken from such patients suggests that immediate hypersensitivity might be involved, although it has in the past been attributed to cell-mediated hypersensitivity to a microbial antigen such as the staphylococci, *Candida* and *Coccidioides*[39].

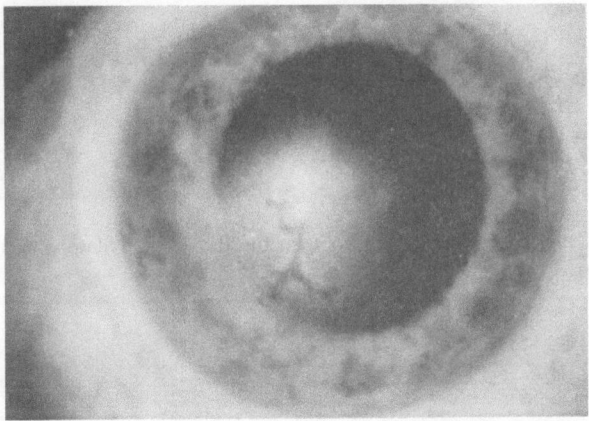

Figure 9.I.26 Ulcerative herpetic keratitis associated with stromal disease

Viruses, in the form of herpes simplex and zoster and adenovirus, may exist and proliferate in the epithelium of the cornea, and may penetrate the corneal stroma in the case of the herpes viruses to produce inflammatory responses in the stroma (Figure 9.I.25), particularly when ocular protective immunity is compromised[10] or systemic immunity is deficient[40]. It is known that the corneal stroma is rich in IgG and it can be shown that specific antibody may be sequestered in the stroma[41]; thus immune complex formation following antigen penetration of the stroma is easily explained with the consequent release of complement and attraction of inflammatory cells followed by tissue damage as in the case of herpetic keratitis[42, 43] (Figure 9.I.26). The stromal responses occurring in infections with herpes zoster or adenovirus (Figure 9.I.27) have not been investigated and so the mechanism of their production is ill-understood.

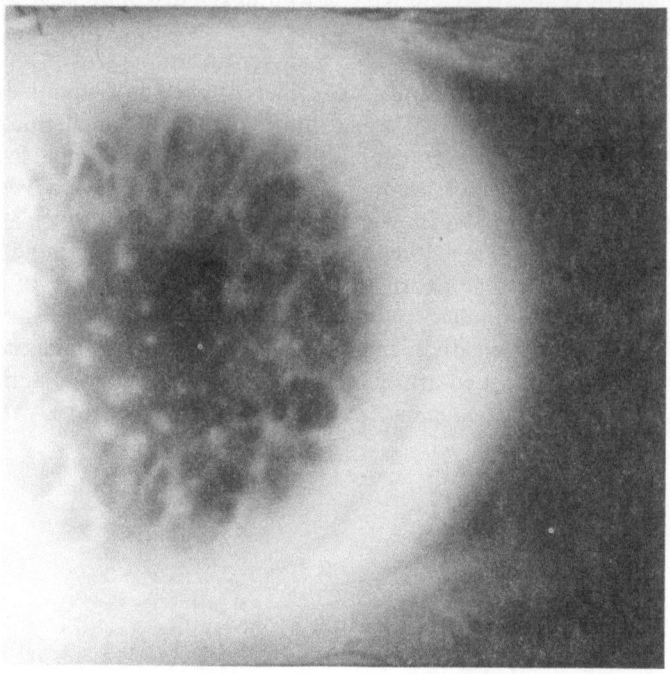

Figure 9.I.27   Punctate corneal opacities situated in the stroma following adenovirus Type 8 infection

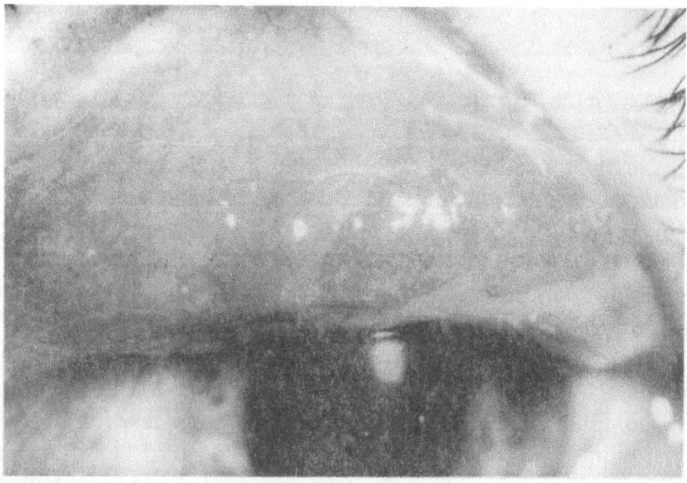

Figure 9.I.28   Follicles in the upper fornix of the conjunctiva in a patient with inclusion conjunctivitis due to *Chlamydia trachomatis*

Infection of the eye with chlamydial organisms may cause a follicular conjunctivitis at birth, childhood or adulthood. In Europe where the organism is transmitted via a venereal route, ocular infections produce a follicular conjunctivitis (Figure 9.1.28), with a spontaneously resolving punctate epithelial keratitis, but in endemic areas where reinfection is frequent[44], corneal damage may ensue with vascularization and opacification of the stroma (Figure 9.1.29). The precise mechanisms of corneal injury in trachoma in contrast to inclusion conjunctivitis are not yet clearly understood, but it seems likely that both humoral and cell-mediated processes are of importance in both immunity and tissue damage[45].

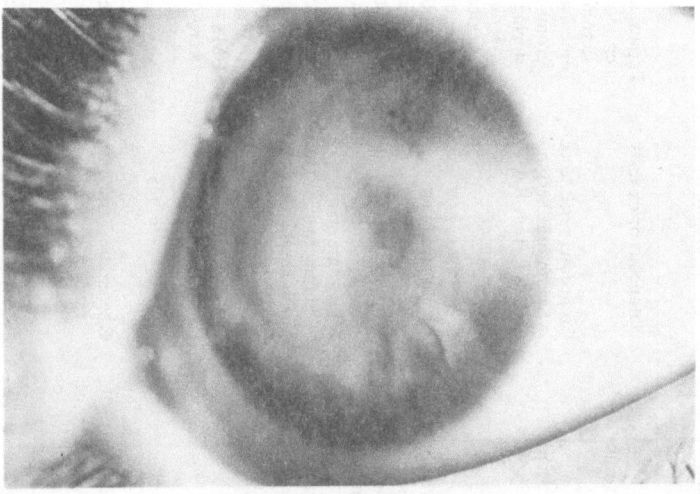

Figure 9.1.29 Diffuse corneal scarring in a patient with hyperendemic trachoma. (Courtesy Dr Sorab Darougar)

ALLERGIC EYE DISEASE ASSOCIATED WITH SYSTEMIC DISEASE

Table 9.1.5 demonstrates how some inflammatory diseases of the external eye, uvea, and the retina may occur in association with systemic disease, in which an immunological process in the mechanism has been invoked, although this has not yet been precisely identified.

Inflammatory disease of the sclera

This may involve the episclera in a simple or nodular form, or the sclera as diffuse, nodular or necrotizing forms. Simple episcleritis occurs in females in their forties with symptoms of redness and grittiness[46]. The onset may be

Table 9.1.5 Allergic eye disease associated with systemic disease

Systemic disease	Associated ocular disease	Immunological mechanisms and features	Investigations	Treatment of eye disease
Hay fever	Papillary conjunctivitis	Immediate hypersensitivity	Cutaneous prick tests	Topical antihistamine, disodium cromoglycate, or short-term topical steroid (i.e. for 1 to 2 weeks)
Atopic asthma or eczema	Vernal disease. Papillary conjunctivitis of variable severity. Occasional secondary keratitis	Immediate hypersensitivity	Cutaneous prick tests. Serum IgE. Serum RAST. Tear RAST	Topical antihistamine, disodium cromoglycate. Topical corticosteroid during exacerbation. If perennial, then low dosage systemic corticosteroid. Surgical removal for corneal plaque formation
Rheumatoid arthritis (adult)	Keratoconjunctivitis sicca (KCS) in 10–15% (If xerostomia = Sjögren's syndrome). Nodular episcleritis, and scleritis. Peripheral corneal melting syndrome (PCMS)	Little known about eye disease. Lymphoid aggregations in lacrimal gland. Some deposition of immune complexes	Rheumatoid factor. Reduced tear production (Schirmer's test). Typical punctate staining of conjunctiva in inter-palpebral strip (with rose bengal). Sedimentation rate raised. ESR +	KCS – Replacement therapy with artificial tears. Episcleritis; short-term topical corticosteroid; oxyphenbutazone. Scleritis; oxyphenbutazone or indomethacin in milder cases; topical corticosteroid and oxyphenbutazone; systemic immunosuppression if threat to vision. PCMS – Topical anticollagenases; topical steroid; if associated with scleritis, removal of conjunctival strip alongside ulcer, systemic immunosuppression if threat to vision
Juvenile (mono- or oligo-articular)	Bilateral chronic iridocyclitis. Band keratopathy. Cataract	Probably different mechanisms of tissue damage according to type	Rheumatoid and anti-nuclear factor. ESR +	Topical corticosteroid and mydriatics; occasional systemic steroid
Ankylosing spondylitis	Recurrent anterior uveitis	Precise immunological mechanisms not identified	Rheumatoid factor – ve; HLA B27 in nearly all. ESR +	Topical corticosteroid and cycloplegics
Reiter's disease	Conjunctivitis and corneal infiltrates. Iridocyclitis	Precise mechanisms not identified	Rheumatoid factor – ve; HLA B27 often found. ESR +	Topical corticosteroid and cycloplegics

Behçet's disease	Recurrent hypopyon. Uveitis. Retinal arteritis. Vitritis	Immunological disease or genetic pre-disposition to a particular virus disease	HLA B5. Antibody against fetal oral mucosa. ESR +	Topical corticosteroid and cycloplegics. Systemic immunosuppression
Systemic lupus erythematosus	Keratoconjunctivitis sicca. Cotton wool exudate and haemorrhages in retina	Circulating auto-antibodies. Decreased serum complement. Immune complexes. T lymphocyte depletion	Autoantibodies. Rheumatoid factors. Cryoglobulins. ESR +	Systemic therapy with corticosteroid and immunosuppression
Polyarteritis nodosa	Retinopathy (hypertensive). Cotton wool exudates. Episcleritis/scleritis. Uveitis. Peripheral corneal melting syndrome	Possible role of immune complexes	Rheumatoid factor. Histology of skin or renal biopsy. ESR +	Corticosteroids and immunosuppression
Wegener's granulomatosis	Exophthalmos. Cotton wool retinal exudates. Uveitis: scleritis: peripheral corneal melting syndrome	Necrotizing granulomatous reaction around small arteries and veins	Leukocytosis. Thrombocytopaenia Eosinophilia. ESR +	Systemic corticosteroid and immuno-suppression
Sarcoidosis	Conjunctival nodules. Episcleritis. Band keratopathy. Irido-cyclitis. Secondary cataract. Retinal exudates. Cystoid macular oedema	Depleted cell-mediated immunity	Hypergammaglobulin-aemia. hypercalcaemia. TB anergy. Kveim reaction +ve. X-ray studies	Topical and systemic corticosteroid cycloplegics
Erythema multiforme	Acute purulent conjunctivitis with membrane formation. Later, conjunctival cicatrization and symblepharon. Entropion trichiasis. corneal vascularization and scarring. Reduction in tear production	Possible role of hyper-sensitivity to drug and micro-organism. forming hapten link with cell surface	Search for *Mycoplasma* organisms	Artificial tears. Topical antibiotic. Cautious topical corticosteroid. Lid surgery

sudden and the redness is diffuse. The aetiology is not known, although there is limited evidence of an association with atopic disease.

Nodular episcleritis presents with symptoms similar to diffuse episcleritis (Figure 9.I.30), but the course of the disease is more protracted and again females are affected more commonly than males[46]. The nodule is composed histologically of mononuclear cells and eosinophils. Diffuse anterior scleritis is associated with systemic immunological disease in approximately 10% of patients, rheumatoid arthritis being the most common. The condition is commonest in females between 40 and 70 years of age, and the onset is insidious and is therefore occasionally misdiagnosed.

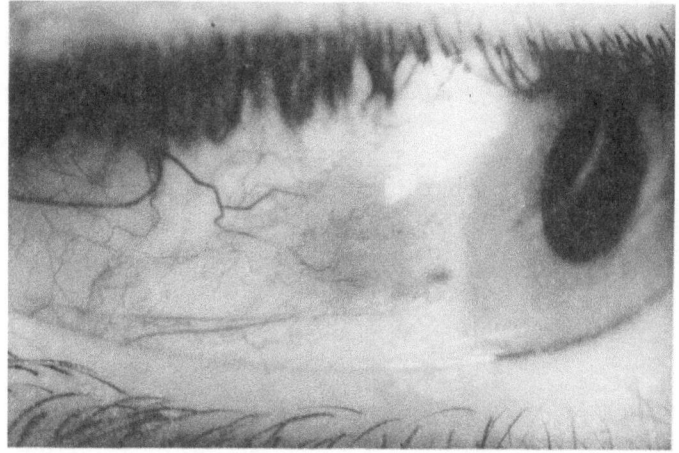

Figure 9.I.30 Nodular episcleritis in a 23-year-old female patient

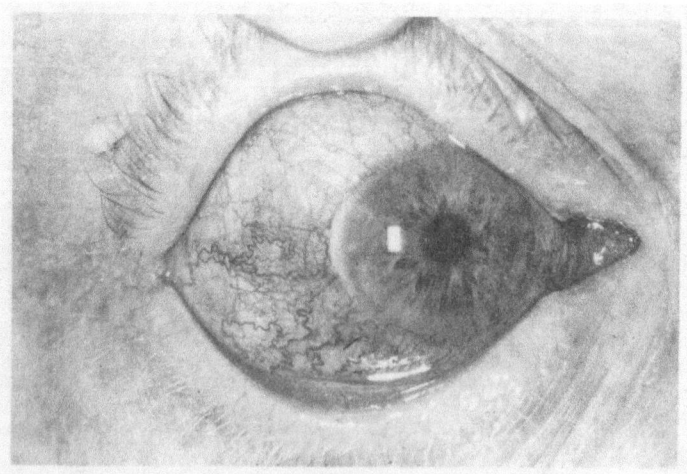

Figure 9.I.31 Nodular scleritis in a 42-year-old male without other systemic disease

Nodular scleritis (Figure 9.1.31) is associated with pain and severe tenderness and has a deep red or violet colour. The condition is associated with systemic disease with immunological features in a low percentage of patients, one of the commonest associations being herpes zoster ophthalmicus[47].

Necrotizing scleritis may occur with or without inflammation and because of its destructive properties may give the greatest difficulty to the clinician. The seriousness of the condition is indicated from the results of a large series[47], where 60% of patients developed ocular or systemic complications, 40% suffered a significant loss of visual acuity and 29% died within 5 years of the onset of the disease. Pain and discomfort are the presenting features and

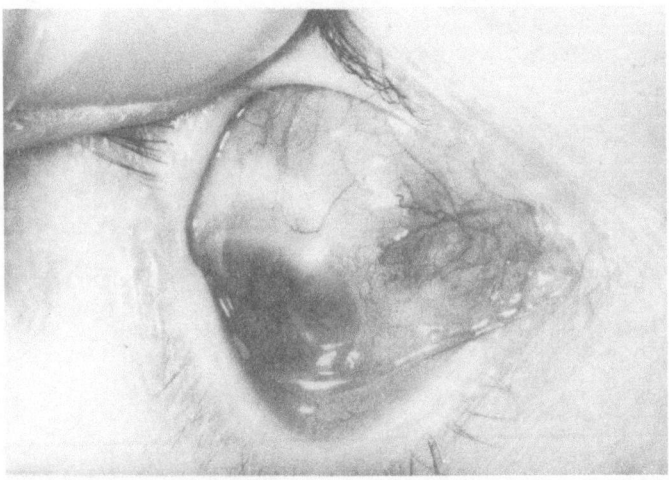

Figure 9.1.32 Scleral thinning following nodular scleritis with exposure of the pigmented tissue of the choroid or ciliary body occurring in a 55-year-old female

examination demonstrates local areas of scleral hyperaemia and necrosis. On occasions the inflammation may be annular around the corneal limbus and following spontaneous regression may leave the appearance of translucent sclera through which the pigmented tissue of the ciliary body can be seen (Figure 9.1.32). Scleritis can be associated with uveitis and corneal opacification often with lipid deposits at the inner edge (Figure 9.1.33). Ischaemia may occur at the centre of a nodule, and in the absence of inflammation may produce a perforation (scleromalacia perforans).

Histologically scleritis shows some of the typical changes found in the inflammatory connective tissue diseases with fibrinoid necrosis, abnormal cellular reactions and fibrin deposition. Vasculitis, endothelial proliferation and fibrinoid degeneration of the vessel wall may lead to thrombosis and infarction of the tissues supplied by the vessel. The cellular infiltration consists of plasma cells and lymphocytes, with the appearance of giant cells and macrophages towards the centre of the lesion. In an area of necrosis, the collagen fibres are not apparent, and mucopolysaccharide and cell morphology are unrecognizable. The association of scleritis with other connective tissue diseases (Table 9.I.5), in which immune complexes appear to have a prominent role, suggests that scleritis may be involved in a similar way. So far, however, the evidence in the various forms of the disease remains speculative and the relative importance of cell-mediated and humoral mechanisms is uncertain. It remains of some relevance that it has been possible to induce a scleritis-like lesion in rabbits sensitized to ovalbumin following local scleral injection[46].

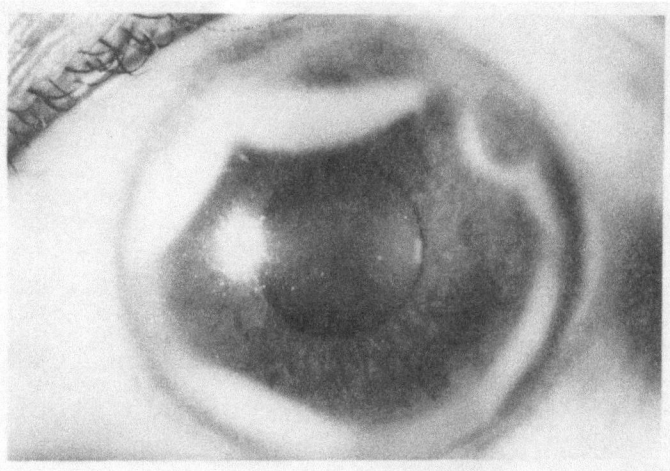

Figure 9.I.33   Immune deposits occurring in the cornea of a 30-year-old male following a series of attacks of nodular scleritis

Oxyphenbutazone ointment is the treatment of choice in episcleritis, as this disease has a high recurrence rate and so topical steroids, if employed, may produce unwanted side-effects.

In the less severe anterior diffuse or nodular scleritis, systemic therapy with oxyphenbutazone may reduce pain and inflammation, and if there is no response, then indomethacin may be helpful. Topical steroid or oxyphenbutazone ointment may be used with benefit at the same time as systemic therapy is employed. If scleritis is very severe, scleral necrosis may follow, and if there is no response to oxyphenbutazone or indomethacin, systemic steroids should be given in immunosuppressive dosage[46].

The peripheral corneal melting syndrome can occur in isolation, following intraocular surgery or in association with systemic disease such as advanced inactive rheumatoid arthritis[48], polyarteritis nodosa, Wegener's granulomatosis, or systemic lupus erythematosus. The periphery of the cornea appears to melt spontaneously (Figure 9.I.34) and in the more severe disease, this may eventually lead to prolapse of uveal tissue (Figure 9.I.35). In the most acute cases the melting process may gradually encroach on to the central area of the cornea, leaving an island of elevated stroma which eventually sloughs away. Undoubtedly the melting is due to the overproduction of collagenase[49], but the mechanisms which produce the unusual response must in themselves be variable and possibly involve either local or systemic events or predominantly humoral or cell-mediated mechanisms. Thus circulating antibodies to both corneal and conjunctival epithelium have been reported[50]

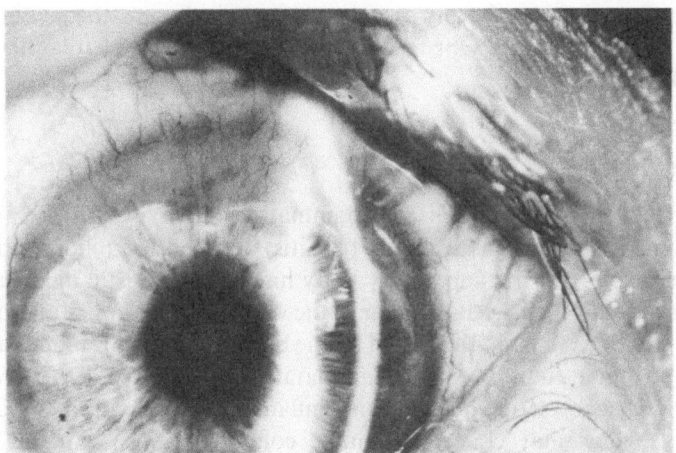

Figure 9.I.34 Peripheral corneal melting syndrome in a 56-year-old male patient with Wegener's granulomatosis

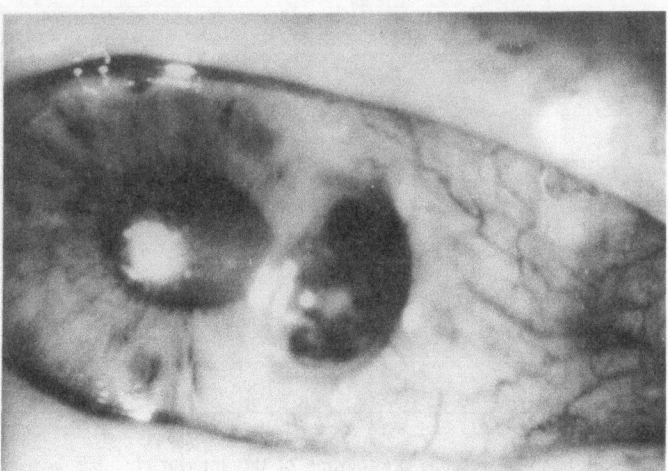

Figure 9.I.35 Corneal perforation following the peripheral corneal melting syndrome occurring in a 69-year-old female with severe rheumatoid arthritis

and by using the leukocyte migration inhibition test evidence of cellular immunity to corneal antigens has been found in six out of seven patients[51].

Because the response to treatment is difficult to evaluate, there is no clear idea as to what this should be. The use of topical corticosteroid should be approached with caution because this may increase the risk of perforation. It has been proposed that the strip of conjunctiva alongside the ulcer should be removed and this has been found to be successful[52]; while in patients with associated systemic disease, systemic immunosuppressive therapy has proved valuable in the occasional patient[53]. However, in certain unfortunate patients, in whom there may not be any associated systemic disease, the melting of the cornea can be relentlessly progressive despite any form of treatment, be it medical or surgical.

Uveitis

The term uveitis should refer to inflammation of the uveal tract and may involve the iris (iritis), ciliary body (cyclitis) and choroid (choroiditis). The blood vessels of the iris and ciliary body have characteristic tight junctions between the endothelial cells, similar to the vessels of the retina. Inflammation of the anterior uvea is characterized by the breakdown of this blood–aqueous barrier. so that in addition to vascular dilatation of the iris vessels, there can be an outpouring of serum protein and inflammatory cells into the anterior chamber, which may collect as minute coin-like deposits on the corneal endothelium to form keratic precipitates which may be either plasma cells or

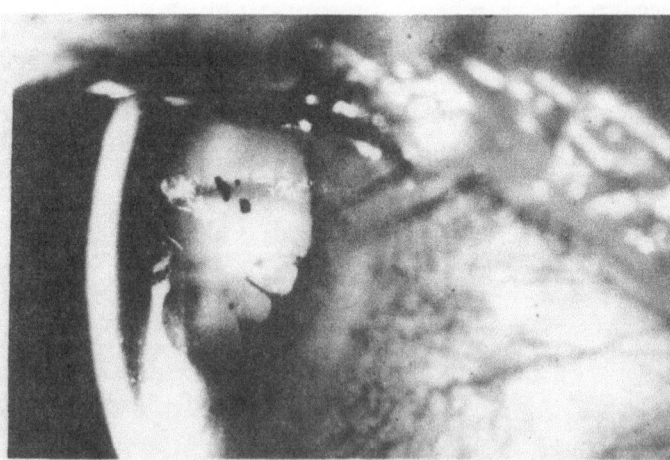

Figure 9.I.36   Slit-lamp microscope photograph of the anterior chamber in a patient with anterior uveitis associated with ankylosing spondylitis. The irregularity of the pupil is due to formation of posterior synechiae. There are some deposits of iris pigment on the anterior surface of the lens. (Courtesy Mr Christopher Dean Hart)

lymphocytes[54]. The inflamed pupil margin may become adherent to the lens, producing posterior synechiae (Figure 9.I.36). Haze in the optic media due to cellular exudation, as seen with the ophthalmoscope, is a valuable way of evaluating inflammatory disease of the eye when the vitreous is involved in the disease. Techniques using the slit lamp microscope, together with a Goldmann contact lens with an attached scleral depressor, has afforded precise and accurate examination of the extreme periphery of the retina and the uveal tissue anterior to the pars plana. Exudates occurring in the peripheral fundus signal three different inflammatory processes[55]. They may provide a concomitant sign of anterior uveitis, a sign of inflammation of the pars plana itself, or a concomitant sign of posterior inflammation. Chronic uveal inflammation can be associated with oedema and cystic changes at the macula with subsequent visual loss (Figure 9.I.37).

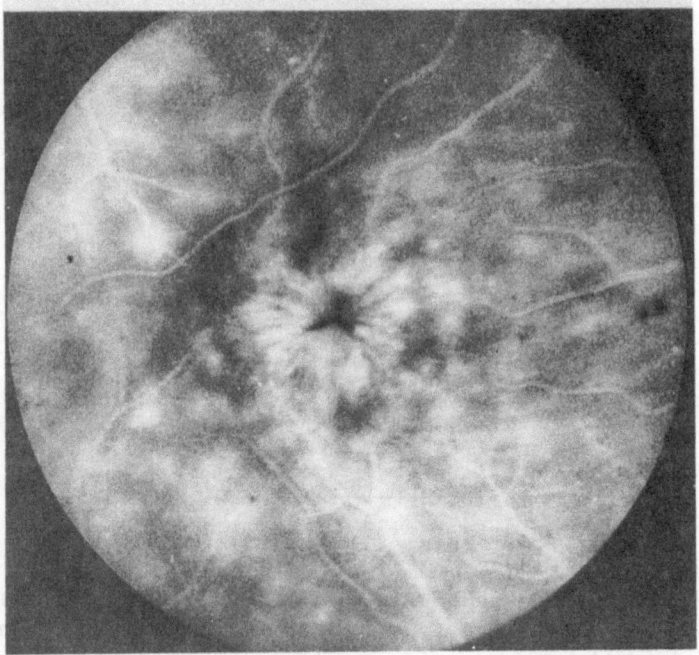

Figure 9.I.37   Cystoid macular oedema demonstrated with fluorescein angiography of the retina in a patient with posterior uveitis. (Courtesy Mr Christopher Dean Hart)

A classification of uveitis with some of the causes is shown in Tables 9.I.6 and 9.I.7. Work with tissue-typing antigens has shown that a high proportion of patients with ankylosing spondylitis possess HLA-B27, a human leukocyte antigen which is only present in 6% of the population. In Reiter's disease in which uveitis may be a complication, a high proportion of patients possess HLA-B27, and similar findings have been made in patients with juvenile

Table 9.1.6   Causes of metastatic uveitis

Infective agent	Ocular disease
Histoplasma capsulatum	focal peripheral and central retinal disease
Toxocara	focal choroiditis
Toxoplasma	peripheral or central choroiditis
Treponema pallidum	congenital retino-choroiditis (pepper and salt); secondary pigmentary degeneration of the retina
	iritis in secondary syphilis
Mycoplasma tuberculosis	focal choroiditis and miliary choroidal tubercles
Mycoplasma leprae	acute serous or nodular iritis
Herpes simplex virus	keratitis
	kerato-uveitis
	uveitis
Herpes zoster virus	uveitis with sectorial iris atrophy

Table 9.1.7   Syndromes associated with uveitis (?non-infectious)

Sarcoidosis	anterior or posterior uveitis; papilloedema
Juvenile rheumatoid arthritis (mono- or oligo-articular group)	bilateral iridocyclitis, cataract and band keratopathy
Ankylosing spondylitis	chronic recurrent iridocyclitis
Reiter's disease	conjunctivitis and anterior uveitis
Colitic arthritis	recurrent iridocyclitis
Behçet's syndrome	recurrent panuveitis with aphthous and genital ulceration
Vogt–Harada–Koyanagi syndrome (uveo-encephalitis)	bilateral panuveitis (associated with poliosis, vitiligo, alopecia, auditory symptoms, and meningo-encephalitis)
Sympathetic ophthalmitis	bilateral panuveitis following trauma
Lens-induced uveitis	acute anterior uveitis following lens capsule rupture as in extracapsular cataract extraction

rheumatoid arthritis. Diseases such as ankylosing spondylitis[56], Reiter's disease[57], juvenile rheumatoid arthritis[58], and acute iridocyclitis[59, 60] may be asssociated with each other in various combinations and can occasionally be seen in distinct family groups. Two possible mechanisms have been suggested by which this histocompatability antigen might influence susceptibility to disease. The antigens simulate the antigens of, say, an invading virus so that the host is unable to produce a suitable immune response to the particular organism, or there may be a linkage between the antigen and the immune response gene, a deficiency in which may allow the initiation of the diseases which are apparently in some way related to HLA-B27.

Because of differing diagnostic criteria and aetiological theories, it is difficult to make valid comparisons between uveitis statistics from different countries; but it is clear that some types of uveitis have a definite geographic distribution. Thus exogenous uveitis due to toxoplasmosis (Figure 9.I.38), accounts for 60% of patients in West Africa and 30% in the West Indies, uveitis associated with sarcoidosis accounts for 16% of patients in the West Indies, rheumatic diseases (ankylosing spondylitis, Reiter's syndrome and Still's disease) affect 16% of patients in India and Pakistan, and uveitis due to Behçet's disease accounts for 25% of cases in Japan and 16% in the Middle East.

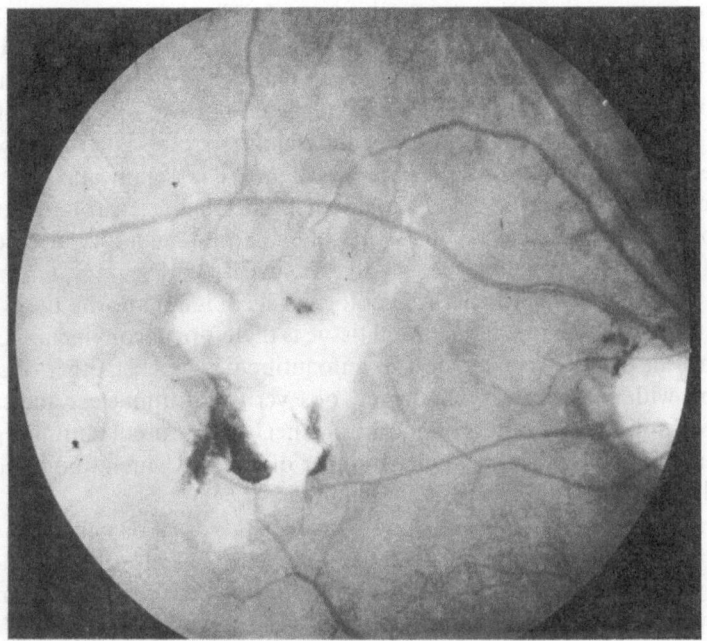

Figure 9.I.38   Active and inactive retinal toxoplasmosis situated at the macula. (Courtesy Mr Christopher Dean Hart)

In patients seen in the United Kingdom, no underlying cause can be recognized in 54% of patients. There are a number of possible mechanisms in which uveitis might occur in the absence of a known aetiological factor. Autoantibody has been located by a number of workers[62, 63] and more recently studies of cell-mediated immunity have demonstrated that uveal antigens can stimulate lymphocytes using the lymphocyte transformation test[64–66] in patients with either sympathetic ophthalmitis or the Vogt–Harada–Koyanagi syndrome. Cross-reactivity between components of the central nervous system and uveal tissue has been proposed and supported experimentally[67]. The possible role of immune complex deposition has been investigated in rabbits[68, 69], following immunization against bovine serum albumin. When non-immune uveal vascular damage was induced in these sensitized rabbits by the intravitreal injection of *Escherichia coli* endotoxin, an intravenous dose of bovine serum albumin was able to induce a recurrence of inflammation. Such a reaction was thought to be due to a permanent alteration in vascular permeability induced by the endotoxin, enabling immune complexes to be deposited in the uveal tract.

The immunological investigation of patients with acute and chronic anterior, chronic posterior and generalized uveal inflammation makes it difficult to suppose these four clinical types of uveitis are due to a single type of reaction causing tissue damage[70]. The serum IgE level was elevated in 28% of patients with acute anterior uveitis, which could imply that immediate hypersensitivity has a role to play in a small proportion of patients with uveitis. Serum IgM has been reported to be elevated in other patients with acute anterior and chronic posterior inflammation, especially in those cases where it is associated with retinal vasculitis. The significance of this is unknown[71]. Although antibody to uveal tissues has been found[72], a high proportion of patients with other types of ocular inflammatory disease show similar antibodies which do not involve the uvea.

In cases of uveitis in which the aetiological agent is not known, the evidence for cytotoxic reactions against uveal tissue is therefore unconvincing. Careful searches have also been made for autoantibodies against other tissues in patients with uveitis of varying degrees of severity[70]. Antinuclear and smooth muscle antibody are both common, together with antireticulin and gastric parietal cell antibody in a smaller number of cases. Rheumatoid factor was slightly raised only in cases of pars planitis.

Treatment of uveitis depends upon whether there is a recognizable causal agent for which specific therapy can be employed. Topical corticosteroids can usually control anterior uveal inflammation, but systemic steroids may be used when there is inflammation in the posterior segment which may lead to loss of vision from cystoid oedema of the macula.

THE LENS

The cornea is offered a considerable degree of immunological protection by the local vascular tissue of the conjunctiva and the corneal–scleral junction, together with the high population of extravascular plasma cells and lymphocytes. In contrast, the lens is the more truly privileged, in that it is in direct contact with the aqueous humour and is protected from the intravascular compartment additionally by the 'tight junctions' which are known to exist between the vascular endothelial cells of both the retinal and iris blood vessels.

Lens-induced uveitis may occur following extracapsular cataract extraction, where the lens capsule is ruptured during the operative procedure and the anterior capsule together with the nucleus and cortex are removed, leaving the posterior part of the capsule *in situ*. Lens remnants have been recognized for a long time as a cause of postoperative inflammation which was initially termed endophthalmitis phacoanaphylactica[73]. The experimental studies in the rabbit indicate that rupture of the lens capsule with escape of the lens contents into the anterior chamber of the eye will excite uveitis in animals which have been pretreated with Freund's adjuvant, but not otherwise. Homologous lens antigens injected into the eye have a minimal effect in the absence of adjuvant[74]. Such findings prompted the search for some natural adjuvant, and streptococcal and staphylococcal antigens were found to potentiate lens reactions[75, 76]. Differentiation between the two broad types of lens antigens, the albinoid and crystalline fractions, showed polymorphonuclear and macrophage infiltration when the former was used as an antigen, while α-crystallin gave rise to a greater degree of lymphocytic response. This suggested that humoral and cell-mediated responses depended upon the particular lens antigen which was predominant in the reaction[77]. It was later demonstrated that lens trauma in previously sensitized animals led to the *in vivo* fixation of IgG and complement, suggesting that lens-induced uveitis was due to the formation of immune complexes.

It is common to find antibodies to lens proteins in patients who are thought to have lens-induced uveitis[78, 79]. These cannot, however, be regarded as diagnostic since antibodies can also be demonstrated in patients with other types of uveitis[80]. The possible mechanism depends upon the formation of immune complexes producing an Arthus-type reaction, which would explain the infiltration with polymorphs in the early part of the reaction[81]. Other investigations into the role of cell-mediated immunity have been reported using the leukocyte migration inhibition test which show that one-third of patients with lens injuries have evidence of T-cell sensitization[82].

RETINAL VASCULITIS

Retinal vasculitis is an inflammatory process predominantly involving the retinal venous system, although it may occasionally affect the arterial system. The vessels of the retina are similar to those of the brain and the anterior uvea in that the endothelial cells possess tight junctions between them which prevent the escape of fluid from the intravascular to the extravascular compartment. Inflammatory disease is able to break down this blood–retinal barrier, producing oedema in the area of retina involved, with the formation of retinal haemorrhages and exudates around the vessels. Changes in vascular permeability may be well demonstrated by means of fluorescein angiography[83] (Figure 9.I.39). A peripheral type of disease which was first described by Eales[84] is found frequently in young adults in association with intraocular haemorrhage. A central retinal vasculitis produces an appearance similar to central retinal vein occlusion[85], but the evidence of inflammation is not accepted by all authorities[86]. The occasional association of retinal vasculitis

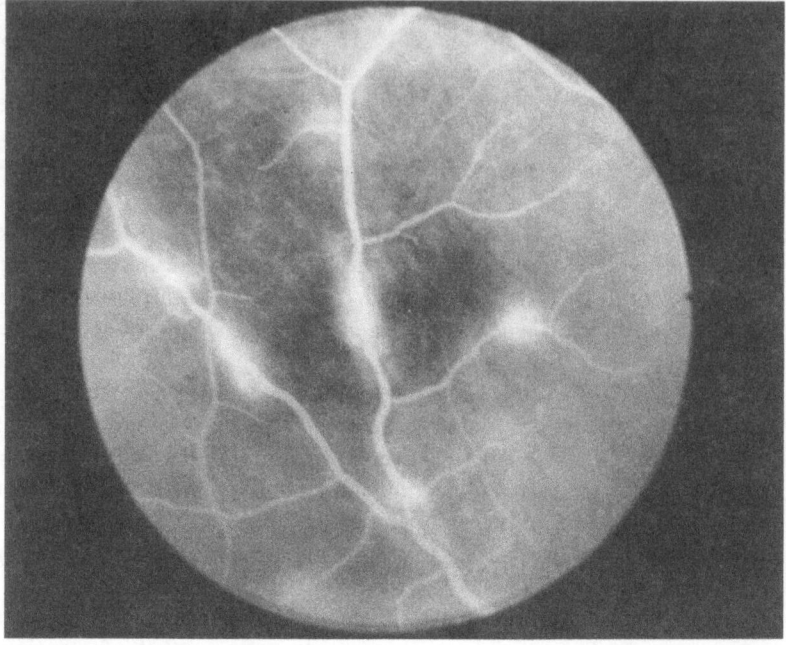

Figure 9.I.39   Fluorescein angiogram demonstrating leakage of dye into the surrounding tissues from the peripheral retina venules, in a patient with retinal vasculitis. (Courtesy Mr Tim ffytche)

with systemic inflammatory disease has suggested that it may be due to deposition of circulating immune complexes. Immunological evidence has been obtained in a small group of patients with vasculitis of both central and peripheral types. Evidence of circulating complexes was found in the serum in 13 out of 17 patients, as judged particularly by chemotactic activity (69%) and inhibition of EA-rosette formation (59%)[87]. Intraocular inflammation associated with retinal vasculitis can usually be suppressed with the use of retrobulbar or systemic corticosteroid[83].

Treatment

Allergic disease of the external eye involving immediate hypersensitivity can be treated with topical antihistamine drops, or disodium cromoglycate drops during less severe attacks, but topical steroid becomes necessary during exacerbations where there is copious production of mucous discharge leading to multiple erosions of the corneal surface. During such episodes a potent corticosteroid such as dexamethazone should be used for short periods until there is a positive response, when a less potent preparation such as prednisolone drops (0.5 mg/100 ml) can be employed for control in the immediate period following the attack. A rebound of inflammation may occur following sudden reduction of medication, and it is wise to taper the medication off over a period of some weeks. On occasions recurrent vernal disease can be of such severity that long periods of schooling are lost, and it is in these patients that low dosages of systemic corticosteroid (e.g. prednisolone 2.5 mg) may be adequate to allow reduction of topical steroids. If used long term these can lead to the production of cataract or glaucoma (Table 9.I.8).

Table 9.I.8 Complications of topical corticosteroid in ophthalmology

---

Elevation of intraocular pressure (causing pathological cupping of optic disc if used for long periods)
Posterior subcapsular cataract
Enhanced proliferation of herpes simplex virus producing geographic ulcer
Reduced immunological protection against secondary invaders
Corneal melting (in high dosage)
Rebound of inflammation if suddenly curtailed

Particular care should be taken in the use of topical steroids in the treatment of infective external eye disease, where immune reactions occur in the corneal stroma. In herpes simplex keratitis, their use can lead to an enhancement of the rate of proliferation of the virus leading to massive ulcer and increased penetration of virus antigen into the corneal stroma and anterior uvea (Figure 9.I.40). In such cases corticosteroid should be avoided at all costs, with the exception of central stromal disease which is thought liable to lead to permanent scarring, where dilute prednisolone drops may be used provided that concomitant antiviral cover is given in the form of idoxuridine, adenine

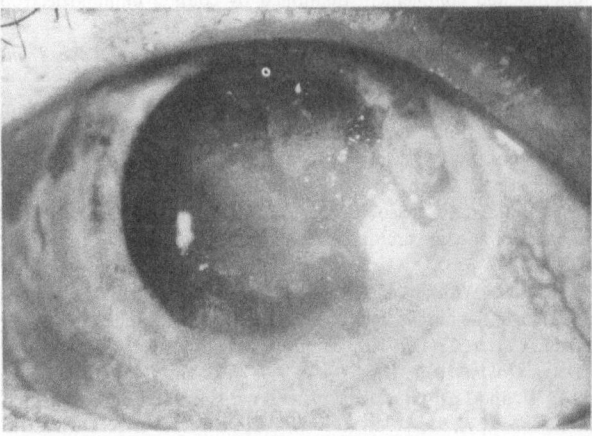

Figure 9.I.40 Massive geographic corneal ulcer in a patient with ulcerative herpetic keratitis who was erroneously treated with topical corticosteroid. (Courtesy Chapman and Hall)

arabinoside, or trifluorothymidine drops. In contrast, it is usually safe to employ corticosteroid therapy in stromal keratitis and anterior uveitis in patients with ocular involvement following herpes zoster infection. In such cases it is necessary to continue topical therapy for some weeks, following which it should be tapered off to avoid a sudden exacerbation. In the case of the superficial punctate keratitis which precedes stromal opacity formation in adenovirus infection, the early use of topical steroid can be of benefit in preventing deep opacities which may take some time to clear.

Corticosteroids should be used with caution in conditions of the external eye associated with systemic manifestations, such as cicatricial mucous membrane pemphigoid and epidermolysis bullosa, together with uveitis associated with systemic diseases. Such diseases require frequent follow-up, to ensure that no secondary invasive organism has caused further disease and at the same time to monitor the intraocular pressure. On occasions where there is little response to topical therapy, and the eye disease is a manifestation of systemic disease, treatment of the latter can result in resolution of the local disease, as in the uveitis of Behçet's disease and in certain patients with the peripheral corneal melting syndrome.

References

1. Allansmith, M. R. (1974). Ocular allergy – diagnosis and management. In Golden, B. (ed.) *Ocular Inflammatory Disease*. (Springfield, Ill.: Thomas)
2. Maurice, D. M. (1969). The cornea and sclera. In Davson, H. (ed.) *The Eye*, pp. 489. (New York: Academic Press)
3. Hodson, S. and Miller, F. (1976). The bicarbonate ion pump in the endothelium which regulates the hydration of rabbit cornea. *J. Physiol.*, **263**, 563
4. Bluestone, R., Easty, D. L., Goldberg, L. S., Jones, B. R. and Pettit, T. H. (1975). Lacrimal immunoglobulins and complement quantified by counter-immunoelectrophoresis. *Br. J. Ophthal.*, **59**, 279
5. Jones, B. R. (1971). Prospects in immunogenic disease of the outer eye. *Trans. Ophthal. Soc. UK*, **91**, 509
6. Allansmith, M. R., Ereiner, J. V. and Baired, R. S. (1978). Number of inflammatory cells in normal conjunctivitis. *Am. J. Ophthalmol.*, **86**, 200
7. Easty, D. L., Birkenshaw, M., Merrett, T., Merrett, J. and Madden, P. (1979). Immunology of atopic eye disease. In *The Mast Cell*. (London: Pitman)
8. Markham, R. H., Carter, C., Scoble, M. A., Metcalf, C. and Easty, D. L. (1977). Double-blind clinical trial of adenine arabinoside and idoxuridine in herpetic corneal ulcers. *Trans. Ophthal. Soc. UK*, **97**, 333
9. Allansmith, M. R., Whitney, C. R., McClellan, B. H. and Newman, L. P. (1973). Immunoglobulins in the human eye. Location, type and amount. *Arch. Ophthalmol.*, **89**, 36
10. Easty, D. L. and Carter, C. (1979). Mechanisms of resistance and hypersensitivity in herpetic keratosis. *Trans. Ophthal. Soc. UK*
11. Frankland, A. W. and Easty, D. L. (1971). Vernal kerato-conjunctivitis: an atopic disease. *Trans. Ophthal. Soc. UK*, **91**, 479
12. Easty, D. L., Entwistle, C., Funk, A. and Witcher, J. (1975). Herpes simplex keratitis and keratoconus in the atopic patient; a clinical and immunological study. *Trans. Ophthal. Soc. UK*, **95**, 267

13. Abelson, M. B., Soter, N. A., Simon, M. A., Dohlman, C. H. and Allansmith, M. R. (1977). Histamine in human tears. *Am. J. Ophthalmol.*, **83**, 417

14. Morgan, G. (1971). The pathology of vernal conjunctivitis. *Trans. Ophthalmol. Soc. UK*, **91**, 467

15. Bloch-Michael, E., Audiòn-Berault, J., Diebold, J., Herman, D., Dry, J. and Campinchi, R. (1977). A study in immunofluorescence of the plasma cells in allergic conjunctivitis in particular of the cells forming immunoglobulin E. *Arch. Ophthalmol. (Paris)*, **37**, 89

16. Tada, T. and Ishizaka, K. (1970). Distribution of E-forming cells in lymphoid tissues of the human and the monkey. *J. Immunol.*, **104**, 377

17. Mackie, I. A. and Wright, P. (1978). Giant papillary conjunctivitis (secondary vernal) in association with contact lens wear. *Trans. Ophthal. Soc. UK*, **98**, 3

18. Easty, D. L., Rice, N. S. C. and Jones, B. R. (1972). Clinical trial of topical disodium cromoglycate in vernal keratoconjunctivitis. *Clin. Allergy*, **2**, 99

19. Rice, N. S. C., Easty, D. L., Garner, A., Jones, B. R. and Tripathi, R. (1971). Vernal keratoconjunctivitis and its management. *Trans. Ophthalmol. Soc. UK*, **91**, 483

20. Friedlaender, M. H. (1979). Ocular allergy and immunology. *J. Allergy Clin. Immunol.*, **63**, 51

21. Furcy, N., West, C., Andrews, T. *et al.* (1975). Immunofluorescent studies of ocular cicatricial pemphigoid. *Am. J. Ophthal.*, **80**, 825

22. Waltman, S. and Yariam, D. (1974). Circulatory autoantibodies in ocular pemphigoid. *Am. J. Ophthal.*, **77**, 891

23. Wright, P. (1979). The enigma of ocular cicatricial pemphigoid. *Trans. Ophthalmol. Soc. UK*, **99**

24. Wright, P. (1975). Untoward effects associated with practolol administration; oculomococutaneous syndrome. *Br. Med. J.*, **1**, 595

25. Garner, A. and Rahi, A. H. S. (1976). Practolol and ocular toxicity. *Br. J. Ophthal.*, **60**, 684

26. Rahi, A. H. S., Chapman, C. M., Garner, A. and Wright, P. (1976). Pathology of practolol induced ocular toxicity. *Br. J. Ophthal.*, **60**, 312

27. Germutch, F. G., Maumenee, A. E., Senterfit, L. B. and Pollack, A. D. (1962). Immunohistologic studies of antigen-antibody reactions in the avascular cornea. 1. Reactions in rabbits actively sensitized to foreign protein. *J. Exp. Med.*, **115**, 919

28. Movat, H. Z., Fernando, N. V., Urjuhara, T. *et al.* (1963). Allergic inflammation. III. The fine structure of collagen fibrils at sites of antigen–antibody interaction in Arthus-type lesions. *J. Exp. Med.*, **118**, 557

29. Silverstein, A. M. and Khodadoust, A. A. (1973). Transplantation immunology of the cornea. In *Corneal Graft Failure*, pp. 105–120. (A Ciba Foundation Symposium)

30. Barker, C. L. and Billingham, R. E. (1977). Immunologically privileged sites. In Kunkel and Dixon (eds.) *Advances in Immunology*, pp. 1–44. (New York: Academic Press)

31. Paufique, L., Sourdille, G. and Offret, G. (1948). *Les Greffes de la Cornée (Keratoplasties)*. (Paris: Masson)

32. Maumenee, A. E. (1955). The immune concept; its relationship to corneal homotransplantation. *Ann. N.Y. Acad. Sci.*, **59**, 453

33. Polack, F. M. (1962). Histopathological and histochemical alterations in the early stages of corneal graft rejection. *J. Exp. Med.*, **116**, 709

34. Maumenee, A. E. (1951). The influence of donor–recipient sensitisation on corneal grafts. *Am. J. Ophthalmol.*, **34**, 142

35. Silverstein, A. M. and Khodadoust, A. A. (1973). Transplantation biology of the cornea. In *Corneal Graft Failure*, pp. 105–120. (A Ciba Foundation Symposium)

36. Polack, F. M. (1973). Corneal graft rejection; clinico-pathological correlation. In *Corneal Graft Failure*, pp. 127–139. (A Ciba Foundation Symposium)

37. Gibbs, D. C., Batchelor, J. R., Webb, A., Schlesinger, W. and Casey, T. A. (1974). The influence of tissue type compatibility on the part of full thickness corneal grafts. *Trans. Ophthal. Soc. UK*, **94**, 101

38. Chignell, A. H., Easty, D. L., Chesterton, J. R. and Thomsitt, J. (1970). Marginal ulceration of the cornea. *Br. J. Ophthal.*, **54**, 433
39. Thygeson, P. (1954). Observations on non-tuberculous phlyctenular keratoconjunctivitis. *Trans. Am. Acad. Ophthalmol. Otolaryngol.*, **58**, 128
40. Easty, D. L., Maini, R. M. and Jones, B. R. (1973). Cellular immunity in herpes simplex keratitis. *Trans. Ophthalmol. Soc. UK*, **93**, 171
41. Felberg, N. T. and Sery, T. W. (1978). The reverse Wessely ring phenomenon: immune corneal rings following systemic immunisation. *Br. J. Ophthal.*, **62**, 831
42. Meyers, R. L. and Pettit, T. H. (1973). The pathogenesis of corneal inflammation due to herpes simplex virus. 1. Corneal hypersensitivity in the rabbit. *J. Immunol.* Vol. III, **4**, 1031
43. Meyers. R. L. and Pettit. T. H. (1974). Chemotaxis of polymorphonuclear leucocytes in corneal inflammation; tissue injury in herpes simplex virus infection. *Invest. Ophthalmol.*, **13**, 187
44. Jones, B. R. (1975). The prevention of blindness in trachoma. *Trans. Ophthal. Soc. UK*, **95**, 16
45. Monnickendam, M. and Darougar, S. (1979). An animal model for hyperendemic trachoma; a study of immunity and hypersensitivity to *Chlamydia*. In Silverstein and O'Connell (eds.) *Immunology and Immunopathology*
46. Watson, P. G. and Hazelman, B. L. (1976). The sclera and systemic disorders. In *Major Problems in Ophthalmology*. Vol. II. (London: W. B. Saunders)
47. Watson, P. G. and Hayreh, S. S. (1976). Scleritis and episcleritis. *Br. J. Ophthalmol..* **60**, 163
48. Jayson, M. I. V. and Easty, D. L. (1977). Ulceration of the cornea in rheumatoid arthritis. *Ann. Rheumatic Dis.*, **36**, 428
49. Brown, S. I. (1975). Mooren's ulcer; histopathology and proteolytic enzymes of adjacent conjunctiva. *Br. J. Ophthal.*, **59**, 670
50. Brown, S. I., Mondino, B. J. and Rabin, B. S. (1976). Autoimmune phenomenon in Mooren's ulcer. *Am. J. Ophthal.*, **82**, 835
51. Mondino, B. J., Brown, S. I. and Rabin, B. S. (1978). Cellular immunity in Mooren's ulcer. *Am. J. Ophthal.*, **85**, 788
52. Brown, S. I. (1975). Mooren's ulcer. Treatment by conjunctival excision. *Br. J. Ophthal.*, **59**, 675
53. Easty, D. L., Madden, P., Jayson, M. I. V., Carter, C. and Noble, B. A. (1978). Systemic immunosuppression in marginal keratolysis. *Trans. Ophthal. Soc. UK*, **98**, 410
54. Inomata, H. and Smelser, G. K. (1970). Fine structural alterations of corneal endothelium during experimental uveitis. *Invest. Ophthal.*, **9**, 272
55. Eisner, G. (1972). Biomicroscopy of the peripheral fundus. *Surg. Ophthal.*, **17**, 1
56. Brewerton, D. A., Caffrey, M., Hart, F., Dudley, J., James, D. C. O., Nicholls, A. and Sturrock, R. D. (1973). Ankylosing spondylitis and HL-A 27. *Lancet*, **1**, 904
57. Brewerton, D. A., Nicholls, A., Oates, J. K., Caffrey, M., Waters, D. and James, D. C. O. (1973). Reiter's disease and HL-A W. 27. *Lancet*, **2**, 996
58. Rachelefsky, G. S., Teraski, P. J., Katz, R. and Stiehm, R. (1974). Increased prevalence of W-27 in juvenile rheumatoid. *N. Engl. J. Med.*, **290**, 892
59. Brewerton, D. A., Nicholls, A., Caffrey, M., Walters, D. and James, D. (1973). Acute anterior uveitis and HL-A W.27. *Lancet*, **2**, 994
60. Ehlers, M., Kissmeyer-Hielsen, O., Kjerbye, K. E. and Lamm, L. U. (1974). HL-A W.27 in acute and chronic uveitis. *Lancet*, **1**, 99
61. Perkins, E. S. (1976). Epidemiology of uveitis. *Trans. Ophthal. Soc. UK*, **96**, 105
62. Ujihara, H. and Kogure, M. (1961). Studies on auto-antigenicity in uveitis. In *Clinical Studies. Acta Soc. Ophthal. Japn.*, **65**, 1060
63. Aronson, S. B., Yamamato, E., Goodner, E. and O'Connor, G. R. (1964). The occurrence of an autoanti-uveal antibody in human uveitis. *Arch. Ophthalmol.*, **72**, 621
64. Hammer, H. (1971). Lymphocyte transformation test in sympathetic ophthalmitis and Vogt–Koyanagi–Harada syndrome. *Br. J. Ophthalmol..* **55**. 850

65. Marav, G. E., Font, R. L., Johnson, M. C. and Alepa, F. P. (1971). Lymphocyte stimulating activity of ocular tissues in sympathetic ophthalmia. *Invest. Ophthalmol.*, **10**, 770
66. Char. D. H.. Brun. J. and West. W. (1977). Thyluns-derived lymphocytes in the Vogt–Koyanagi–Harada syndrome. *Invest. Ophthalmol. Vis. Sci.*. **16**. 179
67. Bullington, S. J. and Waksman, B. H. (1958). Uveitis in rabbits with experimental allergic encephalomyelitis. *Arch. Ophthalmol.*, **59**, 435
68. Gamble, C. N., Aronson, S. B. and Brescia, F. B. (1970). Experimental uveitis. 1. The production of recurrent immunologic (Auer) uveitis and its relationship to increased uveal vascular permeability. *Arch. Ophthalmol.*, **84**, 321
69. Gamble. C. N.. Aronson. S. B. and Brescia. F. B. (1970). Experimental uveitis. II. The pathogenesis of recurrent immunologic (Auer) uveitis. *Arch. Ophthal.*. **84**. 331
70. Rahi. A. H. S.. Holborow. E. J.. Perkins. E. S., Gungen, Y. Y. and Dimming, W. J. (1976). Immunological investigations in uveitis. *Trans. Ophthal. Soc. UK*, **96**, 113
71. Koliopoulos. J. X.. Perkins. E. S. and Seitanides, B. E. (1970). Serum immunoglobulins in retinal vasculitis. *Br. J. Ophthal.*, **54**. 233
72. Aronson. B.. Yamamoto. E., Goodmer, E. and O'Connor, G. R. (1964). The occurrence of an autoanti-uveal antibody in human uveitis. *Arch. Ophthalmol.*, **72**, 621
73. Uhlenhuth. P. and Haendel. L. (1910). Untersuchungen über die praktische verwert barkeit det anaphylaxie zur Erkennung and Unterscheidung verschiedener EiweiBarten. *Z. Immunforsch.*, **4**, 761
74. Muller, H. (1963). Phacolytic glaucoma and phacogenic ophthalmia (lens induced uveitis). *Trans. Ophthalmol. Soc. UK*, **83**. 689
75. Halbert, S. P., Locatcher-Kharazo, D., Swick, L., Witmer, R., Seegal, B. and Fitzgerald, P. (1957). Homologous immunological studies of ocular lens. 1. *In vitro* observations. *J. Exp. Med.*, **105**, 439
76. Burkey, E. L. (1934). Production of lens sensitivity in rabbits by the action of staphylococcus toxin. *Proc. Soc. Exp. Biol. Med.*, **31**, 447
77. Behrems. M. and Mamski. W. (1973). Ocular responses to crystallin and albuminoid in lens sensitized inbred rats. *Ophthalmic Res.*, **5**. 89
78. Witmer. R. (1957). Phacogenic uveitis. *Ophthalmologica (Basel)*. **133**. 326
79. Luntz. M. H. and Wright. R. (1962). Lens induced uveitis. *Exp. Eye Ref.*. **48**. 317
80. Perkins. E. S. and Wood. R. M. (1964). Autoimmunity in uveitis. *Br. J. Ophthal.*, **48**, 61
81. Marak. G. E. (1976). Experimental lens induced granulomatous endophthalmitis. In *Proceedings of the 1st International Symposium on Immunology and Immunopathology of the Eye*. Strasbourg 1974. *Mod. Probl. Ophthal.*. **16** (Basel: Karger)
82. Kincses. E. and Szaso. G. (1976). Humoral and cellular response after injury of the lens. In *Proceedings of the 1st International Symposium of Immunology and Immunopathology of the Eye*. Strasbourg 1974. *Mod. Probl. Ophthal.*. **16** (Basel: Karger)
83. ffytche. T. J. (1977). Retinal vasculitis. A review of clinical signs. *Trans. Ophthal. Soc. UK*, **97** 457
84. Eales, H. (1880). Primary retinal haemorrhage in young. *Birmingham Med. Div.*, **3**, 262
85. Lyk, T. K. and Wyber, K. (1961). Retinal vasculitis. *Br. J. Ophthal.*, **45**, 778
86. Hart, C. D., Sanders, M. D. and Miller, S. J. H. (1971). Benign retinal vasculitis. Clinical and fluorescein angiographic study. *Br. J. Ophthal.*. **55**. 721
87. Andrews. B. S.. McIntoch. J.. Petts. V. and Penny. R. (1977). Circulating immune complexes in retinal vasculitis. *Clin. Exp. Immunol.*. **29**. 23

Additional Recommended References

Aronson. S. B. and Elliott. J. H. (1972). Ocular inflammation. (St Louis: C. V. Mosby)
Rahi. A. H. S. and Garner. A. (1976). *Immunopathology of the Eye*. (Oxford: Blackwell Scientific)

Manski, W. (1973). Immunological studies on normal and pathological lenses in the human lens in relation to cataract. Ciba Foundation Symposium. Elliott and Fitzsimmons (eds.). (Amsterdam: Excerpta Medica)

9 PART II:
Allergic Disorder of the Ear

N. MYGIND and J. THOMSEN

INTRODUCTION

It is well known that allergic contact dermatitis can affect the skin on the auricle and in the ear canal. In principle, signs and symptoms are similar to those of ordinary contact dermatitis, and the reader is therefore referred to Chapter 6.

In the middle ear, atopic allergy has been related to secretory otitis media, which is a very prevalent disease in childhood and a frequent cause of hearing loss. It has also been claimed that allergy can cause disease of the inner ear, i.e. Ménière's disease. This part of Chapter 9 will deal with the evidence for and against a causal relationship between allergy and secretory otitis media and Ménière's disease.

SECRETORY OTITIS MEDIA

Is secretory otitis media an allergic disease?

Secretory otitis media is characterized by the presence of an effusion in the middle ear. It can either be a serum-like fluid or a very viscid mucous substance (glue ear). Eustachian tube malfunction, negative middle ear pressure and plasma transudation, together with proliferation of goblet cells and glands, and hypersecretion, are factors of importance for the formation of effusion[1]. As the lumen of a child's eustachian tube is only 1 mm wide it seems likely that it may become blocked by allergic inflammation of the nasal mucosa. In the American literature[2] allergy is often mentioned as an important cause of secretory otitis media, but the correlation between these two disorders is not so evident that it can be accepted without qualification.

Histological and immunological evidence

In order to demonstrate a causal association between secretory otitis media and allergic reactions in the middle ear mucosa, a cytological examination of middle ear effusion is required. Such studies have shown that there is no eosinophilia in the effusion[3, 4] or in the middle ear mucosa[5]. In the nose the secretion/serum ratio is higher for IgE than for IgG[6], indicating local IgE synthesis, whereas in the middle ear effusion the ratio is higher for IgG than for IgE[7]. Thus, neither cytological nor immunological investigations suggest that IgE-mediated allergic reactions occur in the middle ear lining.

Clinical evidence

Although it is unlikely that allergic inflammation is the direct cause of the formation of middle ear effusion, it is still possible that allergy is of indirect significance, via nasal blockage and eustachian tube malfunction. In a panel discussion of serous effusion of the middle ear[8] the participating allergists, paediatricians and otologists estimated that 20–90% of their cases with secretory otitis media had an allergic aetiology. Such clinical experience is apparently substantiated by reports of a very high frequency of allergy in children with secretory otitis media[9, 10]. However, the children in these studies were not randomly selected from the total population of children with secretory otitis media but were all referred to an allergy clinic. So a high incidence of allergy had to be expected in the patients investigated. The lack of a control group makes the interpretation of the results difficult and such studies have to be regarded with reservation. Palva and Holopainen[4] have reported normal serum IgE levels in children with secretory otitis media. In addition, they showed that 20% of the patients had eosinophilia in the nasal secretions. Murray and Anderson[11] have found the figure to be 17% in normal children.

Controlled clinical evidence

Kjellman and co-workers[12] examined the occurrence of atopic predisposition and of allergic diseases in consecutive children referred to an ear, nose and throat department for adenoidectomy. A meticulous allergy examination was carried out in 154 children; the main cause for surgery was recurrent acute otitis or secretory otitis in 94 children, and nasal symptoms in 60 cases.

Atopic disease in parents or siblings was present in 49%, and in the patient's past or present history in 24%. A total of 40% of the children had two or more laboratory findings which were characteristic of an atopic state. This is an over-representation of allergic predisposition and disease, as atopic disease in the family history was found in 30% in a reference group of newborn children, and the incidence of atopic disease was 15% in a reference group of unselected 7-year-old children in the same region.

The authors conclude that these findings seem to indicate a connection between recurrent otitis media and atopic allergy, and it is further mentioned that measurement of serum IgE may be of value in children who are referred for adenoidectomy. It is suggested that the search for relevant allergens followed by treatment may prevent relapses of acute otitis media and secretory otitis.

Obviously this meticulous investigation is suggestive of an association between atopic allergy and middle ear disease, but it is difficult to distinguish with certainty between causality and coincidence. The children studied were all referred to the hospital for adenoidectomy. In many children who have this operation, pathologically abnormal adenoids are not the real indication[13]; they finally end up in the operation theatre because they visit their doctor with symptoms and signs which are traditionally attributed to enlarged adenoids, without any real evidence that this is so.

Both otitis media and atopic allergy are very prevalent diseases, frequently resulting in visits to the surgery. The allergic child, often visiting the doctor, is at 'greater risk' of being referred to hospital for adenoidectomy than his non-allergic friend without close physician contact, but with a similar degree of trivial ear and nose symptoms, interpreted as 'symptoms and signs of enlarged adenoids'. These considerations are a demonstration of the classical Berkson's fallacy, well known from the statistical epidemiological literature.

While emphasizing this, we nevertheless agree with Kjellman in his cautious conclusion that this controlled study indeed seems to suggest an association between otitis and allergy, but we also wish to emphasize that this is the first controlled study indicating such a relationship.

Tympanometric evidence

For scientific purposes a diagnosis of secretory otitis media, merely based on otoscopy, is unsatisfactory due to a considerable degree of inter-examiner variation. More reliable is the objective and highly reproducible measurement of middle ear pressure provided by tympanometry.

Recently Fernandes and co-workers[14] published the first tympanometric study of children from a paediatric allergy clinic, based on 100 children (aged between 8 months and 17 years), who were suffering from asthma or rhinitis. In six ears from five children (5%) a flat tympanometric curve was found, indicating a middle ear effusion. Unfortunately a non-allergic control group was not included. In non-selected 3-year-old children, Fiellau-Nicolaisen and co-workers[15] found flat curves in 10%, and Tos and co-workers[16] found a similar percentage in 1–2-year-old children. In another study[6] 24% had middle ear effusion 3 months after an uncomplicated acute otitis, and a similar figure was found in non-selected children in a kindergarten[17].

These studies have demonstrated the high prevalence of middle ear effusion in childhood, and in persistent cases a treatment requiring secretory otitis media may develop. It is also obvious that the frequency of flat tympanomograms depends upon age, time of the year and environmental factors (climate, and school conditions). In our opinion these studies also point at such factors being much more important for the development of secretory otitis media than the occurrence of atopic allergy.

The high prevalence of middle ear pathology during childhood may give the allergist, who is aware of a possible connection, the impression that otitis media is over-represented in his allergic patients. In fact, the 5% flat curves found in allergic children[14] is a low figure, considering that 50% of the patients were between 2 and 7 years, at which age children are often afflicted by middle ear diseases. Thus, this first tympanometric study of allergic diseases does not favour the hypothesis of a causal relationship between atopic allergy and secretory otitis media.

Conclusions

In the report from the first conference on recent advances in middle ear effusions[18] there was no hard evidence linking secretory otitis media and allergy. On the contrary, two reports from the second conference on advances in otitis media with effusion have been regarded as disproving such a relationship[19a,b].

In fact, there is no conclusive evidence to support the statement that allergy is the cause of any significant number of secretory otitis media cases. It seems likely that an active nasal allergy can aggravate the ear symptoms via eustachian tube malfunction, but strictly speaking we still do not know whether there exists any causal association between the two disorders. It is mandatory that future studies follow correct epidemiological principles, include a control group, and that objective measurements are used. Before positive evidence is provided in this way, it seems incorrect to recommend topical steroid treatment and 'elimination diets', without any evidence of the offending allergen[2].

MÉNIÈRE'S DISEASE

Ménière's disease was described by Prosper Ménière in 1861[20] as a syndrome of vertigo, tinnitus and hearing impairment, and it has since been recognized as a distinct clinical entity. In 1938 Hallpike and Cairns[21] discovered that the endolymphatic hydrops was a consistent pathological finding in this disease. The vestibular and auditory symptoms may begin simultaneously, or one may precede the other by days or years. The frequency of attacks is variable and long remissions from symptoms are common. The actual incidence of Ménière's disease is unknown, although various estimates are reported in the world literature. The most thorough appears to be the report of Stahle et al.[22], giving a prevalence of 46 cases per 100 000. Rupture of the inner cell layer of the membranous labyrinth and subsequent bulging of the outer layer provides a logical explanation for the episodic vertigo and fluctuating hearing impairment so characteristic for Ménière's disease[20]. While there is general agreement about Ménière's disease being a clinical expression of inner ear changes caused by dysfunction of the endolymphatic sac, there are probably multiple causes for this sac failure. All treatments which aim at a palliative or curative effect are based on some notion of aetiology, among which are metabolic disorders, sympathetic vasomotor disturbances, endocrine diseases, etc., and allergies. In general, the explanation as to how these conditions affect inner ear physiology are hypothetical and lack supporting data.

The first report attempting to link Ménière's disease and allergy was published by Duke[23]. In 1953 Gundrum[24] linked allergy and Ménière's disease together by demonstrating eosinophilia in cytologic smears of the postnasal secretion. Throughout the years there have been additional reports, mainly in the American literature[25-31]. In many of these reports the diagnosis of allergy is based mainly upon the case history and allergy testing by the Rinkle technique of serial dilution titration, and by Lee's provocative food testing method. Satisfactory studies do not support the validity of these tests[32].

The most serious report on the problem of allergy and Ménière's disease has been published by Stahle et al.[23]. These authors examined 56 patients with Ménière's disease and a control group of 50 normal persons, and could not demonstrate any increased levels of serum IgE in Ménière's patients as compared to the normals. The authors conclude that the low total IgE level in Ménière patients indicates that atopic allergy is not of importance in the pathogenesis of this disorder. They also determined IgE antibody activity by the radioallergosorbent test (RAST). They used six common allergens: cow's milk, egg white, hazel-nut, fish, house dust and house dust mite. Blood analysis of IgE antibodies against these six allergens was negative throughout in all patients. Their conclusion was that if Ménière's disease is caused by a reagin-triggered mechanism, the offending allergen is not to be found in the group of common allergens mentioned above. In conclusion, there are no convincing data in favour of a causal relationship between allergy and Ménière's disease.

References

1. Tos, M. and Bak-Pedersen, K. (1972). The pathogenesis of chronic secretory otitis media. *Arch. Otolaryngol.*, **95**, 551
2. Lecks, H. I. (1973). Serous otitis media. In Speer, F. and Dockhorn, R. J. (eds.) *Allergy and Immunology in Children*, p. 521. (Springfield: Thomas)

3. Senturia, B. H., Gessert, C. F., Carr, C. D. and Baumann, E. S. (1958). Studies concerned with tubotympanitis. *Ann. Otol. (St Louis)*, **67**, 440

4. Palva, T. and Holopainen, E. (1976). Secretory otitis media. *Acta Otolaryngol. (Stockh.)*, **81**, 204

5. Hentzer, E. and Jørgensen, M. B. (1972). The submucous layer of the middle ear in chronic otitis media. *Arch. Ohr.-, Nas.- u. Kehlk.-Heilk*, **201**, 108

6. Mygind, N., Meistrup-Larsen, K.-I., Thomsen, J., Thomsen, V. F., Josefsson, K. and Sørensen, H. (1979). Penicillin in acute otitis media. A double-blind placebo-controlled trial. *Clin. Otolaryngol.* (In press)

7. Mogi, G., Honjo, S., Maeda, S., Yoshida, T. and Watanabe, N. (1974). Immunoglobulin E (IgE) in middle ear effusions. *Ann. Otol. (St Louis)*, **83**, 393

8. Schambaugh, G. E. (1975). Panel discussion. Serous effusion of the middle ear. *Laryngoscope*, **85**, 128

9. Lecks, H. I. (1961). Allergic aspects of serous otitis media in childhood. *N.Y. St. J. Med.*, **61**, 2737

10. Dees, S. G. and Lefkowitz, D. (1972). Secretory otitis media in allergic children. *Am. J. Dis. Child.*. **124**. 364

11. Murray, A. B. and Anderson, D. O. (1969). The epidemiologic relationship of clinical nasal allergy to eosinophils and goblet cells in the nasal smear. *J. Allergy*, **43**, 1

12. Kjellman, N.-I. M., Synnerstad, B. and Hansson, L. O. (1976). Atopic allergy and immunoglobulins in children with adenoids and recurrent otitis media. *Acta Paediatr. Scand.*, **65**, 593

13. Hibbit, J. and Tweedie, M. C. K. (1977). The value of signs and symptoms in the diagnosis of enlarged adenoids. *Clin. Otolaryngol.*, **2**, 297

14. Fernandes, D., Gupta, S., Sly, R. M. and Frazer, M. (1978). Tympanometry in children with respiratory diseases. *Ann. Allergy*, **40**, 181

15. Fiellau-Nikolaisen. M. and Lous. J. (1977). Tympanometry in three-year-old children. I. *Scand. Audiol.*. **6**. 199

16. Tos, M., Poulsen, G. and Borch, J. (1978). Tympanometry in 2-year-old children. *ORL*, **40**, 77

17. Meistrup-Larsen, K.-I., Andersen, M. S., Helweg, J., Deigaard, J. and Peitersen, E. (1979). Variations in tympanomograms in children attending group care during a 1 year period. *Acta Otolaryngol. (Stockh.).* (In press)

18. *Ann. Otol. (St Louis)*, 1976, **85** (Suppl.), 25

19a.Virolainen. E.. Pukahha. H.. Aantaa. E.. Tuohimaa. P.. Ruuskanen. O. and Meurman. O. H. (1979). The prevalence of secretory otitis media in 7–8 year old school children. *Ann. Otol. (St Louis).* (In press)

19b.Yamashita, Y., Okazaki, N. and Kumazawa. T. (1979). Relation between nasal and middle ear allergy – An experimental study. *Ann. Otol. (St Louis).* (In press)

20. Schuknecht. H. F. (1968). Correlation of pathology with symptoms of Ménière's disease. *Otolaryngol. Clin. N. Am.*. p. 433

21. Hallpike, C. and Cairns, H. (1938). Observations on the pathology of Meniere's syndrome. *J. Laryngol.*, **53**, 625

22. Stahle, J., Stahle, C. and Arenberg, I. K. (1978). Incidence of Meniere's disease. *Arch. Otolaryngol.*, **104**, 99

23. Duke, W. W. (1923). Meniere's syndrome caused by allergy. *J. Am. Med. Assoc.*, **81**, 2179

24. Gundrum, L. K. (1953). Etiologic analysis of one hundred cases of Meniere's symptom-complex. *Arch. Otolaryngol.*, **57**, 123

25. Rinkle, H. J. (1963). The management of clinical allergy. *Arch. Otolaryngol.*, **77**, 42

26. Godlowski, Z. Z. (1960). Endocrine management of selected cases of allergy based on enzymatic mechanism of sensitization. *Arch. Otolaryngol.*, **71**, 513

27. Lee, C. H., Williams, R. I. and Binkley, E. L. (1969). Provocative testing and treatment for foods. *Arch. Otolaryngol.*, **90**, 87

28. Powers, W. H. and House, W. F. (1969). The dizzy patient. Allergic aspects. *Laryngoscope*, **79**, 1330

29. Endicott, J. N. and Stucker, F. J. (1977). Allergy in Meniere's disease related to fluctuating hearing loss. Preliminary findings in a double-blind crossover clinical study. *Laryngoscope*, **87**, 1650

30. Pulec, J. L. (1977). Indications for surgery in Meniere's disease. *Laryngoscope*, **87**, 542

31. Powers, W. H. (1978). Metabolic aspects of Meniere's disease. *Laryngoscope*, **88**, 122

32. Golbert, T. M. (1975). A review of controversial diagnostic and therapeutic techniques employed in allergy. *J. Allergy*, **56**, 170

33. Stahle, J., Deuschl, H. and Johansson, S. G. O. (1974). Meniere's disease and allergy. *Equil. Res.*, **4**, 22

9 PART III:
Allergy and the Kidney

D. GWYN WILLIAMS

Type I immune reactions causing renal disease are seemingly uncommon, and in only a small number of instances is there some proof more convincing than *post hoc ergo propter hoc* that reaginic antibody has a pathogenic role. In contrast, of course, is the much greater frequency of Type III (antigen–antibody complex mediated) reactions causing glomerulonephritis, either as a result of deposition in glomeruli of circulating complexes, or of glomerular localization of antigen alone and the subsequent combination with specific antibody *in situ*. Type II reactions in the kidney are represented by the lesions caused by antibody directed against antigens in glomerular or tubular basement membranes. The former, with its ability in some cases to cross-react with the basement membrane of pulmonary alveoli, is the primary pathogenetic mechanism in Goodpasture's syndrome. Cell-mediated reactions (Type IV) are prominent in the rejection of grafted kidneys, and may play a part in some forms of glomerulonephritis, particularly interstitial nephritis.

Despite the rarity of recognized Type I reactions, they are of considerable interest for practical and theoretical reasons. Firstly, when suspected or proven, there is the possibility of cure (a rare experience for nephrologists caring for patients with glomerular disease) by desensitization or withdrawal of the allergen. Secondly, since the clinical features (i.e. a relapsing nephrotic syndrome), the histological appearances of the glomeruli, and the response to steroid therapy are indistinguishable from those of the minimal change nephrotic syndrome (MCNS), the question arises of whether Type I reactions are responsible for at least some cases of MCNS, the aetiology and pathogenesis of which are unknown.

TYPE I REACTIONS AND NEPHROTIC SYNDROME

Some details of the small number of cases in which there are reasonable grounds for suspecting Type I reactions to be playing a role are shown in Table 9.III.1.

Table 9.III.1 Details of patients with a nephrotic syndrome due to allergy

Case no. /sex	Age at onset of nephrotic syndrome (years)	Atopic symptoms	Allergen and proof	Treatment and response	Biopsy findings	Author
1 M	39	hay fever	tree and grass pollen; seasonal incidence and remission following desensitization	desensitization; remission	focal thickening of basement membrane and hypercellularity ND*	Hardwicke et al.[1]
2 M	2	rhinitis	moulds; skin test	steroids; remission	ND	Wittig and Goldman[2]
3 M	7	hay fever	ragweed; skin test; remission following desensitization	desensitization; remission	ND	
4 M	14	eczema	grass pollen; skin test	steroids and desensitization; remission	ND	
5 M	8	hay fever	grass pollen; skin test; remission following desensitization	desensitization; remission	ND	Wilkinson[3]
6 M	10	hay fever	grass pollen; skin test; raised serum level of pollen specific IgE	steroids and desensitization; remission	Min. ch.†	
7 M	2	eczema; hay fever later	tree and grass pollen; skin test; raised serum level of pollen specific IgE	steroids and cyclophosphamide; improved	ND	Reeves et al.[4]
8 M	44	eczema, asthma, hay fever	tree and grass pollen, house dust; skin test	steroids; improved	Min. ch.	
9 F	5	eczema, asthma, urticaria	pollens, chicken eggs, animal hairs; raised serum level of specific IgE	steroids; frequent relapse then removal of allergens, desensitization; prolonged remission	ND	Richards et al.[5]
10 M	8	asthma	cow's milk; partial or complete remission on elemental diet, relapse on exposure to milk, further remission on withdrawal of milk positive skin test to milk	see preceding column	Min. ch.	Sandberg et al.[6]
11 F	2	eczema			ND	
12 M	3	asthma, eczema			Min. ch.	
13 F	3	eczema			Min. ch.	
14 M	3	none			Min. ch.	
15 M	4	asthma			Min. ch.	

*ND = not done; †Min. ch. = minimal change

Clinical features

In Table 9.III.1 there is a preponderance of males, and all but two presented during childhood. All patients presented with the nephrotic syndrome and in most this was with a background of atopic symptoms which in many of the cases had preceded the onset of the nephrotic syndrome by several years. A notable and important feature is that in some of these patients relapse of proteinuria could occur at times when they were not exposed to the allergen presumed responsible, e.g. patient 3 with hay fever and sensitivity to grass pollen had relapses during the winter months. The implication of this observation, further discussed below, is that the allergen in question and its reaginic antibody are not the sole factors causing glomerular damage in these patients.

The allergens involved were unremarkable, representing those commonly causing atopic symptoms.

Proof that Type I reactions caused the proteinuria

The most convincing proof lies in two groups of patients. In cases 1, 3, 5 and 9 there was an improvement or cure following desensitization to the allergen to which sensitivity had been found on skin testing. In cases 10–15, each of which had a positive skin test to cow's milk, there was an unequivocal increase in proteinuria on exposure to cow's milk and remission on its withdrawal, albeit unaccompanied by a rise in serum IgE – it was not reported whether there was any rise in the amount of IgE specific for cow's milk accompanying the relapses.

In the remainder of the patients the association of sensitivity to an allergen with nephrotic syndrome provides only circumstantial, albeit strong, evidence that the renal disease is allergic. This evidence is embellished in patients 6 and 7 by the rise in total concentration of serum IgE accompanied by an increase of IgE specific for the allergen at the time of relapse.

The improvement resulting from the use of steroids does not, of course, constitute evidence that Type I reactions were responsible, as idiopathic MCNS is itself steroid-responsive.

Other immunological phenomena

In some patients, usually in association with accompanying hay fever, there has been an eosinophilia. A fall in serum C3 concentration at the time of relapse was noted in patient 6, and in this case and that of patient 7 there were strongly positive C1q precipitation tests during relapse, indicating that there may have been circulating antigen–antibody complexes. As well as IgE specific for pollen, there was a rise in IgG pollen-specific antibody.

Pathology

A renal biopsy was performed in eight patients and in seven the appearances on light microscopy were reported to be consistent with minimal change nephrotic syndrome, i.e. normal glomeruli or at most slightly increased cellularity of the mesangium. Immunoglobulins G, M, A, and in particular E, were not detectable. In patient 2 the biopsy tissue was reported as showing focal thickening of the glomerular basement membrane with slight hypercellularity of the mesangium.

Pathogenesis

In this group of patients the pathogenesis is not known, and indeed it is not understood in idiopathic MCNS itself.

There is no evidence to support a local reaction within the kidney itself analogous to that occurring on mucosal surfaces. IgE has not been detected in renal tissue in these particular patients, and the absence of basophils in affected kidneys also makes a localized reaction hard to accept.

It is more likely that the combination of reaginic antibody, which could include IgG as well as IgE, with basophils and mast cells at sites distant from the kidney causes release of substances such as histamine and slow reacting substance A which circulate and at the glomerulus produce a change in permeability.

Another possible mechanism for glomerular damage is that immune complexes form (as suggested by the fall in serum levels of both IgG and C3) and that complement activation follows with the production of C3a, C5a and C567, All of which can act as anaphylatoxins and hence may alter capillary permeability. In this connection it is of note that allergens producing atopy activate C3 in serum[7], and that antigen–antibody complexes containing IgE have been found in the plasma of individuals suffering atopic symptoms[8]. Yet again, any effect of antigen–antibody complexes in this disorder is presumably remote since immunoglobulins and complement components are not detectable in the kidney.

Two clinical observations in this group of patients emphasize that as well as being unknown, the pathogenesis of this disorder is complicated. Firstly, atopic symptoms precede by years in some patients the onset of nephrotic syndrome, suggesting that a change in the host has allowed the disease to occur, e.g. an alteration in glomerular susceptibility to agents changing permeability, or reduced inhibition of substances causing increased permeability, or, more subtly, a lessened ability to eliminate the allergen, the ensuing persistence of which results in new manifestations of disease.

Secondly, in some of these patients nephrotic syndrome relapses have occurred not only on exposure to allergens, but also following infections, as is well recognized in idiopathic MCNS. Although the infectious agents could behave as antigens for reaginic antibodies, it is more reasonable to assume that they mainly cause a Type III response. In other words, in these particular patients a Type I reaction may not be the only insult to cause proteinuria; the glomeruli can be damaged as a consequence of other modes of immune response. How this happens is not known, either in idiopathic MCNS itself or in this subgroup of patients.

Nonetheless, the cure following desensitization in some patients clearly indicates that reaginic antibody can have a specific role in causing the disease.

Treatment

If the allergen to which the patient has demonstrable sensitivity on intra-dermal testing is indeed responsible through a reaginic mechanism for the renal damage in these patients, then desensitization or removal of the allergen from the environment would be expected to effect a cure if it were the only cause. This seems to have been so quite convincingly in the three patients who were treated by desensitization alone, and in those patients who remitted on withdrawal of cow's milk. Thus, if a patient with nephrotic syndrome is suspected of having an allergic cause, there is a real possibility that cure can be effected without the use of steroids or cyclophosphamide. As can be seen from Table 9.III.1, these drugs have been employed, sometimes in combination with desensitization, and as in MCNS they have proved effective.

NEPHROTIC SYNDROME WITH POSSIBLE TYPE I REACTION AS A CAUSE

There have been several descriptions of a nephrotic syndrome following exposure to various substances which could conceivably have been acting as an allergen, such as bee venom[9], serum, poison oak and poison ivy[10]. In none of these cases was there any evidence that the renal disease was a Type I reaction apart from the circumstantial nature of the case, so they are merely recorded here as possibly allergic renal disease, and not discussed with the cases with fuller documentation described above.

TYPE I REACTIONS AND IDIOPATHIC MINIMAL CHANGE NEPHROTIC SYNDROME

MCNS is the commonest cause of nephrotic syndrome in children, and accounts for approximately 10% of adult nephrotics. One of its most outstanding characteristics is that despite the lack of evidence for its being either inflammatory or due to local immune mechanisms operating in the glomeruli, it responds, either with complete remission or marked reduction in proteinuria, to treatment with drugs commonly regarded as being immuno-suppressive, i.e. steroids, cyclophosphamide and azathioprine. The beneficial effect of these drugs therefore suggests that the immune system is at fault in MCNS, and a number of associated abnormalities have been described. Prominent among these are diminished response of patients' lymphocytes to mitogens[11], the inhibition by patients' sera of a normal lymphocyte response to mitogens[12], and cytotoxicity of patients' lymphocytes against isolated renal epithelium[13]. Although neither hypocomplementaemia nor circulating C3 breakdown products have been demonstrated in minimal change sera, there is some evidence that complement activation has occurred in that sera from patients inhibit uptake by normal lymphocytes of sheep cells coated with antibody and complement[14], and there are raised serum levels of immuno-conglutinin in patients in relapse[15]. Circulating immune complexes have been detected during relapse[16], but they do not activate complement[17]. Added to this direct evidence is the association of MCNS with Hodgkin's disease, which is noted for its alteration in cell-mediated immunity, and the induction of remission of MCNS by measles, which itself produces depression of cell-mediated immunity.

Since, as described above, the nephrotic syndrome occurring with Type I reactions is similar to MCNS, it is possible that in some patients MCNS represents an otherwise unrecognized form of reaginic antibody disease.

In favour of reaginic antibodies playing a role in the pathogenesis of idiopathic MCNS are the following. There is a seasonal increase in the frequency of this condition, which rises in June and July, i.e. at the same time as diseases due to pollen sensitivity. Children with MCNS have a higher incidence of atopy than controls – 38% of 40 patients compared with 18% of controls[18]. The associated atopic disorder was most frequently hay fever, but asthma and eczema were also present. In the same group of patients a high frequency of HLA-B12 was found, and associated with this haplotype was a high frequency of positive skin-prick tests to mixed grass pollen or mites. Serum IgE levels are higher in MCNS[19, 20], and these too are significantly associated with the presence of HLA-B12, both as total IgE and as IgE specifically directed against grass pollen[18]. The marked tendency for relapse of MCNS to follow infections could be interpreted as another sign that these patients are allergic, the infective agent behaving as an allergen.

On the other hand, despite an early report that IgE was detectable by immunofluorescence in the glomeruli of these patients[21], subsequent workers have failed to demonstrate glomerular IgE[22, 23]. It is therefore hard to accept that IgE is involved in causing any direct local glomerular changes and if IgE is responsible for glomerular damage then, as discussed above, it presumably brings about this effect at a distance. The failure of doxantrazole to bring about remission in MCNS in a small uncontrolled study is a point against a Type I reaction causing the proteinuria, but does not exclude it[24].

TYPE I REACTIONS AND OTHER RENAL DISEASE

There is some evidence that reaginic antibody may be playing a role in interstitial nephritis. This is characterized histologically by interstitial oedema, infiltration of the renal interstitium by plasma cells and lymphocytes accompanied by various degrees of tubular atrophy. In the acute form the patient presents with haematuria, proteinuria and in several cases with acute renal failure.

Acute interstitial nephritis is associated with infections, e.g. scarlet fever, diphtheria, mumps, measles, and many drugs, particularly the penicillins (especially methicillin), cephalothin, rifampicin, thiazides, frusemide and phenindione. In the case of interstitial nephritis due to drugs there is clinical evidence that the lesion is a form of hypersensitivity in that the disease is not dose related, occurs in only a minority of patients receiving the drug, and is frequently accompanied by a rash, fever and eosinophilia. That a Type I reaction may be in part responsible is suggested by increased levels of IgE in the serum of some of these patients[25], the presence of plasma cells bearing IgE in one case of interstitial nephritis following phenobarbitone ingestion[26], and the presence of basophils in the interstitium of another case[27].

There is, however, evidence that other immunological mechanisms may operate in drug-induced interstitial nephritis such as cell-mediated toxicity and antibodies against tubular basement membrane generated by a combination of drug and tubular basement membrane which behaves as an antigen[28].

Lastly, some patients with Henoch–Schönlein purpura and nephritis have a history suggestive of sensitivity to food as a precipitating factor for their illness. Although immunochemical studies on the serum[29] and histological studies of renal tissue[30] provide strong circumstantial evidence that the nephritis of Henoch–Schönlein purpura is an immune-complex disease, the food sensitivity in some cases hints that a Type I reaction may be partaking in the glomerular damage.

References

1. Hardwicke, J., Soothill, J. F., Squire, J. R. and Hozti, G. (1959). Nephrotic syndrome with pollen hypersensitivity. *Lancet*, **1**, 500
2. Wittig, J. H. and Goldman, A. S. (1970). Nephrotic syndrome associated with inhaled allergens. *Lancet*, **1**, 542
3. Williamson, D. A. J. (1970). Nephrotic syndrome associated with inhaled allergens. *Lancet*, **1**, 778
4. Reeves, W. G., Cameron, J. S., Johansson, S. G. O., Ogg, C. S., Peters, D. K. and Weller, R. O. (1975). Seasonal nephrotic syndrome. *Clin. Allergy*, **5**, 121
5. Richards, W., Olson, D. and Church, J. A. (1977). Improvement of idiopathic nephrotic syndrome following allergy therapy. *Ann. Allergy*, **39**, 332

6. Sandberg, D. H., McIntosh, R. M., Bernstein, C. W., Carr, R. and Strauss, J. (1977). Severe steroid-responsive nephrosis associated with hypersensitivity. *Lancet*, 1, 388

7. Berrens, L. and Van Rijswijk-Verbeek, J. (1973). Inactivation of complement (C3) in human sera by atopic allergens. *Int. Arch. Allergy Appl. Immunol.*, 45, 30

8. Brostoff, J., Johns, P. and Stanworth, D. R. (1977). Complexed IgE in atopy. *Lancet*, 2, 741

9. Venters, H. D., Vernier, R. L., Worthen, H. G. and Good, R. A. (1961). Bee sting nephrosis – a study of the immunopathologic mechanism. *Am. J. Dis. Child.*, 102, 688

10. Rytand, D. A. (1948). Fatal anuria, the nephrotic syndrome and glomerulonephritis as sequels to dermatitis of poison oak. *Am. J. Med.*, 5, 548

11. Schulte-Wisserman, H., Straub, E. and Funke, P. J. (1977). Nephrotic syndrome of childhood and disorder of T cell function. *Eur. J. Pediatr.*, 124, 121

12. Moorthy, A. V., Zimmerman, S. W. and Burkholder, P. M. (1976). Inhibition of lymphocyte blastogenesis by plasma of patients with minimal change nephrotic syndrome. *Lancet*, 1, 1160

13. Eyres, K., Mallick, N. P. and Taylor, G. (1976). Evidence for cell-mediated immunity to renal antigens in minimal change nephrotic syndrome. *Lancet*, 1, 1159

14. Smith, M. D., Barratt, T. M., Hayward, A. R. and Soothill, J. F. (1975). The inhibition of complement-dependent lymphocyte rosette formation by the sera of children with steroid sensitive nephrotic syndrome. *Clin. Exp. Immunol.*, 21, 236

15. Ngu, J., Barratt, T. M. and Soothill, J. F. (1970). Immunoconglutinin and complement changes in steroid sensitive relapsing nephrotic syndrome of children. *Clin. Exp. Immunol.*, 6, 109

16. Stuhlinger, W. D., Verroust, P. J. and Morel-Maroger, L. (1976). Detection of circulating soluble immune complexes in patients with various renal diseases. *Immunology*, 30, 43

17. Levinsky, R. J., Malleson, P. H., Barratt, T. M. and Soothill, J. F. (1978). Circulating immune complexes in steroid responsive nephrotic syndrome. *N. Engl. J. Med.*, 298, 126

18. Thomson, P. D., Stokes, C. R., Barratt, T. M., Turner, M. W. and Soothill, J. F. (1976). HLA antigens and atopic features in steroid responsive nephrotic syndrome of childhood. *Lancet*, 2, 765

19. Groshong, T., Mendelson, L. and Mendoza, S. (1973). Serum IgE in patients with minimal change nephrotic syndrome. *J. Pediatr.*, 83, 767

20. Sobel, A. T., Intrator, L. and Lagrue, G. (1976). Serum immunoglobulins in idiopathic minimal change nephrotic syndrome. *N. Engl. J. Med.*, 294, 50

21. Gerber, M. A. and Paronetto, F. (1971). IgE in glomeruli of patients with nephrotic syndrome. *Lancet*, 1, 1097

22. Lewis, E. J., Kallen, R. J. and Rowe, D. S. (1973). Glomerular localization of IgE in lipoid nephrosis. *Lancet*, 1, 1395

23. Roy, L. P., Westberg, N. G. and Michael, A. F. (1973). Nephrotic syndrome – no evidence for a role for IgE. *Clin. Exp. Immunol.*, 13, 553

24. Bluett, N. H., Chantler, C. and Hughes, D. T. (1977). Failure of doxantrozole in steroid-sensitive nephrotic syndrome. *Lancet*, 1, 809

25. Ooi, B. S., First, M. R., Pesce, A. J., Pollak, V. E., Bernstein, I. L. and Jao, W. (1974). IgE levels in interstitial nephritis. *Lancet*, 1, 1254

26. Faarup, P. and Christiansen, E. (1974). IgE-containing plasma cells in acute tubulo-interstitial nephropathy. *Lancet*, 2, 718

27. Colvin, R. B., Burton, N. E., Hyslop, N. E., Spitz, L. and Lichtenstein, N. S. (1974). Penicillin-associated interstitial nephritis. *Ann. Intern. Med.*, 81, 404

28. McCluskey, R. T. and Colvin, R. B. (1978). Immunological aspects of renal tubular and interstitial diseases. *Ann. Rev. Med.*, 29, 191

29. Garcia-Fuentes, M., Chantler, C. and Williams, D. G. (1977). Cryoglobulinaemia in Henoch–Schönlein purpura. *Br. Med. J.*, 2, 163

30. Heaton, J. M., Turner, D. R. and Cameron, J. S. (1977). Localisation of glomerular 'deposits' in Henoch–Schönlein nephritis. *Histopathology*, 1, 93

10
Allergy, Insects and Arachnids

A. W. FRANKLAND and M. H. LESSOF

INTRODUCTION

Man has coexisted with insects for millions of years, and more recently the Pharaohs cultivated bees as an industry. We read that six of the ten plagues of Egypt were caused by arthropods of some sort. Assyrian cuneiform depicts insects and the Aztec Indians of Mexico prepared a red dye from them. The insects are characterized by having three body segments, three pairs of legs, usually two pairs of wings and one pair of antennae. Included in this group are the lice, beetles, bugs, caterpillars, fleas, bees, wasps, yellow jackets, hornets, ants, mosquitoes and flies. The arachnids are characterized by having two body segments, four pairs of legs, no wings or antennae and in this group are the spiders, ticks, scorpions and mites. The Insecta and Arachnida should be referred to collectively as 'arthropods'.

TOXICITY VERSUS ANAPHYLAXIS

The toxic reactions caused by the arthropods in man are chiefly associated with the injection of venom; the toxic effects depend upon the composition of the venom and the amount injected. The venom of a scorpion is particularly potent and can cause death in a baby while, in contrast, even multiple stings from wasps, bees and ants may be relatively well tolerated. One sting from a bee can cause death in a subject allergic to bee stings, but over 500 stings from a swarm of bees, although producing severe toxic effects from the introduction into the body of pharmacologically active substances, may not kill the non-allergic adult[1].

The evolution of venoms has endowed stinging insects with an injectable mixture of amines, peptides and enzymes which have remarkable pharmacological effects on their enemies. The many biologically active components of bee, wasp and hornet venoms are shown in Table 10.1. Histamine, serotonin

Table 10.1 Components from venom of wasp, hornet and honeybee (After Habermann, 1972)[2]

	Wasp	*Hornet*	*Honeybee*
Vasoactive amines	histamine	histamine	histamine
	serotonin	serotonin	—
	—	acetylcholine	—
	dopamine	dopamine	dopamine
	noradrenaline	noradrenaline	noradrenaline
	—	adrenaline	—
Peptides	wasp kinins	hornet kinins	apamin
			melittin
			mast cell degranulating peptide (401)
Enzymes	phospholipase A	phospholipase A	phospholipase A
	phospholipase B	phospholipase B	—
	hyaluronidase	hyaluronidase	hyaluronidase
	acid phosphatase	—	—
	histidine decarboxylase	—	—
			acid phosphatase
Free amino acids	many	many	many

and acetylcholine need no special emphasis. The active region of wasp kinin is identical with mammalian bradykinin, and a number of other peptides and protein enzymes are present which are capable of disrupting a wide range of cell mechanisms. Bee venom can produce effects which range from haemolysis (melittin) to neurotoxicity (apamin)[2]. These actions are largely dose related and the main toxic effect derives from melittin, which constitutes 50% of dried venom.

We still do not understand why a relatively small percentage of individuals become anaphylactically sensitized to insect venoms in quantities so small that their pharmacological action is relatively slight. Venoms contain a large variety of pharmacologically active amines and peptides, quite apart from the major allergens. Although these are not responsible for anaphylaxis, they do affect the rate of absorption and could also influence the immunological response in other ways. The main allergens in bee venom appear to be two enzymes, phospholipase A and hyaluronidase, which make up only 12% and 1–3% respectively of the dried weight. Molecular size may be a factor[3], since hyaluronidase (mol. wt. 50 000) and phospholipase A (mol. wt. 15 000) are much larger molecules than melittin (mol. wt. 2840) and apamin (mol. wt. 2038). Melittin can, nevertheless, act as an allergen in some cases[4]. It is also the larger molecules that provide the major allergens of vespid venoms[5], which contain three major proteins, a phospholipase, a hyaluronidase and the most potent vespid allergen, which is a protein of unknown function known as antigen 5. Cross-reactivity between venoms and individual allergens among the vespid species certainly occurs, but these proteins do not appear to cross-react with those obtained from honeybee venom.

Despite earlier views to the contrary[6], allergic reactions to venom seem to occur more frequently in atopic than in non-atopic subjects[7]. Some degree of local hypersensitivity is, however, extremely common even in non-atopic subjects, as may be demonstrated by the frequency with which successive bites by the ubiquitous fleas and mosquitoes produce increasing local reactions.

STINGING INSECTS

Diagnostic methods and IgE

It is amazing how often the person stung cannot identify the stinging insect, but the common honeybee (*Apis mellifera*) is the one that leaves its sting in the wound. Bumble bees (Bombidae), although large and noisy and feared for this reason, are not vicious, but children may be stung if, when barefoot, they tread on a bumble bee that is feeding on clover. There are thousands of species of wasps and not all sting. Those that do include the *Polistes*, hornets and yellow jackets. The common social wasps are the yellow jackets and hornets, contained in the genus *Vespula*, and the *Polistes* wasps, which are of the subfamily Polistinae.

Skin tests, although valuable in confirming the diagnosis of insect allergy, can be difficult to interpret. Intradermal tests with 0.05 ml of a solution containing 1 µg/ml of bee venom (i.e. 50 ng in all) can induce non-specific positive reactions in some non-allergic subjects. Reactions to bee venom can therefore be regarded as significant, positive responses only when the venom concentration is 100 ng/ml or less. Using these criteria, patients with a history of anaphylactic reactions to bee stings within a 3-year period have been reported as having positive tests in 30 out of 34 cases[8]. In such circumstances, the finding of a negative test may indicate that the patient is no longer allergic.

In the past, it has not been possible to demonstrate a positive radio-allergosorbent test (RAST) in all of these patients, which raises doubts about whether these reactions are always IgE mediated. It now appears that the occasional finding of a negative RAST may, however, reflect the difficulty in detecting low levels of specific IgE by this method. Now that improvements in RAST technique have allowed the specific IgE content of undiluted serum to be assayed, it has been shown[9] that anti-bee venom IgE is detectable in all patients who have had anaphylactic reactions to a sting. As a discriminating test this is still less useful than a skin test, for although non-beekeeper control subjects give negative RAST results, 58% of non-allergic beekeepers are also found to have a significant but usually low level of IgE antibody to bee venom. The circumstances in which detectable levels of specific IgE are associated with clinical evidence of allergy or anaphylaxis will be considered below. It seems possible – but so far unproven – that the greater discriminating ability of skin tests is related to the presence, in the non-allergic beekeeper, of additional blocking factors such as IgG antibody, which may prevent both the skin response and clinical anaphylactic reactions.

Despite these minor reservations, there is experimental support for the suggestion that clinical sensitivity to Hymenoptera is related to the IgE antibody response to venom proteins. Serum from allergic patients can be used to sensitize normal basophils, which will then release histamine on venom challenge[10]. Basophil sensitization cannot be effected, however, after the removal of IgE antibody from the serum.

Clinical aspects

There is virtually always some local reaction to a sting, but where this is very marked and persistent there is a danger that subsequent stings may be followed by generalized reactions. In such cases the evidence of an IgE-mediated reaction is largely clinical, but a positive RAST for IgE antibodies to bee venom has been found in 41 out of 43 (95%) beekeepers whose reaction to a sting exceeded 50 mm in diameter[9]. If. in spite of antihistamines, the local reaction is extensive and severe, it may be justified to give 10–20 mg prednisolone for its anti-inflammatory effect.

Together with local and classical anaphylactic reactions after stings, many different syndromes have been described. The serum sickness type of reaction, with joint pains and fever, may develop several days after an immediate reaction has subsided, and this may persist for some weeks[11]. Renal reactions, characterized by haematuria or proteinuria, also occur and are usually short-lived. Local skin reactions of delayed hypersensitivity or more extensive vesicular eruptions have also been described. There may be a delayed onset of peripheral neuropathy, intracranial haemorrhage or oedema, and mental changes and myocardial infarction have been precipitated on occasions. The pathogenesis of these various syndromes is unknown, but immune complex reactions cannot easily be ruled out in these circumstances and immuno-therapy is not necessarily indicated in such cases.

Anaphylaxis

There are varying grades of severity of anaphylaxis. In its mildest form the response appears to be entirely cutaneous, with erythema, pruritis, urticaria and angioedema. In more severe reactions the patient is hypotensive and may complain of faintness and misty vision. Such reactions are nearly always preceded by an aura which the patient comes to recognize. Commonly, this involves pulsating noises in the ears, constriction of the throat, substernal pain and fear of impending death. Following this brief period there may develop further frightening symptoms – respiratory difficulty, laryngeal oedema, nausea, vomiting and acute abdominal pain, sometimes followed by diarrhoea. Unconsciousness can follow in 5 to 30 minutes after the sting. The severely affected will be doubly incontinent but usually, although not always, they are unconscious when this occurs. When a patient becomes unconscious within less than 5 minutes of the sting. the risk of dying from an attack is considerable. A patient who has developed unconsciousness in 15 minutes may note that it develops after another sting in 10 minutes, then in 5 minutes, and then in 3 minutes. The next sting may well be fatal and the patient knows it. Although cardiac arrhythmias occur in the older patient, even children below the age of 10 can die from sting anaphylaxis[12].

After anaphylactic death from an insect sting, it is not unknown for a newspaper to report correctly that the dead person was terrified that he might be stung but to add, incorrectly, that the sting must have been intravenous. One such patient, a female aged 53, who had received high dosage aqueous whole body but not venom immunotherapy, died from a wasp sting in less than 3 minutes. At autopsy, except for minimal microscopic congestion of the lungs, there was no macroscopic abnormality to account for death. The injection of adrenaline, which it was known she could competently give, lay unused by the body. The exact cause of death in such a patient is not easy to explain. and immunological post-mortem studies may be needed[13]. The pathophysiology of anaphylaxis is poorly understood. Plasma histamine levels parallel the degree of hypotension, but other mediators are almost certainly involved and respiratory difficulty and anoxia may play a part[14].

An injection of adrenaline is the emergency treatment of acute anaphylaxis – 0.5 ml of a 1 : 1000 solution can be given by deep subcutaneous injection and repeated in 2–5 minutes. If possible (and if the laws of the land allow) the patients can be taught how to give their own injections. More practical, however, is a pressurized atomizer containing isoprenaline or adrenaline such as asthmatics use. Two puffs of this are given immediately after a sting and repeated every 5 minutes until skilled help can be obtained.

When severe hypotension fails to respond to adrenaline, volume replacement and α-adrenergic agonists will be necessary. In acute anaphylaxis antihistamines and corticosteroids provide no immediate benefit[15]. Some of the later effects following anaphylaxis will, however, be helped by antihistamines and especially by corticosteroids.

Treatment of insect sting allergy

Many thousands of individuals have been treated with whole body extract of bees, which has been considered suitable since Benson and Semenov's report in 1930[16]. But the use of whole body extract is open to many objections, including the fact that it may itself provoke a syndrome resembling serum sickness[17]. A critical review of this treatment has been published by Lichtenstein and his co-workers[18]. Lichtenstein's group found that of 182 patients with a history of an anaphylactic reaction to a bee sting, one-third had negative skin tests. Of the remainder, who gave a history of anaphylaxis and had a positive skin test to venom, 40% did not react to a subsequent sting[19]. Past claims about the effects of whole body treatment therefore need to be balanced against a proper assessment of the natural history of the disease.

The course of bee sting allergy is by no means always benign, as mortality figures clearly indicate[20]. On being stung again 13% of patients have a more severe generalized reaction[21, 22] and for such patients the need for effective treatment is obvious. A case can be made for treating all those with insect sting allergy who give a history of systemic reactions and who have positive skin reactions to venom, given intradermally in concentrations of 0.1 µg/ml or less. The material used should not be whole body extracts but venom, of which a variety of types are now available in the USA, including honeybee, yellow jacket, yellow hornet, the white faced (bald faced) hornet and wasp (Pharmacia Diagnostics, Piscatway, New Jersey 08854).

The availability of venoms for diagnosis and treatment represents an important advance in clinical allergy, since venom immunotherapy has been shown in controlled trial studies to have a highly significant effect in preventing anaphylactic reactions to subsequent stings[19]. The evidence is more clear and unequivocal than for any other form of immunotherapy used in treating allergy. Of 19 patients treated with venom, only one subsequently had a reaction following an in-patient challenge sting. Of the 14 patients who failed to respond to treatment with placebo or whole body extract, 13 subsequently responded to venom immunotherapy and were shown, on subsequent stinging, to have no reaction. Even the two 'failed' cases after venom treatment (one in each group) showed reactions that were much reduced in severity.

A full bee sting provides about 50 µg of venom. Venom therapy can usually start with about 1% of this dose and Lichtenstein advises 0.1 µg as a starting dose, followed by two further doses of 1 µg and 3 µg at 30-minute intervals on the first day[18]. By giving weekly injections subsequently, maintenance doses of 100 µg can usually be reached within about 6 weeks, but some patients cannot go on to monthly maintenance doses until they have increased slowly to this level over 6 months or even a year. Occasionally, patients may require stings or injections of venom every week or two in order to maintain their clinical immunity. If the interval is lengthened, mild systemic symptoms may recur[23]. About one in six patients has a systemic reaction during the course, whatever dosage regime is used. Venom immunotherapy therefore carries some hazards and should perhaps be used only by physicians who are experienced in administering allergens.

Immunological basis for immunotherapy

The experience which has now been accumulated with bee venom treatment has resolved any remaining doubts about the effectiveness of immunotherapy as a technique. The superiority of bee venom over whole body extracts has also emphasized the important requirement, that an effective vaccine for the treatment of allergy should contain a high proportion of relevant allergenic material. As a model for studying the conditions that make for effective immunotherapy, insect allergy thus has a potential importance out of all proportion to its frequency. Even so, the reasons for its effectiveness are poorly understood.

It was hoped that protection was a function of IgG or blocking antibodies against bee venom proteins[24]. In that case, the need for maintenance therapy could be monitored by measuring IgG antibody levels. It is known that IgE antibody induced by stings can persist for up to 20 years, while the IgG antibody has a protective role, it is perhaps not surprising, therefore, that antibody has a protective role, it is perhaps not surprising therefore, that where immunotherapy is not continued, patients may again develop further anaphylactic reactions after bee stings[8]. The current tendency is to continue maintenance injections or bee stings at intervals of 1 to 2 months for a period of years or until IgE antibody can no longer be demonstrated.

There are, however, objections to the use of IgG antibody measurements as an indicator of progress. Although a substantial rise in these antibodies usually accompanies successful immunotherapy, some patients with an increased IgG antivenom antibody level are not improved. Moreover in Germany, in 15 children with bee sting allergy, the effect of immunotherapy was evaluated and no correlation was found between a given IgG titre and the degree of clinical protection[25]. Despite the suggestion that the passive infusion of IgG antibody to bee venom can have a partial protective effect[26] this does not appear to be a very powerful factor. Yunginger and Santrach[27] identified four bee sting patients who were treatment failures after immunotherapy, despite having shown significant rises in serum IgG antibody to phospholipase A. Subsequently they received a plasma transfusion containing high levels of IgG antibody to phospholipase A but, when challenged with a sting on days 2–6 after transfusion, these patients continued to experience sting anaphylaxis. Assuming that their allergic reaction was directed against phospholipase A and not against hyaluronidase or some other component, it appears that IgG antibody – at least to phospholipase A – cannot provide reliable protection against sting reactions. This raises important questions about the part played by other factors still being studied including the stimulation of T cells that have a suppressor action on IgE antibody reactions. More information is needed about the effect of central control mechanisms, both upon antibody regulation and upon cellular reactivity. In other types of allergy the suggestion has been made that the injection of modified allergens, apart from stimulating IgG antibody production, can suppress established IgE reactions in a remarkable way[28]. If current attempts to use 'venomoids' in similar fashion are successful, this could result in an important change in approach for immunotherapy.

Meanwhile, regardless of theoretical considerations, venom immunotherapy is now accepted as being of practical value. A history of anaphylaxis following a sting, together with a positive skin test or RAST, should be regarded as an indication both for immunotherapy and, in the case of beekeepers, for giving up bees. Patients who disregard the advice to give up bees sometimes find that, after immunotherapy, they can nevertheless tolerate further stings or they may even encourage regular stings by way of 'maintenance therapy'. Such patients can nevertheless have further anaphylactic reactions, for example after multiple stings. The protective effect, even in 'satisfactory' cases, is by no means absolute. We still have much to learn about the risk factors which decide whether a patient remains sting sensitive.

INHALANT INSECT ALLERGY

When carrying out air sampling of the air spora and also when looking microscopically at house dust, it is noteworthy how often it is possible to recognize parts of insects. These relatively large particles are unimportant, but the main allergenic threat from insects comes from shed skin scales, dried secretion and particularly dried faecal dust, with a particle size of approximately 1 μm in diameter. Radioimmune studies in dust-mite-allergic subjects, indicate that the mite allergenic activity of the purified mite allergen is concentrated particularly in the mite faecal material[29]. Locust faeces have been found to give the largest skin reaction in locust-sensitive patients and extracts of this material have been used both in diagnosis and for immunotherapy in locust laboratory workers who developed rhinitis and asthma from airborne locust material[30].

Faecal matter is not, however, the only sensitizing substance, as has been noted in a review by Fuchs[31]. In 1929 Figley[32] reported a patient with seasonal asthma occurring during the time that mayflies (Ephemeroptera) swarmed round Lake Erie. The patient knew that his symptoms were caused by the mayflies but the insects produced no emanation or dust. It was then found when studying the life cycle of the mayfly that the excitant was a very thin and delicate skin shed in the final moulting. This stuck to many surfaces, and the dried particles became airborne. As these insects have a world-wide distribution along river banks and lake shores, they may represent unrecognized causes of inhalant respiratory allergy in a number of cases. Another seasonal cause of inhalant respiratory allergy, which affects fishermen and workers in fish food stores, is the maggot. One of the authors of this chapter (AWF), while investigating 'wet inhalant allergens', found 32 patients who used

maggots as bait when fishing, and who developed rhinitis and asthma, as well
as local urticaria and a particularly gross swelling of the penis. The types of
maggots used in this country are usually but not always those of the common
bluebottle (Table 10.2).

Table 10.2   Maggots used in angling

Common	Latin	Angling
Common housefly	*Musca domestica*	squatts
Greenbottles	*Lucilia*	ponkies
Bluebottles	*Calliphora*	gozzers

In 1949, AWF also became interested in the case of a civil airline navigator,
who flew from London to Khartoum. He had mild seasonal hay fever due to
grass pollen in Great Britain, but developed severe asthma in Khartoum
during late June and all July. The patient was sure that the cause of his asthma
was the Nemeti fly, which is found in clouds along the banks of the Nile in the
hot summer, and which, like Osgood's description of the caddis fly[33] 'fill the air
as snow in a storm'. After investigating swarms of the same midge in central
Cairo in 1956, it became possible to skin-test patients and to demonstrate
immediate reactions both in Egypt and the Sudan, among patients who have
developed inhalant allergic problems from the Nemeti fly. Nor is the caddis
fly itself free of suspicion[33]. In this case it is probably the easily detachable
hairs on the wings that cause inhalant allergic problems. Aphids (Hemiptera)
are even more widely distributed throughout the world, with unexcelled
powers of reproduction. It seems likely that they too are responsible for
inhalant allergic problems[34]. The ways in which insect allergy may come to
light are not always straightforward. Families with children who develop
allergic problems from domestic pets are sometimes advised to keep
ornamental fish. This may not be good advice because dried *Daphnia*, a
commonly used fish food, can cause asthma. This seems to be well recognized
in Russia[35]. *Daphnia* have recently been described as causing occupational
allergic rhinitis and asthma in two workers in a fish food store in Germany[36].

Another problem that is easily misinterpreted arises in cases of baker's
asthma in which provocation testing with flour does not produce clinical
symptoms. It has been found that cereals are commonly infested with weevils
and that the infesting wheat weevil – *Sitophilus granarius* – can cause inhalant
rhinitis and asthma[37]. Further studies showed that flour handlers, whether in
the bakery, flour mills, or working on grain ships at the dockside, can develop
chest complaints. Bronchio-alveolitis was shown to be caused specifically by
the grain weevil, and this seems to be a first account of alveolitis caused by an
insect[38]. 'Barn disease' in the Orkney Islands is due to mites in animal feeding
stuffs which can give rise to IgE and/or IgG antibodies in the affected

workers[39]. Winter asthma from food storage mites has been confirmed in such cases, by positive skin tests and RAST, thus correcting the previous tentative diagnosis of farmer's lung[40].

Other occupational inhalant allergic problems have been noted in several circumstances. Beekeepers may be allergic not only to bee stings, but also to honey and to airborne bee material which cause sneezing and wheezing when working on the hive. In Japan, workers in the silk industry can develop rhinitis and asthma from silk worms, and also from moths and butterflies[41].

These numerous examples serve to emphasize the importance of the problem. It would seem that insects in general are strong inhalant sensitizers in 'allergy-prone' man – those with a family or personal history of atopic disease. It is noteworthy that those workers who are already suffering from an inhalant allergic problem are often those who became sensitized, and to take locusts as an example, the longer the exposure, the higher the incidence of either skin test reactions and/or clinical allergy in the insects (Table 10.3). Extrapolating we can argue that the 'allergy-prone' should not work with strong sensitizers or allow them into their environment.

Table 10.3   Analysis of allergic and non-allergic subjects in contact with locusts

Type of patient	Number	Positive skin test to locust	Clinically locust sensitive
Normal non-allergic (no family history of atopy)	12	4	0
Normal with positive atopic family history	6	3	1
Normal but positive skin tests to some common allergens	2	1	0
Known allergic (atopic) patients	12	10	6
Total	32	18	7

House dust and mites

In 1923 Ancona[42] described inhalant allergic problems from mites. But mainly from the many studies of Voorhorst[43] it has been realized that a house dust mite is the main producer of the house dust allergen. Skin testing with dust extracts suggests, however, that patients are more likely to react to dust from their own country, suggesting that the allergens vary from one country to another. The arthropod content between different localities in one country and between different countries is known to differ greatly; for example, cockroach (Blattidae family) is a known allergen[30, 43] which is present in much greater quantities in Cairo house dust compared with that of London. In Finland, on the other hand, cockroaches are uncommon, but the hitherto uninvestigated silver fish or bristle tail (*Lepisma saccharina*) may be the commonest house insect[44]. Skin tests with silver fish have been reported as being positive in dust-sensitive subjects more often than skin test reactions to the house dust mite. In central Germany (Berlin) a beetle, *Trogoderma augustum solium*, has become a common household pest and a potent local environmental allergen[45].

It would seem therefore, that the mites of various kinds are by no means the only allergens in house dust, but numerous skin, RAST and bronchial provocation studies have nevertheless confirmed their importance. It now appears that they also provide the main allergen in damp houses (in which they thrive) rather than the moulds which were previously thought to be important[46].

Miyamoto and co-workers[47] studied the dust collected from nine cities in Japan and showed that its allergenicity largely depended upon the total and very variable number of mites contained in it. The subject of dust and mites was well reviewed by Aas[48]. He tested the effect of house dust immunotherapy in asthmatic children, and showed in a controlled study lasting 2.5 to 3 years that bronchial reactivity to dust extract challenge was markedly lessened. More recently a controlled trial of mite extract immunotherapy was carried out in asthmatic children by Warner and his co-workers[49]. All children had an immediate positive bronchial provocation test and most had also a delayed response. Immunotherapy significantly helped the patients and interestingly those with the best clinical results lost the late reaction to bronchial provocation.

BITING INSECTS

In choosing which human subjects they wish to sting or bite, pests are selective in their approach, presumably because of differences related to temperature, moisture, age, sex, colour, movement and perhaps the emotional state of the victim. Whether some body odours may have a pheromone effect in attracting insects is totally unknown. Of greater clinical interest are the many available and useful repellants, which can provide some limited protection to those who provide an undue attraction for insects.

The Hymenoptera – bees, wasps, hornets and ants, Diptera – mosquitoes and flies, Siphonaptera and Cryoplua – fleas and lice, Hemiptera – bugs, and the Arachnida – mites, ticks, spiders and scorpions, often have a complicated life history. We are not concerned here with their life history, or the good or harm they do, but only with what happens to man when some part of the arthropod is introduced through the skin and sets up a reaction.

It has been estimated that over a million people are bitten by mosquitoes every day. The local reaction that is produced is allergic in nature. Mosquitoes and other blood-feeding insects introduce some of their saliva just before starting their blood meal. The response that follows locally was shown originally by Mellanby[50] to follow a pattern of sensitization which is a highly specific allergic reaction. Not only mosquitoes but other blood-feeding insects, as well as stinging insects, seem to follow a definite pattern of sensitization. We do not know why for some insects and in some people, the response differs greatly from only a small local response to anaphylaxis and even death. Others go through a sequence that starts with sensitization and proceeds to what appears, at least clinically, to be a state of tolerance. Although there have been difficulties in demonstrating IgE antibodies, immediate skin test reactions to flea, for example, have been demonstrated[51] and clinically delayed reactions may also occur – as with the actual bite itself.

One of the authors of this chapter (AWF), an atopic individual, having marked local immediate skin response to many biting insects, decided to observe the effects of a biting insect that he had never encountered before. The insect chosen was *Rhodnius prolixus*, the cone nose or kissing bug from South America. After bites at weekly intervals, a pattern of response was to be observed in sequence and could be photographed[52] – no reaction, delayed reaction, immediate reaction and no reaction. Unfortunately the eighth blood feed produced anaphylaxis. The many different patterns of response that can occur are depicted in Figure 10.1. After the phase of no response to the first

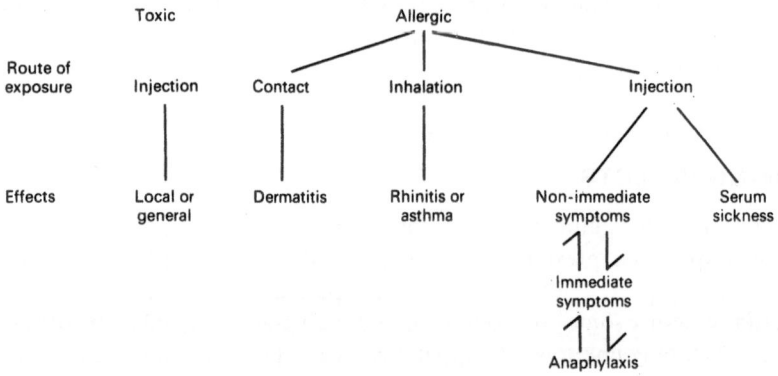

Figure 10.1   Adverse effects of insects in man

sting or bite, there is a local delayed response, which is usually relatively mild and manifests itself, in the case of fleas and mosquitoes, as the condition of papular urticaria. Occasionally this response is severe and lasts for a few days; or there can be a gross delayed response in a patient who subsequently develops an even more marked local or generalized immediate response. The response pattern is very variable, but with frequent stings or bites, the response often develops rapidly to a final stage of no reaction. However, even after the first sting, some patients may develop a typical serum-sickness-like syndrome within a period of 10 to 14 days, with fever, lymphadenopathy, urticaria and polyarthritis[53, 54].

Fire ants. like other Hymenoptera. can not only produce toxins but also cause both local and general allergic reactions. Two patients who lived in Bahrain were recently seen after developing severe local and finally anaphylactic responses to ant stings.

Reactions to different insects may vary in the same patient. A patient of one of us (AWF) had generalized reactions from a wasp sting, a rather similar reaction from many ant stings, but only local pain from a hornet sting. Most ants have stings, but imported fire ants, *Solenopsis richteri*, have recently caused increasing concern because of the allergic reactions which they can cause. This is most notable in the southern states of America, where these insects have spread rapidly and have also caused extensive crop damage. *Solenopsis xyloni* (McCook) and the common fire ant, *S. germinata fabricius*, have a less important role. The 'fire ant' is so-called because it causes an intense burning and fierce pain when it stings. After biting firmly with its jaws, the fire ant pivots round in a circle, inserting its abdominal stinger as it goes. This results within a few hours in the formation of a vesicle. The fluid in the blisters becomes purulent and the pustules last for a week to form scabs and finally scars. In elderly patients, especially if there is a tendency towards varicose veins, the lower extremities may be covered with small fibrotic nodules or areas of infectious eczema. Skin tests have been used for testing for fire ant allergy, but so far immunotherapy has not been successful when attempted. When tested on rabbits, the clinical and pathological course was not altered by antihistamines or steroids given in various ways[55].

SKIN LESIONS

Parasitic mites

We will not mention all the local effects that this class of arthropods produce. The recognition of ascariasis (mite infestation) is often difficult, particularly if a careful superficial examination of the character and distribution of the irritating rash is not carefully undertaken. Some people seem to be very much more sensitive to chigger mites than others, which suggests that there may be an allergic basis to these reactions. In man affected by scabies or 'the itch', the mites burrow in the skin for several weeks without causing any irritation. They are therefore particularly infectious, especially to any close contacts in this presensitizing period. There are 20 or so different varieties of mites each of which has a specific vertebrate host. The one that commonly attacks man is *Sarcoptes scabei* var. *hominis*. The other varieties do occasionally parasitize man. A mangy dog, many laboratory animals, particularly the rat, and the various poultry and bird nest mites have all been seen causing irritating rashes in patients sent for 'allergic' diagnosis and treatment. Scabies occurs commonly during wars but at the time of writing it seems relatively common again in Britain and in some of the Arab states.

Contact dermatitis

More than 50 different caterpillars protect themselves by their irritant hairs. When man comes in contact with these urticating caterpillars, there may be local dermatitis, while some individuals may have systemic reactions. The problem may be easy to diagnose when a boy becomes sensitized while breeding caterpillars for his school biology project, but it may not be so obvious when a local crop of caterpillars causes widespread skin sensitization in a local community as they fall off the trees. They may even sensitize the dermatologist investigating the outbreak[56]. The type of reaction produced may depend on the sensitivity of the individual as well as the amount of toxic material introduced into the skin. The 'puss caterpillar' (*Megalopyge opercularis*) of Texas, North Carolina and Florida, known in Mexico as *el perrito*, can cause particularly severe reactions[57]. Other Lepidoptera cause less trouble than the puss caterpillar, but it may be that the sensitizing properties rather than the toxic effects explain individual differences in response. Sometimes a local effect on the skin is only toxic as with blister beetles. These have an almost world-wide distribution, the best known being the coconut beetles of the Pacific Islands and the 'Spanish fly' of Spain. Cantharides is still collected for medicinal rather than aphrodisiac purposes. Occasionally the amateur or professional beekeeper can develop a contact dermatitis from propolis (bee glue) which bees collect from the sticky secretions of trees and plants.

References

1. Murray, J. A. (1964). Case of multiple bee stings. *Central Afr. J. Med.*, **10**, 249
2. Habermann, E. (1972). Bee and wasp venoms. *Science*, **177**, 314
3. King, T. P., Sobotka, A. K., Kochoumian, L. and Lichtenstein, L. M. (1976). Allergens of honey bee venom. *Arch. Biochem. Biophys.*, **172**, 661
4. Paull, B. R., Yunginger, J. W. and Gleich, G. J. (1977). Melittin: An allergen of honey bee venom. *J. Allergy Clin. Immunol.*, **59**, 334
5. King, T. P., Sobotka, A. K., Alagon, A., Kochoumian, L. and Lichtenstein, L. M. (1978). Protein allergens of white-faced hornet. yellow hornet and yellow jacket venoms. *Biochemistry*. **17**. 5165
6. Settipane, G., Newstead, G. and Boyd, G. (1972). Frequency of hymenoptera allergies in an atopic and normal population. *J. Allergy Clin. Immunol.*, **50**, 146
7. Miyachi, S., Lessof, M. H., Kemeny, D. M. and Green, L. A. (1979). Comparison of the atopic background between allergic and non-allergic beekeepers. *Int. Arch. Allergy Appl. Immunol.*, **58**, 160

8. Miyachi, S., Lessof, M. H. and Kemeny, D. M. (1979). Evaluation of bee sting allergy by skin tests and serum antibody assays. *Int. Arch. Allergy Appl. Immunol.*, **58**, 148

9. Kemeny, D. M., Lessof, M. H. and Trull, A. K. (1980). IgE and IgG antibodies to bee venom as measured by a modification of the RAST method. *Clin. Allergy.* **10**. 413

10. Sobotka, A. K., Valentine, M. D., Benton, A. and Lichtenstein, L. M. (1974). Allergy to insect stings. I. The diagnosis of IgE-mediated Hymenoptera sensitivity by venom induced histamine release. *J. Allergy Clin. Immunol.*, **53**, 170

11. Light, W. C., Reisman, R. E., Shimizu, M. and Arbesman, C. E. (1977). Unusual reactions to bee stings. *J. Allergy Clin. Immunol.*, **59**, 391

12. Jensen, O. M. (1962). Sudden death due to stings from bees and wasps. *Acta Path. Microbiol. Scand.*, **54**, 9

13. McCormick, W. F. (1963). Fatal anaphylaxis reactions to wasp stings: Review with immunological studies of fatal case. *Am. J. Clin. Pathol.*, **39**, 484

14. Kaplan, A. P., Hunt, K. J., Sobotka, A. K., Smith, P., Horakova, Z., Grabuick, H. and Lichtenstein, L. M. (1977). Human anaphylaxis. A study of mediator systems. *Clin. Res.*, **25**, 261A

15. Austen, K. F. (1978). The anaphylactic syndrome. In Samter, M. (ed.) *Immunological Diseases*, Vol. 2, pp. 885–889. (Boston: Little Brown)

16. Benson, R. L. and Semenov, H. (1930). Allergy in its relation to bee sting. *J. Allergy*, **1**, 105

17. Hunt, K., Valentine, M. D., Sobotka, A. K., Yunginger, J. W. and Lichtenstein, L. M. (1976). Serum sickness associated with non-venom protein in mixed Hymenoptera whole body extract. *J. Allergy Clin. Immunol.*, **57**, 246

18. Lichtenstein, L. M., Valentine, M. D. and Sobotka, A. K. (1979). Insect allergy: The state of the art. *J. Allergy Clin. Immunol.*, **64**, 5

19. Hunt, K. J., Valentine, M. D., Sobotka, A. K., Benton, A. W., Amodio, F. J. and Lichtenstein, L. M. (1978). A controlled trial of immunotherapy in insect hypersensitivity. *N. Engl. J. Med.*, **299**, 157

20. Parrish, M. H. (1959). Deaths from bites and stings of venomous animals in the U.S. *Arch. Intern. Med.*, **104**, 198

21. Settipane, G. A. and Chafee, F. H. (1979). Natural history of allergy to Hymenoptera. *Clin. Allergy*, **9**, 385

22. Settipane, G. A. and Boyd, G. K. (1970). Prevalence of bee sting allergy in 4992 boy scouts. *Acta Allerg.*, **25**, 286

23. Yunginger, J. W., Paull, B. R., Jones, R. T. and Santrach, P. J. (1979). Rush venom immunotherapy program for honey bee sting sensitivity. *J. Allergy Clin. Immunol.*, **63**, 340

24. Lessof, M. H., Sobotka, A. K. and Lichtenstein, L. M. (1978). Effects of passive antibody in bee anaphylaxis. *Johns Hopkins Med. J.*, **142**, 1

25. Urbanek, R., Forster, J. and Karitzky, D. (1979). Specific IgG antibodies against bee venom, phospholipase A, melittin and apamin. *J. Allergy Clin. Immunol.*, **63**, 181

26. Lessof, M. H., Sobotka, A. K. and Lichtenstein, L. M. (1977). Protection against anaphylaxis in Hymenoptera-sensitive patients by passive immunization. *Mon. Allergy.* **12**. 253

27. Yunginger, J. W. and Santrach, B. A. (1979). Treatment failures following honey bee venom immunotherapy: Use of passive immunization. *J. Allergy Clin. Immunol.*, **63**, 179

28. Kudo, K., Okudaira, H., Miyamoto, T., Nakagawa, T. and Horiuchi, Y. (1978). IgE antibody response to mite antigen in the mouse. *J. Allergy Clin. Immunol.*, **61**, 1

29. Platts-Mills, T. (1979). Personal communication

30. Frankland, A. W. (1953). Locust sensitivity. *Ann. Allergy*, **11**, 445

31. Fuchs, E. (1979). Insects as inhalant allergens. *Allergol. Immunopathol.*. **7**, 227

32. Figley, K. D. (1940). May fly (Ephemera) hypersensitivity. *J. Allergy.* **11**. 376

33. Osgood, H. (1957). Allergy to Caddis fly (Trichoptera). I. The insect. *J. Allergy*, **28**, 113

34. Gaillard, G. E. (1950). The aphid – an insect allergen. *J. Allergy.* **21**. 386

35. Ado, A. D. (1964). Personal communication
36. Meister, K. (1979). Professional asthma owing to Daphnia allergy. *Abstracts of Annual Meeting of the European Academy of Allergology and Clinical Immunology*, p. 59. (Helsinki: Sandoz)
37. Frankland, A. W. and Lunn, J. A. (1965). Asthma caused by the grain weevil. *Br. J. Ind. Med.*, **22**, 157
38. Lunn. J. A. and Hughes. D. T. D. (1967). Pulmonary hypersensitivity to the grain weevil. *Br. J. Ind. Med.*. **24**. 158
39. Cuthbert, O. D., Brostoff, J., Wraith, D. J. and Brighton, W. D. (1979). 'Barn allergy' asthma and rhinitis due to storage mites. *Clin. Allergy*, **9**, 229
40. Grant, I. W. B., Blyth, W., Wardrop, V. E., Gordon, R. M., Pearson, J. C. G. and Mair, A. (1972). Prevalence of farmer's lung in Scotland: A pilot survey. *Br. Med. J.*, **1**, 530
41. Kino, T. and Oshima, S. (1978). Allergy to insects in Japan. I. The reaginic sensitivity to moth and butterfly in patients with bronchial asthma. *J. Allergy Clin. Immunol.*, **61**, 10
42. Ancona, G. (1923). Asma epidermico 'Pediculoides ventriculosus'. *Policlinico*, **30**, 45
43. Voorhorst, R., Spieksma-Boezeman, M. I. A. and Spieksma, F. Th. M. (1964). Is a mite the producer of the house dust allergen? *Allergie Asthma*, **10**, 329
44. Pajarre, R. (1979). *Abstracts of Annual Meeting of the European Academy of Allergology and Clinical Immunology*, p. 9. (Helsinki: Sandoz)
45. Rudolph, R. (1979). *Abstracts of Annual Meeting of the European Academy of Allergology and Clinical Immunology*, p. 3. (Helsinki: Sandoz)
46. Frankland, A. W. (1972). House dust mites and allergy. *Arch. Dis. Child.*, **47**, 327
47. Miyamoto, T., Oshima, S., Ishizaka, T. and Sato, S. (1970). Allergenic identity between the common flour mite (*Dermatophagoides farinae* (Hughes 1961)) and house dust as a causative antigen in bronchial asthma. *J. Allergy*, **42**, 14
48. Aas, K. (1976). House dust and mites in bronchial asthma. In Weiss, E. B. and Segal, M. S. (eds.) *Bronchial Asthma*. p. 547. (Boston: Little. Brown)
49. Warner. J. O.. Price. J. F.. Soothill. J. F. and Hey. E. N. (1978). Controlled trial of hyposensitization to *D. pteronyssinus* in children with asthma. *Lancet*, **2**, 912
50. Mellanby, K. (1946). Man's reaction to mosquito bites. *Nature (London)*, **158**, 554
51. Feingold, B. F. and Benjamini, E. (1961). Allergy to flea bites: Clinical and experimental observations. *Ann. Allergy*, **19**, 1275
52. Frankland, A. W. (1955). Uber die Entwicklung einer experimentell induzierten Uberempfindlichkeit gegen Insekten (*Rhodnius*). *Allergie Asthma*, **1**, 229
53. Frazier, C. A. (1969). *Insect Allergy. Allergic and Toxic Reactions to Insects and other Arthropods*. (St Louis: Warren H. Green)
54. Loveless, M. H. (1964). Summer hazards: Insect stings. *Curr. Med. Dig.*, p. 733
55. Parrino, J., Kandawalla, N. M. and Lockey, R. F. (1979). Treatment of local skin response to imported fire ant sting. *J. Allergy Clin. Immunol.*, **63**, 135
56. Blair, C. P. (1979). Brown tail moth caterpillars and their rash. *Clin. Exp. Dermatol.*, **4**, 215
57. Hermes, W. B. and James, M. T. (1961). *Medical Entomology*, 5th Edn. (New York: Macmillan)

11
Drug Allergies

H. E. AMOS

INTRODUCTION

Drug allergies are a recognized clinical entity but diagnosis is often based solely on a demonstration that there is an association between drug administration and some clinical event that is unrelated to the known natural history of the disease being treated. Using such a diagnostic criterion has almost certainly led to confusion about the true incidence of drug allergies and reduced confidence in quoted incidence figures. Nevertheless, hypersensitivity reactions induced by drugs are a considerable problem for drug manufacturers, as they are, at present, difficult or indeed impossible to predict by existing toxicological screening procedures.

DRUGS AS ANTIGENS

Drugs, due to their chemical simplicity and small molecular weight cannot activate the immunological system and initiate the sequence of events which lead to production of allergized lymphocytes or antibodies. To induce drug-specific immunological responses, a drug can function as a hapten, which in combination with a macromolecule provides the necessary requirements for stimulating hapten-specific antibodies. This indispensability for macromolecular interaction imposes a number of constraints which influence the immunogenicity of a drug.

Nature of drug–macromolecule binding

Elegant studies by Landsteiner and Jacobs[1] using a halogen-substituted nitrobenzene model, led to the proposition that a hapten must covalently link with a protein before hapten-specific immunological responses are produced.

It is unlikely that covalent binding is an absolute requirement, but evidence that other types of chemical binding, such as electrostatic or hydrophobic interactions, are sufficient to form a 'complete-antigen' from a hapten–protein complex is still very sparse. The main line of argument against Landsteiner's proposition is provided by the demonstration[2] of antibodies to small molecular weight compounds which are structurally incapable of covalent interaction.

Metabolism

It has been accepted for a number of years that one of the reasons for failing to detect antibodies to drugs is that the hapten may be a metabolic product, which will induce cross-reacting antibodies with the parent drug molecule. Drugs are metabolized by a mixed function oxidase enzyme system (MFO) located in the subcellular microsomal complex. Although most cells possess MFO to a varying extent, the main site of metabolism is the liver. The liver hepatocyte is also the synthetic cell for albumin. Thus within the microcosm of the hepatocyte, conditions exist for generating reactive drug intermediates which could couple *de novo* to albumin and leach into the serum as stable hapten–protein complexes. There is no evidence at the moment to support this concept, but there is evidence supporting the idea that reactive metabolites can stimulate antibodies[3].

GENETIC FACTORS WHICH INFLUENCE DRUG HYPERSENSITIVITY

Control genes

It has been firmly established that an individual's ability to respond immunologically to an antigenic stimulus is dependent upon the expression of specific immune response genes (*Ir* genes). These genes are closely allied to the major histocompatibility complex and code for initial antigen recognition[4]. Failure to develop an allergic response however is not necessarily indicative of an absence or depression of the antigen-specific *Ir* gene. There are other inbuilt genetic controls acting at a higher level of complexity, which also influence overall development of immune responsiveness, for example, the genetic control exercised in antigen processing by macrophages[5].

Histocompatibility antigen (HLA) haplotype

An association between the disease ankylosing spondylitis and HLA 27 is well established[6]; similar relationships exist for other diseases[7–9] and attempts are being made in many centres to see whether such correlations can be used to define populations at risk.

In relation to hypersensitivity, it has been shown that positive prick skin tests, interpreted as an IgE-mediated response, correlated with a particular HLA serotype[10] and that the correlation was statistically significant with simple chemical allergens. Attempts to find an association between individuals with a specific adverse drug effect and HLA haplotypes have been disappointing. An intensive study carried out on patients with the oculomucocutaneous syndrome induced by practolol failed to define a common HLA type[11].

Genetic linked disease associations

It is a widely held belief that atopic individuals have a higher propensity to develop drug allergies than normal individuals but data supporting such a general contention are sparse. Most surveys which have been carried out tend to support the contention[12] and studies with specific drugs have shown an increased incidence of allergic drug reactions in atopics, but whether such an increase is related to an immunological event manifest in atopics or whether it is just a reflection of increased drug intake is not resolved.

HYPERSENSITIVITY TISSUE DAMAGE

Coombs and Gell[13] attempted to group immunologically induced tissue damage into four mechanistic types: Type I corresponded to the old notion of immediate hypersensitivity and included clinical anaphylaxis; Type II involved the complement-mediated lytic reactions; Type III encompassed associated tissue damage from antigen–antibody complex formation; and Type IV corresponded to delayed or cell-mediated hypersensitivity. It is possible that most allergic drug reactions can be identified with one or more of these types[14] but two syndromes which are closely linked to drug administration are less easily analysed and require special consideration. These are drug-induced lupus erythematosus and the oculomucocutaneous syndrome.

Clinical manifestations

Drug-induced lupus erythematosus

Many drugs have been reported as causative agents for a lupus-like condition and the two which have received most experimental attention are hydralazine and procainamide.

Since the original reports describing hydralazine lupus[15, 16], much attention has been paid to the relationship of drug-induced lupus with the established clinical entity, systemic lupus erythematosus.

A number of clinical manifestations seems to be common to both diseases, fever, arthralgia, pleuritis, pericarditis, skin rashes and anaemia. An analysis of patients with drug-induced lupus enables a number of generalizations to be drawn about the chief features of the disease. There is, by definition, an association with drug administration but there is no relationship between the disease and dose or duration of treatment. Clinical signs may appear as early as 2 weeks after starting treatment or be delayed as long as 8 years[17, 18]. Drug-induced lupus seems more common in older patients but this is probably a relative finding which reflects the age group of those taking the drug. There does appear to be a sex difference between the two syndromes: systemic lupus occurs predominantly in young women. A second difference is the predilection for the involvement of different organs. Most investigators accept that drug-induced lupus rarely affects the kidney, whereas systemic lupus often causes renal disease. There have been reports of immune complex nephritis induced by hydralazine[19, 20], but it could be argued that since lupus nephritis is a comparatively late manifestation of the disease, it rarely has time to develop before the offending compound is withdrawn.

Oculomucocutaneous syndrome

The syndrome was defined by ICI, in conjunction with the Committee on Safety of Medicines, to encompass the diverse pathological signs induced by practolol. Cardinal features of the syndrome include a skin rash which superficially resembles psoriasis[21], dry eyes, with conjunctival tissue destruction[22] and peritoneal thickening which is often sufficient to cause intestinal obstruction[23]. There have been claims that some of these changes can be brought about in patients treated with beta-blockers other than practolol[24], but the incidence is small and there are differences in pathological detail. The mechanism by which practolol causes a diffuse serositis is unclear, and it is likely but by no means proven that a common mechanism underlies the lesions. However, all attempts to model the condition have so far been unsuccessful.

Adverse phenomena, immunologically inducible by drugs

Anaphylaxis

Acute peripheral vascular collapse with or without respiratory disease, which comes on within minutes of antigen challenge constitutes the anaphylactic syndrome. It is one of the most serious drug-induced allergic responses which can be lethal if not promptly treated and there is no way at present to predict with any degree of certainty whether an individual is likely to experience anaphylaxis in response to drug challenge.

Anaphylaxis is dependent upon the presence of IgE antibodies which have the ability to sensitize mast cells and basophils passively, by membrane interaction through the Fc piece[25]. Bridging two adjacent cell-bound IgE molecules by antigen leads to an allosteric membrane change which initiates a biochemical sequence leading to synthesis and release of preformed, pharmacologically active mediators.

The model most often studied for drug-induced anaphylaxis is the clinical Type I response to penicillin. It has been shown that the major determinant for penicillin, the penicilloyl conjugate, is formed through the β-lactum ring via an amide linkage to proteins[26-28] and that IgE antibodies of penicilloyl specificity are inducible. Skin testing patients with Type I reactions to penicillin using a major determinant reagent will often fail to elicit positive skin responses. It was shown by analysing patterns of skin reactivity in penicillin-sensitive patients that this failure was due to heterogeneity of the penicillin antigen. Positive results could be obtained in patients if a reagent containing two or more of the following was used: penicilloyl conjugate, determinants in the penicilloate–penilloate group and crystalline penicillin[29]. It is not clear what the exact determinant specificity is being expressed in these reagents but clearly minor determinants assume an important role in Type I reactions to penicillin.

Skin manifestations

Damage to dermal vessels

Damage to dermal vessels from any cause will result in skin manifestations which can be divided into distinct dermatological entities.

Exanthematous eruptions – These form the most frequent type of skin rashes produced by drugs. Defined entities such as erythema multiforme and the group known as toxic erythemas are more associated with some drugs than others, e.g. sulphonamides, barbiturates, pyrazolone derivatives, halide derivatives and troxidone[30].

Vasculitis – The group of diseases covered by the term vasculitis have vessel damage mainly on the venous side of the dermal capillaries. Vasculitis is essentially an inflammatory condition and can be caused by deposits of antigen–antibody complexes in the microvasculature which fix complement; complexes must reach a critical size and they are usually deposited in the region of turbulent blood flow. Thus there is probably a mechanical element governing anatomical localization and there is also evidence that the amount of complexes formed can be decreased by antihistamine drugs, suggesting that a leukocyte-dependent histamine release mechanism might also be operating[31].

Polyarteritis nodosa – This condition is a special type of vasculitis which affects the small- and medium-size arterioles. Typical skin lesions consist of dermal or subcutaneous nodules grouped along the course of an artery. A number of drugs have been causally related, chloramphenicol, penicillin, streptomycin, sulphonamides and barbiturates[32], but whether the arteritis is immunologically mediated by drug-specific antibodies is not substantiated.

Purpura – Drugs can damage capillary endothelial cells by toxic mechanisms resulting in purpuric haemorrhages but platelet damage with thrombocytopenia is more likely to be the mechanism of immunologically induced purpura.

The pioneering work on drug-induced thrombocytopenia was carried out by Ackroyd[33]. Working with the hypnotic Sedormid (now withdrawn from the pharmacopoeia), he showed that an antibody was formed which appeared to have specificity for an antigen derived from a Sedormid–platelet combination. Antibody could only be detected if platelets were in a saturated solution of the drug, indicating that antigen was formed by a non-covalent but essential combination of drug and platelet. Complement was fixed by the platelet–drug antibody complex resulting in lysis of the platelets.

An alternative explanation proposed for the mechanism of platelet damage based on experiments with quinidine-induced thrombocytopenia, relegates the platelets to a passive role and considers them specialized cells which are capable of absorbing on to their surfaces a drug antibody complex[34]. It is still not totally clear which of the two mechanisms is responsible for the clinical thrombocytopenia, but whatever the mechanism, platelets are particularly susceptible target cells for Type II tissue damage.

Urticaria – Urticaria is associated with Type I hypersensitivity reactions and is thought to be a skin response to release of vasoactive amines such as histamine. These mediators can be released by immunological mechanisms through production of IgE antibodies or by non-immunological pathways via the cholinergic autonomic system[35]. It is also possible to produce urticarial rashes by a Type III mechanism; allergic complexes fix complement and release biologically active components, anaphylatoxins, which cause basophils to discharge their histamine.

Damage to cellular components of the skin

Eczema or dermatitis – This is the most frequent adverse clinical sign when drugs are applied directly to the skin. The incidence of allergic contact dermatitis to medicaments is high. In one international study 24% of 2000 consecutive patients with eczema were found to be allergic to drugs of which neomycin and benzocaine were the most common[36]. Much experimental work has been done on allergic contact dermatitis and conclusions support the contention that the mechanism is a cell-mediated hypersensitivity.

Photosensitivity – Most dermatologists consider photosensitivity to consist of two components, one phototoxic and the other photoallergic. The latter is thought to be essentially a Type IV contact sensitivity reaction in which light acts to biotransform an inert compound to a contact allergen[37].

Bullous eruptions – Epidermal blistering can be chemically induced by drugs such as penicillamine[38]. In fact, it has been estimated that 7% of patients treated with penicillamine for 6 months or more will develop some type of clinical pemphigus[39]. The mechanism by which the skin changes are brought about is unknown. Although penicillamine has been shown to be immunogenic[40], it is unlikely that the skin changes are a direct consequence of a hypersensitivity reaction. More likely, they result from secondary changes due to either a direct action of the drug on epidermal structures, for example the inhibition of cross-linkages in mature collagen or as a sequel to a primary effect of the drug on T cells.

Drug-specific rashes – Two well-defined drug rashes which may be immunologically mediated are the fixed drug eruption and the ampicillin rash. Fixed drug eruptions originally described by Brocq[41] and known to be caused by many drugs[42], have remained a considerable enigma. There is no definite evidence to incriminate an allergic mechanism, and experiments designed to see if antigen is formed locally in the affected area have proved negative[43].

The maculopapular eruption associated with ampicillin administration is unique among drug rashes in that it appears 10–12 days after starting the drug. It is also invariably produced if ampicillin is given to patients with infectious mononucleosis. So far no clear explanation for the rash is available. The most that can be deduced from the evidence is that the rash may be connected in some way with abnormal lymphocyte function.

Isolated organ damage due to hypersensitivity drug reactions

Liver

Liver, being the site of primary metabolism for the majority of drugs, is particularly vulnerable to damage by antibodies with metabolite specificity. In actual fact, there are very few cases reported which have been adequately examined demonstrating hypersensitivity tissue damage. Chlorpromazine and halothane are often quoted as causing immunologically mediated liver damage, the former producing a cholestatic jaundice and the latter hepatocellular damage, resembling acute viral hepatitis. A detailed analysis of the evidence, however, shows that no drug-specific antibodies have so far been identified and except for one unconfirmed report[44] no *in vitro* antigen-specific lymphocyte interaction has been demonstrated.

Kidney

The kidney is also an organ which can metabolize drugs, in that the cells have microsomal mixed function oxidase activity but, in comparison with liver, the chances of immunogenic complexes being sequestrated from the cells into the blood must be diminished due to the inability of kidney cells to synthesize albumin *de novo*. Thus conditions are less favourable for antigen–antibody interaction within the organ. However, due to the unique vasculature of the kidney, deposits of antigen–antibody complexes can build up to cause a Type III allergic nephritis. Immunoglobulin deposits on the renal basement membrane have been demonstrated in patients with the nephrotic syndrome following penicillamine therapy[45] and since the sera of such patients also contain antibody to penicillamine[40], it is reasonable to assume that the complexes contain penicillamine antigen. Disruption of the functional integrity of the basement membrane following complement fixation by allergic complexes is assumed to be the fundamental lesion causing the nephrotic syndrome. Danger of inducing immune complex nephritis is particularly pertinent during hyposensitization procedures – continued administration of antigen in established allergic states fulfils the necessary condition for the precipitation of antigen–antibody complexes.

The link between renal damage and a concomitant drug allergy may not always be clear. For example, acute oliguric renal failure has been described following *p*-amino salicylic acid (PAS) administration and it has been demonstrated that renal failure is preceded by an intravascular haemolysis due to an acute allergic response induced by PAS[46]. Thus the kidney is damaged indirectly probably by an association of haemoglobinuria with shock from renal ischaemia.

Formed elements of the blood

Type II tissue damage involving formed elements of the blood has been studied extensively. The immunological mechanism leading to haemolytic anaemia following quinidine[47] and penicillin[48] has been worked out and shown to be a complement-dependent interaction between a drug-specific circulating antibody and a drug determinant intimately attached to the red cell membrane.

In cases typified by anaemia induced by α-methyldopa, the mechanism is different in that drug-specific antibodies are not produced. Instead, the drug interacts directly with red cells and creates new determinants which stimulate an autoantibody[49].

White blood cells can also be damaged by immunologically mediated reactions to drugs and the reactions which have been thoroughly investigated are those induced by sulphapyridine[50] and amidopyrine[51]. Leukoagglutinins can be detected in the serum provided free drug is also present. This requirement for free drugs suggests that white cells may be damaged by indirect mechanisms or that a drug–white cell linkage is only effective if the equilibrium favours combination. This is a situation analogous to the conditions necessary for detecting antibodies to Sedormid.

INVESTIGATION OF AN ALLERGIC DRUG REACTION

It must be appreciated that predictive immunological assessment of drugs is still in its infancy. Considerable strides have been made to test whether a drug is likely to be toxic to cells involved in the immune system but little progress has been made in assessing a drug's potential for inducing hypersensitive tissue damage. Thus there is a degree of risk from unforeseen reactions which must be accepted if drugs are to be used in medicine and this throws considerable responsibility on clinical immunologists to be aware of dangers and to appreciate the implications of diagnosing an allergic drug effect. There is no doubt that allergic drug reactions are likely to prove a problem if and when new legislation for product liability comes into force. Definite criteria for diagnosis must be established, which effectively means a systemic pattern of investigation.

Amos[52] suggested that the investigation should be a four-phase study, although it is appreciated that a sequential order might not be possible in every case and that one phase may assume more importance than the others.

Phase I – Clinical investigation

Phase I of the study involves a detailed history of an individual patient or an assessment of epidemiological data if there is more than one. The majority of symptoms from untoward drug reactions develop slowly and allow plenty of time for a careful history before making any decisions on management. Anaphylactic reactions allow no such luxury and the history of these patients must be taken retrospectively and be particularly searching.

In taking a history, special attention should be paid to time of onset and any periodicity of unexpected symptoms. Periodicity is important as signs and symptoms of an allergic drug reaction are likely to reach their maximum following antigenic challenge.

If symptoms differ significantly from the natural history of the disease being treated, attention should be focused on a detailed index of all therapeutic preparations, including proprietary brands that the patient may have taken. Physicians should also be aware that many drugs are put into food and drink as preservatives, flavours or stimulants so the patient's eating and drinking habits may need analysing. By taking detailed drug histories, a possible candidate for the adverse effect may become obvious, and any drug interactions should be evident.

Epidemiological studies relating to adverse reactions are usually conducted in the first instance by the manufacturing company concerned, as they should have access to all available data, both published and confidential. Data available to bureaucratic bodies such as the Committee on Safety of Medicines may not be helpful in trying to answer the type of questions which will decide whether a reaction is idiosyncratic. These organizations rely on a reported diagnosis and are not in a position to evaluate the basis on which a diagnosis is made.

Phase 2 – Detection of a generalized immunological activation

The objective of phase 2 investigation is to demonstrate an association between administration of a particular drug and some immunological phenomena which might be interpreted as signalling a hypersensitivity mechanism.

It is not too time consuming or difficult, using commercially available reagents, to obtain a complete immunological profile on a patient. Measurement of serum immunoglobulins, especially IgE, might be informative; elevated IgM and IgG levels are difficult to relate to specific antigen challenge but a rise in total serum IgE could indicate a possible Type I hypersensitivity tissue damage. It has been claimed that IgE levels are raised in patients with anaphylaxis induced by penicillin[53] and in a reported series of 62 patients with drug allergy, 23 had raised IgE levels[54]. The important point to establish, however, is that any observed elevation in IgE levels is due to drug challenge and does not reflect a normally raised level due to some superimposed atopic condition.

Alteration in complement levels is also a good indicator of immunological activation. A depressed level of total haemolytic complement, indicating complement utilization, is likely to occur when the hypersensitivity reaction involves the formation of circulating antigen–antibody complexes – Type III hypersensitivity damage. It is also important to measure the levels of individual complement components, particularly the early components, C1q, C4 and C2. A drug could conceivably induce complement activation using the alternative pathway, which bypasses the early components but nevertheless produces a form of toxic damage. Activation of complement by antigen–antibody complexes is by the classical route, so measuring the early components can help to distinguish between the two mechanisms.

Autoantibodies are another indication of immunological activation. Finding antinuclear antibodies (ANA), for example, may confirm a possible drug-induced lupus, as all patients with clinical signs of drug lupus have antinuclear antibodies. It is not clear, however, if ANA can be taken to herald the development of overt lupus. In one study[55] 5% of patients with ANA induced by drug treatment eventually developed clinical signs of lupus.

Finding tissue-specific autoantibodies such as the intercellular antibody induced by practolol[56] poses a number of experimental questions to determine which of the various mechanisms of autoantibody production might involve the drug. For example, it might damage tissues by a direct toxic action causing them to become sufficiently antigenic to stimulate autoantibodies, or the drug might interfere with the control T cells exercise on the antibody secretory function of B cells. This latter mechanism has been suggested as an explanation of autoantibodies found in patients with the oculomuco-cutaneous syndrome[57].

In the context of a phase 2 investigation, it is not essential to investigate the detailed mechanism which results in autoantibody production, but it is necessary to define a causal relationship between drug administration and the presence of autoantibodies. As no pretreatment serum sample is likely to be available, defining such a relationship may indeed be difficult.

Phase 3 – Determination of a drug-specific immunological effect

Often the most difficult phase of investigating a drug allergy is to obtain evidence of antibodies or actively allergized cells which have specificity for a drug or some drug product. This information is fundamental in diagnosing an allergic drug reaction and it is unwise to make such a diagnosis in its absence. The methods used in a phase 3 investigation can be divided into two sections; those involving the patient and measuring some type of skin reactivity and those requiring laboratory-orientated techniques.

Skin tests

Various types of skin tests have been used in an attempt to either predict a potential allergic drug reaction or to confirm diagnosis of a suspected allergy.

There is no general agreement on the overall predictive value of skin tests in drug allergy, and there are few data relating to any drug other than penicillin. In one prospective study of 218 patients with past histories of penicillin allergy, skin testing with benzylpenicilloyl-polylysine and a minor deter-minant mixture proved to be of predictive value[58] and this is the general view of most clinical immunologists. But there are considerable problems in routine skin testing which frequently make results difficult to interpret.

The major problem is the form of the antigen used for testing. Injecting diluted solutions of drug is unsatisfactory as it relies on the drug being able to combine with proteins in skin to form an antigen. This is unlikely to happen as dilution will be further increased by tissue fluids and dispersion accelerated. Coupling drugs *in vitro* to carrier molecules has an advantage over using uncoupled drugs as it allows the hapten–protein ratio to be controlled permitting maximum plurivalency. There is some risk attached to injecting haptens coupled to macromolecules as they are liable to actively allergize a non-allergic individual. To minimize this disadvantage, various combinations of drugs coupled to non-immunogenic carriers have been tried but the efficacy of preformed complexes as elicitors of skin reactions decreases as the structure of a carrier approximates more closely to that of an homologous protein.

There is also considerable danger attached to skin testing, particularly for diagnostic purposes. Even when the concentration of test material is kept low, there is much more absorption from an intradermal or a scratch test than there is from a prick test (see Chapter 3). Fatal anaphylactic reactions have been produced by intradermal testing in penicillin-sensitive patients[59] and, as a rule, intradermal injections should not be attempted before a prick or scratch test with an equivalent dilution. However, even a scratch test can introduce sufficient antigen to elicit severe anaphylactic reactions[60].

Patch testing, which is designed to detect a cell-mediated hypersensitivity state, is safer than invasive skin tests, but it is still not without risk. Elucidation of delayed type hypersensitivity responses for detecting cell-mediated immunity can be achieved by monovalent haptens, as there is no requirement for cross-linking antibody molecules. Thus solutions of the drug can be applied on a patch and provided concentrations are adjusted to a strong but non-toxic level, reasonable confidence can be placed in the result.

Provocation tests are sometimes carried out, particularly if various attempts at skin testing have failed. Giving a drug by the same route which produced a reaction has the advantage that it may lead to formation of the same sensitizing determinant. A comprehensive attempt to evaluate test dose procedures was a study of 312 provocation tests in 274 hospital patients with cutaneous manifestations of drug allergy; 63 different drugs were administered and 86% of the tests gave positive results[61]. The conclusion drawn from this study was that provocation tests were reliable when performed with caution and the test dose carefully chosen for each individual patient.

In conclusion, judicious use of skin tests and carefully controlled provocation procedures can provide valuable information on the nature of an inducing allergen and the specificity of the response. Decision, however, to use these techniques must always be tempered by a careful risk–benefit analysis, and the axiom, 'first do no harm', should be a prominent thought for any investigator.

In vitro tests

Laboratory procedures currently used to detect antibodies to drugs are basic immunological techniques which are documented in laboratory manuals of immunology but certain entities make detecting drug antibodies particularly difficult.

Drug antibodies are transient species which reach maximum serum levels at the height of an adverse reaction. On stopping the drug they rapidly disappear from serum, so reducing chances of detecting them by *in vitro* techniques. The optimum serum sample to test, therefore, is one taken when clinical manifestations of the adverse effect are florid. When planning a laboratory investigation of an allergic drug reaction an early decision has to be made on how the drug is to be presented to the antibody. Choice of indicator particle and method of linkage are two variables which may necessitate preliminary investigation.

The type of indicator will dictate the test end-point but passive haemagglutination, phage neutralization and various forms of radioprecipitation assays are the systems most commonly used. Whatever the indicator particle, the drug has to be chemically linked to it in order to effect antibody interaction. Obviously drug structure will impose constraints on linkage, and often a drug can be linked in more than one way. Thus the projected antigenic determinants which can be presented to antibody are limited and may differ from the antigen formed *in vivo*. It is therefore important to establish the immunological specificity of any positive result. This is usually achieved by inhibition experiments using the drug and compounds modelled on the drug.

For Type I reactions, indirect methods for detecting antibody–antigen interactions are available. Mast cells and basophils, sensitized with IgE will, in the presence of specific antigen, release histamine, which can be assayed either spectrophotometrically or by bioassay. Direct basophil degranulation has also been used, and claims have been made that degranulation of basophils can be detected in 90% of immediate type allergies[62].

In vitro methods for detecting cell-mediated hypersensitivity induced by drugs are of less value than *in vitro* procedures for identifying drug-specific antibodies. Measurement of lymphocyte proliferation following specific antigen has been applied to the study of many drug allergies[63], but opinion is divided on its efficacy. Moreover correlation with cell-mediated immunity is not absolute. Subpopulations of lymphocyte can be identified by selective proliferation induced by different mitogens, but the proliferative response following antigen stimulation is non-selective. Nevertheless specific stimulation of allergized lymphocytes by a drug-antigen can be interpreted as indicating the presence of an existing specific allergic state.

Macrophage migration inhibition as described by David *et al.*[64] is a more reliable indicator of a cell-mediated immune state, but the test is difficult to standardize and it has yet to find a place in the scheme for investigating drug allergies.

Recently the possibility of reactive drug metabolites having antigenic properties has received increasing attention. The problem is how to detect antibodies without characterizing the metabolite determinant. One approach is to metabolize a drug *in vitro* using the mixed function microsomal oxidases and add a carrier protein which can act as a scavenger molecule to bind any reactive metabolic product. The carrier protein can then be extracted from the system and used in either haemagglutination assays[3] or radioprecipitation techniques[65].

This approach makes two basic assumptions (1) a drug is metabolized by liver microsomal enzymes; and (2) generated metabolites will bind to proteins. For the majority of drugs these two assumptions will be valid.

The system has been successfully used to detect antibodies to a practolol metabolite but awaits further evaluation with other drug allergies. Clearly much more work is needed to refine methods of detecting antibodies to drug metabolites before their significance in drug allergy can be assessed.

Phase 4 – Clinical relevance of phase 2 and phase 3

Data generated during phase 2 and phase 3 investigations would not normally provide a sufficient data base on which to make a confident diagnosis of an allergic drug reaction. If criteria for allergenicity are fulfilled by the haptenic drug, antibody production will be the likely result. But it does not always follow that hypersensitivity tissue damage will arise. There are no data available relating the incidence of drug antibodies with the overall incidence of drug-induced hypersensitivity reactions. Antibodies to drugs are not usually measured unless there is some clinical reason for doing so, but it is known that IgM antibodies to penicillin have been found in patients who have never experienced any adverse effect from the drug.

To establish diagnostic significance of drug-specific antibodies it is necessary to demonstrate that antibodies relate in some way with the clinical signs of an adverse effect. In some cases this will not create a problem. Demonstration of drug-dependent haemolytic antibodies in cases of acute haemolytic anaemia is a convincing cause and effect relationship; but where tissue damage is less well defined, it becomes imperative to prove that the presence of drug-specific antibodies is involved in the pathogenesis of an adverse effect. There is no absolute procedure for doing this. A case must be built up against the drug, using both clinical and laboratory methods, until accumulated evidence justified a definitive diagnosis. The cardinal feature in a phase 4 investigation is relating antibody titres to the disease state. A fall in titre and amelioration of clinical signs following drug withdrawal is one form of circumstantial evidence which should be relatively easy to obtain. However, harder data could emerge from a well-controlled challenge study in which immunological responses to drug challenge follow secondary immune kinetics and parallel any exacerbation of tissue damage. A challenge study of this type for patients with adverse reactions to practolol revealed an interesting finding: only one of six patients investigated developed tissue damage on challenge, and this patient had high levels of antibody at the time of challenge[65]. The significance of such a result is that an antibody–antigen reaction could be causally related to pathological events in the oculomucocutaneous syndrome.

FUTURE TRENDS

There is no doubt that proposed legislation relating to product liability will set new challenges to biologists concerned with drug safety evaluation. The emphasis must be on an understanding of those factors which govern the idiosyncratic nature of hypersensitivity reactions. Mention has already been made of genetic constraints which operate in forming an antigen from drugs and in the response of an individual to the antigen. It is expansion of experimental effort in these two areas which offers the best chance of defining populations at risk of an allergic drug reaction.

At present, a candidate drug in an early stage of development is given to volunteers for pharmacokinetic and pharmacodynamic studies. No attempt is made, however, to determine metabolic profiles of volunteers, but it is well established that the half-life of antipyrine differs in different groups of subjects and that studies with the hypotensive agent debrisoquine have characterized metabolically different genetic groups[66]. It should be possible using experimental animals to define a number of 'marker drugs' which are metabolized by different sets of mixed function microsomal enzymes. Such 'marker drugs' could then be given to volunteers to screen for extremes of biological variation in metabolism. Once a volunteer panel has been established, it could be used to evaluate a candidate drug realistically and determine the metabolite variability. Moreover, it would be possible to measure immunological responses in each individual and investigate a correlation with the defined metabolic profile. Acquiring these data in volunteers would enable the significance of any adverse drug effect to be rapidly appreciated.

A disappointment so far is that monitoring of patient HLA types has not proved to be of any value in predicting populations at risk to allergic drug reaction. Furthermore there is no foreseeable application of basic knowledge on genetics of the immune response to the investigation or control of drug allergies. Undoubtedly a greater understanding of genetics may eventually lead to such an application, but at present much more work is needed.

Data on structural activity relationship can make it possible to predict protein binding and perhaps specific binding to functional groups. This is an increasingly valuable tool in toxicology, but its use in predicting potential immunogens needs exploiting. Emphasis on defining the relationship between macromolecules which link covalently to a drug *in vivo* and the immunogenic potency of the complex could result in a structural activity analysis on which to base a predictive assessment of a potential immunogen.

Advances in methodology leading to improved retrospective investigations of adverse drug effects must be an absolute priority and will inevitably assume an increasingly important role in medicolegal judgements.

Finally treatment of drug allergies is likely to become more specific. Withdrawal of the drug and systematic treatment will always be the main clinical approach, but with pharmacologically novel and therapeutically valuable compounds such treatment may not be acceptable. The interest which has been shown in developing specific monovalent haptenic inhibitors for IgE-mediated response could well develop into a recognized form of treatment. In fact it may well be in the interest of pharmaceutical companies to think about developing such compounds in parallel with the proposed therapeutic agent!

References

1. Landsteiner, K. and Jacobs, J. (1935). Studies on the sensitisation of animals with simple chemical compounds. *J. Exp. Med.*, **61**, 643
2. Plescia, O. J., Braun, W. and Palczuk, N. C. (1964). Production of antibodies to denatured deoxyribonucleic acid. *Proc. Nat. Acad. Sci. (Wash.)*, **52**, 279
3. Amos, H. E., Lake, B. G. and Atkinson, H. A. C. (1977). Allergic drug reactions: An *in vitro* model using a mixed function oxidase complex to demonstrate antibodies with specificity for a practolol metabolite. *Clin. Allergy*, **7**, 423
4. McDevitt, H. O. and Chinitz, H. (1969). Genetic control of antibody response: relationship between immune response and histocompatibility (H-2) type. *Science*, **163**, 1207
5. Biozzi, G., Stiffel, C., Mouton, D., Bouthillier, Y. and Decreusfond, C. (1972). Cytodynamics of the immune response in two lines of mice genetically selected for high and low antibody synthesis. *J. Exp. Med.*, **135**, 1071
6. Brewerton, D. A., Caffrey, M., Hart, F. D., James, D. C. O., Nichols, A. and Sturrock, R. D. (1973). Ankylosing spondylitis and HLA 27. *Lancet.* **1**. 904
7. Bertrams, J., Kuwert, E. and Liedtke, U. (1972). HLA antigens and multiple sclerosis. *Tissue Antigens*, **2**, 405
8. Falchuk, Z. M., Rogentine, G. N. and Strober (1972). Predominance of histocompatibility antigen HLA 8 in patients with gluten sensitive enteropathy. *J. Clin. Invest.*, **51**, 1602
9. Grumet, F. C., Konishi, J., Payne, R. O. and Kriss, J. P. (1973). Association of Graves Disease with HLA 8. *Clin. Res.*, **21**, 493
10. Marsh, D. G., Bias, W. B., Wsu, S. H. and Goodfriend, L. (1973). Association between major histocompatibility (HL-A) antigens and specific reaginic antibody responses in allergic man. In Goodfriend, L., Sehon, A. H. and Orange, R. R. (eds.) *Mechanisms in Allergy. Reagin mediated Hypersensitivity*, p. 113. (New York)
11. Dick, H. M., Wright, P., Chapman, C. M., Zacharias, J. J. and Nicholls, J. T. (1978). Adverse reactions to practolol: some observations on the possible relevance to immune mechanisms. *Allergy*, **33**, 71
12. Hurwitz, N. (1969). Predisposing factors in adverse reactions to drugs. *Br. Med. J.*, **1**, 536
13. Coombs, R. R. A. and Gell, P. H. G. (1963). Classification of allergic reactions responsible for clinical hypersensitivity and disease. In Gell, P. H. G. and Coombs, R. R. A. (eds.) *Clinical Aspects of Immunology*, **1**, 575. (Oxford: Blackwell Scientific Publications)
14. Amos, H. E. (1976). Hypersensitivity mechanisms responsible for tissue damage. In *Allergic Drug Reactions*, p. 9. (London: Edward Arnold)
15. Perry, H. M. J. and Schroeder, H. A. (1954). Syndrome simulating collagen disease caused by hydrallazine (Apresoline). *J. Am. Med. Assoc.*, **154**, 670
16. Dunstan, H. R., Taylor, R. D., Corcoran, A. C. and Page, I. H. (1954). Rheumatic and febrile syndrome during prolonged hydrallazine treatment. *J. Am. Med. Assoc.*, **154**, 23
17. Kosowsky, B. D., Taylor, J., Lawn, B. and Ritchie, R. F. (1973). Long term use of procainamide following acute myocardial infarction. *Circulation*, **47**, 1204
18. Blomgren, S. E., Condemi, J. J. and Vaughan, J. H. (1972). Procainamide induced lupus erythematosus. Clinical and laboratory observations. *Am. J. Med.*, **52**, 338
19. Alarcon-Segoria, D., Wakin, K. G., Worthington, J. W. (1967). Clinical and experimental studies on the hydrallazine syndrome and its relationship to systemic lupus erythematosus. *Medicine*, **46**, 1
20. Dammin, G. J., Nora, J. R., Reardon, J. B. (1955). Hydrallazine reaction: Case with L.E. cells antimortem and postmortem and pulmonary renal splenic and muscular lesions of disseminated lupus erythematosus. *J. Lab. Clin. Med.*, **46**, 806
21. Felix, R. H., Ive, F. A. and Dahl, M. G. C. (1974). Cutaneous and ocular reactions to practolol. *Br. Med. J.*, **2**, 68
22. Wright, P. (1975). Untoward effects associated with practolol administration: oculomuco-cutaneous syndrome. *Br. Med. J.*, **1**, 595

23. Brown. P.. Baddeley. H.. Read. A. E.. Davies. J. D. and McGarry. J. (1974). Sclerosing peritonitis – an unusual reaction to a beta-adrenergic blocking drug (practolol). *Lancet*. **2**. 1477

24. Jensen, A. H., Mikkelsen, H. I., Wadskov, S. and Sondergaard, J. (1976). Cutaneous reactions to propranolol ('Inderal'). *Acta Med. Scand.*, **199**, 363

25. Stanworth, D., Humphrey, J. H. and Bennich, H. (1962). Specific inhibition of the Prausnitz-Kustner reaction of an atypical myeloma protein. *Lancet*, **2**, 330

26. Levine, B. B. and Ovary, Z. (1961). The N(D-benzyl) penicilloyl group as an antigenic determinant responsible for hypersensitivity to penicillin G. *J. Exp. Med.*, **114**, 875

27. De Weck. A. L. (1962). Studies on penicillin hypersensitivity 1. The specificity of rabbit anti-penicillin antibodies. *Int. Arch. Allergy*, **21**, 20

28. Parker. C. W.. Shapiro. J.. Kern. M. and Eisen. H. N. (1962). Hypersensitivity to penicillinic acid derivatives in human being with penicillin allergy. *J. Exp. Med.*, **115**, 821

29. Levine, B. B. and Redmond, A. P. (1969). Minor haptenic determinant specific reagins of penicillin hypersensitivity in man. *Int. Arch. Allergy*, **35**, 445

30. Assem, E.-S. K. (1977). Drug allergy. In Davies, D. M. (ed.) *Textbook of Adverse Drug Reactions*, p. 389. (Oxford University Publications)

31. Kniker. W. T. (1972). Prevention of immune complex disease. In Lepow, I. H. and Ward, P. A. (eds.) *Inflammation – Mechanism and Control*. p. 343. (New York: Academic Press)

32. Felix. R. H. and Stevenson. C. J. (1977). Skin disorders. In Davies. D. M. (ed.) *Textbook of Adverse Drug Reactions*, p. 298. (Oxford University Publications)

33. Ackroyd, J. F. (1949). The pathogenesis of thrombocytopenic purpura due to hyper-sensitivity to Sedormid. *Clin. Sci.*, **7**, 249

34. Shulman, N. K. (1958). Immunoreactions involving platelets. A steric and kinetic model for formation of a complex from a human antibody, quinidine as a hapten and platelets, and for fixation by the complex. *J. Exp. Med.*, **107**, 665

35. Calnan, C. D. (1964). Urticarial reactions. *Br. Med. J.*, **2**, 649

36. Cronin, E., Bandmann, H. J., Calnan, C. D., Fregert, S., Hjorth, N., Magnusson, B., Maibach. H. I., Malten, K., Meneghini, C. L., Pirala, V. and Wilkinson, D. S. (1970). Contact dermatitis in the atopic. *Acta Derm-venereol. (Stockholm)*, **50**, 183

37. Willis. I. and Kligman, A. M. (1968). Mechanism of photo allergic contact dermititis. *J. Invest. Derm.*, **51**, 378

38. Hewitt, J., Lessana-Leibowitch, M., Benveniste, M. and Saporta, L. (1971) Un cas de pemphigus induit par la D-penicillamine. Le pemphigus iatrogene existe-t-il? *Ann. Med. Intern.*, **122**, 1003

39. Marsden, R. A., Ryan, T. J., Vauhegan, R. T., Walshe, M., Hill, H. and Mowat, A. G. (1976). Pemphigus foliaceus induced by penicillamine. *Br. Med. J.*, **4**, 1423

40. Amos, H. E. (1968). Defection of antibodies in penicillamine sensitivity. *Postgrad. Med. J. Suppl.*, **27**

41. Brocq. L. (1894). Eruption erythemato pigmentée fixe due a l'antipyrine. *Ann. Dermatol. Syphiligr.*. **5**. 308

42. Pashricka, J. S. (1978). Drugs causing fixed eruptions. *Br. J. Dermatol.*, **100**, 183

43. Porter, D. I. and Comaish, S. (1969). Fixed drug eruption: An autoradiographic study of exchange graphs. *Br. J. Dermatol.*, **81**, 171

44. Paronetto, F. and Popper, H. (1970). Lymphocytic stimulation induced by halothane in patients with hepatitis following exposure to halothane. *N. Engl. J. Med.*, **283**, 148

45. Lachmann, P. J. (1968). Nephrotic syndrome from penicillamine. In *Penicillamine. Postgrad. Med. J. Suppl.*, **27**

46. MacGibbon. B. H.. Loughbridge. L. W.. Hourihane, D. O. B. and Boyd, D. W. (1960). Auto immune haemolytic anaemia with acute renal failure due to phenacetin and p-amino salicylic acid. *Lancet*. **1**. 7

47. Freedman, A. L., Barr, P. S. and Brody, E. A. (1967). Haemolytic anaemia due to quinidine: observations on its mechanism. *Am. J. Med.*, **20**, 806

48. White, J. M., Brown, D. L., Hepner, G. W. and Worlledge, S. M. (1968). Penicillin induced haemolytic anaemia. *Br. Med. J.*, **3**, 26

49. Worlledge, S. M., Carstairs, K. C. and Dacie, J. V. (1966). Auto-immune haemolytic anaemia associated with α-methyldopa therapy. *Lancet*, **2**, 135

50. Moeschlin, S. (1954). Weitere Beobachtunger unver Immunoleukopenien und Agranulo-cytosen. *Schweiz. Med. Wschr.*, **84**, 1100

51. Moeschlin, S. and Wagner, K. (1952). Agranulocytosis due to the occurrence of leukocyte-agglutinin (Pyramidon) and cold agglutinins. *Acta Haemat. (Basel)*, **8**, 29

52. Amos, H. E. (1979). Immunological aspects of practolol toxicity. *Int. J. Immunol. Pharmacol.*, **1**, 9

53. Wide, L. and Juhlin, L. (1971). Detection of penicillin allergy of the immediate type by radio-immunoassay of reagin (IgE) to penicilloyl conjugates. *Clin. Allergy*, **1**, 171

54. Assem, E.-S. K. (1972). The passive sensitization of human lung as a test for drug allergy. In Dash, C. H. and Jones, H. E. H. (eds.) *Mechanisms in Drug Allergy*, p. 179. (Edinburgh and London: Churchill Livingstone)

55. Hope, R. R. and Bates, L. A. (1972). The frequency of procainamide induced systemic lupus erythematosus. *Med. J. Aust.*, **2**, 298

56. Amos, H. E., Brigden, W. D. and McKerron, R. A. (1975). Untoward effects associated with practolol: demonstration of antibody binding to ephithelial tissue. *Br. Med. J.*, **1**, 598

57. Allison, A. C., Denman, A. M. and Barnes, R. D. (1971). Cooperating and controlling functions of thymus-derived lymphocytes in relation to autoimmunity. *Lancet*, **2**, 135

58. Levine, B. B. and Zolov, D. M. (1969). Prediction of penicillin allergy by immunological tests. *J. Allergy*, **43**, 231

59. Driagin, G. B. (1966). Anaphylactic shock with fatal outcome following intradermal test for sensitivity to penicillin (Russian). *Terarky*, **38**, 118

60. Dogliotti, M. (1968). An instance of fatal reaction to the penicillin scratch test. *Dermatologica (Basel)*, **136**, 489

61. Kauppinen, K. (1972). Cutaneous reactions to drugs; with special reference to severe bullous mucocutaneous eruptions and sulphonamides. A clinical study. *Acta Derm. (Kyoto)*, **52** (Suppl. 68), 1

62. Monoret-Vautrin, D. A., Grilliat, J. P. and Pupil, P. (1972). Basophil degranulation in drug allergy. In Dash, C. H. and Jones, H. E. H. (eds.) *Mechanisms in Drug Allergy*. (Edinburgh and London: Churchill Livingstone)

63. Halpern, B., Ky, N. T. and Amache, N. (1969). *In vitro* lymphoblast transformation test (L.T.T.) as a tool for the study of drug hypersensitivity. In *Proceedings of the European Society for the Study of Drug Toxicity*, **10**, 27

64. David, J. R., Al-Askari, S., Lawrence, H. S. and Thomas, L. (1964). Delayed hypersensitivity *in vitro*. I. The specificity of inhibition of cell migration by antigens. *J. Immunol.*, **93**, 264

65. Amos, H. E., Lake, B. G. and Artis, J. (1978). Possible role of antibody specific for a practolol metabolite. *Clin. Allergy*, **7**, 423

66. Idle, J. R., Mahgoub, A., Lancaster, R. and Smith, R. L. (1978). Hypotensive responses to debrisoquine and hydroxylation phenotype. *Life Sci.*, **22**, 979

12
The Effect of Antibacterial Antibiotics on Immune Reactions and Host Resistance to Infection

J. M. DEWDNEY

INTRODUCTION

There are many examples of drugs which influence the development and expression of specific immune responses or which affect non-specific host defences. Some, such as the immunosuppressives and immunostimulants are used in the clinic to this end. For others, including many cytotoxic agents, drugs used in cancer chemotherapy, and anti-inflammatory agents, these effects accompany or may be secondary to the drug's intended therapeutic action.

In some instances, such drugs may be found to have a beneficial effect on the outcome of infection in treated patients. In others, an adverse effect may result and recurrent or persistent infection episodes may be added to the presenting disease.

Antibacterial antibiotics are widely prescribed for the treatment of infection and have proved to be highly effective in providing broad-spectrum anti-bacterial therapy. Impressive though the results of modern antibacterial chemotherapy are, it is acknowledged that cure is effected most readily if host defence mechanisms are normal. In circumstances where integrity of these mechanisms is impaired, even an optimal chemotherapeutic regimen may fail to control bacterial disease. Thus, patients with defects in the afferent or efferent pathways of specific immune responses, or who have defects in cellular or humoral factors involved in non-specific host resistance, are at risk from persistent, recurrent, severe infections which often respond inadequately to antibiotic therapy.. For detailed reviews of the factors affecting susceptibility to infection in compromised hosts, reference should be made to Allen[1], Lachmann and Rosen[2], Pahwa et al.[3] and Quie et al.[4].

Attempts have been made to explore the interaction of infecting organism, host response and antibiotic therapy in experimental situations.

One type of approach is reported by Esplin and Marcus[5]. Under conditions of suboptimal treatment with benzyl penicillin it was shown that adrenal-ectomized mice were less able to deal with an experimentally induced pneumococcal infection compared with sham operated controls; mortality of the mice was higher and the number of viable organisms recovered from peritoneal fluids was greater.

Others have tackled the problem by studies in vitro. It has, for example, been shown that the presence or absence of polymorphonuclear leukocytes has a significant effect on the bactericidal activity of antibiotics in bacterial cell cultures[6, 7].

In general it seems, that during the short time period of a culture experiment, the presence of leukocytes enhances the bactericidal action of the antibiotic-containing culture, whether the bacterium used is sensitive to the antibiotic[6] or resistant[7]. Interpretation of results obtained over longer periods of incubation is difficult, as it is necessary to take into account the viability of the leukocytes, antibiotic penetration into the leukocytes, and intracellular killing by leukocytes. In general, at least for benzyl penicillin[6], methicillin and gentamicin[7], no synergistic activity is noted once the bacterium is taken up by the leukocyte. Only where antibiotic is known to penetrate the cell, as in the case of rifampicin and vancomycin, could the influence of leukocytes be shown over these longer periods[7].

These experiments exemplify the evidence that in vivo host defences or individual components of non-specific resistance, as in the in vitro work, have a significant effect on infection or on bacterial killing. They also highlight a topic that will be referred to several times in this review. Because few antibiotics readily penetrate cells, and even those that do so may not be able to kill bacteria in the stationary phase within the cell, intracellular killing must be a direct and important responsibility of phagocytic cells. If these cells are functioning normally adequate protection is ensured. If, however, there are defects in the ability of these cells to respond to chemotactic stimuli, or to phagocytose and kill organisms, then intracellular killing will not be sufficient to ensure survival of the host. As has been pointed out[8], failure of the polymorphonuclear cell (PMN) to effect intracellular killing may be of less significance than failure of the mononuclear phagocyte. The PMN has a short life span, approximately 7 hours, and bacteria within the cell at death will be released and subjected to attack from alternative defence systems. A more serious threat to health arises if there is persistence of viable organisms – for example Brucella, Listeria or Salmonella – in the macrophages, as these cells have a significantly longer life span. Vigorous antibiotic therapy with high doses of bactericidal antibiotics, if given as early as possible in infections of this kind, will help to ensure interaction of antibiotic and bacterium in the extracellular environment and therefore successful therapy.

Thus under normal circumstances, in the therapy of bacterial disease, cure is effected through the dual actions of antibiotic and host resistance.

Clearly, the major role of the antibiotic is directed against the bacterial pathogen, but it is important to consider whether the antibiotic has an additional ability to influence the host's response, either beneficially or adversely, qualitatively or quantitatively.

THE EFFECT OF ANTIBIOTICS ON THE MONONUCLEAR PHAGOCYTIC SYSTEM

In this section, the effect of antibiotics on blood monocytes, tissue macrophages and the fixed macrophages of the spleen and liver is considered.

Micro-organisms gaining access to the bloodstream or to the lymphatics will in most instances be removed by fixed macrophages of the mononuclear phagocyte system. Blood monocytes migrate from the circulation into sites of tissue inflammation and there mature into macrophages, thus providing a population of dividing cells with a high capability for phagocytosis, protein synthesis and intracellular killing of bacteria.

The effect of antibiotics on phagocytic capacity, as measured by the rate of clearance of intravenously administered colloidal carbon or other particulate matter, has received limited attention. In general, it seems that antibiotics have a minimal effect only, although there are reports that the tetracyclines, possibly because of their preferential distribution to lymphoid tissues, the spleen and Küpffer cells of the liver, may reduce phagocytosis under certain experimental conditions, notably when phagocytosis is stimulated by lipopolysaccharide[9]. It is difficult to establish the mechanism by which an antibiotic might influence phagocytic clearance rates. It is known that infection increases the functioning of cells of the mononuclear phagocyte system, for example Küpffer cells and macrophages of the spleen. It has been shown[10] that the normal increase in systemic phagocytic activity (K value) of rats with undefined respiratory infection can be substantially reduced by treatment with tetracycline at 12 mg/rat/day, and that the resistance of infected rats to shock is thereby overcome. It seems probable that the role of the antibiotic was the elimination, at least in part, of the infective stimulus to phagocytosis. A similar explanation could be offered for the results of another study[11] in which it was shown that oxytetracycline reduced the phagocytic index of rabbits given typhoid vaccine.

A more direct attempt to show any effects antibiotics may have on phagocytic clearance rates was reported by Sewell and Nichol[12]. They showed that the clearance of colloidal carbon was reduced in mice treated orally with any of several tetracyclines, chloramphenicol, neomycin, streptomycin or dihydrostreptomycin. Benzyl penicillin had some enhancing effect, whether given orally or subcutaneously. The fact that suppression was only observed after oral therapy might suggest a possible explanation, in that it seems likely that the antibacterial agents interfered with the normal gut flora and so diminished stimuli to phagocytosis.

Although there is no evidence that the mononuclear phagocyte system is involved, it is appropriate to consider studies which have shown that antibiotic therapy can enhance susceptibility to infection or increase virulence. It seems likely that these too may be explained by an action of the antibiotic on the enteric flora.

It has been found that even single oral doses of one of several antibiotics, benzyl penicillin, dihydrostreptomycin, and to a lesser extent bacitracin or oxytetracycline, enhanced the susceptibility of mice to oral infection with *Salmonella enteritidis*; subcutaneous antibiotic had no effect, again raising the possibility that interference with the normal gut flora might be responsible[13]. Gorczyca and McCarty[14] suggested a similar explanation for the finding that treatment with oxytetracycline increased mortality in *Candida*-infected goats. Untreated goats and those treated with benzathine penicillin survived the infection, whereas four of five goats treated with oxytetracycline died. The authors postulated that the oxytetracycline had upset the balance of enteric flora and that products of *Escherichia coli* cell lysis were responsible for increasing the virulence of the *Candida*. That this may not be the full explanation is suggested by Seelig[15] who, in reviewing this work, points out that it might equally have been due to a lowering of β_1-globulins and α-globulins in the serum of the oxytetracycline-treated goats, for apparently the *Candida*-killing activity of normal serum resides in these serum fractions.

In experiments involving aerosol infection of guinea-pigs with tetracycline-resistant staphylococci, it has been shown that 50 mg of tetracycline given orally twice daily, before and following infection, prolonged the duration of the infection as measured by isolation of staphylococci from nasal washings; but it resulted in no dissemination of disease[16]. It is of interest that, after several months during which it was not apparent, the organism could be re-isolated following further treatment with tetracycline. Again, perhaps the explanation is that the antibiotic upset normal microflora in the nasal airways, allowing staphylococci to multiply.

Returning to the question of the effect of antibiotics on fixed macrophages of the mononuclear phagocyte system, there is no unequivocable evidence of any direct effects. Clearly, effects on opsonins, which are known to facilitate clearance of intravenously administered particulate matter, will have an important influence on the performance of these cells. This is discussed later. Only in extreme cases is it likely that the functioning of this basic, high-capacity system will be sufficiently disordered to cause problems in the control of infection. Protection against bacteria with polysaccharide mucoid capsules, such as the pneumococci and *Haemophilus influenzae*, is dependent upon optimal splenic function, as shown in experimental studies in splenectomized rats and also in splenectomized patients who, like those with sickle cell anaemia in which the spleen architecture and function is destroyed, are prone to infections with these organisms[8]. By and large though, the capability of the system, especially through the Küpffer cells of the liver, ensures adequate protection, and both non-specific and antigen-specific host defence mechanisms will proceed.

It has been shown that the phagocytic activity of human blood monocytes, as measured by the uptake of labelled *Listeria*, is increased by ampicillin, the tetracyclines and chloramphenicol at concentrations lower than the minimum inhibitory concentrations of each antibiotic against this strain of *L. monocytogenes*[17]. The effect was not directly on the cell, as preincubation of monocytes with antibiotic, followed by the addition of the bacteria, was without effect. Several other antibiotics, gentamicin, polymyxin B and dihydrostreptomycin, all increased the rate of ingestion and intracellular killing by mouse peritoneal macrophages, when added to cell cultures at less than the minimum inhibitory concentration (MIC)[18, 19]. The suggestion is that the antibiotic altered the surface structure of the bacteria in such a way as to encourage both uptake, and when within the cell, the action of bactericidal processes, in effecting bacterial killing. At concentrations relevant to therapeutic administration, Ødegaard and Lamvik[20] found that chloramphenicol had no effect on the ability of cultured human monocytes to ingest labelled *Candida*, although at very high concentrations (5 mg/ml) it caused a moderate decrease in attachment and ingestion, and slight effects on intracellular digestion. It is known that rifampicin penetrates mouse peritoneal macrophages and human blood monocytes and can thus kill intracellular organisms[21, 22], and therefore it might be expected that antibiotics of this class would affect monocyte function. In fact, it has been shown that rifampicin may impair macrophage function. Mice were infected with a rifampicin-resistant *Mycobacterium tuberculosis* strain. Those treated with rifampicin died sooner than untreated controls, suggesting an immunosuppressive effect of some kind[23]. Other reports have identified immunosuppressive properties of this antibiotic. Rifamycin s.v., the rifampicin nucleus, inhibits macrophage cytotoxicity to syngeneic erythrocytes although it seems to have no effect on endocytosis by mouse macrophages[24, 25] at concentrations of 50 µg/ml.

THE EFFECT OF ANTIBIOTICS ON SPECIFIC IMMUNE RESPONSES

The possibility must be examined that antibiotics could influence the development of specific immunity to infecting organisms.

The most obvious influence relates to antigen mass. An effective antibiotic will eliminate the infecting organism and therefore, as a function of its antibiotic efficacy, eliminate the source of antigenic determinants responsible for initiating a specific immune response. In many early studies[26] in which attempts were made to measure the effects of antibiotics on the immune response to infection it seems most likely that suppression was caused in this way.

In work designed to measure more unequivocally a direct effect of antibiotics on the primary immune response of rabbits, [^{131}I]bovine serum albumin was injected together with either benzyl penicillin, chlortetracycline, dihydrostreptomycin or oxytetracycline subcutaneously, starting 24 hours before antigen and continuing throughout the immunization period[26]. Each of the antibiotics depressed the immune response although there was marked variation between individual animals. The possibility that anorexia was responsible for this variation was ruled out.

Slanetz[27] reported the result of pretreatment of rats and mice with antibiotics, either chlortetracycline, chloramphenicol or oxytetracycline added to their diet. A short 2-day pretreatment period led to enhanced antibody production; but a 14-day period of pretreatment led to a depressed antibody response to killed *Salmonella* antigens. In another study[28] chlortetracycline had no effect on the development of immunity to a non-viable antigen when given to mice intraperitoneally over a 6-day period, and Averlianova[29] concluded that tetracyclines and penicillin G given for up to 3 years to dogs had no effect on the development of antibodies to typhoid vaccine.

These results suggest that antibiotics can influence the antibody response directly, although it is impossible to judge the possible pathways by which they do so. As suggested earlier, the antibiotic treatment might alter the gut flora and so affect the phagocytic ability of macrophages. These cells are of course non-specific, in the sense that they do not carry receptors capable of antigen recognition nor do they synthesize antibody. They are, however, critical to the development of a specific immune response by selective antigen handling and presentation of antigen to appropriate lymphocyte populations and any diminution of their role would lead to an impaired immune response.

A more readily explicable effect of antibiotics on antibody production is exemplified by the antitumour antibiotics, and by chloramphenicol and rifampicin. These antibiotics depress protein synthesis or interfere with the processes of translation and transcription or with messenger RNA function. Chloramphenicol has not surprisingly therefore been shown to depress the antibody response[30]. The secondary antibody response to bovine serum albumin or to diphtheria toxoid by rabbit lymph node explants was markedly inhibited at only 5 μg/ml chloramphenicol present in the cultures over the whole incubation period. An effect at the level of messenger RNA was felt to be most likely, in view of the requirement for antibiotic to be present during the early stages of synthesis.

There are no reports that antibiotics affect the specific immune response by an effect on the T or B-lymphocyte populations or subsets of them. However, it has been shown recently that a number of cephalosporins inhibit the response *in vitro* of lymphocytes to three mitogens, PHA, Con A and pokeweed, suggesting that, at clinically relevant concentrations, these antibiotics could be immunosuppressive although there is no clinical or animal evidence in support of this[31]. The mechanism is not clear but it seems unlikely from the data presented that it is due to binding of the antibiotic to the mitogen, as has been recorded for polymyxin B and lipopolysaccharide mitogen[32]. The fact that several of the cephalosporins inhibited the response to all three mitogens makes inhibition of the receptor on the lymphocyte an unlikely mode of action. In the studies quoted, neither penicillin, streptomycin nor chloramphenicol had any inhibitory effect.

Although the effects are not dramatic, antibiotics can thus affect the specific immune response, and this should be borne in mind in the therapy of patients compromised with respect to their immunological performance. The susceptibility to infection of patients with primary immunodeficiency disease is well known and has recently been well reviewed[3, 33, 34]. In general it seems clear that B-cell deficiency syndromes, associated with hypogammaglobulinaemia, are characterized by severe, recurrent bacterial infections due to pneumococcus, meningococcus, streptococcus, pseudomonas and *Haemophilus influenzae*. The antibiotic therapy of these patients requires special consideration. Bacterial infection is not of prime concern in the T-cell deficiency syndromes; patients characteristically suffer severe virus diseases, rubella, varicella, or cytomegalovirus for example, and severe fungal infections.

THE EFFECT OF ANTIBIOTICS ON COMPLEMENT-DEPENDENT HOST RESISTANCE

In counterbalance to the more deleterious effects of complement activation in human disease, for example, in bacteraemic shock, in the disseminated intravascular coagulation syndrome and in immune complex disease, complement components have a key role in many biological processes involved in host resistance to bacterial infection. Serum is also known to possess non-specific, bactericidal properties, and this activity seems to reside in the products of activation of the alternate complement pathway.

Neutrophil chemotaxis is strongly influenced by complement components. In addition, attachment of bacterium to phagocytic cell usually requires serum components; these factors, opsonins, include complement-derived products which thus enhance phagocytosis[35].

Where deficiency of individual complement components exists, it might be expected that there will be an increased susceptibility to infection. Primary, presumably genetic, defects of complement components are rare. C1, C3 and C5 deficiency states have been recognized and severe bacterial infections have been experienced in these patients [2,3,36,37]. Deficiencies of opsonins, complement and IgM are also quite common in neonatal and particularly in premature, infants and it has been noted that the bactericidal activity of their sera against Gram-negative organisms is suboptimal[38]. However, most changes in complement levels are due to immunological reactions in tissues and to severe infections. An example is seen in malaria, in which large amounts of complement can be bound by antigen–antibody complexes and eliminated from the bloodstream.

The association of increased susceptibility to bacterial infection in complement-depleted states makes it important to consider whether the antibiotic chosen for therapy might influence the complement system directly.

Roth and Goldstein[39] tested the serum of patients, after they had received oral tetracycline at recommended doses for 12 days, for its ability to inhibit the growth of *Candida albicans*; no inhibition of normal killing was observed. Forsgren and Gnarpe[40] have considered this topic again in relation to the bactericidal properties of serum. Four tetracyclines, tetracycline HCl, oxytetracycline, doxycycline and lymecycline, were shown to inhibit the normal bactericidal action of human serum towards *E. coli*. A maximum of 30% inhibition was observed using 10 µg/ml doxycycline; lower concentrations had only small effects. Evidence was presented that this action of tetracyclines was a consequence of their ability to chelate divalent cations; the addition of magnesium ions almost fully restored the serum bactericidal activity. This conclusion is in line with work which suggests that the bactericidal properties of non-immune serum are a function of activation of the alternate complement pathway, activation which requires Mg^{2+}. This is also in agreement with recent evidence[41] that the inhibiting action of tetracyclines on polymorphonuclear leukocyte chemotaxis is due to chelation of the intracellular divalent cation pool.

Forsgren and Gnarpe[42] extended their study to evaluation of serum derived from volunteers who had been given a single dose of doxycycline, 200 mg or 300 mg orally. Bactericidal activity of the serum taken some 5 hours after the antibiotic was significantly reduced, and enhanced survival of added *E. coli* was observed.

THE EFFECT OF ANTIBIOTICS ON POLYMORPHONUCLEAR LEUKOCYTES

Cells of the polymorphonuclear leukocyte series, and in particular the neutrophil, play a role which is second to none in the control of bacterial infection. It is a short-lived cell, with a half-life in the bloodstream of 6–7 hours, and large reserves of mature cells ready for mobilization are to be found in bone marrow.

In order to fulfil its critical role in defence of the host, it is important that several functions of the neutrophil are intact. It must be present in adequate numbers. Severe granulocytopenia, whether of bone marrow origin or originating in the periphery, will lead to inadequate control of bacterial infection. Quie[43] has reviewed the conditions under which neutropaenia leads to increased susceptibility to infection by staphylococci, *E. coli*, *Klebsiella* and other organisms. He makes reference to neutropaenia due to drugs such as nitrogen mustard and chlorambucil, due to disease, as in rheumatoid arthritis or lupus, and due to congenital abnormality.

The neutrophil must also be capable of movement. Becker[44] has pointed out that the important functions of this cell type all relate to movement of one kind or another. The neutrophil must be capable of responding to chemotactic stimuli if it is to achieve an antibacterial effect in tissues. It must be capable of effective phagocytosis, a process involving movement of part of the cell membrane, and it must be able to bring lysosomal enzymes in intracellular organelles to the phagocytic vesicle, if the antimicrobial systems are to be effective. These antimicrobial systems include both oxygen-dependent and oxygen-independent systems and these have been reviewed[45].

There are a number of disease states in which defects of neutrophil functions are recognized and in which an increased susceptibility to bacterial infection is noted.

Defects of chemotaxis have been regularly reported in Chediak–Higashi's disease, in Job's syndrome associated with hypergammaglobulinaemia of the E class, in rheumatoid arthritis, in juvenile diabetes and in the 'lazy-leukocyte syndrome' in which it seems that mature neutrophils are reluctant to leave the bone marrow[43,46]. It has been suggested that in some of these cases the problem is one of a lack of deformability. For a variety of reasons, it can be seen that neutrophils in some of these conditions lack the normal neutrophil's fluidity of movement. Bacterial infection can be a clinical problem in many of these patients.

Phagocytosis and the metabolic activation of the cell consequent upon uptake of particles are responsible for the intracellular killing of bacteria. These processes increase oxygen consumption and production of hydrogen peroxide, and activate the hexose monophosphate shunt. This can be defective in chronic granulomatous disease (CGD), in Chediak–Higashi's syndrome, in burns and, transiently, in severe acute bacterial infections[47,48]. All are characterized in the clinic by severe and frequently life-threatening episodes of bacterial infection. The detailed analysis of the underlying neutrophil defect has led to an understanding of their normal function and of the control mechanisms that lead to bacterial death. For example, the role of H_2O_2 in bacterial killing has been better understood by the finding that CGD neutrophils fail to accumulate the host-derived H_2O_2 which kills bacteria such as staphylococci. Conversely, infections with H_2O_2-producing bacteria, streptococci and pneumococci are rare in these patients as the cells' ability to accumulate H_2O_2 is less important in defence against these species.

In view therefore of the key role played by the polymorphonuclear leukocyte in host defence against bacterial infection, the effect of antibiotics on the numbers or the function of these cells is important.

Granulocytopenia

Drug-induced granulocytopenia or agranulocytosis can arise from a direct toxic effect of the drug on bone marrow cells or by a peripheral effect on circulating leukocytes[49]. It is a rare complication of the use of antibiotics. Chloramphenicol is known to give rise to erythroid suppression and associated leukopenia and more rarely to aplastic anaemia and pancytopenia. In this serious, irreversible condition, septicaemia is a major cause of death[50].

Other antibiotics have been reported as causes of granulocytopenia, for example benzyl penicillin[51], nafcillin[52, 53], methicillin[54], oxacillin[55] and gentamicin[56]. In some cases, it has been concluded that it results from maturation arrest in the granulocyte series due to an effect on the bone marrow, which is usually normal or hyperplastic in appearance[52, 54].

There is very little evidence that granulocytopenia results from peripheral destruction of granulocytes by antigranulocyte antibodies. Using leukocyte agglutination assays no such antibodies have been found. However, a recent paper has reported[57] the presence of antineutrophil antibodies, which are capable of opsonizing normal neutrophils, in the serum of neutropenic patients who had received either an isoxazole penicillin or a cephalosporin and vancomycin.

Although these are rare complications of antibiotic therapy, they should be borne in mind in relation to any patient who remains febrile in the face of apparently adequate antibiotic therapy.

The effect of antibiotics on neutrophil chemotaxis

Experimental studies have been carried out in modified Boyden chambers, using methods which allow discrimination between random mobility and directional movements towards a concentration gradient generated by chemotactic factors. These studies have shown that certain antibiotics affect these two forms of neutrophil movement. It is possible that antibiotics could have their effect in one of several ways. The antibiotic could directly inhibit a biochemical pathway required for the neutrophil's adequate functioning, it could perturb the cell membrane resulting in depression or excitation of function, or it could mask important receptor sites. By interacting with and destroying chemotactic factors antibiotics might also remove the stimulus to cell migration. They could themselves be chemotactic or could influence true chemotaxis adversely by stimulating the random mobility of the cells.

In the studies reported in this section, there is some experimental evidence which suggests that certain antibiotics act by these mechanisms on poly-morphonuclear leukocyte chemotaxis. Variations in methodology, chemo-tactic stimuli, cell source and methods of assessment make overall conclusions difficult, but it does seem that at least one group of antibiotics, the tetracyclines, have notable effects on leukocyte chemotaxis.

It has been shown that tetracycline HCl inhibits both random migration and the chemotaxis of human neutrophils towards *Mycoplasma pneumoniae*, at concentrations in the 0.01–10 μg/ml range, whereas concentrations in excess of 100 μg/ml stimulated mobility[58]. Directional movement of human neutro-phils may be inhibited by similar concentrations of tetracycline, both when antibiotic is added to the neutrophils prior to incubation and when added to the chemoattractant side of the chamber[59]. In these studies low concentrations of erythromycin and clindamycin HCl had an inhibitory effect, whereas no inhibition was observed with benzyl penicillin. Majeski[60–62] and co-workers have evaluated a range of antibiotics in a similar experimental system and confirmed the inhibitory effects of the tetracycline group of antibiotics. Inhibition was modest (20% inhibition) at 10 μg/ml and marked at 100 μg/ml. Erythromycin was found also to be inhibitory at low concentrations and methicillin also, although only at very high levels. It was of interest that some antibiotics apparently stimulated chemotaxis at clinically relevant doses; chloramphenicol did so, as did nafcillin at levels of 1–10 μg/ml. Oxacillin, gentamicin and cephalothin were without effect. Goodhart[63] has provided further evidence of the inhibitory effect of tetracycline HCl on human polymorph chemotaxis at concentrations of 10 μg/ml and greater.

Analysis of the results of these studies suggests that tetracyclines may have an effect both on the neutrophil itself and on the generation of chemotactic factors. An agarose plate method has been used in which neutrophils preincubated with antibiotic were placed in inner wells and measurements made of migration towards an *E. coli* culture filtrate mixture in the outer wells. Using this method it has been shown that relatively high concentrations, 25–100 μg/ml, and preincubation with antibiotic are essential for inhibition to be obtained[64, 65].

These results suggest that tetracyclines might act directly on the neutrophil to inhibit its chemotactic responses and this would not be unreasonable in view of what is known about the distribution and localization of tetracyclines.

Tetracyclines are taken up by neutrophils and other blood cells[66, 67] and the more lipid-soluble tetracyclines, for example doxycycline, have a greater inhibitory effect on neutrophil chemotaxis[64]. This suggests the possibility of an intracellular or membrane effect. It has been shown that tetracyclines have the ability to inhibit the activity of certain enzymes, for example the synthesis of cytochrome oxidase[68]; and at least some of the antienzyme effects of these antibiotics are due to binding of divalent cations[69]. Gnarpe and Leslie[70] attribute the inhibitory effect of tetracyclines on chemotaxis and phagocytosis to this chelating effect, as these ions are necessary for both these functions. This has been confirmed also by Goodhart, whose work suggested that the tetracyclines inhibit leukocyte chemotaxis by chelation of the intracellular divalent cation pool[41]. It may be therefore that chelation accounts for many of the effects of tetracyclines on neutrophil function, on the bactericidal effects of serum, and on the generation of chemotactic factors from serum.

Analysis of results using other antibiotics suggests that those antibiotics which have a marked inhibitory effect on neutrophil chemotaxis are those which inhibit protein synthesis or transcription; thus fusidic acid, chloramphenicol, actinomycin D, puromycin and rifampicin were strongly inhibitory. It is possible therefore that proteins necessary for the chemotactic response are synthesized on contact of the cell with chemotactic factors, and that this is blocked by antibiotics which interfere with transcription, translation or protein synthesis[64].

Guinea-pig polymorphonuclear leukocyte chemotaxis can be inhibited by several antibiotics[71]. The results obtained in this study introduced the concept that some antibiotics can also be chemoattractants: cloxacillin appeared to be so under the experimental conditions used.

The clinical relevance of the effects of antibiotics on neutrophil chemotaxis is not clear. It has been shown for some antibiotics, in particular the tetracyclines, that inhibition can occur at clinically achieved tissue levels. This is underlined by Martin et al. who have shown that for 24 hours after a 1 g dose of tetracycline, neutrophils taken from each of two volunteers had a significantly reduced capacity to respond to chemotactic stimuli. At a peak serum concentration of $10.2 \mu g/ml$ 4 hours after dosing, there was a 90% reduction in response[58]. It seems unlikely that in the normal, infected person these effects could be important. In the compromised host, however, with dysfunction of host responses, it could well be that the additional inhibitory action of the antibiotic might influence the outcome of the infection adversely. Clinical benefit could equally be expected. Esterley et al.[59] have put forward the view that the inhibitory activity of tetracyclines on neutrophil chemotaxis is of benefit in certain inflammatory conditions, for example acne, a view shared by Plewig and Schopf who found that oral or systemic tetracyclines suppressed inflammation caused by topical potassium iodide application[72].

Effect of antibiotics on phagocytosis and intracellular killing of bacteria by polymorphonuclear leukocytes

Antibiotics might affect the processes of phagocytosis and intracellular killing of micro-organisms in polymorphonuclear leukocytes by an effect on the bacteria, on membrane function or metabolic processes of the cell, or on the interaction of bacterium and cell.

There is some evidence that certain antibiotics can render bacteria more susceptible to phagocytosis or more liable to be killed rapidly in the intracellular environment. Staphylococci which have been pretreated with benzyl penicillin, erythromycin or chloramphenicol are more readily phagocytosed by guinea-pig peritoneal exudate cells than untreated staphylococci[73]. Alexander and Good similarly found that bacteria preincubated with benzyl penicillin or streptomycin at concentrations which damaged but did not kill the organisms, were more rapidly phagocytosed and then more rapidly killed than intact organisms[6]. A later study[74] did not confirm this effect with benzyl penicillin, or oxacillin but did find that nafcillin, another β-lactam antibiotic, increased the susceptibility of some bacteria to phagocytosis. Phagocytosis of spirochaetes can be enhanced by antibiotic therapy with tetracycline, erythromycin or benzyl penicillin[75]. Minocycline, a tetracycline antibiotic, had a similar effect[76]. It appears from these studies that alteration, perhaps even of a minor kind, to the surface integrity of the bacteria can render them more attractive to the phagocyte.

Antibiotics can interfere with the critical absorption phase of phagocytosis, so that adherence may occur but ingestion may be halted. Downey and Pisana[77] have demonstrated this effect with bacitracin, using guinea-pig polymorphs and either latex or staphylococci. This effect seems to be of some importance with the tetracycline group of antibiotics. Numerous workers have shown that tetracyclines can inhibit the phagocytosis of bacteria and yeasts, both *in vivo* and *in vitro*[12, 70, 78-80]. Others, however, have failed to show significant effects at reasonable dose levels[40, 42, 81, 82], or have even demonstrated stimulation[83].

The tetracyclines are, as noted earlier, chelating agents, and it is possible that it is this activity which, by interference with divalent cations, prevents the interaction of bacterium and leukocyte[41]. The more lipid-soluble tetracycline doxycycline might in this manner be expected to be the more inhibitory as borne out by the studies of Melby and Midtvedt[79]. Scanning electron microscopy results[70] showed that, in the presence of doxycycline, the polymorph surface morphology was smooth, with few pseudopodia and many adherent *E. coli*. In the absence of drug, very few adherent bacteria were seen and the polymorph surface was rough, with long, numerous pseudopodia. It is known that divalent ions are important for phagocytosis of Gram negative organisms and possibly also for latex particle engulfment[77], whereas for staphylococci they do not appear to be necessary[84]. As discussed earlier in this chapter, the inhibitory effect of tetracyclines on other host defence mechanisms is similarly mediated. It should be noted that in some but not all of the studies above, in which tetracyclines inhibit particle ingestion, yeasts or Gram negative organisms were used rather than staphylococci.

Antibiotics might equally affect the metabolic pathways involved in intracellular handling of micro-organisms. Rifampicin penetrates leukocytes both *in vitro* and *in vivo* and can kill intracellular organisms, but this antibiotic does not seem to have a significant effect on the phagocytic or killing functions of the cell[81]. High levels of chloramphenicol have been shown to impair activation of the hexose monophosphate shunt, through partial inhibition of NADH oxidase in polymorphonuclear leukocytes. Under these circumstances the normal postphagocytic increase in oxygen consumption fails to occur[85-87]. Kitani and Kokubun have also studied the effects of chloramphenicol on phagocytic function[88]. Leukocytes from patients treated with chloramphenicol were shown to have reduced phagocytic activity, as measured by uptake of *Candida*, for 2–6 hours after antibiotic. By 24 hours the phagocytic activity had returned to normal. A similar impairment was demonstrated for leukocytes taken from rabbits pretreated with either 100 mg/kg or 500 mg/kg chloramphenicol for 7 days. In earlier work[77] polymyxin B was found to partially inhibit the burst of respiratory activity which accompanies phagocytosis.

There is very limited information on any effect antibiotics may have on other intracellular enzymes. Zabirov and Shchepetkina showed that predosing of rats with benzyl penicillin or oxacillin for 5–7 days increased phagocytosis and killing of staphylococci by polymorphonuclear leukocytes. This was associated with increased level of intracellular lysozyme[89]. A recent study throws a little more light on this topic[90]. The authors studied the interrelationships between Gram negative bacteria, the β-lactam antibiotic carbenicillin, and rabbit leukocytes. Sonicated leukocytes lost bactericidal activity but this could be restored by the addition of subinhibitory levels of carbenicillin to the supernatant culture fluids, suggesting that there could be interaction between the antibiotic and enzymes involved in the intracellular killing of bacteria. The importance of this finding could be that, on the death of polymorphs, any live bacteria which had been protected from antibiotic activity, due to their intracellular location, might be subjected to an enhanced bactericidal attack in the extracellular tissue fluids. It was of interest that in this study neither polymyxin B nor the aminoglycosides had this effect.

The nitroblue tetrazolium dye reduction test has proved of value in related studies. This test is used to identify leukocytes with oxidase activity, that is those that have responded to phagocytosis by increased oxygen uptake, increased hexose monophosphate shunt activity and hydrogen peroxide production. The basis of the test is that phagocytosis is an anaerobic process in which the required energy is supplied by glycolysis. Oxidized NBT is colourless, but when reduced it forms a blue formazan precipitate. The dye therefore substitutes for oxygen as a hydrogen acceptor in those leukocytes in which an increased oxygen uptake has occurred.

Rubinstein and Pelet, in an evaluation of the NBT test in infections, found that patients under intensive therapy with a number of antibiotics had a transient decrease in maximum NBT reduction capacity. *In vitro* incubation of normal granulocytes with tetracyclines, at clinically relevant concentrations, showed a significant decrease in NBT reduction by these cells.

Inhibition *in vitro* occurred with rifampicin, ampicillin and gentamicin but only at concentrations far in excess of therapeutic levels[91]. This provides additional evidence for the ability of tetracyclines to inhibit intracellular oxidation processes, and further work recently published is in agreement[92]. These authors showed that doxycycline had an effect upon the number of human polymorphonuclear leukocytes able to reduce NBT in the presence of *Haemophilus influenzae* in an *in vitro* system; the number of cells reducing NBT was lower than the control at 0.1 µg/ml and substantially lower at 10 µg/ml. This study is of interest also from the point of view of the β-lactam antibiotics. In the majority of studies, this group of antibiotics has been found to have little or no effect on the function of polymorphonuclear leukocytes. However, Thomke and Burgi[92] first demonstrated the inhibitory effects of doxycycline and then showed that under the same conditions amoxycillin at concentrations above 0.1 µg/ml caused a significant increase in the number of polymorphonuclear leukocytes reducing the NBT dye. These results seem to be of some clinical significance. The same authors showed that the sputum of bronchitic patients treated with amoxycillin stimulated an increase in the number of NBT-reducing normal leukocytes, whereas sputum from patients treated with doxycycline or cotrimoxazole had no stimulatory effect[92]. Stimulation of leukocyte function has also been demonstrated by Szauer and Schwartz[93] in a model system involving the production of *E. coli* sepsis in the dog; they found that the β-lactam antibiotic cephalothin increased both dye uptake and reduction.

These studies on the stimulatory effect of β-lactam antibiotics on polymorphonuclear leukocytes are in agreement with earlier work[12,94] which demonstrated increased phagocytic activity in antibiotic-treated animals, and more recently it has been shown that two α-carboxy substituted penicillins, carbenicillin and sulbenicillin, can increase phagocytosis and killing of *Pseudomonas* strains at *in vitro* concentrations as low as one-sixteenth of the MIC for the bacterium used[90,95]. In comparative studies, the aminoglycosides had no effect, and polymyxin B achieved an effect only at the MIC. In a later paper[96], it was shown that this effect could be significant in terms of chemotherapy in experimental infections. Two strains of *Proteus mirabilis*, which had similar MIC values determined in broth, were found to differ with respect to susceptibility to carbenicillin in the presence of rabbit polymorphonuclear leukocytes. The more susceptible strain showed a reduced ability to invade the mouse bloodstream following *in vitro* carbenicillin treatment, and it was cleared more rapidly from the blood of carbenicillin-treated rabbits.

The situation is by no means clear and in other studies some degree of inhibition of function has been recorded. Raeburn *et al.* have reported that polymorphs from volunteers given 500 mg ampicillin orally showed a transient depression of bactericidal properties[97]. Earlier data of Raeburn[98] albeit from individual patients, stresses that variable effects are obtained and the role of the antibiotic itself is difficult to interpret. For example, measurements were made of the bactericidal properties of polymorphs obtained from chronically ill patients, both during therapy with benzyl penicillin or ampicillin and when receiving no therapy. In one patient, bactericidal activity was decreased on therapy with benzyl penicillin. In another patient, bactericidal activity markedly increased while on ampicillin therapy.

In view of the critical role played by the polymorphonuclear leukocyte in the control of bacterial infection, these studies should now be extended in an attempt to define the basis of antibiotics effects on cell function and to try to establish their clinical importance.

SUMMARY

Successful chemotherapy of bacterial infections depends upon both antibiotic therapy and host-derived factors. Experimental and clinical studies have shown that these are not unrelated, but that antibiotics can interact with host cells or with serum factors to influence the outcome of infection. Antibiotics have been shown to affect the mononuclear phagocyte system, polymorphonuclear leukocyte chemotaxis and phagocytosis, and the bactericidal activity of serum, all immunologically non-specific events. They can also affect the development of antigen-specific immune responses.

Experimental findings suggest that these effects are modest. Only in clinical situations in which host defence mechanisms are impaired does it seem likely that they would be of clinical relevance. Further study, using carefully standardized modern techniques might, however, reveal properties which would be of value in the selection of novel antibiotics for progression to clinical use or bring to light unexpected activities of existing antibiotics.

References

1. Allen, J. C. (1976). Infection complicating neoplastic disease and cytotoxic therapy. In Allen, J. C. (ed.) *Infection and the Compromised Host*, pp. 151–171. (Baltimore: Williams & Wilkins Company)
2. Lachmann, P. J. and Rosen, F. S. (1978). Genetic defects of complement in man. In Miescher, P. A. and Mueller-Eberhard, H. J. (eds.) *Springer Semin. Immunopathol.*, 1, p. 339
3. Pahwa, R., Pahwa, S., O'Reilly, R. and Good, R. (1978). Treatment of the immunodeficiency diseases – progress towards replacement therapy emphasizing cellular and macromolecular engineering. In Miescher, P. A. and Mueller-Eberhard, J. J. (eds.) *Springer Semin. Immunopathol.*, 1, p. 355
4. Quie, P. G., Mills, E. L., McPhail, L. C. and Johnston, R. B. (1978). Phagocytic defects. In Miescher, P. A. and Mueller-Eberhard, H. J. (eds.) *Springer Semin. Immunopathol.*, 1, pp. 323–337
5. Esplin, D. W. and Marcus, S. (1954). Relation between antibacterial action of penicillin and mouse host defenses in systemic pneumococcus infection. *Antibiot. Chemother.*, 4, 123

6. Alexander, J. W. and Good, R. A. (1968). Effect of antibiotics on the bactericidal activity of human leukocytes. *J. Lab. Clin. Med.*, **71**, 971

7. Vaudaux, P. and Waldvogel, F. A. (1978). Combined bactericidal activity of leukocytes and antibiotics against methicillin-resistant *Staphylococcus aureus*. In Siegenthaler, W. and Luthy, R. (eds.) *10th International Congress of Chemotherapy*, Zurich. *Current Chemotherapy*, **1**, 319 (Washington D.C.: Am. Soc. Microbiol.)

8. Drachman. R. H. (1976). Splenic and reticuloendothelial function and infection. In Allen. J. C. (ed.) *Infection and the Compromised Host*, pp. 103–131. (Baltimore: Williams & Wilkins Company)

9. Snell, J. F. (1960). The reticuloendothelial system: I. Chemical methods of stimulation of the reticuloendothelial system. *Ann. N.Y. Acad. Sci.*, **88**, 56

10. Altura, B. M., Hershey, S. G., Ali, M. and Thaw, C. (1966). Influence of tetracycline on phagocytosis, infection, and resistance to experimental shock: Relationship to microcirculation. *J. Reticuloendothel. Soc.*, **3**, 447

11. Mashimo. K. and Harada, T. (1962). Effect of antibiotics on phagocytosis and killing of *Pseudomonas aeruginosa* by polymorphonuclear leukocytes, II. Effect of some antibiotics, and interaction between carbenicillin and PMN-intracellular active material. *Proc. Jpn. Soc. Reticuloendothel. Syst.*. **2**. 24

12. Sewell, I. A. and Nichol, T. (1958). Effect of antibiotics on the phagocytic activity of the reticuloendothelial system. *Nature (London)*, **181**, 1662

13. Bohnhoff, M. and Miller, C. P. (1962). Enhanced susceptibility to *Salmonella* infection in streptomycin-treated mice. *J. Infect. Dis.*, **110**, 117

14. Gorczyca, L. R. and McCarty, R. T. (1959). Effects of prolonged low dosage antibiotic administration and superimposed *Candida albicans* infection on goat serum proteins. *Antibiot. Chemother.*, **IX**, 587

15. Seelig, M. (1966). Mechanisms by which antibiotics increase the incidence and severity of candidiasis and alter the immunological defenses. *Bacteriol. Rev.*, **30**, 442

16. Simon, H. J. (1963). Epidemiology and pathogenesis of staphylococcal infection. I. An experimentally induced attenuated staphylococcal infection in guinea-pigs and its modification by tetracycline. *J. Exp. Med.*, **118**, 149

17. Adam, D., Schaffert, W. and Marget, W. (1974). Enhanced *in vitro* phagocytosis of *Listeria monocytogenes* by human monocytes in the presence of ampicillin, tetracycline, and chloramphenicol. *Infect. Immun.*, **9**, 811

18. Adam, D., Philipp, P. and Belohradsky, B. H. (1971). Studies on the influence of host defence mechanisms on the antimicrobial effect of chemotherapeutic agents. Effect of antibiotics on phagocytosis of mouse peritoneal macrophages *in vitro*. *Arzneim. Forsch.*, **25**, 181

19. Adam, D., Staber, F., Belohradsky, B. H. and Marget, W. (1972). Effect of dihydrostreptomycin on phagocytosis of mouse peritoneal macrophages *in vitro*. *Infect. Immun.*, **5**, 537

20. Ødegaard, A. and Lamvik, J. (1976). The effect of phenylbutazone and chloramphenicol on phagocytosis of radiolabelled *Candida albicans* by human monocytes cultured *in vitro*. *Acta Pathol. Microbiol. Scand.*, **84**, 37

21. Lober, M. C. and Mandell, G. L. (1973). The effect of antibiotics on *Escherichia coli* ingested by macrophages. *Proc. Soc. Exp. Biol. Med.*, **142**, 1048

22. Mandell, G. L. (1973). Interaction of intraleukocyte bacteria and antibiotics. *J. Clin. Invest.*, **52**, 1673

23. Hurd, E. (1977). Drugs affecting the immune response. In Holborow, E. J. and Reeves, W. G. (eds.) *Immunology in Medicine*, pp. 1067–1099. (London: Academic Press)

24. Melsom, H. (1975). The inhibitory effect of rifamycin-SV on macrophage mediated erythrocyte lysis. *Exp. Cell. Res.*, **95**, 1

25. Melsom, H. and Seljelid, R. (1974). Rifamycin – a potent inhibitor of macrophage cytotoxicity. *Exp. Cell. Res.*, **86**, 415

26. Stevens, K. M. (1953). The effect of antibiotics upon the immune response. *J. Immunol.*, **71**, 119

27. Slanetz, C. A. (1953). The influence of antibiotics on antibody production. *Antibiot. Chemother.*, **6**, 629

28. Allen, G. A. and Cooper, M. S. (1955–56). The effect of chlortetracycline on the immune response. In Welch, H. and Marti-Ibanez, F. (eds.) *Antibiotics Annual*, pp. 354–357. (New York: Medical Encyclopedia Inc.)

29. Averlianova, L. L. (1957). The influence of antibiotics on the immunological reactivity of the body. *J. Microbiol. Epid. Immun.*, **28**, 501

30. Ambrose, C. T. and Coons, A. H. (1963). Studies on antibody production. VIII. The inhibitory effect of chloramphenicol on the synthesis of antibody in tissue culture. *J. Exp. Med.*, **117**, 1075

31. Chaperon, E. A. and Sanders, W. E. (1978). Suppression of lymphocyte responses by cephalosporins. *Infect. Immun.*, **19**, 378

32. Jacobs, D. M. and Morrison, D. C. (1975). Dissociation between mitogenicity and immunogenicity of TNP – lipopolysaccharide, a T-independent antigen. *J. Exp. Med.*, **141**, 1453

33. Biggar, W. D. (1976). Analysis and treatment of immunodeficiency diseases. In Allen, J. C. (ed.) *Infection and the Compromised Host*, pp. 1–27. (Baltimore: Williams & Wilkins Company)

34. Provost, T. (1976). Infections associated with T-cell dysfunction. In Allen, J. C. (ed.) *Infection and the Compromised Host*, pp. 49–79. (Baltimore: Williams & Wilkins Company)

35. Müller-Eberhard, H. J. (1975). Complement and phagocytosis. In Bellanti, J. A. and Dayton, D. H. (eds.) *The Phagocytic Cell in Host Resistance*, pp. 87–99. (New York: Raven Press)

36. Alper, C. A., Stossel, T. P. and Rosen, F. S. (1975). Genetic defects affecting complement and host resistance to infection. In Bellanti, J. A. and Dayton, D. H. (eds.) *The Phagocytic Cell in Host Resistance*, pp. 127–141. (New York: Raven Press)

37. Provost, T. and Allen, J. C. (1976). Susceptibility to infection related to deficiencies in the complement system. In Allen, J. C. (ed.) *Infection and the Compromised Host*, pp. 133–149. (Baltimore: Williams & Wilkins Company)

38. Miller, M. E. (1975). Developmental maturation of human neutrophil motility and its relationship to membrane deformability. In Bellanti, J. A. and Dayton, D. H. (eds.) *The Phagocytic Cell in Host Resistance*, pp. 295–307. (New York: Raven Press)

39. Roth, F. J. and Goldstein, M. I. (1961). Inhibition of growth of pathogenic yeasts by human serum. *J. Invest. Dermatol.*, **36**, 383

40. Forsgren, A. and Gnarpe, H. (1973a). Tetracyclines and host-defence mechanisms. *Antimicrob. Agents Chemother.*, **3**, 711

41. Goodhart, G. L. (1978). Further evidence for the role of divalent cations in granulocyte locomotion: Recovery from tetracycline-induced inhibition in the presence of cation ionophores. In *18th Interscience Conference on Antimicrobial Agents and Chemotherapy*, Atlanta, Georgia. Abstract No. 448

42. Forsgren, A. and Gnarpe, H. (1973b). Tetracycline interference with the bactericidal effect of serum. *Nature (London) New Biol.*, **244**, 82

43. Quie, P. G. (1976). Infection associated with phagocytic cell deficiencies. In Allen, J. C. (ed.) *Infection and the Compromised Host*, pp. 81–101. (Baltimore: Williams & Watkins Company)

44. Becker, E. L. (1975). Enzyme activation and the mechanism of polymorphonuclear leukocyte chemotaxis. In Bellanti, J. A. and Dayton, D. H. (eds.) *The Phagocytic Cell in Host Resistance*, pp. 1–14. (New York: Raven Press)

45. Klebanoff, S. J. (1975). Antimicrobial systems of the polymorphonuclear leukocyte. In Bellanti, J. A. and Dayton, D. H. (eds.) *The Phagocytic Cell in Host Resistance*, pp. 45–59. (New York: Raven Press)

46. Gallin, J. I. (1975). Abnormal chemotaxis: Cellular and humoral components. In Bellanti,

J. A. and Dayton, D. H. (eds.) *The Phagocytic Cell in Host Resistance*, pp. 227–248. (New York: Raven Press)

47. Baehner, R. L. (1975). The growth and development of our understanding of chronic granulomatous disease. In Bellanti, J. A. and Dayton. D. H. (eds.) *The Phagocytic Cell in Host Resistance*, pp. 173–200. (New York: Raven Press)

48. Root, R. K. (1975). Comparison of other defects of granulocyte oxidative killing mechanisms with chronic granulomatous disease. In Bellanti, J. A. and Dayton, D. H. (eds.) *The Phagocytic Cell in Host Resistance*, pp. 201–226. (New York: Raven Press)

49. Hartl, P. W. (1973). Drug induced agranulocytosis. In Girdwood, R. H. (ed.) *Blood Disorders due to Drugs and Other Agents*, pp. 147–186. (Amsterdam: Excerpta Medica)

50. Yunis, A. A. (1973). Chloramphenicol toxicity. In Girdwood, R. H. (ed.) *Blood Disorders due to Drugs and Other Agents*, pp. 107–126. (Amsterdam: Excerpta Medica)

51. Forsgren, J. (1968). Penicillin-induced granulopenia. *Br. Med. J.*, **II**, 184

52. Markowitz, S. M., Rothkopf, M., Holden, F. D., Stith, D. M. and Duma, R. J. (1975). Nafcillin-induced agranulocytosis. *J. Am. Med. Assoc.*, **232**, 1150

53. Sandberg, M., Tuazon, C. U. and Sheagren, J. N. (1975). Neutropenia probably resulting from nafcillin. *J. Am. Med. Assoc.*, **232**, 1152

54. McElfresh, A. E. and Huang, N. N. (1962). Medical intelligence. Bone-marrow depression resulting from the administration of methicillin. *N. Engl. J. Med.*, **266**, 246

55. Passoff, T. L. and Sherry, H. S. (1978). Oxacillin induced neutropenia. *Clin. Orthop. and Related Res.*, **135**, 69

56. Chang, J. C. and Reyes, B. (1975). Agranulocytosis associated with gentamicin. *J. Am. Med. Assoc.*, **232**, 1154

57. Weitzman, S. A., Stossel, T. P. and Desmond, M. (1978). Drug-induced immunological neutropenia. *Lancet*, **1**, 1068

58. Martin, R. R., Warr, G. A., Couch, R. B., Yeager, H. and Knight, V. (1974). Effects of tetracycline on leukocytaxis. *J. Infect. Dis.*, **129**, 110

59. Esterly, N. B., Furey, N. L. and Flanagan, L. E. (1978). The effect of antimicrobial agents on leukocyte chemotaxis. *J. Invest. Dermatol.*, **70**, 51

60. Majeski, J. A. and Alexander, J. W. (1977). Evaluation of tetracycline in the neutrophil chemotactic response. *J. Lab. Clin. Med.*, **90**, 259

61. Majeski, J. A., McClellan, M. A. and Alexander, J. W. (1975). Evaluation of leukocyte chemotactic response in the presence of antibiotics. *Surg. Forum*, **26**, 83

62. Majeski, J. A., McClellan, M. A. and Alexander, J. W. (1976). Effect of antibiotics on the *in vitro* neutrophil chemotactic response. *Am. Surg.*, **42**, 785

63. Goodhart, G. L. (1978). Effects of aminoglycosides on neutrophil chemotaxis. In Siegenthaler, W. and Luthy, R. (eds.) *10th International Congress of Chemotherapy*, Zurich. *Current Chemotherapy*. **1**. pp. 320–321. (Washington D.C.: Am. Soc. Microbiol.)

64. Forsgren, A. and Schmeling, D. (1977). Effect of antibiotics on chemotaxis of human leukocytes. *Antimicrob. Agents Chemother.*, **11**, 580

65. Forsgren, A., Schmeling, D. and Banck, G. (1978). Effect of antibiotics on chemotaxis of human polymorphonuclear leukocytes *in vitro*. *Infection*, **6** (Suppl. 1), 102

66. McQueen, J. K. (1972). Localization and metabolic effects of drugs in leucocytes. In MacPhee, T. (ed.) *Host Resistance to Commensal Bacteria*, pp. 239–245. (Edinburgh and London: Churchill Livingstone)

67. Park, J. K. and Dow, R. C. (1970). The uptake and localization of tetracycline in human blood cells. *Br. J. Exp. Pathol.*, **51**, 179

68. Pious, D. A. and Hawley, P. (1972). Effect of antibiotics on respiration in human cells. *Pediatr. Res.*, **6**, 687

69. Malek, P., Rokos, J., Burger, M., Kolc, J. and Prochazka, P. (1958–59). The effect of antibiotics of the tetracycline group on enzymes and the practical clinical significance thereof. In Welch, H. (ed.) *Antibiotic Annual*, pp. 221–224. (New York: Medical Encyclopedia Inc.)

70. Gnarpe, H. and Leslie, D. (1974). Tetracyclines and host defence mechanisms, doxycycline interference with phagocytosis of *Escherichia coli*. *Microbios*, **10A**, 127

71. Kuratsuji, T., Kagawa, J., Yamamoto, M. and Iwata, T. (1977). Influence of antibiotics on neutrophil chemotaxis. In Siegenthaler, W. and Luthy, R. (eds.) *10th International Congress of Chemotherapy*, Zurich. *Current Chemotherapy*, 1, p. 322 (Washington D.C.: Am. Soc. Microbiol.)

72. Plewig, G. and Schopf, E. (1975). Anti-inflammatory effects of antimicrobial agents: an *in vivo* study. *J. Invest. Dermatol.*, **65**, 532

73. Zalman, M. V., Frasinel, N. and Neagoe, N. (1963). Phagocytose des staphylocoques pathogènes sous l'action des antibiotiques. *Arch. Roum. Pathol. Exp. Microbiol.*, **22**, 919

74. Friedman, H. and Warren, G. H. (1974). Enhanced susceptibility of penicillin-resistant staphylococci to phagocytosis after *in vitro* incubation with low doses of nafcillin. *Proc. Soc. Exp. Biol. Med.*, **146**, 707

75. Butler, T. (1978). Phagocytosis of *Borrelia recurrentis* after antibiotic treatment. In *18th Interscience Conference on Antimicrobial Agents and Chemotherapy*, Atlanta, Georgia. Abstract No. 449

76. Rayburn, J., Barnwell, P. A. and Raff, M. J. (1976). The effect of minocycline on *in vitro* phagocytosis of staphylococci by human leukocytes. *Clin. Res.*, **24**, 607A

77. Downey, R. J. and Pisano, J. C. (1965). Some effects of antimicrobial compounds on phagocytosis *in vitro*. *J. Reticuloendothel. Soc.*, **2**, 75

78. Forsgren, A., Schmeling, D. and Quie, P. G. (1974). Effect of tetracycline on the phagocytic function of human leukocytes. *J. Infect. Dis.*, **130**, 412

79. Melby, K. and Midtvedt, T. (1977). The effect of eight antibacterial agents on the phagocytosis of ^{32}P-labelled *Escherichia coli* by rat polymorphonuclear cells. *Scand. J. Infect. Dis.*, **9**, 9

80. Munoz, J. and Geister, R. (1950). Inhibition of phagocytosis by aureomycin. *Proc. Soc. Exp. Biol. Med.*, **75**, 367

81. Hoeprich, P. D. and Martin, C. H. (1970). Effect of tetracycline, polymyxin B, and rifampin on phagocytosis. *Clin. Pharmacol. Ther.*, **11**, 418

82. Kernbaum, S. (1974). Pouvoir candidacide des polynucleaires neutrophiles humains et chimiothérapie antibacterienne. *Pathol. Biol.*, **22**, 789

83. Koshik, T. F. (1967). Changes in the phagocytic reaction and in organs of the reticulo-endothelial system in albino mice following administration of tetracycline. *Byul. Ekap. Biol. Med.*, **61**, 168

84. Bryant, R. E. (1969). Effect of divalent cation depletion on phagocytosis of staphylococci. *Yale J. Biol. Med.*, **41**, 303

85. Kaplan, S. S. and Finch, S. (1970). Studies on the mechanism of chloramphenicol impairment of human leukocyte function. *Proc. Soc. Exp. Biol. Med.*, **134**, 287

86. Kaplan, S. S., Perillie, P. E. and Finch, S. C. (1969). The effect of chloramphenicol on human leukocyte phagocytosis and respiration. *Proc. Soc. Exp. Biol. Med.*, **130**, 839

87. Lehrer, R. I. (1973). Effect of colchicine and chloramphenicol on the oxidative metabolism and phagocytic activity of human neutrophils. *J. Infect. Dis.*, **127**, 40

88. Kitani, N. and Kokubun, Y. (1976). Effect of chloramphenicol on phagocytic activity in human polymorphonuclear cells. In Williams, J. D. and Geddes, A. M. (eds.) *9th International Congress of Chemotherapy*, London. *Chemotherapy*, **4**, 321. (London and New York: Plenum Press)

89. Zabirov, I. S. and Shchepetkina, L. V. (1973). Effect of penicillins on phagocytic activity of blood leukocytes of albino rats. *Antibiotiki*, **18**, 1029

90. Nishida, M., Mine, Y., Nonoyama, S. and Yokota, Y. (1976). Effect of antibiotics on the phagocytosis and killing of *Pseudomonas aeruginosa* by rabbit polymorphonuclear leukocytes. *Chemotherapy*, **22**, 203

91. Rubinstein, A. and Pelet, B. (1973). False negative N.B.T. tests due to transient malfunction of neutrophils. *Lancet*, **1**, 382

92. Thomke, E. T. and Burgi, H. (1978). The influence of antibiotic therapy for acute exacerbations of chronic bronchitis on phagocytic nitrobluetetrazolium reduction. *Pharm. Acta Helv.*, **53**, 24

93. Szauer, J. S. and Schwartz, S. A. (1976). Effects of preventive antibiotics on neutrophil phagocytosis as measured by the nitroblue tetrazolium dye test. *Surg. Gynecol. Obstet.*, **142**, 725

94. Hewes, C. G. and Shay, D. E. (1955). Antibody formation in the guinea-pig as a result of oral administration of chlortetracycline and penicillin. *Antibiot. Chemother.*, **5**, 101

95. Mine, Y., Nonoyama, S. and Nishida, A. (1974). Effect of antibiotics on phagocytosis and killing of *Pseudomonas aeruginosa* by polymorphonuclear leucocytes. II. *Jpn. J. Antibiot.*, **27**, 122

96. Nishida, M., Mine, Y. and Nonoyama, S. (1978). Relationship between the effect of carbenicillin on the phagocytosis and killing of *Proteus mirabilis* by polymorphonuclear leukocytes and therapeutic efficacy. *J. Antibiot.*, **XXXI**, 719

97. Raeburn, J. A., Watson, E., Hanson, E. J. and Johnston, T. (1976). Antibiotic activities inside leucocytes. In Williams, J. D. and Geddes, A. M. (eds.) *9th International Congress of Chemotherapy*, London. *Chemotherapy*, **4**, 17 (London and New York: Plenum Press)

98. Raeburn, J. A. (1972). Bacterial killing by leucocytes *in vivo* and *in vitro*. In McPhee, T. (ed.) *Host Resistance to Commensal Bacteria*, pp. 253–261. (Edinburgh and London: Churchill Livingstone)

Index